Do Vaccines Cause That?!

A GUIDE FOR EVALUATING VACCINE SAFETY CONCERNS

Do Vaccines Cause That?!

A GUIDE FOR EVALUATING VACCINE SAFETY CONCERNS

**Martin G. Myers, M.D.
and Diego Pineda**

Galveston, Texas
www.i4ph.org

Do Vaccines Cause That?!
A Guide for Evaluating Vaccine Safety Concerns
Copyright © 2008 by Martin G. Myers and Diego Pineda
www.DoVaccinesCauseThat.com

Cartoons copyright by Sidney S. Harris, used with permission.

i4ph Immunizations for Public Health

301 University Blvd.
Galveston, TX 77555-0351
nnii@i4ph.org
www.i4ph.org

Some sections in this book were first published online at the NNii Web site, *www.immunizationinfo.org*.

Notice: This book provides information about vaccine safety questions but it is not intended to be an immunization guide for parents. The information contained in this book should not be used as a substitute for the medical care and advice of your health care provider. There may be variations in treatment that your physician may recommend based on individual facts and circumstances.

ISBN-13: 978-0-9769027-1-3
ISBN-10: 0-9769027-1-0

Cover and interior design by Diego Pineda

Printed in the United States of America

For our children and yours

Contents

Immunity; Diabetes; Guillain-Barré Syndrome; multiple sclerosis; low blood patelets; inflammatory bowel disease; arthritis.

Foreword

The development and implementation of vaccines over the past five decades have increasingly provided the American population with freedom from nearly all those infectious diseases that caused major morbidity and mortality in years past. It is therefore paradoxical that the need for a publication such as this has become essential. Most parents and physicians are unfamiliar with the serious vaccine-preventable diseases (paralytic polio, diphtheria, measles encephalitis, pneumococcal pneumonia, and *Haemophilus influenzae* meningitis, among others) that have been eliminated or markedly reduced in the country; and most are unaware that these same diseases are only a jet plane ride away from their infants and children. For example, there have been repeated importations of measles in recent years with resultant spread to unimmunized children in contact with the infected traveler.

The authors of this volume have recognized the absolute need to provide parents with clearly understandable, science-based information about vaccines, immunization, and vaccine safety.

Martin Myers is a pediatrician who has devoted his distinguished career to the prevention of infectious diseases in children. In addition to chairing a university department of pediatrics, he directed the National Vaccine Program Office under the assistant secretary of health from 2000 to 2002 and since then has been director of public health policy and education at the Sealy Center for Vaccine Development of the University of Texas Medical Branch. Since 2003 he has served as executive director and editor for the National Network for Immunization Information (NNii)—an affiliation of the Infectious Diseases Society of America, the Pediatric Infectious Diseases Society, the American Academy of Pediatrics, the American Academy of Family Physicians, the American College of Obstetrics and Gynecology, the American Nurses Association, the American Medical Association, the National Association of Pediatric Nurse Practitioners, and the Society for Adolescent Medicine. The NNii remains independent and accepts no funding from either government or industrial sources in order to assure freedom from any charge of conflict of interest. His collaborator, Diego Pineda, has been a science writer and associate editor at the NNii since 2004. In their roles at NNii, Dr. Myers and Mr. Pineda manage the website *www.nnii. org*, which publishes up-to-date information about vaccines and vaccine safety. Their decision to write this book expanding on the information from the website was made partially in response to the many parents who asked for such a book to help them understand all the confusing information in the media today about vaccine safety.

In the era of the Internet, and the widespread coverage of medical events by the media, it is difficult, if not impossible, for parents without a sophisticated scientific background to distinguish between information and misinformation. The initial chapters of the book offer careful, articulate explanations to the reader as to how best to weigh and evaluate what they read or hear about vaccine safety and immunization. How a scientist distinguishes temporal from causal events and relationships is critical to these explanations. With this background, the reader is then prepared to proceed through additional chapters that deal specifically with concerns relating to possible vaccine-related adverse events. Exhaustively and convincingly, they discuss specific vaccine safety concerns that have been paramount in recent years. The processes that are described in the initial chapters are then used to assist in evaluation of these concerns and to enable the reader to assess what is published in the media. The overall theme is to arrive at conclusions based on science. Where scientific evidence is not available or is inconclusive, the authors frankly admit this and encourage the acquisition of further knowledge.

One hopes—anticipates—that besides a broad lay audience, health care personnel at every level will take advantage of this book to augment their own perspectives so they can discuss vaccines more comfortably and convincingly with the families for whom they are responsible.

Samuel L. Katz, M.D.
W.C. Davison Professor
Chairman Emeritus of Pediatrics
Duke University

Louis W. Sullivan, M.D.
President Emeritus
Morehouse School of Medicine

SECTION I
WEIGHING
THE EVIDENCE

Vaccines—Victims of their Own Success: Why Do We Give Vaccines for Diseases We Don't See?!

In 1736 I lost one of my sons, a fine boy of 4 years old, by the Small Pox... I long regretted bitterly and I still regret that I had not given it to him by inoculation; This I mention for the sake of parents, who omit that operation on the supposition that they should never forgive themselves if a child died under it; my example showing that the regret may be the same either way, and that therefore the safer should be chosen.
Benjamin Franklin, Autobiography, 1791

Our children are our most precious assets. As parents, we want to protect them in the best ways possible. Indeed, most parents agree that vaccinations are the best way to protect children against disease—even though they may be unfamiliar with the diseases that vaccines prevent and are troubled that the immunizations are painful.[1] But some wonder if vaccinations are really necessary and are concerned because some parents believe that their children have been harmed by vaccines. Perhaps you are confused about contradictory information about vaccine safety.

Because modern biomedical technology has made—and continues to make—new vaccines available, it is only natural for parents to also worry about whether all those vaccines "are really needed" (yes, they are, as we describe later in this chapter), and whether a child's immune system can "handle so many vaccines" (yes, it can, as we discuss in Chapter 9).

New parents have lots of questions—about feeding, sleeping, rashes, diaper frequency, and the child's development, as well as about the need for shots and the safety of vaccines. Most parents get information about all these issues from a trusted doctor or nurse, but they may still have more questions. Often parents will also obtain health information from TV, radio, newspapers, and the Internet. As we will discuss later in this section, the news media often present contrasting view points, which creates interesting stories, but stories that might not reflect the best available science. Information found on the Internet can be reliable—or it can be cleverly packaged misinformation. It is important to know how to distinguish reliable information about vaccine safety from misleading materials that could lead to poor decisions for our children's health.

Since 2004, we have managed an evidence-based Web site about vaccines and vaccine safety (*www.immunizationinfo. org*). Every article on this Web site is reviewed for accuracy by other experts and for clarity by nonscientists. Not surprisingly, we get many questions from parents, students, journalists, nurses, physicians, and others about the benefits and risks of vaccines. We have tried to incorporate answers to many of those questions in this book.

THE INCREDIBLE IMPACT OF 100 YEARS OF VACCINES

During the 20th century, infectious diseases began to be better controlled thanks to the availability of clean water and pest control. But it was not until vaccines became widely used in the 1950s that the rate of the vaccine-preventable diseases dropped dramatically in the United States.[2]

For example, before the measles vaccine was licensed in 1963, there were about 500,000 reported cases and 500 deaths from measles each year. In 2005, only 66 cases were reported. Also, since the *Haemophilus influenzae* type b (Hib) vaccine was introduced in 1985, serious Hib disease among children younger than 5 years of age—an important cause of brain damage, deafness, and other long-term problems—has declined from about 20,000 cases per year to 9 cases in 2005.

There was a large epidemic of rubella in 1964 and 1965, 4 years before the rubella vaccine was licensed. This epidemic affected 12.5 million people. Of the 20,000 infants born with congenital rubella syndrome, infection caused 11,600 to be born deaf, 3,580 to be born blind, and 1,800 to be born mentally retarded. In modern times, with widespread use of rubella vaccine, there have been only four cases of congenital rubella from 2003 through 2006.

In 1952, polio paralyzed more than 21,000 people in the United States, mostly children. Polio left a body part such as a leg unusable because of nerve damage. In modern times, with widespread use of polio vaccine, there have been no cases of natural polio in this country in almost 30 years.

IF THE DISEASES ARE GONE, WHY DOES MY CHILD STILL NEED THE VACCINE?

Decades ago, when thousands of children and adults in the United States contracted smallpox, diphtheria, poliomyelitis, or measles each year,[2] parents feared these diseases. Because of the success of vaccines, the situation is very different today: the diseases aren't seen and some people have developed a false sense of security.

High immunization rates have lowered the number of cases of these illnesses to nearly zero in the United States. Most parents have never seen a child paralyzed by polio, or choking to death from diphtheria, or brain damaged by measles, congenital rubella, or Hib. As a result, fear of these diseases does not—but should—haunt parents just as it did historically. These diseases seem to be gone. But they are not!

Except for smallpox, the diseases that vaccines can prevent are still here. For example, tetanus—which does not spread from person-to-person—is still in the soil. Cases of mumps and rubella (and congenital rubella) continue to occur.

Do Vaccines Cause That?!

VACCINE-PREVENTABLE ILLNESSES BEFORE AND SINCE ROUTINE CHILDHOOD VACCINATION BEGAN IN THE UNITED STATES.

	Number of Cases Before Vaccine Was Widely Used*	Year Vaccine Recommended for Routine Childhood Vaccination	Number of Cases			
			2003*	2004*	2005*	2006*
Smallpox	48,164	Early 1900s	0	0	0	0
Diphtheria	175,885	Mid-1940s	1	0	0	0
Pertussis[j]	142,271	Mid-1940s	11,647	25,827	25,616	15,632
Tetanus	1,314	Mid-1940s	20	34	27	41
Paralytic Polio	16,316	1955	0	0	0[‡]	0
Measles	503,282	1963	56	37	66	55
Mumps	152,209	1967	231	258	314	6,584
Rubella	47,745	1969	7	10	11	11
Congenital rubella	823		1	0	1	1
Invasive Hib[†]	20,000	1985	32	19	9	29
Invasive S. pneumoniae[†]	17,240	2000	845	1,162	1,495	1,861
Hepatitis A (acute)	26,796	1995	7,653	5,683	4,488	3,579
Hepatitis B (acute)	26,107	1986	7,526	6,212	5,119	4,713
Varicella	4,000,000	1995	20,948	32,931	32,242	48,445
Deaths	105		2	9	3	0

[j] Numbers of cases of pertussis were at a historic low of 1,010 in 1976. The rise in cases since then probably involves reduced immunity over time (time elapsed since last vaccination or infection), plus an increased awareness of whooping cough in teenagers and adults for whom there is now a booster vaccine.

[†] Children less than 6 years of age.

[‡] In 2005, there was one case of imported, vaccine-associated paralytic poliomyelitis.

* Data obtained from Centers for Disease Control and Prevention. See references 2-6.

And measles—the most contagious disease—is active in many places in the world, repeatedly arriving in our midst by airplane.

Although it is reasonable to worry about vaccine side effects, we must carefully examine each claim about safety and consider it in light of the known benefits of vaccination.

First, we need to compare safety concerns to the risk of the disease prevented by the vaccine. We need to recognize that almost all vaccine-preventable diseases are still "out there" and are capable of infecting our children and their friends. With global air travel, for example, measles, mumps, rubella, diphtheria, and polio are just a plane ride away.

Second, we need to understand the science of vaccine safety, and use available tools—like the ones offered in this book—to evaluate the information presented in the media and by those who voice vaccine safety concerns.

VACCINE-PREVENTABLE DISEASES ARE UNSEEN BUT NOT GONE: ONE WEEK'S HEADLINES

Measles Cases Now Total 11, *San Diego Union-Tribune* (02/16/08)
Chicken Pox Outbreak Spurs Call for Vaccinations, *Wichita Eagle* (02/12/08)
NSW: Measles Warning as Five Cases Reported, *Australian Associated Press* (02/11/08)
Whooping Cough Is Making a Comeback, *Louisville Courier Journal* (02/07/08)

This book will help you sort through the conflicting information about vaccines. We hope to provide the facts you need to make informed decisions about vaccines. Our goal is to give parents who have questions a means to understand the merits and limitations of vaccines, based on the available evidence.

THE BOTTOM LINE: WHY DO WE STILL NEED TO GIVE VACCINES FOR DISEASES WE DON'T SEE?!

Vaccines prevent disease and death. They have been so effective that the absence of disease in our communities has made us feel safe. However, the infecting germs are still lurking and can come back to our communities. When parents stop vaccinating their children, the unseen diseases can return. That is why we need to continue giving vaccines, even if we don't see the diseases they prevent. To not immunize a child can have tragic consequences for the child, the child's family, and for the child's classmates and friends.

IF YOU WANT TO READ MORE:

Centers for Disease Control and Prevention. 1999. Achievements in public health, 1900-1999. *Morbidity & Mortality Weekly Report* 48:621-8. Available online at *www.cdc.gov/mmwr/ PDF/wk/mm4829.pdf.*

Offit PA, Bell LM. 2003. *Vaccines: What You Should Know* (3rd ed). Hoboken, NJ: Wiley & Sons, Inc.

Vaccine Side Effects and Risk Perception: What if My Child is the One in a Million?!

Aunt Josephine was giving them a tour of their new home and so far appeared to be afraid of everything in it, from the welcome mat—which, Aunt Josephine explained, could cause someone to trip and break their neck—to the sofa in the living room, which she said could fall over at any time and crush them flat.
Lemony Snicket, A Series of Unfortunate Events, Book 3

During one of her child's pediatric visits, Diane was reading the doctor's handout about the DTaP (diphtheria-tetanus-acellular pertussis) vaccine. It had a section about serious but rare adverse reactions to the vaccine. One bullet read, "Serious allergic reaction (less than 1 out of a million doses)."

She knew that immunization was "the right thing to do," but the handout was pretty scary. As she watched her son play in the waiting room, she couldn't help but wonder, "What if he *is the one* in a million?"

Although Diane's concern about her son being "the one in a million" who experiences a serious reaction to the vaccine is understandable, she misses the point that the probability is extremely low: 999,999 children who receive the vaccine do not have the reaction. A risk of one in a million is equivalent to 30 seconds in a year, 1 inch in 16 miles, or 1 drop in 16 gallons. If one million people were lined up one foot apart the line would be 189 miles long! A one in a million risk means that of the 4.1 million children born in the United States every year, four of those children across the country could be affected.

You can also put the probability into perspective with other risks: A child has 1 chance in 6,666 of dying in a car crash (in any given year); 1–4 chances in 1,000 of dying of measles if infected; and 1 chance in 2 of dying of tetanus if contracted.

Many well-educated and intelligent people are innumerate,[1] which means they have difficulty with mathematical concepts and methods. They have no problem identifying with the language of poets and philosophers who write about life's tragedies. But the language of scientists, who call such tragedies "adverse events," leaves most parents cold.

This book is an attempt to translate the language of scientists for today's parents.

ASSESSING RISKS OF VACCINE SAFETY

The expression "less than one in a million will experience the side effect" is a statement of risk. It is calculated by dividing the number of reported cases of a side effect by the total number of doses of vaccine given.

The risk of "less than one in a million" is actually so low that scientists may not be able to tell whether the event was in fact caused by the vaccine or not.

For example, scientists argue whether Guillain-Barré (GHEE-yawn BAR-ay) syndrome—a polio-like form of paralysis—occurs after influenza immunization by coincidence or is caused by the vaccine. This syndrome occurred after the swine influenza vaccine program in 1976 at a rate of about 1 per 100,000, but it isn't clear whether annual influenza vaccine causes Guillain-Barré at a rate of about one in a million or occurs by coincidence.[2] (See page 188.)

Most serious complications that occur after influenza vaccination occur even less frequently than that. The experts agree that there are some real complications of the vaccine, but they are so rare that it is not possible to calculate the true rate of the risk—such as the risk of developing encephalitis after measles vaccination.[3] (See page 202.)

Relative Risk of Vaccine Side Effects

1 in 1
- Local reactions after influenza (up to 65/100)
- Pain and swelling at injection site after Hib (25/100)
- Local reactions after Hepatitis A (21/100)

1 in 10
- Fever, aches & pains after influenza (15/100)
- Rash after measles, fever after MMR (5-15/100)
- Pain after HBV or placebo (3/100)

1 in 100

1 in 1,000
- Febrile seizure after MMR (3/10,000)

1 in 10,000
- Severe allergic reaction after MMR
- Low platelet count after measles (1/22,300)

1 in 100,000
- Severe allergic reaction after Hepatitis B (1/600,000)

1 in 1,000,000
- Severe allergic reaction after measles (1/1,000,000)

Note: To show both common and rare reactions, these are shown on a $\log_{10}$ scale. Reactions are for rates discussed in reference 3.

Pain when the shot is given and then local reactions—such as pain, swelling, redness—with or without fever, and generally feeling crummy, concern all parents. Depending on the vaccine and which dose the child just got, these types of reactions can occur fairly often (fever 5-15% of the time after measles vaccine, for example). In some cases they even occur most of the time (for example, local reactions after the first dose of influenza vaccine occur as often as 65% of the time). These reactions pass in a day or two, but no one likes to have their child not feeling well. This is why doctors and nurses often recommend something for fever and discomfort when they give the vaccines.

In some children, fever can sometimes cause a "febrile seizure"–for example, 3 per 10,000 after the measles, mumps, and rubella combination vaccine (MMR). Although a febrile seizure can be the first seizure that a child with a seizure problem has, most of the time the seizures go away as the child gets older. Although it took many years to collect the data to prove it, *none* of the routine childhood vaccines cause ongoing seizure problems (see page 201).

PERCEPTIONS OF RISKS ABOUT VACCINE SAFETY

While risk can be measured, risk perception–what we think about risks–often cannot be. Despite the fact that many health risks are at their lowest levels ever, perceived health risks are the center of attention for the media–especially in regard to vaccines.

Media reports about the alleged vaccines–autism link, for example, are published almost every week. Scientists say they have been disproved, but some parents insist they have been proven.

These media reports often cite both sides of the story with equal emphasis. Although one conclusion may be based on scientific evidence, the other may not. These contradictory reports generate uncertainty among parents considering immunizations for their children–thus possibly affecting their perceptions of risk and their decision to vaccinate their child.[4]

Research shows that people respond better to some types of risk than others.[5] For example, natural risks (such as infectious diseases) are better tolerated than manmade risks (such as vaccine side effects) and risks that affect adults are better tolerated than risks affecting our children. Risks that are perceived to have unclear benefits are less tolerated than risks where the benefits are clearly understood. Take, for example, measles and the MMR vaccine. Because measles is no longer epidemic in the United States, some parents *incorrectly* believe that the risk of contracting the disease is lower than the risk of their child experiencing a serious side effect from MMR. If they think that there is little benefit from immunizing their child, they may conclude that there is no reason to take the risk of experiencing an adverse event.

Perception of risk depends on people's experiences and knowledge. A person who experienced an adverse event after vaccination—or thinks that someone else did—would likely think that vaccines are riskier than a person who has not. Conversely, someone who has survived a vaccine-preventable disease—or a physician who has treated that disease—will likely be an advocate for vaccines.

Antivaccine activists and immunization advocates are both responding to risk perceptions. For instance, in the 1980s a mother reported that she believed that her child's "minimal brain damage, learning disabilities, and attention deficit disorder" were caused by whole-cell pertussis (whooping cough) vaccine. As a consequence, she did not give the vaccine to her next two children, both of whom developed whooping cough—one of them severe, according to her account—because she *incorrectly* thought the risk to be lower from the illness than the vaccine.

On the other hand, the mother of a teenage boy who died suddenly of meningococcal meningitis in 1998 is an equally outspoken advocate for the meningococcal vaccine, urging other families to vaccinate their teenagers, because she wants to help others avoid what she went through with the loss of her son.

In the same way, many older pediatricians are assertive advocates for vaccine use because they vividly recall caring for children with vaccine-preventable diseases. They watched these children die or become permanently damaged and they don't want to see today's children suffer those dreaded diseases.

Taking extreme positions after dramatic life experiences is understandable, but it may not be the wisest choice. We must define a middle ground where risks and benefits are objectively evaluated and properly balanced.

The media is always eager to report differences in opinion. Reporters call it "balance" when they quote contrasting thoughts. What parent would not sympathize more with a distraught mother convinced that her child was harmed by a vaccine than with a scientist who dismisses that concern? While the mother's words sound warm and compassionate, the scientist's words often seem cold and technical.

Emotional arguments versus facts may make good two-sided stories, but may not be accurate—they may even be misleading.

This sympathy for the subjects of emotional stories may be reinforced by the medical community. Some physicians may not take time to address parents' concerns adequately, dismissing them too quickly. A few may even become annoyed when parents question their recommendation to immunize their child. Such experiences may strengthen the hesitant parents' concerns, predisposing them to believe new claims about vaccine side effects.

VACCINE SIDE EFFECTS AND ADVERSE EVENTS

Soon after being diagnosed with a common type of childhood leukemia (cancer of the blood), 5-year-old Ronald began treatment with the drug doxorubicin. Within an hour of receiving the first injection, Ronald felt nauseous and vomited. This was the first of a series of well-known side effects of doxorubicin, which not only kills cancer cells but normal cells as well.

HEALTH RISKS AND THE MEDIA

Journalists are in the business of informing the public, whether about politics, local news, or health risks.

Although we are surrounded by health risks, only a handful of risks will be featured at any given time in the media, and the content and emphases are not driven by public health issues. Rather, a health risk is more likely to become a major news story if these triggers are present:

1. Questions of blame.

2. Alleged secrets and attempted cover-ups.

3. Human interest through identifiable heroes, villains, or victims.

4. Links with existing high-profile issues or personalities.

5. Conflict.

6. Signal value: *What's next?*

7. Many people exposed to the risk, even if at low levels (*It could be you!*).

8. Strong visual impact (pictures of suffering).[6]

After a week, Ronald had sores in his mouth and lips, gastrointestinal ulcers, and a low blood cell count—all because of the drug, which later would also cause him to lose his hair.

Despite these very unpleasant side effects, Ronald's parents knew there was no other option. Without the treatment, Ronald would die. On the other hand, leukemia is cured, on average, 80% of the time following chemotherapy.

Like doxorubicin, most available drugs cause side effects—ranging from mild through life-threatening. Nevertheless, people will tolerate those side effects if they can expect a benefit.

As with any drug, there are risks and side effects with vaccines, although serious side effects—those that involve hospitalization, severe illness, or death—are mostly rare. For instance, the oral polio vaccine can cause paralysis in a small number of recipients. And smallpox vaccine can cause a rare side effect that leads to serious illness and death. When polio and smallpox were common in the United States, people tolerated these side effects because the risk of being paralyzed or killed was much greater from the disease than the vaccine. Things changed when polio and smallpox were eliminated from the country—cases of paralysis after the oral polio vaccine and deaths from smallpox vaccine became more common than natural smallpox and polio. Killed polio vaccine (IPV)—without the side effect of paralytic disease—was substituted for oral polio vaccine (instead of stopping immunization altogether because children could still be exposed to polioviruses imported from other areas of the world). Use of smallpox vaccine was stopped because the disease had been eradicated.

SIDE EFFECTS (OR SIDE REACTIONS) are symptoms and signs that occur either locally—such as pain or redness at the injection site—or in other parts of the body—such as headache or fever—because of a particular immunization or dose of a drug. A mild measles-like rash after measles vaccine is fairly common, for example. Serious, life-threatening allergic reactions can be side effects of vaccines, but occur very rarely. The symptoms of a serious allergic reaction include:

- Difficulty breathing
- Hoarseness or wheezing
- Hives
- Paleness
- Weakness
- Fast heart beat
- Dizziness
- Swelling of the throat

AN ADVERSE EVENT is something quite different from a side effect. A *side effect* is "caused by" the vaccine, whereas an *adverse event* is something that occurred at about the time a vaccine was given, but which could have been caused by the vaccine or could have just occurred at that time by coincidence. Although fever is a side effect of many vaccines, not all occurrences of fever after vaccines are caused by the vaccine. This book discusses how scientists determine whether an adverse event is actually a side effect—that is, caused by the vaccine. Thus, when an adverse event occurs after vaccination, it needs to be determined whether the adverse event was caused by the vaccine or whether it was just coincidental—that is, it was going to happen anyway.

VACCINE-ASSOCIATED PARALYTIC POLIO (VAPP)

Poliomyelitis ("polio") is caused by intestinal viruses that spread from person to person in stool and saliva. When polioviruses are present in a community, most infected people have few or no symptoms. Less than 1% of poliovirus infections result in paralysis. In some cases of paralysis, the muscles used to breathe may be weakened, leaving the victim unable to breathe on his or her own. Some who develop paralytic polio die, some recover completely, but many are left with some lingering paralysis, often involving one or more arms or legs.

Before invention of the polio vaccine, 13,000 to 20,000 people were paralyzed by polio, and about 1,000 people died from it each year in the United States.[7] Two main types of polio vaccination have been used: injection with killed polioviruses (inactivated polio vaccine or IPV) or oral—swallowing weakened (attenuated) polioviruses (oral polio vaccine or OPV). Widespread vaccination has eliminated polio from the United States and much of the Western Hemisphere, although it remains a threat in some countries in Africa and south central Asia. IPV works by causing the child to make antibodies (immunity) that protect against paralytic illness if the child should later become infected with a poliovirus.

OPV increases the immunity of the community to polio because the weakened vaccine virus causes infection without symptoms. It also can be spread by those who have been immunized to others, immunizing them as well.

Although no drug—including vaccines—is 100% safe, there is a much higher standard of safety expected of preventive vaccines than for drugs because

- ◆ Vaccines are generally given to many people, most of whom are healthy.
- ◆ Most children born in the United States begin receiving vaccinations shortly after birth and continue to receive vaccines during their first 2 years of life—with additional immunizations and booster doses years later.

The rapid reduction of cases of polio worldwide has largely resulted from using OPV because it is easy to use in mass campaigns, provides long-term immunity, and rapidly reduces the spread of the polioviruses when many in the community are immunized.

Most people vaccinated against polio have no adverse reactions. However, about 1 out of 2.4 million doses of OPV distributed in the United States caused vaccine-associated paralytic polio (VAPP). This is because OPV contains live-attenuated viruses that sometimes can become neurovirulent again—that is, they can cause paralysis. Immune-compromised people are at increased risk for VAPP and may shed neurovirulent viruses for years. Continuous circulation of OPV-derived viruses in populations with poor hygiene and low immunity levels can lead to rare outbreaks of polio. Because OPV has a serious but rare side effect (paralysis) and because children in the United States will rarely be exposed to polioviruses, a new polio vaccine schedule was recommended in 1997 using both IPV and OPV.[7] Then, in 2000, an all-IPV schedule was recommended. OPV is no longer recommended and is not available for routine use in the United States. IPV has been continued in order to protect our children from introductions of polioviruses from other parts of the world.

OPV continues to be used in countries where polio infections still occur—and would likely be used if there were to be an outbreak in the United States—as OPV is the preferred vaccine to contain an outbreak. Between 250 and 500 cases of VAPP occur each year worldwide.

+ Many vaccines are given to children at the ages when developmental and other problems are being recognized for the first time (birth to 36 months of age). Stories about bad things happening to children after a vaccination circulate widely on the Internet, are discussed on radio and TV, and are described in magazines and newspapers. Scientists take these reports of adverse events very seriously, but they recognize that just because something happened at about the same time that a vaccine was given does not mean that the vaccine *caused* the problem.

These facts—the time when vaccines are given and their widespread use—make them perfect "suspects" to be blamed for causing diseases of unknown or poorly understood causes (such as the diseases in Section II of this book).

COMMUNITY IMMUNITY

Public health officials know that vaccines are most effective when almost everyone has been immunized: the infectious agent cannot spread in a community with a lot of immune people and those who are not immune will be protected by the immune people around them. This is called community (or herd) immunity.

With community immunity, vaccinated people help those who don't or can't receive a vaccine.

WHO NEEDS TO BE PROTECTED BY COMMUNITY IMMUNITY?

PERSONS TOO YOUNG FOR VACCINATION
+ children under 6 months are not given influenza vaccine, because they have a poor immune response to this vaccine
+ children under 12 months do not respond well to

measles vaccine, but can be vulnerable to severe disease

PERSONS WITH COMPROMISED IMMUNE SYSTEMS—children being treated for certain other diseases cannot usually receive live virus vaccines, such as measles or chickenpox vaccines. For example, children being treated

- for certain forms of cancer
- for immune deficiency diseases
- with certain medicines, such as steroids

PERSONS WITH OTHER MEDICAL REASONS

- pregnant women are not given rubella vaccine

PERSONS WHO DID NOT BECOME IMMUNE WHEN THEY WERE IMMUNIZED BUT WHO CANNOT BE EASILY IDENTIFIED

- such as occurs about 5% of the time after measles vaccine

PERSONS WHO INTENTIONALLY DID NOT GET VACCINATED

A child who has never had measles or the MMR vaccine is susceptible to measles. In other words, if exposed to measles virus, the child could become infected and develop the measles along with its potential complications. However, if everyone in proximity to the susceptible child (like in a classroom) is immune to measles, the susceptible child can be protected—unless the child is in contact with the case of measles elsewhere. Because everyone else is immune, measles cannot spread through the classroom.

However, measles vaccine only makes 95% of vaccinees immune—which is the threshold for measles virus to spread in classrooms—so a second dose of a measles-containing vaccine is recommended. Because 95% were immune after the first measles vaccine, after the second dose almost all the children will be immune, blocking the transmission of the infection to the susceptible classmates.

Imagine, for example, a community of 100 people where 98% were immunized once against measles:

- Two people are susceptible because they are not immunized
- Five others are susceptible because the vaccine fails (it is estimated that the measles vaccine does not work 5% of the time)

Thus, 93 people (95% of 98) in that community are immune against measles—but 7 are still susceptible. If measles were introduced into the community, these seven people might develop measles. People who don't understand these numbers might say that the vaccine didn't work—because most of those who got measles got the vaccine (5 of the 7). Of course, they neglect to point out that 93 did not!

With a second dose of measles vaccine, those in whom the first dose failed have a better chance of becoming immune. After the two doses, only the two unimmunized, and perhaps one of the others, might develop measles if they were exposed—and most of these would be protected by community immunity because measles doesn't spread well in communities where more than 95% of people are immune.

Community immunity is achieved when the vast majority of the population is immune. In other words, a population needs high immunization rates to reap the benefits of community immunity. Thus, a city or town with many unimmunized children and young adults is at higher risk for the introduction and the sustained spread of vaccine-preventable diseases. The same is true at the neighborhood, church, or day care level, too. Whenever and wherever a community has many unimmunized people, the entire community is at risk.

MANDATORY IMMUNIZATIONS FOR SCHOOL ATTENDANCE

Some vaccines are required by state law so that the number of children who are immunized is big enough to achieve community immunity. This helps protect the health of the public. The goal of these laws and policies is to increase immunization rates.

However, some people think that vaccine requirements violate their civil rights because they object to vaccines for religious or philosophical reasons.

Many states permit exemptions for these people despite the fact that avoiding vaccination puts others in the community at risk.

Different states require different vaccines and have different exemptions. For listings of requirements by state, see *www.immunizationinfo.org.*

In 2001, 63% of U.S. children 19 to 35 months of age were fully immunized with all the vaccines recommended at that time. It was estimated that of the remaining 37% of these children, 3 children per 1,000 had never received any vaccines, while the others were incompletely immunized.[8]

States that allow philosophical exemptions to immunization laws have many more unvaccinated children than states that do not have philosophical exemptions. Indeed, unvaccinated children tend to cluster in certain states and communities, increasing the risk of transmitting vaccine-preventable diseases to others in those communities—to the incompletely vaccinated children as well as to the small number whom vaccination did not protect.

Children who had received exemptions are 35 times more likely to contract measles and, of course, are more likely to spread measles to others.[9]

Although the number of unvaccinated children in the United States is small, it has been increasing. Unvaccinated children tend to cluster in certain states—California, Illinois, New York, Washington, Pennsylvania, Texas, Oklahoma, Colorado, Utah, and Michigan—and their parents tend not to consider the advice of physicians or other health professionals.

VACCINE REQUIREMENTS FOR SCHOOL ENTRY

All states require some immunizations for school and day care entry (see *www.immunizationinfo.org* for an up-to-date state-by-state list of requirements).

- These types of laws became widespread in the 1960s and 1970s because not enough children were immunized to prevent outbreaks of vaccine-preventable illnesses—communities had not achieved "community immunity." These outbreaks often started among school children and spread to the unimmunized and some of the fully immunized children (especially outbreaks of measles).
- The goal of such laws is to protect the health and welfare of the public by having a high proportion of children immune to these diseases when they congregate in schools—the perfect setting for the spread of infectious agents.
- Some people cannot be immunized because of an underlying medical condition, so the states permit exemptions from the required vaccines for medical reasons—hopefully these people will be protected by community immunity.
- Many states also permit exemptions for religious reasons and some others permit exemptions from immunizations for philosophical reasons—these people may be protected by "community immunity" too, except when there are so many of them that community immunity no longer works.

THE BOTTOM LINE: WHAT IF MY CHILD IS THE ONE IN A MILLION?!

In summary, vaccines have greatly reduced the risks from many serious infectious diseases, rendering them unknown to the public. Fear about vaccine side effects has replaced fear of the diseases. Meanwhile, vaccine safety concerns have negatively affected immunization rates, opening a door for infectious diseases to return and harm our children.

This scenario brings up some important questions: Are parents who do not vaccinate their children making informed decisions? Are they able to distinguish misinformation about vaccines from reliable information? Or are they missing some information—such as the risks of the diseases and the importance of community immunity? Do physicians and nurses understand the concerns of parents about vaccine safety?

The next chapter deals with the problem both parents and scientists face when little or no information is available to answer whether or not a vaccine is causing a serious side effect.

IF YOU WANT TO READ MORE:

Ropeik D, Gray G. 2002. *Risk: A practical guide for deciding what's really safe and what's really dangerous in the world around you.* New York: Houghton Mifflin.

Centers for Disease Control and Prevention. 2007. *Parents' guide to childhood immunizations.* Available online at *www.cdc. gov/vaccines/pubs/parents-guide/.*

"I STOPPED TAKING THE MEDICINE BECAUSE I PREFER THE ORIGINAL DISEASE TO THE SIDE EFFECTS."

Missing Information and Technical Jargon: Why Can't Medical Researchers Talk Normally?!

Whatever you have been told, science is not about certainty. And this creates problems for those health professionals who are charged with interpreting and relating data to the general public. We are expected to refute wholesale misunderstandings, in a popular forum, to people who may well be intelligent but who know nothing of evidence-based medicine, in soundbite format.
Ben Goldacre, The Guardian, Nov. 2, 2005

Asthma, autism, and type 1 diabetes rates seem to have increased dramatically since the 1980s. Some media reports are even talking about asthma and autism "epidemics."

What are the reasons behind these boosts? Are there changes in the inheritance of genes in our population? Does living in the city or suburbs make a difference? Are there environmental contaminants in our air, water, food, or vaccines? Are we recognizing illnesses differently?

Some people believe that the parallel increase in the number of vaccine doses given to children in the past two decades is to blame for these "epidemics." In the early 1980s, children in the United States received 5 shots and 3 oral doses of vaccines in their first 2 years of life; in the 2000s, they could receive more than 20 shots.

Is there a cause-and-effect relationship between more vaccines and the increasing numbers of cases of asthma, autism, or diabetes? Or is it just coincidence? How do you decide?

What about other things that have also increased in the past 20 years such as cell phones, personal computers, microwave ovens, fast food restaurants, and soft drink consumption? Do they have something to do with the increase in many childhood diseases or is it merely coincidental?

When a vaccine safety concern is suggested, the necessary data to support or reject the hypothesis may not yet have been collected—in fact sometimes this may take several years of research. This was the case with the whooping cough vaccine some years ago.

Although whole-cell pertussis (whooping cough) vaccines were first licensed in 1914, they were not widely available for use until later. From the 1920s to the 1940s, between 115,000 and 270,000 whooping cough cases were reported each year in the United States, with 5,000 to 10,000 deaths per year.

In 1948 the pertussis vaccine was combined with vaccines against tetanus and diphtheria and this combined DTP vaccine soon began to be routinely used in the United States. By the 1970s, whooping cough cases had decreased 99%, with only 1,010 cases reported in 1976. The same happened in other countries where routine DTP immunization was implemented.[1]

With whooping cough almost gone, attention shifted from the disease to the vaccine's associated adverse events.

Common DTP side effects included redness, pain, and swelling at the site of injection; fever; irritability; and drowsiness. Some less common reactions were seizures caused by fever (febrile seizures)—scary but self-limited seizures that occur in young children because of fever—and prolonged, inconsolable crying.

These reactions seemed too much to the eyes of young parents who had never seen a child choking with pertussis or coughing until his or her ribs were broken.

In the early 1980s, some parents claimed that the DTP vaccine caused their child to develop brain damage (see Chapter 5), infantile spasms, or sudden infant death syndrome (SIDS). They argued that the vaccine was dangerous and no longer necessary because whooping cough had largely disappeared.

This resulted in lower immunization rates in many countries. In the following years, pertussis epidemics broke out in the United Kingdom, Sweden, Japan, and the Russian Federation. Vaccine manufacturers, especially in the United States, faced multimillion-dollar lawsuits for alleged personal injuries; a number of manufacturers stopped producing DTP.[2]

In the midst of it all, scientists looked for evidence that would either prove or disprove the claims about the safety of the DTP vaccine. They began epidemiological and laboratory studies, but a number of years would pass before the results became available. Meanwhile, policy makers and public health officials had to take action to ensure that the public was protected and that lawsuits would not threaten the nation's vaccine supply.

In 1986, Congress passed the national Childhood Vaccine Injury Compensation Act, which established the national Vaccine Injury Compensation Program (VICP) to compensate children who the court considers to have been injured by vaccines—that is, it does not require or mean scientific proof of injury. The VICP covers complications from vaccines that have been recommended for all children by the Centers for Disease Control and Prevention (CDC). It is funded from a tax on each dose of a vaccine.

The 1986 act also specified that the Institute of Medicine (IOM)—part of the National Academy of Sciences—review the medical literature on health problems or injuries occurring after vaccination with pertussis or rubella vaccines. The IOM formed a panel of 11 experts that examined 18 possible adverse events following the pertussis vaccine.[3]

The IOM panel used five categories to organize the strength and direction of their conclusions. Of 18 adverse events examined, 10 fell in the categories "insufficient evidence" and "no evidence available"—illustrating the problem of how to make a scientific report when the information was not available or was insufficient. In fact, the panel's report stated that during the review, they found many gaps and limitations. This creates a setting of "scientific uncertainty"—the scientists may believe that there is no cause-and-effect association between the vaccine and the concern, but intellectually they must equivocate because the definitive data must still be collected.

Besides the studies searching for an association between DTP and reported adverse events, researchers also tried to develop new pertussis vaccines with fewer side reactions. As a result, in 1991 the Food and Drug Administration (FDA) licensed the DTaP vaccines (diphtheria-tetanus-acellular pertussis).

While DTP was made using whole cells of the pertussis germ, DTaP was made using only small, purified snippets of the germs. Fewer side effects—soreness, swelling, and redness at the injection site, crying, fever, and febrile seizures—have been reported with DTaP than with DTP.

As we will see later, the concerns about brain damage, infantile spasms, and SIDS were excluded when more data became available. However, initially—until that missing information was obtained—the VICP made awards to children who the court thought might have been brain injured by the DTP vaccine.

The DTP vaccine has been completely replaced in the United States by the DTaP vaccine, but it continues to be extensively used elsewhere in the world.

The history of whooping cough vaccines contains some elements common to the evolution of many vaccine safety issues:

1.   A vaccine safety concern is suggested through case reports (observations of *possible* associations) or by an increase of reports of *possible* reactions.

2.   Scientists say they don't know whether the vaccine

caused the adverse event or it was just coincidental in time—the information is insufficient (missing) to permit reaching a conclusion.

3. Public health officials compare the possible risk from the adverse event of concern with the known risk of the disease, based on whatever available data there are. The results of their analyses guide policy recommendations—which still must be made to protect the public health, even in the absence of all the desired information.

4. The media reports the scientific "uncertainty" as scientists conduct the needed research.

5. Many parents may become confused about vaccine benefits and risks.

6. Immunization levels may fall and outbreaks of disease may occur if community immunity declines.

Consistently, there is a period of uncertainty, a period of missing information. And people respond differently during these periods.

♦ Some parents react with fear and do not immunize their children.

♦ Other parents dismiss the concerns as speculative and trust that their doctor will know what to do.

♦ Still others—perhaps because their children have the condition attributed to the vaccine—decide that the vaccine caused the adverse event, despite the lack of scientific evidence one way or the other.

When all the available scientific information is not sufficient to prove a relationship between an adverse event and vaccine administration—or to favor coincidence—scientists will often state that "the data are insufficient to either accept or reject the hypothesis." To be accurate, they equivocate even when they believe that no causal association will be found.

NICK'S STORY: DEALING WITH SCIENTIFIC UNCERTAINTY

In the early 1990s, the Morris family from Columbus, Georgia, saw the news about the scary adverse events supposedly happening after DTP vaccination. Thinking they were making an informed, educated decision, they chose not to complete the series of shots for their son, Nick—who had only had one dose by then.

At age four, Nick contracted whooping cough. Violent coughing attacks made him vomit and his face turn blue. He had to be hospitalized with pertussis complications that almost took his life away.

Nick's parents dealt with the uncertainty about the safety of the DTP vaccine by not immunizing him. Mr. Morris later said that the media frightened him by stating the risks of the vaccine without noting the risks of whooping cough.[4]

Without complete and scientifically valid information about vaccines, parents cannot make informed decisions. They need to have access to accurate evidence-based information so that they understand the importance of community immunity, and what the actual risks of disease complications are. Without this information many may develop a false sense of security and regard immunizations as unimportant.

SEARCHING FOR MISSING INFORMATION

How do you determine if a new vaccine is going to be safe? Basically, scientists vaccinate volunteers and then wait. If no adverse reactions occur, no health problems arise, the vaccine is considered safe.

Of course, before being tested in humans, vaccines are tested for safety in animals. However, because mice and humans do not always respond in the same way to a drug or treatment, a candidate vaccine may look safe in animal studies but later cause health problems in humans. For this reason, human studies are both required and strictly regulated.

Scientists ensure the safety of a vaccine by closely monitoring increasing numbers of people and then watching carefully for the appearance of any adverse event(s).

The FDA, through its Center for Biologics Evaluation and Research (CBER), regulates all aspects of the testing and licensure of vaccine products intended for humans. All products regulated by the FDA, including vaccines, undergo a rigorous review of laboratory and clinical data to ensure the safety, efficacy, purity, and potency of these products.

Before licensure, vaccines must be tested in clinical trials. A clinical trial is a human research study done to determine whether a vaccine (or drug or treatment) works and whether it is likely to be safe.

Clinical trials are conducted in phases. Phases I, II, and III describe the regulatory steps in vaccine development and testing before the vaccine is licensed.

> **Phase I:** Researchers test the safety and immune response of the vaccine in a small number of people (20 to 80 people).
>
> **Phase II:** The vaccine is tested in more people (100 to 300) to establish what dosages are most likely to be effective as well as safe.
>
> **Phase III:** The vaccine is now tried in thousands of people. During this phase, researchers gather data on the effectiveness and safety of the vaccine by comparing two groups—one receives the vaccine being tested and the other receives a different vaccine or a placebo.

A placebo is an inert compound identical in appearance to the material being tested, which may or may not be known to the investigator and/or patient. For example, in a controlled clinical trial, a control group might receive salt water—the placebo—instead of the actual vaccine. If neither the person giving the vaccine nor the person receiving the vaccine knows whether it is vaccine or placebo the study is said to be "double blinded."

Safety concerns may arise at any stage of the animal studies or clinical trials. When this happens, the FDA may request that more information be provided. If data show that the vaccine is causing serious adverse events, the manufacturer or FDA may suspend the trials.

Common adverse events can be identified by comparing the number of cases of those events in vaccine recipients with the number of cases in placebo recipients. If many more adverse events occur in the vaccine recipients, the vaccine may be the cause of the reaction.

However, side effects that are rare (for example, 1 in 10,000 or lower) may not be detected because the numbers of participants in the prelicensure trials are not large enough to find these rare events.

For example, to identify a rare adverse event that occurs 1 time per every 10,000 vaccinees may require 30,000 vaccinees plus 30,000 controls or more to be studied. Hundreds of thousands or even many millions of doses of vaccine may need to be administered to determine whether a vaccine causes a very rare adverse event. The FDA may require the manufacturer to collect data on this many vaccine recipients after a vaccine is licensed as a condition for granting the license (so-called "Phase IV postlicensure studies").

Following licensure, the FDA and CDC monitor reported adverse events to detect possible unexpected very rare adverse events.[5]

Thus vaccine safety research often requires very large studies.[6]

In addition to the required Phase IV trials—or post-licensure evaluations—adverse events are sought after the vaccine is licensed through large populations of patients, such as the Vaccine Safety Datalink project as well as spontaneous reporting systems such as the Vaccine Adverse Event Reporting System (VAERS)—see Chapter 4.

THE RSV VACCINE TRIALS

In the 1950s, an effective vaccine against polio was created by inactivating (killing) polio virus with formalin—the chemical formaldehyde diluted in water.

When introduced into the body, the dead or harmless virus in the vaccine causes an immune response without causing the disease. The immune system develops antibodies that will effectively kill or neutralize the virus if the person is exposed to it in the future.

The success of the inactivated polio vaccine led scientists to try to develop other vaccines through the same method of inactivation.

In a 1966–1967 prelicensure, placebo-controlled trial, scientists tested a formalin-inactivated vaccine against respiratory syncytial virus (RSV)—a very common cause of lower respiratory infections, such as pneumonia, in young children.

Each year in the United States, it is estimated that between 70,000 and 126,000 infants are hospitalized with RSV pneumonia or bronchiolitis—inflammation of the bronchioles (small airways) that causes wheezing.

The vaccine or placebo was administered to infants and children between 2 months and 9 years of age. However, the vaccine did not protect against RSV infection when a natural outbreak occurred some time later; in fact, the children had worse lower respiratory illnesses—80% of the children who received the RSV vaccine had to be hospitalized, whereas only 5% of children in the control group were hospitalized.

In other words, those vaccinated had more severe RSV disease than those who did not receive the vaccine. Two of the vaccinated infants died.[7]

The formalin-inactivated RSV vaccine from the 1960s was never licensed because of these safety concerns, which were identified in the prelicensure studies. There is still no licensed RSV vaccine.

The reason for the problem with the original RSV vaccine is now understood and new RSV vaccines are under development.

PUBLIC HEALTH POLICY DECISIONS IN THE FACE OF MISSING INFORMATION

Unfortunately, public health policy recommendations often must be made in the face of incomplete information: health professionals and parents want guidance as to what to do while the missing information is being collected.

The CDC must recommend what to do. Their recommendations are based on the information that is available and the input from public health authorities, the scientists who are most directly involved, members of industry, the other branches of government, as well as from interested citizens.

At times, agencies of the U.S. government (like the CDC or NIH or Congress itself) ask the IOM to advise them about data interpretation.

TECHNICAL JARGON

The late Carl Sagan said during a 1995 speech, "We have designed our civilization based on science and technology and at the same time arranged things so that almost no one understands anything at all about science and technology. This is a clear prescription for disaster."

Even when information is available, scientists often have trouble communicating their findings to the public. Not only do they communicate with technical terms, but often their words may mean something completely different from the same words when used in everyday conversations.

In the following table are some words or expressions that, when used by vaccine safety researchers, have a different meaning than when used in plain conversational English. On page 219, you will find a glossary with definitions of common vaccine research terms.

Expression/ Word	What it means for vaccine scientists	What it means for the public
Vaccine adverse event	Something that occurred at about the same time as vaccination, which may or may not be caused by the vaccine.	Something caused by the vaccine (vaccine reaction or side effect).
Bias	Systematic error that could lead to the wrong conclusion. For example, selection bias means the manner by which subjects were selected could have influenced the results.	Not having an open mind.
Controversy	There are different but plausible interpretations of the same data within the scientific community.	There is a difference in opinion.
The patient "denies xyz"	The patient says she doesn't have the symptoms or hasn't had the disease.	The patient reacts defensively to an accusation.
Epidemiology	The study of how disease is distributed in a population and of the factors that influence that distribution.	Number crunching.
Favors rejection of the hypothesis	The data suggest that the hypothesis should be rejected (but you can't prove a negative).	We still don't know.
The finding won't go away	We couldn't find an alternative explanation.	We're fudging the data.
Inadequate to accept or reject the hypothesis	The data do not allow a definitive statement.	We don't know.
Naive	The person or animal has not previously been exposed to a particular infection, drug, or vaccine.	Unsophisticated, lacking experience or training.
Paralysis	Loss of the ability to move a body part usually as a result of nerve damage.	Inability to act, helpless inactivity.
Plausible	Theoretically possible.	Appearing worthy of belief, factual.
Positive	The results of the study concur with the hypothesis; having a value greater than zero.	Good.
Power	The likelihood of a study finding an effect, if there was one. Or, the number of times a number is multiplied by itself.	Energy, strength, control.
Probably a small risk	The association is likely real but very infrequent. Or, uncertainty.	Likely that it is a risk.
Relative risk	The ratio of two rates of risks, often used to compare risks.	The risks are related.
Safe	Remote or insignificant risk	No risk or zero risk.
Significant	This may not be a chance difference.	Important.
Not significant	Likely due to chance.	Not important.
Uncertainty	When the available scientific information is not sufficient to prove a relationship or is not sufficient to favor rejection of a relationship.	They don't know.

THE BOTTOM LINE: WHY CAN'T MEDICAL RESEARCHERS TALK NORMALLY?!

Talking about the results of their studies on vaccine safety, scientists use expressions such as "favors rejection" or "inadequate to accept or reject the hypothesis." As much as we would like them to say plainly, "vaccines do not cause that," the nature of the scientific method does not allow them to say it—at least if they are honest scientists.

This is because all scientific knowledge is provisional and subject to change when more information is available. As evidence accumulates and it is reproduced once and again, certainty increases, and scientists start talking about facts.

In this book, we evaluate several vaccine safety concerns asking, "Do vaccines cause that?" As you read the next chapter, you will find that it is easier to prove that a vaccine caused an effect than to show that it did not cause the effect.

A quote attributed to Albert Einstein says, "No amount of experimentation can ever prove me right; a single experiment can prove me wrong." Regarding some of these concerns, there is still a lot of missing information, so a definitive "yes" or "no" is not possible. The available evidence, however, can provide us sufficient information to assess the safety of the vaccines currently administered to our children.

IF YOU WANT TO READ MORE:

About Vaccine Safety. *www.cdc.gov/vaccinesafety/.*

Cause or Coincidence: How Do I Tell Whether or Not a Vaccine Caused That?!

A tendency to drastically underestimate the frequency of coincidence is a prime characteristic of innumerates, who generally accord great significance to correspondences of all sorts while attributing little significance to quite conclusive but less flashy statistical evidence.
John Allen Paulos, Innumeracy: Mathematical Illiteracy and its Consequences, 1988

Daniel is a curious one-year-old who loves to play with the TV's remote control. He learned that by pressing the buttons he could change the images in the big gray box. This causes his older brother to jump off the sofa very annoyed. Daniel is amused by his brother's reaction. The funny thing is that it doesn't work when he points the remote at his big brother—nothing happens.

Like Daniel, we all make associations between events that follow each other in time. We call them "cause" and "effect" and expect them to occur always in the same way. That usually works just fine (that's why we don't put our hands on a hot stove).

Sometimes, however, our temporal associations are not enough to determine the true causes of our daily experiences. For example, a couple that discovers that their toddler has diarrhea may blame it on the pizza they let her eat the night before, while the true cause of her diarrhea may be a virus she caught at day care. The cause of the diarrhea could have been the pizza if it was contaminated in the cooking process—but that would probably have resulted in the parents also getting sick from eating the pizza. On the other hand, germs that cause diarrhea and vomiting spread easily in day care centers, particularly when many children have diapers to be changed. For the parents, however, the association could be

48

limited to what they observe—the pizza leftovers—and their knowledge of the subject—that young children are unable to digest some foods.

There is more than meets the eye when establishing causality—as Daniel realized when, unbeknownst to him, his brother took the batteries out of the remote control. Now it didn't cause his brother to jump up no matter where he pointed the remote.

No Such Thing as a Simple Cause

In the late 1990s researchers discovered that virtually all the women with cervical cancer in the world had something in common: they were all infected with certain types of human papillomavirus (HPV). By then it was already recognized that many women with cervical cancer were also infected with genital herpes simplex virus (HSV). Both genital HSV and HPV infections were associated with cervical cancer, but were they the actual cause of the disease?

Association and causation are not the same. While an "association" is an identifiable relationship between an exposure (HSV or HPV infection) and a disease (cervical cancer), "causation" implies that there is a true mechanism that leads from exposure to disease.

The observed association between HPV and cervical cancer was corroborated by the finding that cervical infection with certain types of HPV is necessary for a woman to develop cancer of the cervix: all of the cervical cancers and precancers contain one of these viruses. Furthermore, an HPV vaccine protects against both infection and the cancer caused by the HPV types in the vaccine, but not against other HPV types not in the vaccine. This evidence suggested that there was more than an association; HPV was indeed the cause of cervical cancer.[1]

Although the concept and definition of causation have been matters of debate among philosophers for centuries, medical researchers have adopted working definitions to study the causes of disease.

In general, a disease is caused by an event or condition that precedes the disease and without which the disease would not have occurred. Many diseases have more than a single cause. Understanding all the causes of an illness may appeal to many scientists, but public health (and vaccine safety) researchers are more concerned about *necessary* and *sufficient* causes that can be prevented or treated effectively.

A necessary cause *must* be present for the disease to occur, but other factors may be present too; a sufficient cause alone will inevitably produce the disease.

Infection with a "high-risk" type of HPV is *necessary* for cervical cancer to develop, yet it is not sufficient for the cancer to occur. In other words, a woman will not develop cervical cancer without a high-risk type HPV infection, but the infection alone will not always result in cancer—other factors must be present. In fact, most high-risk HPV infections go away on their own and do not cause cancer. Scientists still don't know why some HPV-infected women develop cancer of the cervix and others don't. They have identified, however, some risk factors that—in combination with a high-risk HPV infection—increase the chances of developing cervical cancer, such as smoking, a diet low in fruits and vegetables, long-term use of oral contraceptives, and a family history of cervical cancer, among others. Still, none of these factors is necessary for the progression of high-risk HPV infection to cancer.[2]

Coming back to Daniel: The TV is turned on, the remote has batteries and is pointing at the TV, and his brother is present in the room—these are all necessary factors to get the desired reaction. With those present, Daniel pushing the button becomes the sufficient cause to provoke his brother.

How Scientists Establish Causality

Below are some factors that scientists consider when trying to determine whether a vaccine is the cause of an adverse event or disease.[3]

TIME OF ONSET: The onset must follow vaccination. If symptoms occurred before vaccination, then the vaccine is not the cause.

VIRUS ISOLATION: Some vaccines are made with a live but weakened virus. If the vaccine virus is found in a part of the body where it normally would not be found (for example, blood or cerebrospinal fluid), then the vaccine may have caused the adverse event.

UNIQUENESS OF THE CLINICAL SYNDROME: Causation may be inferred if the adverse event or disease only occurs following vaccination and does not occur in persons who did not receive the vaccine. Causation may also be inferred if the adverse event occurs a second time after receiving the same vaccine.

BIOLOGICAL MECHANISMS: There must be biological mechanisms that could potentially explain how the vaccine might cause the adverse event. Demonstration of a possible mechanism does not prove that the vaccine caused the problem. However, when there is other evidence of an association, such as epidemiological studies (see explanation below), biological mechanisms that could explain the association might help in establishing whether the vaccine caused the problem.

EPIDEMIOLOGICAL STUDIES: Epidemiological studies often provide the most important evidence as to whether a vaccine caused the problem because most adverse events are not unique clinical syndromes (that is, they also occur in people who did not receive the vaccine). Epidemiological studies determine whether the risk (rate) of the illness of concern is higher in vaccinated persons compared to unvaccinated persons. A higher risk among vaccinated persons could mean that the vaccine caused the adverse event.

BIOLOGICAL PLAUSIBILITY

When establishing causality, an association between the vaccine and the adverse event should be consistent with the biology and the natural history of the disease. In other words, there should be a biological explanation as to how the adverse event could have occurred after exposure to the vaccine.

But the fact that something has such "biological plausibility" doesn't establish causality—it only means it is conceivable.

For example, both HSV (herpes) and HPV (human papillomavirus) have plausible mechanisms by which they could cause cervical cancer. HPV's genetic material is incorporated into the cell it infects, and HSV persists permanently in the infected person.

But scientists now know that women do not have to have genital HSV infection in order to develop cervical cancer. Unlike HPV, which is present in virtually all cases of cervical cancer, HSV is not always present.

Even if biological mechanisms can be demonstrated, it is unlikely to be sufficient evidence to establish causation of an adverse event. Consider a murder trial, for example. The victim was shot. It is easy to demonstrate a mechanism by which a gunshot can kill a person. But that alone is not evidence that the suspect fired the gun.

Other evidence, such as the account of an eyewitness might be needed. Both types of evidence—the known mechanism and the witness's observation—strengthen each other.

On the other hand, if the prosecutor claims that the suspect killed the victim by wishing it, there is no mechanism to support that claim although it might provide a motive.

EPIDEMIOLOGY AND CAUSALITY

Epidemiology is the study of how disease is distributed in a population and of the factors that influence or determine that distribution. Epidemiological studies can help to identify the causes and risk factors of a disease in a community. Causality is often inferred from epidemiological studies by using the following criteria:[4]

STRENGTH OF ASSOCIATION: The greater the difference in rates between the vaccinated and unvaccinated, the more likely there could be a causal relationship.

CONSISTENCY OF ASSOCIATION: The more studies that show similar results using different populations and different study methods, the more likely there is a causal relationship.

DOSE RESPONSE: When it can be shown that there is increasing risk for the adverse event with increasing dose, the more likely that there could be a causal relationship. If the vaccine—or a vaccine component—is the cause of an adverse event, removal of the vaccine or the component should decrease the occurrence of more adverse events.

CESSATION EFFECTS: Discontinuing a drug and having the adverse response go away suggests a causal effect. This is usually more of a consideration for chemicals or drugs and is not often relevant for vaccines.

STATISTICAL SIGNIFICANCE: The likelihood that the results of a study were due to chance is measured by the P value—the smaller the P value, the higher the statistical significance of the study, thus, the more likely the results were not found by a chance occurrence. If the P value is 0.6, there is a 60% chance that the difference is coincidental. By convention, a P value of 0.05 or less is considered a "significant difference" because the probability that the difference is due to chance is only 5% (or less). For example, if you toss a coin twice, the most likely outcome is one head and one tail. If you actually got heads twice you wouldn't think there was a problem with the coin or how you tossed it, because that is the result you would expect to find 25% of the time that you tossed the coin twice. On the other hand, if you tossed it 1,000 times and got heads every time, you would be very suspicious that there was something very wrong with the coin. That's where P values come in; they are a mathematical estimate of the probability of a difference of finding 1,000 heads—instead of the expected 500—just by chance alone (luck) or because it may be a real difference (perhaps because of the coin being heavier on one side).

When scientists refer to "selection bias," they mean that a systematic problem may have occurred in a study that could have led to an erroneous—but statistically significant (small P value)—conclusion. For example, children who frequently visit their physician for a problem such as asthma are more likely to receive a new vaccine than those who don't have to see their physician as frequently. Thus, a study of a large pediatric practice might find that more children with pre-existing asthma are vaccinated. But, because asthmatic children are more likely to be seen for episodes of wheezing, this type of study could erroneously conclude that wheezing occurs more commonly among vaccinated children.

Epidemiological studies help identify the cause of a disease in the general population. But it is harder for these studies to find the cause of rare diseases that occur in only a very small proportion of the population. They can't prove the negative (that is, conclude that a vaccine does not cause a disease); they can only show it is very unlikely to have caused disease.

EVALUATING THE QUALITY OF EPIDEMIOLOGICAL STUDIES

Not all types of epidemiological studies carry the same weight in establishing causality. Every individual study—independent of its type—has to be evaluated based on its merits. Quality depends on the study design, its statistical power (likelihood of being able to find a difference between groups), the presence of selection or information biases (which might lead to finding the incorrect result), what is being measured, and the objectivity of the observer.

When evaluating the safety of a vaccine, all the relevant studies need to be evaluated in this manner before reaching a conclusion about accepting or rejecting a theoretical concern. For instance, in 2001 the Institute of Medicine's Vaccine Safety Committee was unable to reach a conclusion about whether there could be an association between thimerosal preservative in vaccines and the development of autism because there weren't enough good studies. Three years later, however, there were enough studies looking at many groups of children in different communities and using multiple epidemiological tools that the committee was able to state that the data favored the rejection of the theory.[5]

The following are some types of epidemiological studies often performed to examine adverse events.

Clinical trials are large studies that test the safety and effectiveness of vaccines, usually involving two groups randomly selected and assigned—one of which receives the vaccine and the other a placebo (a substance such as saline water or a different vaccine).

Case-control studies compare a group of individuals affected by a disease with a similar group of people who do not have that disease, to seek possible associations. The controls need to be similar in as many ways as possible: year of birth, sex, socioeconomic status, and general practice attended among other things. The proportion of cases who are vaccinated is compared with the proportion of controls with a history of vaccination.

In **cohort studies** researchers look for samples of immunized and unimmunized children who are otherwise similar to see if the adverse effect occurs more commonly among the vaccinated group.

Ecological studies, also known as correlational studies, use data from entire populations (such as countries or cities) to compare the frequency of a disease in that population to another population measure—such as the proportion of the children in that population who have been immunized. This type of study is not as powerful as the previous types because it cannot provide information about the individuals within the population. In other words, researchers cannot tell whether the people with the disease were also the ones who received the vaccine or not.

Case-series reports are descriptions of people with a similar illness. These types of observations are not epidemiological studies but clinical observations about a group of patients. They can lead to suggestions of possible causes or mechanisms for the findings, but because there is no comparison group they can only form the basis of a theory that then needs to be tested. Also, these types of studies do not control for other things that may be happening in the population at the same time.

AN EXAMPLE: ROTAVIRUS VACCINE (ROTASHIELD)

The process to determine whether an adverse event is caused by a particular vaccine is usually prompted by observations or reports of that adverse event. Then researchers conduct epidemiological studies to determine the risk of the event for vaccinated people compared to unvaccinated people. Still other researchers will try to determine potential biological mechanisms that might explain how the vaccine might cause the event.

This process is well illustrated with the history of the first rotavirus vaccine.[6] Rotavirus is an intestinal virus that infects virtually all children by 3 years of age. It is the most common cause of diarrhea in children. The disease can last a week or longer. Most rotavirus infections are mild, but about 1 in 50 cases develops severe dehydration. Each year in the United States, rotavirus results in the hospitalization of 50,000 infants younger than 2 years of age. In developing countries, rotavirus leads to an estimated 480,000 to 640,000 deaths each year.

The FDA licensed the first rotavirus vaccine, RotaShield (RRV-TV), in August 1998. In July 1999, after approximately 1 million children had been immunized with the vaccine, the Centers for Disease Control and Prevention (CDC) recommended that people temporarily stop immunizing infants with RotaShield. The CDC was concerned that the vaccine might be causing a serious bowel disease called intussusception, because an unexpected number of cases of this condition (15) had been reported in children who had received the vaccine. Subsequent epidemiological studies reported that 1 out of every 10,000 to 12,000 infants could be at risk of developing intussusception due to receiving RotaShield.

The clinical trials to evaluate the safety and efficacy of this vaccine involved 17,963 infants in the United States, Venezuela, and Finland. During these trials almost 7,000 infants received the vaccine and the rest a placebo. In retrospect, this number was not large enough to detect an adverse event such as intussusception at a rate of about 1 in 10,000. The CDC recommendations in 1998 noted that:

> In all studies of rhesus rotavirus vaccines combined, intussusception was noted in five of 10,054 (0.05%)

recipients of any reassortant rhesus vaccine (two of these five children received [RotaShield]) compared with one of 4,633 placebo recipients. The difference between the rates of intussusception in these groups was not statistically significant (p = 0.92 for children receiving vaccine; p = 0.45 for children receiving placebo), and the rates observed among vaccinated children were similar to those seen in comparison populations. Although the association of these events with [RotaShield] appears to be temporal rather than causal, postlicensure surveillance is needed for these and other rare adverse events that might occur.[7]

In other words, the trials were unable to show that vaccinated infants were at a higher risk of intussusception than unvaccinated infants. The lesson learned from the first rotavirus vaccine led to later trials of other types of rotavirus vaccines using larger numbers of children. The rotavirus vaccines licensed in 2006 (RotaTeq) and 2008 (Rotarix), for example, were tested in almost 72,000 and more than 63,000 children, respectively, because researchers wanted to have the ability to detect (called "power") cases of intussusception at a rate of about 1 per 10,000. The trials suggest that these new vaccines do not cause intussusception.[8]

To determine whether RotaShield was causing intussusception, four different epidemiological studies—using very different methodologies (case control, retrospective cohort, ecological) and each with different strengths and weaknesses—were employed to look for an increased risk of intussusception occurring predominantly during the first week after the first dose of the vaccine. For example,

• The case-control study—which included 429 infants with intussusception and 1,763 healthy control infants (matched for age and birth hospital)—showed that those who received the rotavirus vaccine were 37 times more likely to have intussusception 3 to 7 days after the first dose than infants who did not receive the vaccine.[9]

- The retrospective cohort study—which included 463,277 children in managed care organizations—showed that those who received the vaccine were 30 times more likely to have intussusception 3 to 7 days after the first dose than infants who did not receive the vaccine.[10]
- The ecological studies, however, did not show an increase in overall rates of intussusception after the introduction of RotaShield.

The timing of the adverse event, the biological plausibility (the virus infects the gut), and the strength and consistency of the evidence led scientists to conclude that there was a cause-and-effect association between RotaShield and intussusception. This example shows the types of evidence used to establish causality and the importance of multiple avenues of evaluation.

Notwithstanding, there has also been an intense scientific debate about this adverse event. While there is consensus among scientists about the cause-and-effect association between the RotaShield vaccine and intussusception, some scientists have hypothesized that because the number of cases of intussusception in the population did not increase, perhaps the vaccine triggered the disease in intussusception-prone infants—that is, these children might have developed intussusception later in infancy anyway.[6,11] This demonstrates the complexity of interpreting causal associations. It also illustrates true scientific controversy and debate in contrast to what the media often calls a controversy or debate—when some are convinced that a vaccine caused an adverse effect, but there is scientific consensus that an association doesn't exist.

RotaShield vaccine was withdrawn from the market by the manufacturer in October 1999. By late 2007, the new rotavirus vaccine RotaTeq, which was licensed in 2006, had been given to more than 4 million children without evidence for an elevated risk of intussusception.

VAERS AND CAUSALITY

The process that led to the suspension of the use of the RotaShield vaccine in 1999 began with an observation from the Vaccine Adverse Event Reporting System (VAERS). VAERS is a national system for reporting any possible adverse reactions after any U.S.-licensed vaccine is administered. VAERS is operated by the CDC and the FDA.

VAERS accepts voluntary reports from everyone—physicians, nurses, parents, patients, or anyone else. They are encouraged to report any untoward event that occurs after a vaccination (from a mild fever to hospitalization to death) whether they believe that the vaccination was the cause or not. Vaccine manufacturers are required to report to the FDA all potential adverse events of which they become aware.[12]

The CDC established Clinical Immunization Safety Assessment centers in 2002 to follow up on specific cases of adverse events reported to VAERS.

The CDC and FDA use VAERS to detect early warning signals. They generate hypotheses about possible unrecognized adverse events that might be caused by a vaccine and look for possible changes in the frequency of recognized side effects.

However, when analyzing data from VAERS, researchers, the public, and the media need to take into account the system's limitations. The information in a VAERS report is not necessarily complete, nor is it checked for its accuracy in most cases. Reports of particular interest, including all deaths and hospitalizations, are followed up by epidemiologists at the CDC or FDA. Sometimes follow-up of these reports reveals serious mistakes and errors in the information, such as reports of events that occurred before the immunization. Also, in 24% of VAERS reports the causes of death on follow-up were different from what was originally reported. In one case a vaccinee who had been reported dead on the VAERS form, had in fact not died.[12]

One wrong assumption when interpreting VAERS data is that all VAERS reports represent side effects caused by vaccines. Rather, it is a system designed to look for adverse events—things that occurred about the same time as vaccination—that then may require additional investigation to see if in fact there is an association with vaccine administration.

In some media reports and on some Web sites, VAERS reports are misrepresented as verified cases of vaccine-caused injuries.

Whereas some events reported to VAERS are likely caused by vaccines (for example, injection-site swelling), others may be related to an underlying disease or condition, or due to drugs being taken—or it may be something that occurred simply by chance shortly after the vaccine was administered.

Adverse events are reported to VAERS in a biased manner. Because VAERS reporting is voluntary, reports are more likely to be submitted for those untoward events that the observer considers more likely to have been caused by the vaccine.

The number of reported adverse events is also influenced by publicity. Thus reports to VAERS of a particular adverse event may be the result of parents or physicians having heard about it in the media, independent of any possible causal relationship between the vaccine and the event in question. For example, in Canada—which has a similar reporting system—media reports of a mild allergic-type reaction after influenza vaccine resulted in a 3- to 5-fold increase in reports of all types of adverse events following influenza immunization compared with the previous year.[13]

In spite of its many limitations, VAERS data have proven to be very useful in ongoing vaccine safety monitoring, especially looking for signals of unexpected or rare adverse events. People trying to use this data to perform causation studies fail to understand the limits of the system, however, and often arrive at unwarranted conclusions.

THE VACCINE SAFETY DATALINK

The Vaccine Safety Datalink project was created in 1990 by the CDC and, as of mid-2007, involves partnerships with eight large health maintenance organizations (HMOs) that continually monitor vaccine safety.[14] The patients' complete medical records at these HMOs are used to analyze vaccine-related information pertaining to more than 5.5 million people in Washington, Oregon, California, Colorado, Minnesota, and Massachusetts.

This large database allows researchers to access already gathered data on:
- all medical visits
- vaccine type
- date of vaccination
- concurrent vaccinations (those given during the same visit)
- the manufacturer
- lot number
- injection site
- potential adverse events

Studying this large group of patient records has several advantages over the other methods of post-licensure vaccine safety monitoring. First, it is a comprehensive medical database. All medical illnesses, whether vaccine related or not, are already in the database. Second, all or almost all information on vaccination is also available.

What kind of studies can be done with this type of large database?

COMPARE VACCINATED CHILDREN TO UNVACCINATED CHILDREN. Investigators can look at data from two different groups—one of vaccinated children and another of unvaccinated children—and determine how many children in each group experience a particular illness. If more children in the vaccinated group have the illness than those who did not receive the vaccine, then the vaccine may be causing the illness. On the other hand, if in both groups the number of ill children is similar, the vaccine is unlikely to be the cause of the event. VAERS does not have the capacity to make these types of comparisons.

COMPARE DIFFERENT POINTS IN TIME. When there is concern that a vaccine may be causing an illness in a certain time frame after vaccination, the number of new cases during this period can be compared with the number of cases at other times to see if it is significantly higher in the period of concern.

For example, the large database was used to study the rate of sudden infant death syndrome (SIDS) after anecdotes (case reports) suggested a possible link to the DTP vaccine. The risk of SIDS was found to be the same for vaccinated children as for unvaccinated children enrolled in the participating HMOs.[15]

RAPID CYCLE ANALYSIS. Unlike VAERS, rapid cycle analysis[16] is used to look for specific adverse event signals in an active, hypothesis-driven process rather than in a passive "data mining" process. That is, this system asks if a particular vaccine safety concern is more frequent or not in those who got the vaccine.

Then, if a signal is detected, the analysis can be refined into a more specific study. Here's how it works for a newly introduced vaccine:

* A specific vaccine safety concern is selected.
* *Each week*, the database is examined for that specific adverse event in vaccinated persons.
* The rate of that adverse event in a comparison group is determined (this becomes the "expected rate").
* The observed frequency of the adverse event after vaccine is then compared weekly to the expected frequency from the comparison group.
* Statistical tools allow the researchers to set a "threshold" for when the number of cases in the vaccinated group should be recognized as greater than expecteda (it is a "signal").

This type of analysis looks for more cases than might be expected for specific conditions of concern. But not all signals turn out to be caused by the vaccine, as was the case with RotaTeq, the rotavirus vaccine introduced in 2006. Researchers looked for bleeding from the intestinal tract (an early sign of intussusception) after vaccination. They compared the rate of children who had bleeding in the stool after vaccination with the expected rate from before the vaccine was introduced and found a signal. The researchers then examined the rate of intestinal bleeding in children who were getting vaccines (except RotaTeq) at the same age as the children who got vaccines that included RotaTeq. The signal disappeared. It turns out, intestinal bleeding was related to the child's age, the season of the year, and which HMO cared for the child (where in the United States the child lived), but was not related to receipt of RotaTeq.[17]

More than 30 studies have used or are using these large HMO databases to examine vaccine safety issues, including the safety of inactivated influenza vaccine among children, and the association between vaccines and asthma or neonatal death.[18,19]

The HMO-based project, however, has some limitations:

- The population in the participating HMOs is not wholly representative of the United States in terms of geography, ethnicity, or socioeconomic status.

- Vaccine coverage rates for most vaccines are very high in the participating HMOs, and thus there are usually few non-vaccinated people available for comprehensive comparisons. One way that researchers address this problem is by using the patient as his or her own control. For instance, fever after MMR vaccine appears between 6 and 12 days after the vaccine is given in 5 to 15% of vaccinees. If not enough non-vaccinated children are available for comparison, researchers could compare the rates of fever in children 2 weeks before and 2 weeks after vaccination. Higher rates in the after-vaccine period would suggest that the vaccine might be causing the fever.

- It is difficult to assess mild or short-term adverse events that may escape medical attention, such as fever.

- The project is not large enough to examine the risk of extremely rare events (one in a million vaccinees) such as Guillain-Barré syndrome after influenza vaccine.

- Because the database contains patient records, it can only be accessed under circumstances that maintain the confidentiality of the individuals and requires prior approval of an Institutional Review Board—

that is, the database cannot be made available to just anyone who wishes to study it.

Despite the above caveats, the HMO-based database project provides a powerful and cost-effective tool for the constant monitoring of vaccine safety. Studies performed using these data sets—along with many other studies—were used by the Institute of Medicine's Vaccine Safety Review Committee to evaluate some vaccine safety concerns.[20]

ARE EPIDEMIOLOGICAL STUDIES "REAL SCIENCE"?

A common misconception—often made by those who oppose vaccines—is that epidemiological studies are not real science.

Scientists, however, expect each other to evaluate all types of studies whether laboratory based, epidemiological, or other. When evaluating the safety of a vaccine, all the relevant studies need to be evaluated before accepting or rejecting a theoretical concern. In addition to epidemiological studies scientists often need to consider important laboratory studies.

Evidence from laboratory experiments can rarely—if ever—establish causality between a vaccine and an adverse event. But laboratory evidence can certainly strengthen epidemiological evidence both by suggesting how the disease develops and by generating new theories.

For example, a landmark finding at the beginning of the 20th century was the discovery by Landsteiner that he could reproduce poliomyelitis in monkeys by injecting them with filtered materials from people with poliomyelitis. Landsteiner's discovery paved the way for the studies that ultimately led to the development of polio vaccines—monkeys were used to show that the live virus vaccine strains in the oral polio vaccine were sufficiently weakened to be safe.

On the other hand, epidemiological studies were crucial

in determining what happened in 1955 when children were developing poliomyelitis after receiving the killed polio vaccine made by Cutter Laboratories.

In his book, *The Cutter Incident*, Paul Offit, writes:

> Langmuir [an epidemiologist] and his team determined the incidence of paralysis in children who had received vaccine from each of eight production pools made by Cutter Laboratories. They found that for children receiving vaccine from six of the pools the incidence of paralysis was the same as the average incidence of paralysis in children in the spring of the preceding five years. But for children receiving vaccine from two of the production pools (lots 19468 and 19764), the incidence of paralysis was almost ten times greater than expected.[13]

It was later shown in the laboratory that the vaccine in these lots contained live viruses—the polio viruses had not been completely inactivated (killed) during manufacture.

In summary, epidemiological studies are as important as other types of scientific studies—such as the following:

IN VITRO SYSTEMS. *In vitro*, which means "in glass," refers to experiments performed outside the body—perhaps in test tubes or petri dishes. Scientists may use in vitro techniques to analyze the effects of vaccine components—chemicals or viruses—on human cells or neurons. These studies help identify what chemicals damage a human organ and to question how an event might occur.

In vitro studies include the growth of viruses in test tubes containing cells from humans or animals. These studies led to the development of polio, mumps, rubella, and chickenpox vaccines, for example.

A 1998 National Institute of Environmental Health Sciences review stressed the difficulties of extrapolating results obtained in a test tube to human beings:

> Because of the complexity of the nervous system,
> multiple functions of individual cells, and our lim-
> ited knowledge of biochemical processes involved
> in neurotoxicity, it is not known how well any in
> vitro system would recapitulate the in vivo [animals
> or humans] system.[21]

ANIMAL MODELS. Experimental studies in animals allow researchers to control the quantity and timing of
vaccine doses and to carefully monitor adverse events.
Animal models of human diseases help researchers
understand how illnesses could be caused. Animal
studies have often provided the first "proof of principle" that a vaccine might work in humans.

When evaluating studies in animal models we need
to consider that

◆ It may not be possible to extrapolate the results to
  humans—different species may not react similarly
  and their sensitivity to the vaccines or its components may be different.

◆ The manifestations of the disease in the animal
  species may not accurately reflect the process in
  humans.

◆ The number of animals may be too small to be able
  to make comparisons.

As the late science writer Victor Cohn said, "Cor-
tisone causes cleft palate in mice but not in humans.
A dose of morphine that can kill a human merely
anesthetizes a dog. Arsenic doesn't induce cancer in
animals but does in man."[22]

Sometimes, the effectiveness of a vaccine cannot
be initially tested in humans. In such instances, the
FDA permits the use of animal models to show that
the vaccine would protect humans. Nonetheless, the

safety of the vaccine must always be tested in humans—after it has been shown safe in vitro and in animals, of course.

HUMAN STUDIES. Some vaccines can only be studied in humans. For example, varicella (chickenpox) virus is very difficult to study in animals because it only naturally infects humans (and a few protected species of primates, like lowland gorillas). As a consequence, the vaccine had to be tested in humans earlier in development than usual. Several attempts to produce a vaccine didn't work because the candidate vaccine viruses either caused chickenpox or because they were so weakened that they did not provide protection.

Similarly, to test whether the chickenpox vaccine would be safe to give to immunocompromised children—such as children being treated for leukemia, who can become ill if they contract chickenpox—the vaccine had to be tested for safety in these patients. These human tests showed that the vaccine virus was still too dangerous for them. Children with these conditions are best protected by community immunity—that is, by not being exposed to wild-type chickenpox. The best way to protect them then is immunizing all their classmates.

COINCIDENTAL ASSOCIATIONS

Coincidence is the observation of two things happening at about the same time. While epidemiological studies can help establish that a vaccine caused an adverse event, they cannot prove with absolute certainty that an adverse event following immunization represents only a coincidence. These tools can only infer that coincidence is the most likely explanation.

Epidemiological studies cannot absolutely prove coincidence (reject causation) because there can always be very rare occurrences that were not detected in the study population, or because the vaccine only accounted for a very small proportion of the adverse events. This is why rather than saying, "the study suggests that the problem was just a coincidence," a scientist will say, "the evidence favors rejection of causation" when the risk for vaccinated children cannot be distinguished from the risk for unvaccinated children.

Thus, the Institute of Medicine (IOM) uses two expressions when they believe there is evidence of causation: one favoring causation—"the evidence is supportive but not definitive"; and one stating causation—"the evidence is definitive." On the other hand, because negative epidemiological evidence can never be 100% certain, there is only the one category for favoring coincidence—that is, "the evidence favors rejection of a causal relationship."

Another element that may help infer coincidence is the finding of alternative causes for the disease or absence of the disease. For example, a few years ago it was noticed that as rates of hepatitis B immunization at birth were increasing, cases of SIDS were decreasing. However, the hepatitis B vaccine was probably *not* protecting against SIDS; rather, increasing use of the vaccine was just coincidental with a successful campaign aimed at persuading parents to place their infants on their backs to sleep.

THE GOLD STANDARD IN VACCINE SAFETY ANALYSIS: THE IOM VACCINE SAFETY REPORTS

The IOM is a nonprofit organization that is part of the National Academy of Sciences (NAS). Congress created the NAS to advise the federal government on scientific and technological matters. However, the academy and the IOM are private, nongovernmental organizations.

The IOM provides science-based advice on matters of biomedical science, medicine, and health. The IOM's mission is to serve as adviser to the nation to improve health. When a government agency wants the IOM to consider an issue, the agency contracts with the IOM to provide a review of the science and to make a report based upon the evidence. The specifics of what the IOM is to evaluate are specified and a fee to reimburse the IOM for its expenses—such as travel for the committee members, salaries for IOM staff, publication expenses, and so on—is agreed upon in advance. Once a contract has been agreed upon, the contracting agency's only input is as one of the sources of scientific data.

The IOM next selects scientists to serve on a committee to review the issue requested by the federal agency. The committee is independent and is expected to provide an evidence-based report that is subject to both internal and external peer review. The committee, however, may accept or reject the reviewers' critiques but must explain why to the IOM's satisfaction.

The IOM Committee on Immunization Safety Review was convened in the fall of 2000 to review and assess a number of vaccine safety concerns. They were expected to review three vaccine safety concerns per year for three years. The 15 committee members that the IOM selected had expertise in pediatrics, internal medicine, immunology, neurology, infectious diseases, epidemiology, biostatistics, public health, risk perception, decision analysis, nursing, genetics, ethics, and health communications.

To assure no conflicts of interest (real or perceived) the IOM excluded from the committee any scientists with financial ties to vaccine manufacturers or their parent companies, or who had served on any federal vaccine advisory committees, or provided expert testimony about vaccines, or who had published papers on issues of vaccine safety.

For each hypothesis to be examined, the committee was charged to assess both the scientific evidence and the significance of the issue for society.

The scientific assessment had two components: an examination of the epidemiological and clinical evidence regarding a possible causal relationship between the immunization and the adverse event, and an examination of experimental evidence for any biological mechanism(s) relevant to the hypothesis.

In the significance assessment, the committee considered the health burden of both the vaccine-preventable disease and the adverse event in question, including the level of public concern about the safety issue.

The committee used five categories of causal conclusions:

1. NO EVIDENCE: There is a complete absence of clinical or epidemiological evidence.

2. EVIDENCE IS INADEQUATE TO ACCEPT OR REJECT A CAUSAL RELATIONSHIP: The evidence is not reasonably convincing either in support of or against causality—in other words, the evidence is sparse, conflicting, of weak quality, or merely suggestive.

3. EVIDENCE FAVORS REJECTION OF A CAUSAL RELATIONSHIP: This is the strongest category in the negative direction. Because epidemiological evidence can never be 100% certain, the conclusion that "the vaccine does not cause the adverse event" or that "the adverse event observed was coincidental" would not be consistent with scientific precepts.

4. EVIDENCE FAVORS ACCEPTANCE OF A CAUSAL RELATIONSHIP: The evidence is strong and generally convincing, although not firm enough to be described as unequivocal or established.

5. EVIDENCE ESTABLISHES A CAUSAL RELATIONSHIP: The

evidence is unequivocal in showing a causal link between the vaccine and the adverse event.

The committee began their assessments from a neutral position—no assumptions were made regarding the association between the vaccine and the adverse event. For each vaccine safety concern they reviewed relevant literature and presentations, including unpublished data, by scientists and interested groups during open scientific meetings. The committee evaluated all the types of evidence available to determine whether the vaccines caused the adverse event or not.

Based on their conclusions, the committee made recommendations for future activities regarding the safety concern.

The eight reports from the IOM's Committee on Immunization Safety Review are listed below. They are technical and sometimes hard to read and understand; however, they are considered to be the most authoritative and reliable documents on vaccine safety currently available. They are available at *www.nap.edu/catalog*.

- Measles-Mumps-Rubella Vaccine and Autism (April 2001)
- Thimerosal-Containing Vaccines and Neurodevelopmental Disorders (October 2001)
- Multiple Immunizations and Immune Dysfunction (February 2002)
- Hepatitis B Vaccine and Demyelinating Neurological Disorders (May 2002)
- SV40 Contamination of Polio Vaccine and Cancer (October 2002)
- Vaccinations and Sudden Unexpected Death in Infancy (March 2003)
- Influenza Vaccines and Neurological Complications (October 2003)
- Vaccines and Autism (May 2004)

THE BOTTOM LINE: HOW DO I TELL WHETHER OR NOT A VACCINE CAUSED THAT?!

The first step when evaluating a vaccine safety concern is to recognize that association and causation are not the same. In other words, if a child experiences an adverse event at about the same time as a vaccination, that does not necessarily mean that the vaccine caused the event—it could be just co-incidence. Here are some questions you can ask to help tell whether it was cause or coincidence:

- Did the first symptoms appear after vaccination?
- If a live virus vaccine was used, was the vaccine virus isolated?
- Does the disease or condition occur only in people who receive the vaccine and not in others?
- Is there a known biological mechanism that could explain how the vaccine might cause the adverse event?
- Are there other possible explanations for the adverse event besides the vaccine (coincidence)?

Many times you will read news reports about scientific studies regarding vaccine safety—or you may read the journal articles themselves. You can use the information in this chapter to evaluate those studies. Ask these questions:

- If some studies suggest a causal relation and others do not, which studies carry more weight? (For example, case-control studies are more powerful than ecological studies.)
- Are there potential flaws in how the study patients were selected?
- Do the conclusions follow from the findings?
- Is the association statistically significant?
- Have respected scientists in the field expressed an opinion?

IF YOU WANT TO READ MORE:

Cohn V, Cope L. 2001. *News & numbers: a guide to reporting statistical claims and controversies in health and other fields,* 2nd ed. Ames, IA: Iowa State University Press.

Offit P. 2005. *The Cutter incident.* New Haven, CT: Yale University Press.

"WE'LL JUST MILL AROUND TILL HE'S ASLEEP, AND THEN SEND HIM BACK UP. THIS OPERATION IS ACTUALLY FOR A PLACEBO EFFECT."

Misinformation and the Return of Infectious Diseases: Does it Matter if Other Parents Don't Immunize their Child?!

We must stop tolerating the rejection and distortion of science. We must insist on an end to the cynical use of pseudo-studies known to be false for the purpose of intentionally clouding the public's ability to discern the truth.
Al Gore, The Assault on Reason, 2007

So far we have seen that the suggestion of a vaccine safety concern is often followed by a period of uncertainty because of the need to gather data. We also looked at how researchers collect the missing information and evaluate the accumulating evidence.

Even after scientists accumulate enough evidence to "favor rejection" of the concern, some people will not be convinced. Among them, some will promulgate their beliefs despite the evidence. They will spread misinformation; they will become misinformers.

Misinformation comes in many guises. Many who unwittingly misinform are themselves uninformed or misinformed, but well meaning. Others may have an incorrect opinion (that is, a subjective judgement). But others may profit by disseminating and popularizing misinformation.

While many journalists, lawyers, and politicians try to provide useful information, some may fail to check the reliability of their sources and others may—knowingly or unwittingly—profit by disseminating misinformation. These profits may come from book sales, movie rights, political support, tort precedents, inches of news space, or minutes of news time.

Additionally, some self-anointed "experts" may profit by

giving testimony in court, making speeches, or publishing pseudoscience.

Misinformation is often spread through the Internet, but it also finds its way into:

- **Mainstream media.** In an attempt to present opposing opinions, journalists can make misinformers appear credible and provide them much exposure.
- **Scientific communications.** Because they often require careful scrutiny and evaluation to understand what has been done and how it needs to be interpreted, these publications can be easily misconstrued. In addition, data—even data published in the most prestigious journals—always need confirmation by others.
- **Pseudoscientific communications.** Some publications have been created specifically to disseminate misinformation.

THE CONSEQUENCES OF MISINFORMATION

Parents who are convinced that their child has been harmed by vaccines may frighten and confuse other parents. This confusion results in more parents withholding vaccines from their children, sometimes leading to disease outbreaks.

Outbreaks of vaccine-preventable diseases often begin among the unimmunized and underimmunized and then spread to the fully immunized in the community—a portion of whom remain susceptible because no vaccine is 100% effective. In other words, *misinformation can cause disease outbreaks*, as history has shown.

The concerns about the whole-cell pertussis vaccine and the development of neurodevelopmental disorders—whether caused by or just temporally associated with vaccine administration—illustrate how vaccine safety concerns can give rise to very real outbreaks of disease.*

In January 1974, a case-series report was published describing 36 children admitted to a hospital in London—over an 11-year period—with "neurological complications" after receiving the diphtheria, tetanus, and whole-cell pertussis (DTP) vaccine.[3] Although the authors cautioned that these were merely observations, the media interpreted the report as evidence that whole-cell pertussis immunization (at that time the only vaccine available to prevent whooping cough) caused brain damage. These cases were later reconsidered. In only 12 of the original 36 cases did the manifestations of brain damage occur close to the time of vaccination and 2 of the children included in the report had never actually received the DTP vaccine.[4,5]

Several studies considered the hypothesis suggested by these case reports. For example, the British National Childhood Encephalopathy Study estimated that brain damage after DTP could have occurred in a small number of children—perhaps as many as one in every 310,000 doses.[5] But other studies could not confirm any association between the whole-cell pertussis vaccine and brain damage (see Chapter 10).

With the introduction of the Vaccine Injury Compensation Program and then the switch from whole-cell to acellular pertussis vaccines in the United States and many other countries, many of these issues resolved, although the whole-cell vaccine continues to be widely used elsewhere in the world—making a recent case-control study that found no evidence for a causal relationship between whole-cell pertussis vaccine and the onset of encephalopathy particularly important.[6]

---

* From the mid 1970s through the mid 1990s many other related events occurred as a consequence of confusion over what the data showed, the interpretation of new evidence as it became available, the development and testing of a new acellular pertussis vaccine, and the maturation of the Vaccine Injury Compensation Program. These events are well described in references 1 and 2.

Interestingly, a 2006 study also showed that some children with alleged severe brain injury that developed after DTP immunization (so-called "vaccine encephalopathy") in fact had a genetic disease[7] that—by coincidence—first became apparent at about the time that vaccine had been administered.

COMMON CLAIMS MADE BY MISINFORMERS ABOUT VACCINES

Claims	Facts
Natural methods of enhancing immunity are better than vaccinations.	The only "natural way" to be immune is to have the disease. Immunity from a preventive vaccine provides protection against disease when a person is exposed to the germ in the future. That immunity is usually similar to what is acquired from natural infection, although several doses of a vaccine may have to be given for a child to have a full immune response.
Vaccines are ineffective.	Vaccines have spared millions of people the effects of devastating diseases.
Vaccines are not needed any more; the diseases are gone.	Because vaccines work so well, we don't see many of these illnesses any more but—except for smallpox—the germs are still very much "out there."
Before the use of vaccinations these diseases had begun to decline due to improved nutrition and hygiene.	Vaccine-preventable diseases only began to drop dramatically after the vaccines for those diseases were licensed and were given to large numbers of children. It is true that in the 19th and early 20th centuries some infectious diseases began to be better controlled because of improvements in sanitation, clean water, pasteurized milk, and pest control.
Giving multiple vaccines at the same time causes an "overload" of the immune system.	Vaccination does not overburden a child's immune system; the recommended vaccines use only a small portion of the immune system's "memory" (see Chapter 9).
Epidemiology—often used to establish vaccine safety—is not science but number crunching.	Epidemiology is a well-established scientific discipline that, among other things, identifies the cause of diseases and the factors that increase a person's risk for a disease (see Chapter 4).
Contaminated vaccination lots (or "hot lots") are more likely to cause an adverse reaction.	The Food and Drug Administration regulates the production of vaccines very carefully to ensure the potency, purity, and safety of vaccines—including their lot-to-lot consistency.

During the period of uncertainty, however, immunizations against pertussis declined in a number of countries—especially where the antivaccine movements were very active[8]—despite public health officials re-emphasizing that brain damage was more common when young children developed whooping cough than the hypothesized vaccine concern.

Because of the concerns about whole-cell pertussis vaccine, immunization rates had dropped in 1978 from 80% to 30% in the United Kingdom—and whooping cough epidemics soon followed. Indeed, between 1977 and 1979 the United Kingdom experienced 102,500 cases of whooping cough with 36 deaths, as shown in the ecological study in the figure below.[3]

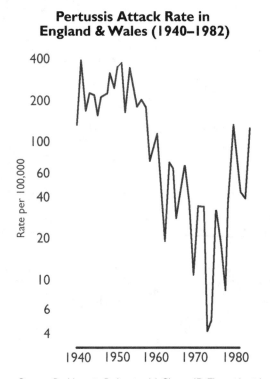

Pertussis Attack Rate in England & Wales (1940–1982)

Adapted from Current Problems in Pediatrics, 14, Cherry JD. *The epidemiology of pertussis and pertussis immunization in the United Kingdom and the United States: A comparative study*, page 12, Copyright (1984), with permission from Elsevier.

In Japan a national debate resulted in the Ministry of Health and Welfare changing the recommended age for immunization because of concerns about the whole-cell pertussis vaccine's safety and claims that it was no longer necessary to immunize because pertussis was not present in the community any more. Vaccine coverage for infants fell from about 85% in 1974 to 14% in 1976.[4] Then, in 1979, a whooping cough epidemic resulted in 13,105 cases and 41 deaths. In the early 1980s Japan re-introduced pertussis-containing vaccines—using the newer acellular pertussis vaccines that cause less fever and local reactions—and the number of cases of whooping cough went down.[8]

Sweden had a similar experience. After discontinuing pertussis vaccine, rates of whooping cough returned to the levels seen in the prevaccine era. Of 2,282 who were hospitalized for whooping cough in 1981–1983, 4% had brain injury from the illness.[4]

The role of misinformation on pertussis outbreaks is hard to define, because it isn't clear when missing information evolved into misinformation. However, a 1998 study examined the impact of the whole-cell pertussis anti-vaccine movements on the number of whooping cough cases in different countries.[8] The researchers divided the countries into those where the anti-vaccine movements had limited impact on the amount of vaccine administered (Hungary, the former East Germany, Poland, and the United States) and countries whose immunization programs were disrupted by these movements (Sweden, Japan, the United Kingdom, Ireland, Italy, Australia, the former West Germany, and the Russian Federation). The study found that whooping cough incidence was 10 to 100 times higher in countries where immunization programs were compromised by anti-whole-cell pertussis vaccine movements than in countries where high vaccine coverage was maintained.

Two decades after the DTP frenzy, another vaccine scare began in the United Kingdom.

In February 1998, a headline in the *Daily Telegraph* read, "Vaccination may trigger disease linked to autism." Thousands of news outlets around the world told the same story, causing panic among many parents, particularly in the United Kingdom. The *Telegraph*'s article was based upon a series of case reports published in the medical journal *The Lancet* by Andrew Wakefield and his colleagues. The study suggested that children who received the measles, mumps, and rubella (MMR) vaccine might have suffered damage to the bowel as a result, which in turn allowed absorption of chemicals from the gut that then injured the brain—thus causing autism.

Although Wakefield's report did not provide any evidence of a link between MMR and autism, media coverage was extensive, giving the theory credibility in the eyes of many in the public.

Wakefield and others then claimed to have found fragments of measles virus in the guts of children with inflammation of the intestine and "vaccine-strain" measles virus in cerebrospinal fluid samples from children with autism. The findings of measles virus in children with autism not only could not be verified by others, but the reported results were shown to have been a consequence of the inaccurate assays employed to detect measles virus.[9]

Not surprisingly, many frightened parents feared the vaccine more than the infections—which were not occurring then in the United Kingdom. In the following years MMR vaccination rates fell from 93% to 79% by 2003, with measles and mumps outbreaks as a consequence. In fact, the decrease in MMR vaccine use as a consequence of this vaccine safety concern coincided with the onset of measles outbreaks.[10]

In 2004 and 2005, the United Kingdom experienced a mumps epidemic with more than 63,500 cases (see figure below). In 2006 there was a mumps outbreak in 11 states that was caused by the same strain of mumps virus causing the epidemic in the United Kingdom,[11] suggesting that the outbreak in the United States came from there. In 2006, the United States had 6,584 cases of mumps compared to the more typical 200 to 300 cases in prior years (see table in Chapter 1).

Cases of Mumps in the United Kingdom

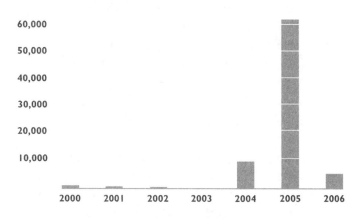

In 2005, there were more than 63,500 cases of mumps in the United Kingdom (data obtained from *www.who.int/countries*; accessed October 5, 2007).

Consider this statement by health officials in the United Kingdom:

> The Health Protection Agency has received reports of 449 confirmed cases of measles in England and Wales to the end of May 2006. This compares to 438 cases for the whole of 2003 and will therefore represent the highest number of cases in one year since our current method of monitoring began in 1995. In the year that MMR was introduced there were just over 86,000 notifications of measles.[12]

Many careful epidemiological studies have now fully refuted Wakefield's suggestions.[13] Indeed, in 2004, 10 of the 13 authors of the initial report formally retracted their suggestion of a possible link between the measles vaccine and autism.[14] Additionally, *The Lancet* published an account of financial conflicts of interest that Wakefield had.[15] Even though the theory has no scientific credibility, a number of groups in the United Kingdom continue to assert that measles-containing vaccines have caused "an autism epidemic." However, as one study after another found no evidence of the link, some people claimed that the vaccine did cause autism, but in too few cases to be picked up by epidemiological studies!

Misinformation can lead to outbreaks of serious vaccine-preventable diseases.

THE NATURAL HISTORY OF MISINFORMATION

The timing and widespread use of vaccines make them easy scapegoats to be blamed for all sorts of serious illnesses.

In spite of the substantial available evidence that allows rejection of some vaccine safety concerns, some people continue to state that vaccines are causing the alleged adverse events. These claims—which were once based on observations when there was insufficient information available—now fall into the category of misinformation. Not all vaccine safety concerns are misinformation—only those that persist despite the evidence against them. Even when the concern stops being an issue for most in the scientific community, it may remain an issue for people with vested interests—whether politicians, lawyers, journalists, or the group that concerns health professionals the most: well-intentioned but misinformed parents trying to understand and alleviate their child's afflictions.

Many media stories use faulty reports and parental concerns to depict a "controversy" about vaccines, failing to mention that the scientific community does not feel that a controversy exists.

Misinformation's natural history usually follows this course:

1. A vaccine safety concern is suggested based on anecdotes or case reports (usually about diseases whose causes are not completely understood).

2. Multiple epidemiological studies using different methods and studying different populations find no evidence to support the concern. Nevertheless, some studies may identify possible mechanisms by which the vaccine might cause the adverse effect.

3. Pseudoscience supporting the theory is put forward—and is often quoted in the media—but is disregarded by most in the scientific community.

4. Because the accumulating evidence appears to not support the hypothesis, the scientific community begins to state that the vaccine likely does not cause the adverse event.

5. Misinformers deny the evidence and discredit those who do not agree with them—scientists, manufacturers, or governments—sometimes suggesting cover-ups and conspiracy theories.

6. Alternative explanations are found to explain the illness and coincidence with immunization is ultimately accepted.

During this process, as new data become available, the concern shifts to being misinformation—the concern has been widely disseminated through the Internet, magazine articles, and talk shows. Many parents are confused and some wonder if vaccinations are the best thing to do.

A couple in Tennessee, for example, confused about vaccine safety because of what a friend had told them, decided to delay their daughter's vaccinations. Some time later, the baby girl was stricken with a form of meningitis (inflammation of the brain) that could have been prevented by the *Haemophilus influenzae* type b (Hib) vaccine.[16]

On the other hand, when the scientific evidence shows the vaccine safety concern to have been caused by the vaccine, there is little room for misinformation. Take for example the first rotavirus vaccine introduced in 1999:

1. The VAERS passive reporting system received several reports of a serious—and sometimes fatal—bowel problem after rotavirus immunization (the suggestion of the concern).

2. Researchers began epidemiological and laboratory studies.

3. As the preliminary results suggested the link with the vaccine might be causal, CDC decided to temporarily suspend the recommendation for use of the vaccine.

4. Multiple epidemiological studies using different methods and studying different populations supported a causal association (although several did not detect an association).

5. The scientific community reached a consensus that the vaccine likely caused the adverse event.

6. Although not noticed by the media, discussion within the scientific community was intense as there was true scientific controversy as to how to interpret some of the data.

7. The CDC withdrew its recommendation for universal immunization. The manufacturer then withdrew the vaccine from the marketplace.

In contrast to the above, when no causal association is found, the collection of sufficient data to conclude that "the data favors rejection of the hypothesis" takes much longer than it did to determine causation as with the rotavirus vaccine.

IDENTIFYING MISINFORMATION

How can you distinguish good information from misinformation? Misinformation often includes one or more of the following elements:

- Invalid assumptions
- Logical fallacies
- Ad hoc hypotheses
- False experts or experts who lack the needed expertise
- Pseudoscience
- Unstated conflicts of interest

INVALID ASSUMPTIONS

An invalid assumption is something you treat as if it were known to be true or false, when in fact it is not.

For example, some parents regard hepatitis B immunization as unnecessary, assuming that this is a disease for which their children are not at risk. These parents think that hepatitis B is a disease mainly of intravenous drug users, sex workers, or men who have sex with men. While it is true that these groups of people are at a *greatly increased* risk for hepatitis B infection, as many as 16–30% of hepatitis B cases have no identifiable source of infection. Unvaccinated children in families with no known risk factors may still be at risk of infection through normal play activities.[17-19] Hepatitis B infection as a child carries with it an increased risk for chronic infection that can lead to cirrhosis of the liver and liver cancer. Thus, the assumption that children whose families seemingly are not at risk of hepatitis B infection—and therefore may not need hepatitis B vaccine—is wrong, as there is no way to know which child will eventually be exposed.

Another common invalid assumption is that "natural"

immunity is better than vaccine-induced immunity.* In other words, that it is better to be naturally infected than vaccinated. The truth is that it is much better to gain immunity from a vaccine because vaccine-preventable diseases can kill or cause permanent disabilities such as paralysis from polio, liver damage or liver cancer from hepatitis B infection, and deafness from meningitis caused by several bacteria (Hib, pneumococci, and meningococci). Immunity from a vaccine offers protection against future disease that is similar to immunity acquired from a natural infection, although several doses of a vaccine may have to be given for a child to have a full immune response. In fact, for some vaccines such as tetanus and Hib, the vaccine is *better* at creating immunity than a natural infection would be.

Invalid assumptions can lead to wrong conclusions. Some invalid assumptions often underlying misinformation claims are listed below.

- Vaccines can and should be 100% safe and effective (the opposite—illness in a vaccinated person proves that the vaccine doesn't work—is also invalid)
- Association is the same as causation
- Epidemiology isn't real science
- Scientists do research only to make a profit

LOGICAL FALLACIES

Misinformers often use rhetorical appeals to make their case about vaccine safety. Their techniques of persuasion, however, are filled with logical fallacies. A logical fallacy is a flaw in an argument that makes the argument illogical or invalid.

The following are some common fallacies used in misinformation about vaccines.

---

* Some misinformers call vaccine-induced immunity "artificial immunity."

Post hoc argument ("after this, therefore because of this"). This is a common fallacy that assumes that just because an event follows vaccination, it must be caused by the vaccine. As described previously (Chapter 4), just because a vaccine is given at about the same time as something is first recognized or happens does not mean that the vaccine is the cause.

For example, this fallacy is commonly seen in online discussion forums, where people say matter-of-factly that a vaccine harmed a child because certain symptoms appeared a few days or weeks after vaccination.

Argument against the person (the "ad hominem" fallacy). This fallacy involves replying to an argument by attacking those presenting the argument rather than the argument itself.

For example, unable to respond with factual arguments to the scientific evidence showing no link between MMR and autism, misinformers attacked those scientists and health officials in Great Britain who said that the vaccine was safe because—in the past—they had been wrong about their initial assessments about "mad cow disease." This was an *ad hominem* fallacy because they claimed that both British scientists and the government were wrong about the safety of MMR simply because they once erred. The critics did not address the evidence about the safety concern.

Although it is reasonable to doubt or reject evidence if the only source of evidence lacks credibility, it is a fallacy to deny evidence based solely on who said it. In the case of MMR, the British health officials were not the only ones showing the safety of MMR—researchers around the world were also publishing evidence of the safety of the triple vaccine.

The *ad hominem* argument takes many forms in the discussion of vaccine safety. From alleged government cover-ups to conspiracy theories describing secret alliances between pharmaceutical companies and the scientific community, misinformers try to discredit those who do not agree with them. Such allegations were made about scientists whose data and analyses refuted the alleged association of thimerosal and autism, for example.[20]

Studies that examined the content and characteristics of antivaccination Web sites, for example, found that these sites said that:

> Doctors were presented as either willing conspirators cashing in on the vaccine "fraud," or pawns manipulated by the shadowy vaccine combine; parents' love and compassion whose intuition about vaccination harms was considered a stronger force than cold, analytical science.[21]

APPEAL TO PITY (ARGUMENTUM "AD MISERICORDIAM"). This fallacy involves misinformers trying to win support for their arguments by appealing to feelings of sympathy or guilt. Misinformation discussions often feature anecdotes (personal stories about individual sick persons) describing children said to have been killed or maimed by vaccines.[21,22]

One example is ThinkTwice.com, which introduces its anecdotes section with the title: "Human Sacrifices (Personal Stories of Vaccine Damage and Death)."

Anecdotes are not necessarily inappropriate—they may serve to illustrate a point or to raise a concern. However, the fallacy is to try to prove causality by using a touching story.

ARGUMENT FROM IGNORANCE. This fallacy claims that a statement is true only because it has not been proven false, or that it is false only because it has not been proven true.

For example, Generation Rescue—a parent-led group that claims that it has found the cause (thimerosal) and the cure (chelation) for autism—commits this logical fallacy when it says:

> There is no evidence to suggest that autism is genetic. No autism gene has ever been found and the search will be endless—how can you have a gene for a mythical condition? Autism is mercury poisoning.[23]

This statement suggests that it is false that autism is genetic because it has not been proven true, which is an argument from ignorance. It erroneously assumes that the lack of evidence for an "autism gene" proves that autism is not genetic; indeed, most autism investigators recognize the importance of genetic factors but do not seriously expect that autism is caused by a single gene. Furthermore, the Generation Rescue statement makes the equally improbable assumption that autism has a proven cause—mercury poisoning. (More about mercury and the genetics of autism in Chapter 8.)

GUILT BY ASSOCIATION. This fallacy claims that a theory or an argument must be false simply because of who supports the argument.

For example, if you distrust pharmaceutical companies, this fallacy would imply that you should disregard a scientist whose analysis reaches the same conclusion as the vaccine manufacturer.

Another example, in *Evidence of Harm: Mercury in Vaccines and the Autism Epidemic: A Medical Controversy*

(published in 2005), freelance journalist David Kirby attempts to make a guilt-by-association case about
vaccine expert and advocate Paul Offit, who wrote a
book about vaccines and vaccine-preventable diseases. Kirby noted that pharmaceutical company Merck
bought 20,000 copies of Offit's book for distribution
around the nation. He cites a lay reviewer from Am-
azon.com who said, "Everyone should proceed with
caution when a multi-billion dollar conglomerate gives
their stamp of approval on a book."[24]

Association between persons or groups does not
mean that they share the same characteristics or motivations; that, of course, does not mean that all data
should not be examined critically.

The power of logical fallacies resides in their ability to
appeal to emotions and distract us from the real arguments
at hand.

CHANGING THE THEORY BECAUSE THE DATA DON'T WORK ("AD HOC" HYPOTHESES)

An *ad hoc* hypothesis adjusts a theory just for the purpose of
salvaging it from being refuted. *Ad hoc* explanations try to
explain findings that do not fit the original theory.

For instance, some activists have charged that the vaccine
preservative thimerosal or measles vaccine are the cause of
an "autism epidemic."

However, when large studies in many countries found
that autism was as common in children immunized with
thimerosal-containing vaccines as in children who did not
receive those vaccines (or were immunized with measles vaccine or not), some of these activists countered with an *ad
hoc* hypothesis: that those studies did not find a difference
because thimerosal causes autism only in genetically suscep-

tible children, a proportion of the population too small to have been detected.

Another *ad hoc* hypothesis combines the thimerosal and measles vaccines hypotheses into a new hypothesis: that together, measles vaccine and the preservative thimerosal (which is not present in measles-containing vaccines) cause autism.[25]

While such theories would need to be tested, these arguments did not originate as the result of molecular evidence from genetic studies but as *ad hoc* hypotheses—to try to argue away the data that failed to support their claims.

FALSE EXPERTS OR "EXPERTS" WHO LACK EXPERTISE

Experts are reliable sources of knowledge, people who have gained recognition through experience and education in their field. Medical experts are increasingly sought as witnesses in legal proceedings, including vaccine injury trials. According to the American Medical Association's (AMA) Code of Medical Ethics, the education, training, and occupational experience of expert witnesses should be specifically in the field discussed in the case.

The AMA states "that the occupational experience should include active medical practice or teaching experience in that same field and that the active medical practice or teaching experience must have been within five years of the date of the occurrence giving rise to the claim."[26]

None of the expert vaccinologists in the world would claim to also be experts in *all* the fields that, in one way or another, are related to vaccine safety.

For this reason, the IOM Committee on Immunization Safety included experts in pediatrics, neurology, immunology, internal medicine, infectious diseases, genetics, epidemiology, biostatistics, risk perception and communication, decision analysis, public health, nursing, and ethics.

Indeed, a curious observation has been that, although some in the vaccinology community criticized the IOM for excluding experts with prior vaccine research from this committee, no experts in vaccinology were included because the IOM wanted to ensure that there would be no perceptions of potential conflicts of interest among the experts.

In the discussions about vaccine safety, some who claim to be experts turn out to be:

EXPERTS IN A SCIENTIFIC FIELD NOT RELATED TO VACCINE SAFETY. An expert in one field may be completely ignorant in another field. For instance, an endocrinologist may be an expert on diabetes but is not likely to be expert about vaccine safety or immunology. Unfortunately, some people eagerly make claims about things outside their field of expertise.

Such is the case of Dr. Mark Geier, who has frequently testified in vaccine injury cases—especially in those involving vaccines and brain damage or neurodevelopmental disorders. In one case, the Special Master—a judicial authority appointed by the VICP court—dismissed Dr. Geier's testimony because of his lack of expertise on the subject of his affidavit:

> Dr. Geier's expertise, training, and experience is [sic] in genetics and obstetrics. He is, however, a professional witness in areas for which he has no training, expertise, and experience.[27]

JOURNALISTS WHO HAVE WRITTEN ARTICLES OR BOOKS ABOUT VACCINE SAFETY. Although many journalists do a good job writing about scientific and medical issues in ways that make this information understandable and informative to the general public (for example, *Vaccine* by Arthur Allen), they are usually specialized medical or science reporters at large news organizations. Good science journalists let the experts speak through their articles instead of purporting to be experts themselves.

Often, however, stories—particularly published by smaller news organizations and local TV stations—have not been checked for the reliability of the facts, and present "controversies" that pit parents or others with an opinion against scientific experts, as if opinions and facts have similar value.

Others simply misinform, whatever is their motivation.

Writing an article or a book does not instantly make someone an expert. The word "author," however, carries some social prestige that many people may equate with "expert."

On March 30, 2006, activist groups organized a "panel briefing on the growing evidence of a link between mercury, vaccines, and autism, and important new developments on Capitol Hill, in major universities and within the mainstream media."[28] The four speakers included the CEO of an autism advocacy group, a congresswoman, and two journalists. None of the speakers would be considered expert at evaluating epidemiological or other scientific data. But these events attract a great deal of publicity and do little to further vaccine safety discussion.

One of the journalists was David Kirby, author of a book *Evidence of Harm*, mentioned previously. His book cleverly portrays the antithimerosal activists in the role of heroes on a mission, representing their views of science and events, implying a cover-up by respected scientists. Despite his lack of scientific background or expertise in any field related to vaccinology or autism, Kirby has been frequently invited as a speaker to discuss scientific studies at events where scientific discourse is not on the agenda, speaking for antivaccine and antithimerosal activists.

The other journalist was Dan Olmsted, the author of *The Age of Autism*, which used to be a regular column from United Press International (UPI). Olmsted said that autism does not occur in unvaccinated Amish children in Pennsylvania. Although his reports have no scientific merit—his research methods included asking a man who sells water purifiers in Amish communities if he had seen autistic Amish— Olmsted is often cited by misinformers to support their arguments.

It is important to remember that exposure and controversies sell books and attract readers.

POLITICIANS WHO CLAIM TO BE EXPERTS. Many politicians do great service by bringing diverse groups together, including parents with opinions and scientists with expertise in order to understand the concerns and the issues.

However, there is little in a politician's training that would be of value for interpreting scientific data. Even congressmen who hold a medical degree may not qualify as experts because they are not actively involved in research or medical practice.

Political scientists define politics as a process of conflict resolution in which support is mobilized and maintained for collective projects. It is important to recognize that politicians gain support—and votes— sometimes by taking on the causes of different interest groups and seeking solutions to these groups' problems.

Between 1999 and 2004 more than 10 vaccine/thimerosal/autism hearings were held before the U.S. Congress—mostly before the Committee on

Government Reform of the U.S. House of Representatives, which serves as Congress's chief investigative and oversight committee.

Representative Dan Burton chaired this committee from 1997 to 2002. His claims to expertise come from being the grandfather of a child who he believes has autism as a consequence of vaccines. When the IOM Vaccine Safety Review Committee said in 2004 that the body of scientific evidence favored rejection of a causal relationship between thimerosal-containing vaccines and autism, Rep. Burton got together with antithimerosal activists to refute the report:

> Unfortunately, I believe the findings announced in the May 18th IOM report are heavily biased, and unrepresentative of all the available scientific and medical research ... I think it is highly irresponsible for the IOM Immunization Safety Review Committee to purport definitive findings to the American public, which are based on selective scientific studies that are greatly flawed to begin with.[28]

We are not trying to imply that whatever politicians or lawyers or journalists say about vaccine safety is wrong just because they are not scientific experts—that would be an ad hominem fallacy—but rather that journalists, lawyers, and politicians are not authoritative scientific experts. Nonetheless, they are often widely quoted by those who can find no real experts to support their beliefs.

What these individuals are really doing is expressing their opinions. Opinions are ideas or thoughts that people have about something. Opinions are personal, subjective judgments. Sometimes false experts present their opinions as facts; sometimes other people take their opinions as facts. But opinions are not facts, which can be observed and verified.

Both journalists and politicians can form opinions and

many of them have contributed in a very positive way to the public discussion of immunization policy and vaccine safety. Nonetheless, they are not scientific experts, and readers should be wary if they are quoted by those who can find no real experts to support their beliefs.

PSEUDOSCIENCE

Science differs from other disciplines in that it has established norms and techniques known as the scientific method. The scientific method has four basic steps:

- Observation—description of an event or disease.
- Hypothesis—proposal of a possible explanation or cause for the event or disease.
- Prediction—use of the hypothesis to predict when the event or disease will occur.
- Experimentation—performance of experiments or studies to test the predictions.

Pseudoscience ("false knowledge") presents itself as scientific but fails to use the scientific method. One common example of pseudoscience is astrology, which portrays itself as scientific by using star charts but then predicts a person's future with vague language and subjective interpretations of the positions of the planets.

Pseudoscientific claims cannot be verified by other researchers because they are usually ambiguous and not measurable. In most cases, these claims are not submitted to peer review (that is, review by experts) before making them public and their methods are difficult to understand, their observations difficult to replicate.

Often, data may be represented to show one outcome when another is the case. Other times the methods that are used are likely to give a predetermined outcome. Only data purporting to support the claims are presented while conflicting data are ignored or discarded. For example, the CDC noted about a study trying to link Hib vaccine and type 1 diabetes that:

> It appears that Dr. Classen may have conducted his statistical analysis after seeing the results and noting that the largest difference was apparent by 7 years. The validity of this type of 'post-hoc' statistical testing, however, is highly questionable. When the full 10 years of follow-up was evaluated the differences were not statistically significant, which is also what was found by Karvonen and colleagues.[29]

The review process of most respected scientific journals tries to ensure that only carefully conducted science is published, but sometimes poorly run studies slip by the most careful editor. Because of the vetting process, however, most pseudoscientific claims about vaccine safety are published in obscure journals or in the alternative medicine press, or as letters to the editor.

Mark Geier (mentioned above) and his son, David Geier, have published a number of reports implying a link between vaccines and neurodevelopmental disorders. One way they have tried to show a link between vaccines and autism utilizes data from the Vaccine Adverse Event Reporting System (VAERS). VAERS data cannot be used to establish causality because reports can be entered by anyone and are not always verified (see Chapter 4).

One amusing, but telling, anecdote comes from Dr. James R. Laidler who demonstrated this by entering a report in VAERS that an influenza vaccine had turned him into *The Hulk*—which was accepted and promptly entered into the database.

According to Dr. Laidler,

> because the reported adverse event was so ... unusual, a representative of VAERS contacted me.

> After a discussion of the VAERS database and its limitations, they asked for my permission to delete the record, which I granted. If I had not agreed, the record would be there still, showing that any claim can become part of the database, no matter how outrageous or improbable. Indeed, since at least 1998 (and possibly earlier), a number of autism advocacy groups have, with all the best intentions, encouraged people to report their autistic children—or autistic children of relatives and friends—to VAERS as injuries from thimerosal-containing vaccines. This has irrevocably tainted the VAERS database with duplicate and spurious reports.[30]

The purpose of VAERS is to tabulate possible adverse events in order to look for "signals" that should be explored systematically.

The Geiers' reports failed to describe methods, important statistical figures were not defined accurately, and data sets overlapped.[31]

In addition to pseudoscience, misinformers often misquote legitimate research claiming that studies support their views, when in fact the original data do not.

The November 14, 2005, issue of the *New York Times* included a full-page advertisement by the group Generation Rescue thanking the researchers who did "groundbreaking research on the connection between mercury and autism."

The ad listed 19 citations of articles—including one by the Geiers.[32] None of the 19 articles shows that mercury causes autism. Although some of them did explicitly examine a possible link between mercury and autism, others were about autism in general with no mention of mercury.

In fact, one of the papers cited in the ad was by Andrew Wakefield, about MMR (not mercury) and autism.

Interestingly, an autism weblog (autismdiva.blogspot.

com) posted a letter to the *New York Times'* editor—which apparently was never published—from five of the researchers listed in the ad.

In the letter, the researchers stated that they do not believe there is a proven connection between mercury and autism. They worried that the ad "may actually mislead the public into thinking that the mercury-autism hypothesis has stronger support in the scientific literature than it actually does."[33]

CONFLICTS OF INTEREST

Most organizations, government agencies, universities, and businesses have definitions of conflicts of interest that differ slightly. We use the following definition for our discussion on how to distinguish between information and misinformation:

> A conflict of interest is a situation in which financial or other personal considerations may directly and significantly affect, or have the appearance of affecting, a person's judgment or responsibility, or the conduct or reporting of any type of research. Owning stock of a vaccine manufacturer, profiting from book sales, profiting from frequent testimonies, or soliciting votes might all be considered—or be perceived as—conflicts of interest.

Many misinformers charge federal employees and vaccine researchers with having conflicts of interest. The federal government has strict ethics rules that require divulging potential conflicts of interest for federal employees (including part-time federal employees, which is the category that most university professors serve in while on federal advisory committees) and their families. If the government ethics review committees feel that a stock in a retirement portfolio of a spouse, for example, could be construed as a conflict of interest, the federal employee (or spouse) must get rid of it if they want to participate, whether or not they could influence any action that would alter the stock.

There is a particular conundrum to consider about vaccine researchers, particularly those in academia. Researchers need funding from outside their universities to support each research program. Without external funding there would be little research support from the university. Although the NIH and other government organizations fund much of the biomedical research in U.S. universities, a lot of research on vaccine development, vaccine preclinical testing, and clinical trials has been funded by grants to the universities from the vaccine industry. It is hard to imagine how an expert in certain aspects of vaccinology could develop expertise without this type of support. However, it is important to note that grant money does not usually go to the investigator but rather to the university that agrees to do the research—although universities often require grants to reimburse the university for a portion of the investigator's salary. These agreements between academia and industry contain stringent rules as to who owns the data and how much control a researcher has over study design. Often the university retains complete control (including ownership of intellectual property) except for clinical trials conducted for regulatory purposes when industry requires more control because all the data must be reviewed by the FDA. Because of the nature of what vaccine researchers do, it is not surprising that some hold patents for their intellectual property, that they may be asked to consult for vaccine companies, or that part of their salary may come from vaccine companies paying the university. Nevertheless these do in fact represent potential conflicts of interest.

For participation in federal advisory committees, *all* these real or perceived conflicts must be divulged and there are specific rules about what an expert may advise about and what they may not advise about because of their potential conflicts.

Misinformers make much ado about industry-funded vaccine research and support for vaccine research. But they know of conflicts of interest because the experts themselves divulge these associations out of the need and desire that their colleagues are fully aware and consider their perspectives accordingly. Few vaccine experts outside government (the authors among them) have no real or perceived conflicts of interest.

Misinformers also have potential conflicts of interest. However, they have no obligation to divulge them. Authors do not need to divulge their book sales income; investigative reporters (or their spouses) do not need to expose their retirement portfolio; and pseudoscientists do not need to divulge their funding sources nor the income they receive from testimony.

Scientific journals also require notification of potential conflicts of interest and publish them to be considered by the readers.

Sometimes, however, researchers do not report their conflicts of interest to journals.

For instance, in March 2004, Richard Horton, editor of *The Lancet*, wrote a statement regarding "serious allegations of research misconduct concerning an article by Dr. Andrew Wakefield and colleagues published in *The Lancet* in February, 1998, [that] were brought to the attention of senior editorial staff of the journal." Horton revealed that by the time of the report in *The Lancet*, Wakefield was conducting another study "with the aim of investigating the grounds for pursuing a multi-party legal action on behalf of parents of allegedly vaccine-damaged children, the existence of which was not disclosed to the editors of *The Lancet*."

In other words, Wakefield was helping lawyers find evidence that the children involved in the lawsuit against manufacturers were harmed by vaccines—and he apparently was paid £55,000 for his services.[34]

The Lancet editors implied that, had they known about this conflict of interest, they may not have published the article.[15]

According to data released in December 2006 by the U.K. Legal Services Commission, up to that year Wakefield was reported as having been paid more than £400,000 in legal fees by lawyers trying to prove that MMR caused autism.[34]

MISINFORMATION ABOUT THIMEROSAL: THE EXAMPLE OF ROBERT KENNEDY JR.

In June 2005, *Rolling Stone* magazine and Salon.com published an article titled "Deadly Immunity" by lawyer Robert Kennedy Jr.[35] The article is a classic example of misinformation. It is unclear what qualifications he brings to his analyses.

Kennedy wrote: "The CDC paid the Institute of Medicine to conduct a new study to whitewash the risks of thimerosal, ordering researchers to 'rule out' the chemical's link to autism," an opinion presented as fact.

The fact is that the IOM is a private, nongovernmental organization, which does not receive direct federal appropriations for its work. Studies undertaken for the government by the IOM usually are funded out of appropriations made available to federal agencies such as the CDC—so, of course the CDC (and NIH) paid for the study. However, IOM reviews are conducted by committees of volunteer scientists, selected by the IOM, who serve without compensation. The funds are used to pay for their travel and meeting expenses and the expenses of the IOM for overhead. Members of the committee were selected for their lack of conflicts of interest—they had never conducted vaccine safety research. They were not paid to find a predetermined result.

In Kennedy's article:

- **He attacks the individuals (ad hominem fallacy) and applies the guilt-by-association fallacy**—"The story of how government health agencies colluded with Big Pharma to hide the risks of thimerosal from the public is a chilling case study of institutional arrogance, power and greed."

- **He appeals to pity**—"our public-health authorities knowingly allowed the pharmaceutical industry to poison an entire generation of American children."

- **He promotes arguments from ignorance**—quoting Boyd Haley, who believes that the increase of autism cases must be caused by vaccines because there are no autistic adults: "If the epidemic is truly an artifact of poor diagnosis, then where are all the 20-year-old autistics?" This is in fact wrong; there are many autistic adults (see Chapter 8).

- **He provides faulty arguments**—"In 1930, the company [Eli Lilly] tested thimerosal by administering it to 22 patients with terminal meningitis, all of whom died within weeks of being injected—a fact Lilly didn't bother to report in its study declaring thimerosal safe." Of course they died, they had terminal meningitis, which means they were going to die.

- **He cites false experts**—the Geiers, Dan Burton, and Dan Olmsted among others, discussed above.

- **He cites pseudoscience and ignores valid science**—he quotes the VAERS studies by the Geiers and dismisses the IOM's rigorous review.

Kennedy charges a cover-up by using out-of-context quotes from transcripts[36] of the so-called Simpsonwood meeting that the CDC convened in 2000 (see page 169). Allegations of a cover-up were dismissed by a 2007 U.S. Senate report.[20]

The meeting was a consultation among several scientists to consider the initial findings of a study in progress looking for possible signals between thimerosal and neurodevelopmental disorders, including autism. One of the authors of this book (Myers) participated in this consultation, presenting the opening paper.

Although only preliminary data were available, there were unexpected neurodevelopmental findings that the CDC wished to have considered.

It is important to note that at no time were there any data suggesting an association with autism in these studies, before or afterward. Indeed, transcripts were made from the meeting (they were not needed by the participants nor required by law) specifically so there would *not* be charges of a cover-up. The discussions focused on how to rapidly collect more data to confirm or reject the findings.

Be that as it may, the more complex issue to address is that Kennedy (as well as Mr. Kirby in his book) misinterpreted—perhaps because of a lack of scientific background—the scientific data and discussions, often interpreting jargon as used in the common vernacular rather than the manner in which scientists speak to each other (see Chapter 3).

Similarly, in quoting from an improperly obtained transcript of a 2001 meeting of the members of the IOM's Immunization Safety Review Committee,[37] Kennedy wrote:

> [The CDC] also instructed the Institute of Medicine, an advisory organization that is part of the National Academy of Sciences, to produce a study debunking the link between thimerosal and brain disorders. The CDC "wants us to declare, well, that these things are pretty safe," Dr. Marie McCormick, who chaired the IOM's Immunization Safety Review Committee, told her fellow researchers when they first met in January 2001.

From Kennedy's article, one might conclude that the CDC *told* the IOM committee what their results should be. Recall that the first report (2001) about thimerosal reported insufficient evidence to accept or reject the hypothesis. When the quote is taken in context, however, it is clear that Dr. McCormick was discussing how the committee should consider the longer-term issues from the parents' perspective—that they should distinguish between the risk for the population and the risk for each individual child:

> I took away actually an issue that we may have to confront, and that is actually the definition of what we mean by safety. It is safety on a population basis, but it is also safety for the individual child. I am wondering, if we take this dual perspective, we may address more of the parent concerns, perhaps developing a better message if we think about what comes down the stream as opposed to CDC, which wants us to declare, well, these things are pretty safe on a population basis. (IOM meeting transcript, page 33)[37]

While the CDC wanted to know if the vaccines were safe for the population as a whole, parents wanted to know the risk for their individual children. Dr. McCormick was simply proposing that besides looking at what the CDC wanted the committee to consider, they should more broadly address parents' concerns. Kennedy continued:

> According to transcripts of the meeting, the committee's chief staffer, Kathleen Stratton, predicted that the IOM would conclude that the evidence was "inadequate to accept or reject a causal relation" between thimerosal and autism. That, she added, was the result "Walt wants"—a reference to Dr. Walter Orenstein, director of the National Immunization Program for the CDC.

The actual text of the transcript shows that Stratton was not predicting that their conclusion would be the outcome. Instead, her point was that Dr. Orenstein hoped that the group would *not* decide that the evidence was "inadequate to accept or reject a causal relation" because such an outcome would not help the CDC set vaccine policy (such as stopping the use of vaccines if a link was found).

Indeed the committee report in 2001 found that the evidence *was* "inadequate to accept or reject a causal relation," despite Dr. Orenstein.

However, 3 years later, in 2004—when there was much more information available—the committee found that the evidence favored rejection of an association between vaccines and autism.

This is the actual text from the transcript:

> I know they are worried about ... saying something is category two, ... that is inadequate to accept or reject a causal relation. What he said is, telling me that it is still a category two isn't enough to tell me what to do. ... What Walt has said is, just telling me it is here isn't enough. That is where he started to call what he wants, what everybody wants in the vaccine safety field is, break this one out for me. (IOM meeting transcript, page 123)[37]

This article by Robert Kennedy Jr. had many inaccuracies. Nevertheless, the piece continues to be a favorite of the antithimerosal activists.

Many of these issues were debunked by a report by Senator Enzi to the U.S. Senate Committee of Health, Education, Labor and Pensions in 2007.[20]

The Bottom Line: Does it Matter if Other Parents Don't Immunize Their Child?!

Misinformation about vaccine safety has tragic consequences—immunization rates decrease and the diseases we were once free from, return. If other parents don't immunize their child, they put your child and the community at risk of terrible diseases. Next time you come across alarming information about the safety of vaccines, ask yourself these questions:

- Are these claims based on valid assumptions?
- Are there any logical fallacies in the information I hear or read about vaccine safety?
- Are those attacking or advocating vaccinations focused on the scientific merits of the issues or on those who do not agree with them?
- Are the claims supported by people with real expertise? What do experts whom I trust think about the claims?
- Is the concern based on good scientific studies or could it be pseudoscience?
- Do the hypotheses originate from evidence or are they *ad hoc* hypotheses?
- Does the source of information have perceived or real conflicts of interest? Have they divulged them? How likely is it that the conflicts of interest affect the information or research?

Identifying reliable information about vaccine safety can seem a daunting task. Some approaches are outlined in the next chapter.

IF YOU WANT TO READ MORE:

Bausell RB. 2007. *Snake Oil Science: The truth about complementary and alternative medicine.* Oxford University Press: New York.

Huber P. 1993. *Galileo's revenge: Junk science in the courtroom.* Basic Books: New York.

Chapter 6

Reliable Information: How Do I Find the Right Information in the First Place?!

A lie gets halfway around the world before
the truth has a chance to get its pants on.
Winston Churchill

Often, it is easier to just start with reliable information than to try to sort out the misinformation from information. The first step is to start with an information source that you **know** is reliable. For many parents this is usually the pediatrician, family physician, or nurse practitioner, but other families want to search further. Unfortunately, many of the places where parents go to find information about vaccine safety are not reliable sources of information.

According to a 2000 study[1] parents obtain vaccine information from the following sources:

- Doctor   84%
- Nurse   8%
- Health clinic   8%
- Friends or family members   7%
- Newspapers or magazines   18%
- Books or journals   12%
- Internet   7%

Most traditional health providers can provide reliable information. Pediatricians often have materials approved by the American Academy of Pediatrics, for example, which convenes groups of experts to prepare materials for parents.

Many parents obtain information about vaccines from well-meaning friends or family members, but they too may be uninformed or misinformed sources.

Television news reaches almost every American home and

influences what Americans know and consider important.

WHEN THE DOCTOR IS CONFUSED: LINDA'S CASE

Even health providers may have misconceptions—or be confused—about the most publicized vaccine safety issues. In Linda's case, her doctor's confusion had grave consequences.

Linda is a 3-year old who has asthma. Her parents know that every year she needs a flu shot. In the winter of 2006 they took Linda to her primary care provider for the influenza vaccine, but the doctor told them he could not immunize her because he did not have the influenza vaccine without thimerosal preservative. So she went home without getting the vaccine.

Influenza vaccine is recommended for children under 18 years of age and children with chronic conditions like asthma. The only available vaccine for Linda at that time would have been the trivalent, inactivated influenza vaccine (TIV) that is given by injection. The only manufacturer of TIV that is licensed for children produces the usual TIV and also one without thimerosal preservative as an alternative for *parents* who do not want to use the vaccine containing thimerosal (see Chapter 8). Neither the CDC nor the American Academy of Pediatrics have expressed a preference for either vaccine because there are no scientific data that would favor one over the other. Also, the reduced thimerosal TIV costs substantially more than the standard vaccine. In other words, Linda should have been given the thimerosal-containing version because it was available.

Two weeks after the clinic visit, Linda was hospitalized for pneumonia resulting from influenza type A infection. She had a 2-day stay in the intensive care unit because of respiratory failure that required her to be intubated (a tube placed in her wind pipe) so she could be mechanically ventilated.[2]

Although health stories account for a great deal of local TV nightly news broadcasts, they can be an unreliable source of health information. These health stories are usually broadcast because they are "hot topics," not because they are of public health importance. Often reporters may make recommendations without citing their data sources, and occasionally they may make egregious errors that could harm viewers who rely on that information.[3]

THE INTERNET AS A SOURCE OF HEALTH INFORMATION

Two-thirds of adults in the United States use the Internet to find health information (all topics). Although the Internet can be a valuable resource, the quality of health information on the Web is extremely variable and difficult to assess. For example, search engines like Google, Yahoo, or MSN only identify topics and provide lists of Web sites, with no guarantee as to whether the content of those Web sites is accurate or not. A search for a vaccine safety term is as likely (and sometimes more likely) to take a person to misinformation as to reliable information.

Always start with a Web site that you know you can trust to give you reliable information. Following are some suggestions.

TRUSTWORTHY HEALTH INFORMATION

THE NATIONAL LIBRARY OF MEDICINE'S MEDLINE PLUS (*www. medlineplus.gov*). This is one of the best places to begin a search about just about any health matter.
THE CENTERS FOR DISEASE CONTROL AND PREVENTION (CDC) (*www.cdc.gov/vaccines*). This is the lead federal agency for protecting the health and safety of Americans at home and abroad. Its Web site provides a wealth of information about health, travel, the environment, and disease prevention.
THE NATIONAL INSTITUTES OF HEALTH (NIH). Because NIH

is the steward of medical and behavioral research for the United States, the newest information can often be found at *www.health.nih.gov*, as well as the Web sites of the various institutes and centers at *www.nih.gov/icd*.

THE AMERICAN ACADEMY OF PEDIATRICS (AAP) (*www.aap. org*). The AAP is the professional organization representing 60,000 pediatricians. Its Web site is aimed at parents and child health professionals and covers a wide range of information about children's health.

TRUSTWORTHY INFORMATION ABOUT VACCINES

THE NATIONAL NETWORK FOR IMMUNIZATION INFORMATION (NNII) (*www.immunizationinfo.org*). Our NNii Web site is designed to provide parents, health care professionals, the media, policy makers, and others with up-to-date, science-based information on immunizations. The site features a searchable database of information on diseases prevented through immunization, essays about immunization issues (the topics are largely suggested by our readers), a listing of all state vaccination requirements, and weekly Immunization Newsbriefs, which highlight vaccine issues in the news. It also includes background on vaccine development and vaccine safety, guidelines for how to evaluate health information on the Internet, and an image gallery of the effects of vaccine-preventable diseases.

CDC's VACCINES AND IMMUNIZATIONS Web site (*www.cdc.gov/ vaccines*). This Web site features publications and fact sheets, including vaccine recommendations, designed for the public as well as for health providers.

CDC's INFORMATION FOR TRAVELERS (*www.cdc.gov/travel*). This Web site is very useful to travelers and their health providers because it is frequently updated and provides information that is useful no matter where you are traveling.

THE WORLD HEALTH ORGANIZATION'S GLOBAL ADVISORY COMMITTEE ON VACCINE SAFETY (*www.who.int/immunization_safety/safety_quality/vaccine_safety_websites/en/index.html*). This site will help you find reliable information on vaccine safety by providing a list of Web sites that meet the criteria of the Global Advisory Committee on Vaccine Safety. This site is particularly helpful for learning about immunization programs in other countries.

WHEN YOU GO TO A SITE LOOK FOR THESE CHARACTERISTICS:

* A good health Web site will display who is responsible for the site. Also, there will be a way to contact the information provider or Webmaster.
* Information should not be slanted in favor of a Web site's sponsor or source of funding. Health information should be accurate and unbiased.

THEN ASK THE FOLLOWING QUESTIONS:

* Do scientific experts review the medical information before it is posted on the Web site? What are their credentials? Remember that credentials are difficult to assess on the Internet and experts in one field may not be experts in another area. It is important to look for sponsoring organizations that allow their name and prestige to be displayed. For example, notice the organizations that allow the NNii Web site (*www.immunizationinfo.org*) to display their names and logos.
* Does the information display the date of last revision, and is it kept up to date?
* What is the scientific evidence for claims made? The original source of facts and figures should be shown. For example, the Web site should provide citations of medical articles or other sources of information. You should be able to distinguish facts from opinions. Also, facts are more reliable if they

come from a published scientific study on humans rather than from unpublished accounts or from reports of a single person or of animal studies. One needs to recognize, however, that many of the antivaccine sites appear legitimate and cite articles from the CDC and other reliable sources but either misquote or take statements out of context. Some Web sites may inaccurately cite published literature.

◆ Does the Web site feature anecdotes (stories about individuals) about purported serious adverse events instead of scientific evidence? If so it is likely not a credible source of information.

◆ How is the Web site funded?

Next, consider the *purpose* of the Web site. The purpose should be to provide accurate and unbiased information about that topic. If the purpose is to advertise a health care product, be skeptical about the information provided. If much of the material on the Web site emphasizes stories about individual children, it may be an antivaccine Web site.

Finally, discuss with your health professional the information that you find on the Web. Health information found on the Web should supplement rather than replace the information or advice given by your physician or nurse.

The Bottom Line: How Do I find the Right Information in the First Place?!

In the midst of a sea of misinformation, trustworthy sources of information are still available. Instead of relying on a search engine to find health information, use authoritative guides and Web sites such as the ones listed in this chapter.

The next section of the book will examine some vaccine safety concerns in detail, evaluating the available evidence for causality and identifying misinformation elements.

IF YOU WANT TO READ MORE:

Wolfe RM, Sharp LK, Lipsky MS. 2002. Content and design attributes of antivaccination web sites. *Journal of the American Medical Association* 287:3245-3248. This technical report is summarized on the NNii web site at *www.immunizationinfo.org/immunization_science_detail.cfv?id=51.*

SECTION II
BLAMING VACCINES

Do Vaccines Cause Asthma?!

*The prevalence of asthma has increased dramatically over the last
25 years in the United States and in other nations as a result of
ill-defined changes in living conditions in modern Western society.*
MaryJane Selgrade et al, Environmental Health Perspectives,
April 2006

Sarah has been waking nearly every day around three in the morning. Breathing is hard—her chest feels tight and she cannot stop coughing. Sarah suffers from asthma, a chronic inflammatory disease of the airways that causes her to wheeze, cough, and have difficulty breathing.

Sarah is a five-year-old African-American with a long history of allergies. Dust, pollen, cats, dogs, cigarette smoke, and even strong smells can trigger asthma attacks. When exposed to these allergens, Sarah's immune system overreacts, causing the muscles around her airways (bronchial tubes) to tighten, and the walls to swell and produce extra mucus. Thus her airways narrow, reducing airflow in and out of the lungs.

Her first attack of asthma hit when she had a nasty cold at one year of age. Late that night she received several shots at the emergency room and since then, Sarah sees her doctor often. A couple of times she had to stay in the hospital overnight because of the wheezing attacks.

Sarah lives with her mother—who also had asthma as a child—in downtown Houston, near a busy interstate highway. The child uses an inhaler for coughing spells and takes medicines every day to control the wheezing. Her asthma cannot be cured, only controlled.

Like Sarah, millions of children in the world suffer from asthma. Indeed, over the past two decades the prevalence of childhood asthma has been increasing in many (but not all) countries, including the United States.

According to the American Lung Association statistics for 2002, over 20 million Americans, of whom 6.1 million were children, had asthma.[1]

Some people think vaccines cause asthma.

In this chapter we will consider what we know about the causes of asthma and then we will consider whether there is any evidence that might support a causal link between vaccinations and the development of asthma.

WHAT IS ASTHMA?

Asthma is a chronic disease characterized by repeated episodes of wheezing, breathlessness, chest tightness, and coughing.

Researchers find it difficult to precisely define asthma because of its varied clinical patterns. For example, not all wheezing illnesses are asthma and sometimes people with asthma don't wheeze. Also, there is no specific clinical test for asthma.

There are a number of tests, however, used to help diagnose asthma, such as showing that the airway obstruction (the cause of the wheezing) is reversible with drugs.

The small airways of the lung have an exaggerated narrowing response to certain stimuli that is considered characteristic of asthma, as is the ability to reverse this narrowing with certain drugs.

Therefore, epidemiological studies are hampered by differences in how physicians diagnose asthma and they often must rely on questionnaires that ask about asthma symptoms or whether a doctor has ever made the diagnosis of asthma.

Without a standard diagnosis for asthma, researchers find it difficult to estimate the actual incidence of the disease in a particular population (they may underestimate or overestimate the incidence), among other problems.

WHAT CAUSES ASTHMA?

We do not fully understand the causes of asthma, which is probably not a single disease and therefore it is probably not due to a single cause (etiology). Sarah's asthma was probably the result of the interaction of genetic, environmental, and social factors. Several of these factors probably combine to trigger her recurring asthma attacks.

GENETIC FACTORS. Studies have found that if a person has a parent with asthma, he or she is three to six times more likely to develop asthma than a person who does not have a parent with asthma.

Many scientists have tried to identify specific genes that make someone susceptible to asthma. They do this by looking for differences in the genetic code between people with asthma and people without asthma. When a gene is more commonly found in groups of people with asthma, it suggests a possible role in the development of asthma. For instance, a literature review published in 2006 identified 25 genes that have been associated with asthma in 6 or more populations and 54 genes that have been associated in 2 to 5 populations.[2] Other factors associated with asthma that may be influenced by genetics are

- ◆ GENDER: Before age 10, boys are almost three times more likely to develop asthma than girls. During adolescence, both males and females have similar rates. In adulthood, however, asthma is more common—and severe—in women.[3]
- ◆ RACE/ETHNICITY: Race/ethnicity affects the risk for developing asthma, although it is not clear whether this is because of a genetic or socioeconomic risk or both. African-Americans have higher rates of asthma than whites and Hispanics (except for Puerto Ricans, whose rates are higher than the others).[4]

ENVIRONMENTAL FACTORS. Some of the things in the environment that could have contributed to Sarah's asthma are[5]

- Tobacco smoke exposure in the home as well as being exposed to smoke during her mother's pregnancy
- Exposure to air pollutants (car exhaust, industrial chemicals, ozone)
- Exposure to indoor allergens and biologics (cockroaches, dust mites, mold, and rodents)
- Severe lower respiratory infections early in life (such as infection with the respiratory syncytial virus, or RSV)

One study of inner-city children with asthma found that short-term increases in air pollutant concentrations—even when below the National Ambient Air Quality Standards—were associated with more frequent asthma symptoms and asthma-related school absences.[6]

Although not an issue for Sarah, adults exposed to sensitizing agents at work—which is known as occupational asthma (in detergent plants, for example)—are also at risk of developing asthma.

SOCIAL FACTORS. Epidemiological studies have also identified some social factors associated with asthma.

It is not clear whether these are really risk factors for asthma or whether these social factors simply make these children more likely to be exposed to the environmental factors discussed above.

For instance,

- Children in poor, urban families (14%) are more likely to have been diagnosed with asthma than children in families that are more affluent (12%)[1]
- Children from single-parent families (16%) are more likely to have been diagnosed with asthma than children in two-parent families (11%)[1]

Asthma is a complex condition (perhaps conditions). Its causes are not solely genetic or environmental, but the result of what some researchers call a gene–environment interaction. A mini-monograph by the Environmental Protection Agency (EPA) summarizes it this way:

> It is likely that the risk of developing asthma is greatest when both genetic and environmental risk factors are present simultaneously. Evidence to date suggests that asthma induction is the result of complex interactions between specific exposures and the genes that interact with such exposures during crucial periods in the natural history of the disease. The current "epidemic" of asthma cannot be explained by genetic factors, but genetic factors may still be important with regard to susceptibility.[7]

MISSING INFORMATION AND THE "ASTHMA EPIDEMIC"

The prevalence of asthma in children has increased over the past 25 years in many countries. Mostly this has been seen in developed countries. In the Unites States, the prevalence increased from 36 per 1,000 children in 1980 to 58 per 1,000 in 2003.[5] According to the World Health Organization (WHO), by 2006, between 100 and 150 million people around the world suffered from asthma.[8]

Although scientists understand many of the pathologic processes and many of the risk factors for developing the disease, they still don't know why asthma is more common now than 25 years ago and why it is more common in countries with a "Western life style." Because changes in the genetic makeup of a population take several generations to occur, most think that it is more likely that changes in the environment and lifestyle differences, rather than genetic changes, account for the increased rates observed. No single environ-

mental factor or lifestyle cause has been shown to be responsible for the increase in the prevalence of asthma.

The increased rates of asthma have been blamed on many
of the changes in modern society such as global warming and
climate change, decreased exercise, changes in diet, oral contraceptives, pet ownership, and the use of air humidifiers. Two
of the most plausible contributors to this increase of asthma
are obesity and tobacco smoke exposure. A third explanation,
the "hygiene hypothesis," also offers some clues.

Let's look at these explanations in detail.

OBESITY. The number of overweight and obese children
in the United States nearly doubled from 1976 to 1994. One
out of every five children is overweight. Obese children suffer
from many health problems including type 2 diabetes, high
blood pressure and cholesterol, sleep apnea, liver disease, and
asthma. For instance, studies have found that

- More than 75% of people visiting emergency departments in the United States and Canada for asthma
  were overweight or obese.[9]
- Girls who became overweight or obese between 6 and
  11 years of age were seven times more likely to develop new asthma symptoms at age 11 or 13.[10]
- The risk of developing asthma for children 6–14
  years of age increases as their body mass index
  (weight) increases.[11]
- The severity and symptoms of asthma decrease when
  obese women lose weight.[12]

The biological plausibility of obesity as one of the causes of
asthma has been well studied in animal models—especially
in mice and rats. Based on these animal studies and the epidemiological evidence in humans, it is very likely that childhood obesity is one of the reasons why more children have
asthma today than 20 years ago.[7]

TOBACCO SMOKE EXPOSURE. Statistical studies consistently

demonstrate that children exposed to tobacco smoke have more respiratory tract illnesses—including asthma and recurrent wheezing episodes—than other children. Also, studies show that adolescents and adults who smoke have a greater risk of developing asthma. The data have been so consistent that the relationship is considered causal—even though asthma occurs in children who have not been exposed to tobacco smoke, and children exposed to tobacco smoke do not always develop asthma. Therefore tobacco smoke exposure is neither a necessary nor a sufficient cause of asthma (see Chapter 4).

A number of other air pollutants affect lung functions and can cause recurrent attacks of wheezing, including particulate matter in air, ozone, and motor vehicle exhaust. However, the evidence favoring exposure to these sources as a risk factor for developing asthma is not as strong as for tobacco smoke.

THE HYGIENE HYPOTHESIS. In 1989, David Strachan observed that hay fever was less common in British families with lots of children. In his paper, Strachan proposed what later would be called the hygiene hypothesis:

> These observations ... could be explained if allergic diseases were prevented by infection in early childhood, transmitted by unhygienic contact with older siblings, or acquired prenatally ... Over the past century declining family size, improved household amenities and higher standards of personal cleanliness have reduced opportunities for cross-infection in young families. This may have resulted in more widespread clinical expression of atopic [allergic] disease.[13]

Since the theory was first proposed, several studies confirmed that children who have frequent contact with other children during childhood are at a lower risk of developing hay fever and allergen sensitization (having a bad reaction to an allergen). In the case of asthma the evidence is conflicting.

While some studies showed that having older siblings and attending a day-care center seemed to protect some children from asthma, this protection was limited to those with a family history of asthma—emphasizing the role of genetics.[14]

Children who grow up on farms—particularly those who have contact with livestock and poultry—have a lower risk of allergies and asthma than children in the same rural areas who do not live on farms. This protection has been hypothesized to be because these children may have more exposure to bacterial components such as endotoxin.[15]

How would endotoxin exposure provide protection? Endotoxin is known to be a powerful immune stimulant so it is plausible that endotoxin could stimulate the young immune system, creating an immune response that limits the body's response to allergens and other environmental exposures.

The protective effect of endotoxin against allergies was also tested in urban areas by researchers from the University of Colorado. They compared concentrations of endotoxin in house dust with allergen sensitization in infants at high risk for developing asthma. Children exposed to higher concentrations of endotoxin had fewer allergic reactions to local allergens.[16]

Thus, there is evidence that living in a cleaner environment could alter an infant's immune response. Like obesity, however, the hygiene hypothesis could account for some—but not all—of the increase in asthma cases seen over the past two decades.

In summary, there is still much missing information about the causes of the "asthma epidemic" in many countries. What we know is that obesity, exposure to tobacco smoke, and reduced immune stimulation in the environment—possibly by bacterial components like endotoxin—seem to have contributed to the increase of asthma.

COMMUNISM AND THE HYGIENE HYPOTHESIS

After World War II, Germany was divided into the German Democratic Republic (East Germany) and the Federal Republic of Germany (West Germany).

East Germany was communist; West Germany was capitalist. The differences in political systems were also manifested in their economies and lifestyles. Although both countries were genetically similar, they were environmentally different. Among other things, East Germany was characterized by high levels of environmental pollution and small living spaces.

In 1990, East and West Germany were reunited. Epidemiologists then began to conduct studies of allergic diseases, comparing the former East with the West German populations.[16] Surprisingly, they found that children in West Germany had higher rates of asthma and allergies than those raised in East Germany. For some, this ecological evidence supports the hygiene hypothesis. Interestingly, immunization rates in East Germany reached 95%, whereas 60-70% of children were immunized in West Germany.

ASTHMA AND VACCINES

Some have suggested that perhaps immunizations have contributed to the increased rates of asthma. The vaccine most commonly blamed was the whole-cell pertussis vaccine (which is no longer used in the United States).

Could exposure to a specific vaccine—or to many vaccines—be related to the subsequent development of asthma as some have suggested? How could vaccines increase the risk of asthma and allergic diseases?

One suggestion is that vaccines might change the balance of immunity toward allergic responses in a couple of ways. To understand these theoretical mechanisms let's look at what happens to little Sarah.

HYPOTHESIS #1: Vaccines might stimulate a harmful immune response. Sarah's body sees things in the environment (such as dust and mold) as threatening and makes an immune response. Other children without asthma do not react in that way to dust or mold.

When Sarah was immunized against measles (and other infections), her body was "trained" to make an immune response against the measles virus. Could the vaccines have also trained the body to make an immune response to things other than the virus—such as dust?

In 2002 the Institute of Medicine's (IOM) Immunization Safety Committee reviewed the issue of multiple immunizations and immune dysfunction (see Chapter 9), including the potential link between asthma and vaccines.[18]

HOW VACCINES WORK

Every day, the body is bombarded with bacteria, viruses, and other germs. In fact, the immune system keeps under control billions of bacteria in the intestine alone.

When a person is infected with a disease-causing germ, the immune system mounts a response to it. The pus that develops several days after a dirty skin scrape—after a fall from a bike, for example—results from the normal immune responses.

After most infections, the body develops immune memory—such as antibodies—against every specific germ. The next time the person encounters that germ, the immune memory cells and antibodies quickly recognize it and eliminate it before any sign of infection.

This is why a child who has had measles (or a measles virus-containing vaccine) will only rarely develop the disease again if exposed to the measles virus. The immune system remembers.

They considered whether bystander activation—a complex process that favors some immune responses over others—could be a plausible biological mechanism by which immunizations might cause a heterologous allergic response, such as asthma.

According to the IOM, although there was some evidence that might support such an association, the data were weak—that it was not very likely that this mechanism was an important contributor to causing asthma and other allergic diseases.

HYPOTHESIS #2: Vaccines might suppress a beneficial immune response.

An indirect mechanism by which vaccines might affect the tendency to develop allergic responses, such as asthma, might be by preventing the infection.

The next time the child encounters the virus that causes measles, the immune system will destroy the virus before it can cause symptoms. The immune system can recognize and effectively combat hundreds of thousands, probably millions, of different organisms.

A vaccine works in a similar way. However, instead of one natural infection, it may take several doses over several months or years for immunity to develop after a vaccine.

Some vaccines contain an inactivated (killed) or an attenuated (weakened) form of the germ, or just a piece of the germ. When introduced into the body, the vaccine causes a memory immune response to the germ without causing the illness. This memory immune response, being like the natural one after infections, will combat the germ if the person is exposed to it in the future.

Thus, vaccination protects the child against infection with a germ without the child ever developing the illness.

This would cause an imbalance in the immune responses later in life—in a manner similar to that suggested by the hygiene hypothesis.[19] According to this reasoning, if Sarah had not been vaccinated against a particular disease, but instead had gotten the natural infection, perhaps she would not have developed asthma.

In 2002, the IOM Vaccine Safety Committee concluded that there was only weak evidence for the existence of any biological mechanisms by which multiple immunizations—either collectively or individually—under the U.S. infant immunization schedule could possibly influence an individual's risk of allergy.

WHAT ABOUT THE EPIDEMIOLOGICAL EVIDENCE? The IOM committee reviewed one ecological study and five controlled epidemiological studies that looked at possible connections between allergic disease and asthma. The ecological study found that population data did not show an increased risk of asthma due to DTP vaccination. The five epidemiological studies[20-24] found variable results as to whether various vaccines were associated with increased risk of allergic diseases or asthma or not; however, all of these studies had methodological limitations. As a consequence, the IOM committee considered that the evidence from these six studies was weak and not helpful in establishing whether vaccines caused asthma:

> The committee concludes that the epidemiological and clinical evidence is inadequate to accept or reject a causal relationship between multiple immunizations and an increased risk of allergic disease, particularly asthma.[18]

ADDITIONAL STUDIES SINCE THE IOM COMMITTEE'S REPORT WAS PUBLISHED:

◆ One large cohort study involving 167,240 children from four large health maintenance organizations in Washington, Oregon, and California found no increased risk of developing childhood asthma associated with diphtheria, tetanus, whole-cell pertussis vaccine, measles, mumps, rubella vaccine, or oral polio vaccine.[25] This study did find a weak associations for *Haemophilus influenzae* type b and hepatitis B vaccines with the risk of developing asthma—but this finding may only reflect the fact that children with asthma go to the doctor more often, hence they have a greater chance of being immunized (that is, the weak association may have been because of selection bias—see page 54).

- A relatively small case-control study of full-term infants examined whether immunizations received before 18 months of age were related to asthma later in childhood. The investigators found that asthma was not associated with hepatitis B vaccine or the age when the first dose of hepatitis B vaccine was given; the number of doses of whole-cell pertussis, *Haemophilus influenzae* type b, or oral polio vaccines; having received the MMR vaccine; or the total number of doses of vaccinations received. On the other hand, asthma in later childhood was associated with the number of wheezing episodes during infancy.[26]
- A British study of 13,810 children found no association between vaccination with the whole-cell pertussis vaccine and asthma by 7 years of age.[27]
- A Dutch study of 1,201 children 8–12 years of age found no indication for a higher risk of reported physician-diagnosed asthma or allergies after *Haemophilus influenzae* type b vaccination in the first year of life.[28]
- Another Dutch study of 1,872 children, found that diphtheria, tetanus, whole-cell pertussis vaccine, and

inactivated polio vaccination were not related to reported allergies at elementary school age.[29]
◆ An analysis of all the studies that had looked at DTP
vaccine and asthma found no association with the
risk of asthma in childhood or adolescence.[30]
These recent studies have consistently shown that vaccines
do not appear to increase the risk of developing childhood
asthma. In fact, vaccines are very important for children with
asthma who are at increased risk of complications of respiratory infections like influenza.[31,32]

ANAPHYLACTIC (LIFE-THREATENING) ALLERGIC REACTIONS TO VACCINES, INCLUDING ASTHMA

Anaphylaxis is the medical term for a serious allergic reaction that results
in hives, breathing difficulty (asthma and sometimes upper airway swelling), fast heart beat, vomiting, and even death. Anaphylaxis in children
is a rare, but serious allergic reaction that can be caused by proteins, antibiotics, vaccines, vaccine components, or other things in the environment. More commonly, it is caused by tree nuts and peanuts.

The risk of anaphylaxis after vaccination is very low. A Vaccine Safety
Datalink study in four West Coast HMOs identified five cases of potentially vaccine-associated anaphylaxis after administration of 7,644,049
vaccine doses—that is a risk of 0.65 cases per million doses. None of the
five cases resulted in death.[34] Two vaccine components have been identified as the main causes of these rare but serious allergic reactions after
vaccination: gelatin or egg protein.

GELATIN. Modern vaccines sometimes contain stabilizers—substances
that prevent changes in their chemical composition. One such stabi-
lizer is gelatin. People allergic to gelatin may have an allergic reaction
to vaccines that contain gelatin, such as: diphtheria, tetanus, and
acellular pertussis (DTaP); influenza; measles, mumps, and rubella
(MMR); rabies; chickenpox; or yellow fever vaccine.

The recent recommendation for routine immunization of young children with influenza vaccine is projected to be cost-effective for all children but is expected to be cost-saving for young children with asthma.[33]

MISINFORMATION ABOUT ASTHMA AND VACCINES

SPECULATION, INVALID ASSUMPTIONS, AND POST HOC FALLACIES. A frequent misinformer about vaccines and vaccine safety speculated this way:

EGG PROTEIN. The influenza viruses used to make the influenza vaccine are grown in the fluids surrounding chicken embryos, thus the vaccine may contain egg protein.

The measles and mumps vaccines [and therefore also MMR vaccine and the MMR vaccine containing varicella vaccine (MMRV)] may also contain some residual traces of egg protein; although children with severe egg protein allergy seem to tolerate measles vaccine.

The immune system of a person allergic to eggs overreacts to the proteins in the eggs, no matter how they enter the body—either through a breakfast omelet or a flu shot.

A person with asthma who is also allergic to eggs may have an asthma attack as part of the reaction to the egg protein.

Because anaphylactic symptoms include respiratory problems, it is not uncommon that an anaphylactic reaction to a vaccine component results in an asthma attack.

This does not mean that vaccines exacerbate asthma, but simply that they may cause an asthma attack as part of the anaphylactic reaction.

Other potential allergens present in some vaccines are the antibiotic neomycin and baker's yeast.

For a list of possible allergens in each vaccines see:
www.vaccinesafety.edu/components-Allergens.htm.

> Asthma, like autism, is mysteriously on the rise and out of control. An autoimmune disorder that 25 years ago was experienced by some children is now a chronic disease epidemic in our child population. What has changed in the past 25 years?
>
> Could the nearly doubling of doses of vaccines our children get in the first three years of life when their immune systems are most rapidly maturing have anything to do with it?[35]
>
> ... the numbers of children who are suffering from chronic immune and brain dysfunction has sky-rocketed in the past 25 years at the same time that the numbers of doses of vaccines children receive has doubled.[36]

The post hoc fallacy (after this, therefore because of this) here is to try to associate increased use of vaccines with increasing numbers of cases of autism or asthma just because both seem to be increasing at about the same time. One could as easily associate it with the increase in the number of computers and DVD players being used and French fries being eaten today.

While the increase in the rate of childhood asthma over the past three decades is real, the increase in the number of cases of autism that is being observed may be an artifact of reporting. As we will see in the next chapter, increasing recognition of autism probably accounts for much of that change.

Also, there is no evidence that asthma is an autoimmune disease so this also is also an invalid statement. While an asthma attack does involve an abnormal immune response, this is a response to outside agents (allergens), not the body's own cells.

Examples of autoimmune diseases are lupus, type 1 diabetes, and multiple sclerosis, where the immune system attacks the person's own kidney, pancreas, or nervous system.

The 2002 IOM review[18] about multiple immunizations and immune dysfunction distinguished between autoimmune and allergic diseases. Asthma is an allergic disease, not an autoimmune disease (see Chapter 9 for more discussion about autoimmune diseases).

OTHER MISINFORMATION AND LOGICAL FALLACIES. Here is an argument against the person (the ad hominem fallacy) as well as an appeal to pity (the argumentum ad misericordian fallacy):

> At this point, ... 1 in 8 children has asthma. Public health officials, who can't come up with anything better than "dust, mold, cockroaches and smoke," which have been around for centuries, should be held accountable for their failure to give parents a credible explanation as to why so many of our highly vaccinated children are stuck on sick.[36]

Another misinformer wrote:

> Vaccines are destroying our immune systems. Amazingly, the medical profession ignores the incriminating evidence against vaccines, and continues to inflict more unnecessary and harmful vaccines on our nation's infants.[37]

To support this last claim, the misinformer cited a 1996 study of 13 HIV-infected patients who temporarily had higher levels of the virus after being immunized against tetanus—an observation that hardly implies that "vaccines are destroying our immune systems."[38]

THE BOTTOM LINE: DO VACCINES CAUSE ASTHMA?

Asthma is a complex disease without a single cause. Risk factors for asthma include being born in a family with other allergic individuals and/or exposure to certain irritants or allergens.

Based on the available evidence, we conclude that vaccines do not appear to cause asthma.

Could vaccines be a contributor to the current "asthma epidemic" like obesity and tobacco smoke exposure? The evidence shows that this is unlikely. So far, the scientific evidence does not suggest a role of vaccine exposures in the development of asthma. While all the causes of the increasing incidence of asthma in the past two to three decades are not fully known, there are many things—other than the number of vaccines given to children—that have also increased during that time period.

Finally, children with asthma also need vaccines, because they are at increased risk of some vaccine-preventable diseases compared to other children.

"GRANTZ IS CHARTING HIS LIFE BASED ON GENETIC VS. ENVIRONMENTAL FACTORS."

Chapter 8

Do Vaccines Cause Autism?!

Parents who cite the evidence of their own eyes that their children became autistic after receiving ... vaccine are in the grip of one of the oldest of commonsensical fallacies—that association proves causation .... It is the responsibility of scientists to tell them that intensive scientific research in a number of disciplines indicates that the evidence of their own eyes is not true.
Michael Fitzpatrick (physician and father of an autistic boy),
Spiked Online, November 11, 2005

Brandon has no friends. He never goes out to play with other kids. Although he is almost four years old, he doesn't speak yet—he just makes indistinct guttural sounds. Every day, Brandon runs in circles in front of the TV and follows repetitive patterns for hours. Any change in his daily routine, any stranger in the house, would wreak havoc.

Brandon has autism, also known as autistic spectrum disorder (ASD) or pervasive developmental disorder (PDD). His parents have tried everything in their power to cure Brandon, from behavioral therapy with a psychiatrist to gluten-free/casein-free diets and multivitamin/multimineral preparations. So far, they have had little success.

WHAT IS AUTISM?

Autism spectrum disorders are a group of developmental disabilities—autistic disorder; pervasive developmental disorder-not otherwise specified (PDD-NOS); and Asperger syndrome. These diagnostic categories have some of the same symptoms: poor social interactions and communications, and unusual behaviors and interests. People with these disorders vary from the gifted to the severely challenged. These conditions—plus Rett syndrome and childhood disintegrative

139

disorder—make up a broad category known as pervasive developmental disorders. Here we will refer to all these categories together as autism.

Autism occurs in all demographic groups. CDC estimates that about one of every 152 children across the United States had autism in 2002. Autism occurs 4 to 5 times more frequently in boys than in girls[1] and it's more common among the brothers and sisters of an affected child and among persons with certain other hereditary syndromes.[2]

CDC's prevalence studies[3] (the total number of cases detected at one point in time) have looked at children 8 years of age. This is because almost all cases should have been detected by that age, either in children's medical records or within the educational system, or both. However, autism can often be detected as early as 18 months, which is important because early interventions provide more opportunity for children with autism to learn and have their symptoms treated.[4]

Despite misinformation to the contrary,[5] autism is now being recognized in many adults[6,7] who were not identified before.

WHAT CAUSES AUTISM?

The causes of autism are unknown. Most evidence, however, suggests that genetic factors are among the main causes of autism. Family studies have shown that if one non-identical twin has autism, the other will also have it about 10% of the time; for identical twins the chance may be as great as 92%.[8] Despite family and twin studies, the majority of cases of autism occur in individuals without other recognizable genetic conditions. Some individuals, with some other hereditary medical conditions—such as the fragile X syndrome, tuberous sclerosis, Prader Willi syndrome, disorders of mitochondrial function—can also have features of autism.[2,9]

Disorders of Mitochondrial Function

Mitochondria are the power factories within each cell in the body. Mitochondria are essential for survival as they provide the energy to drive all the cell functions. To maintain and increase power production requires coordination between the genes in the nucleus—that we inherit from our mothers and fathers—and tiny bits of genetic material in the mitochondria—inherited just from our mothers. The inheritance of genetic changes in mitochondria is complex because there are hundreds to thousands of mitochondria in every cell.

Over the past 15–20 years, researchers have increasingly recognized disorders of mitochondrial function. Children with a mitochondrial disorder may develop normally for a while, but when stressed—perhaps by infection or fever—they may be unable to make all the energy that they need. The brain requires a large amount of energy. So, when these children are stressed, the brain is the place most often affected; brain injury of this type is often called mitochondrial encephalopathy. Children with mitochondrial encephalopathy may develop a number of symptoms of brain injury: altered mental state, seizures, problems with walking, poor language skill, attention deficit disorder, and others. Although there is little compelling evidence that mitochondrial disorders are linked with autism, features of autism have been reported in some patients with mitochondrial disorders; mitochondrial abnormalities have also been found in some children with autism.[10]

In 2007, the National Vaccine Injury Compensation Program (VICP) (see page 37) conceded a case concerning a child with a mitochondrial disorder. Two days after being immunized, she developed fever, lethargy, irritability, prolonged screaming, decreased response to stimuli, and she refused to walk. During the next 10 days, these symptoms of encephalopathy continued, she could not climb stairs, and she had periods of arching backwards when she screamed. Over months, her symptoms evolved to include muscle weakness and some features of autism. Six years later she developed seizures.[11,12]

The VICP is a "no-fault alternative to the traditional tort system for resolving vaccine injury claims."[13] A family can be compensated if the child received a vaccine on the VICP list, had an injury recognized by the VICP (such as encephalopathy), and the vaccine either caused the injury or "caused an existing illness to get worse." We think that the VICP conceded this case without a court ruling because the intent of the law is to compensate families without challenge when a case meets these preset statutory criteria, whether or not scientific causation has been established.

It is not possible to determine whether the onset of this child's mitochondrial encephalopathy occurred coincidental in time with vaccination (for example, if she had an unrecognized viral illness) or whether the stress of vaccination unmasked the mitochondrial disorder.

There is no evidence that vaccines cause mitochondrial disorders. No practical tools for screening for rare mitochondrial disorders exist at the moment.

At this time, our knowledge about mitochondrial disorders is incomplete, but we do know that children with mitochondrial disorders are at risk for encephalopathy after stress such as infections that can be prevented by vaccines.

In addition to genetic predispositions, there could be some as yet unknown environmental factors contributing to the development of autism. However, except for congenital rubella infections,[14] epidemiological studies have failed to find a link between specific environmental exposures and increased risks of autism.

Except for Rett syndrome, which has been shown to be caused by changes in one gene, scientists don't expect to find a single gene associated with autism—indeed they expect that as many as 10 or more genes or chromosome abnormalities may relate to the various symptoms of autism. Recent reports, for example, demonstrated that CNTNAP2 was an autism-susceptibility gene in one group of autistic children.[15] Another study of children with autism in both the United States and

Iceland showed that some other changes in chromosomes[16] might account for about 1% of cases of autism.

Because adults with autism have reduced rates of repro-duction, many scientists assume that the high rate of preva-lence of autism may be due to new mutations in genes and chromosomes.

Read more about autism at *www.medlineplus.gov/autism*.

IS THERE AN AUTISM EPIDEMIC?

Is autism more common now than it was two or three decades ago? Is the rate of new cases of autism really increasing or are children previously classified with other disorders now being diagnosed as autistic? It is clear that more cases of autism in recent years are being recognized, but it is not clear whether more cases of autism are occurring as well.

The U.S. Department of Education reported a many-fold increase in the number of children with autism receiv-ing educational support for the disorder between 1991 and 2001.[17] Other reports seem to show a continuing increase in the number of cases of autism.[3] CDC has embarked upon systematic studies to examine whether there are increasing numbers of cases occurring and whether there are differenc-es in the geographic distribution of cases.[1] It is too early to determine from the CDC studies whether the rate of new cases of autism is increasing, but in their initial comparisons the rates did differ in different areas of the United States and there were increased rates in some states—but not in others— between 2000 and 2002. The apparent increased prevalence of autism could have two different explanations.

- One explanation might be that the number of new cases has remained about the same but more peo-ple than before are now being diagnosed as having autism.

- ◆ Another explanation might be that the number of new cases has increased and more cases are being identified.

It is clear from many studies that changes in the diagnostic criteria for autism have greatly expanded the recognition of autism by broadening the definition of what is considered autism. For example, before 1980 there were no standard diagnostic criteria for autism in the Diagnostic and Statistical Manual (DSM) of the American Psychiatric Association; any diagnosis made during that time period was based on the definition of each individual psychiatrist. In addition, only two of the five types of autism now recognized were then considered to be autism. For instance, a study in England found that two forms of autism not recognized in the earlier diagnostic categories—Asperger disorder and pervasive developmental disorder not otherwise specified—accounted for almost three -fourths of the autism diagnoses in 1998-1999.[18]

A 2008 study found that some adults who were diagnosed as children with developmental language disorders, would be diagnosed as having autism using the diagnostic tools available today.[19]

In addition, the diagnosis of autism now allows financial coverage for some specialized services from many healthcare payors and school systems that were not available before, providing an incentive to use this diagnostic category both in the medical centers and in the schools.

To make things more difficult, most of the numbers for autism prevalence in the United States previously came from data of children who were receiving either 1) medical care or 2) special education services, sources of data that overlap but which by themselves may be incomplete. That is why the new CDC studies now look at both, correcting for those children identified in both datasets.[1]

Some think that better diagnosis alone cannot account

for the entire increase in the prevalence of autism. They believe that, when more epidemiologic data become available, the third explanation will prove to be true—that there has been a large increase in prevalence because of changed definition/recognition of autism but also that there has been a true increase in the number of cases of autism.[20]

VACCINES AND AUTISM

Some have hypothesized that vaccines have caused an increase in autism. Autism symptoms are usually first noticed between the ages of 12 months and 4 years of age. Of course, these are about the same ages when children receive a number of vaccines. In addition, we give many more vaccines to infants and toddlers now than we did in the past. Although the vaccine-preventable diseases have decreased remarkably as new vaccines have been introduced, the timing of their administration has led some to believe that one or more of the immunizations could cause autism.

Two main hypotheses linking vaccines and autism have been suggested. One involves measles vaccines—usually given as the measles-mumps-rubella vaccine (MMR). The other involves the mercury-containing preservative, thimerosal—previously used in many vaccines. These are separate issues although they have sometimes been confused in some media reports. Despite what you may have heard, neither the MMR or MMRV vaccine have ever contained thimerosal because the weakened vaccine viruses would have been inactivated by the preservative.

MEASLES VACCINES AND AUTISM

An association between measles-containing vaccines and autism was first suggested in a series of case reports in 1998 by

Andrew Wakefield and his colleagues.[21] They described 12 children with pervasive developmental disorders and gastrointestinal (GI) symptoms. In eight of the cases, the parents or physicians reported that the symptoms began within two weeks after the children received the MMR vaccine. The authors of the study hypothesized that this might be a new type of autism characterized by GI symptoms and developmental regression caused by the MMR vaccine.

Although this report contained no proof of a link between MMR vaccine and autism, a headline in London's *The Daily Telegraph* said "Vaccination may trigger disease linked to autism,"[22] a theme that was picked up by many news media.

In 2004, 10 of the 13 authors of the Wakefield study formally retracted their hypothesis by saying of the results:

> We wish to make it clear that in this paper no causal link was established between MMR vaccine and autism, as the data were insufficient. However, the possibility of such a link was raised and consequent events have had major implications for public health. In view of this, we consider now is the appropriate time that we should together formally retract the interpretation placed upon these findings in the paper, according to precedent.[23]

Between the publication of the Wakefield study in 1998 and the retraction in 2004, many research studies looked for evidence for an association between measles vaccine and autism. For instance, the 2004 Institute of Medicine (IOM) report (see page 70) on vaccines and autism reviewed 16 such studies, including 9 controlled observational studies, 3 ecological studies, and 2 studies based on a passive reporting system in Finland. *All of these studies consistently showed no association between MMR and autism.*[24]

Wakefield and his team also claimed that measles virus lodged in the intestines, releasing toxins that affected the brain, thus causing autism. Not only could other researchers not replicate Wakefield's reports of measles virus genetic material in the guts of autistic children, but the methodologies that Wakefield and his collaborators used were also shown to have been flawed.[25-28] According to a British investigative reporter, Wakefield was paid handsomely to try to prove that the MMR vaccine was unsafe.[29]

The IOM concluded that the data "favored the rejection of the hypothesis"—in other words, the evidence failed to show a link between measles vaccines and the development of autism. After the IOM report, additional reviews have also shown no association.[30]

The theory that measles vaccine causes autism has been fully discredited.[27] Nevertheless, the MMR scare attracted so much media attention that MMR immunization rates fell in a number of countries—at least in part, if not completely, because of misinformation about this safety concern.

Subsequently, there have been outbreaks of measles in Great Britain, the Netherlands, Germany, and Switzerland; and an epidemic of mumps in Great Britain (which was the likely source of an outbreak in the United States in 2006).[31]

The story of Andrew Wakefield and the scare about MMR vaccine causing autism have been summarized in the medical literature and the popular media.[27, 32]

THIMEROSAL-CONTAINING VACCINES AND AUTISM

In Great Britain and parts of Europe the alleged vaccines-autism link focused on the MMR vaccine, but in the United States the culprit of debate has been thimerosal, a mercury-containing preservative used in vaccines worldwide since the 1930s.

WHAT IS THIMEROSAL?

Thimerosal is a compound made up of ethylmercury attached to a chemical similar to aspirin. In the body, it is split apart, releasing the ethylmercury.

Thimerosal is 49.6% mercury by weight. It was a preservative for many (but not all) vaccines in use in the United States until 2001. It is still used as a preservative in many parts of the world. Thimerosal is also used as a preservative in some eye, ear, and other topical solutions, antivenins, immune globulins, and skin test antigens.*

Historically—in high concentration—thimerosal was used as an antiseptic (merthiolate) for wound management. Thimerosal is currently used in vaccines for two purposes:

- as a preservative to prevent bacterial and fungal contamination of multiple dose vials of vaccines during their clinical use. In this case, thimerosal is added at the end of the production process either to the liquid vaccine itself or—in the case of dry powder vaccines—to the liquid used to dilute the vaccine.
- as a part of the manufacturing process to kill the bacteria and fungi that might enter the vaccine during the vaccine production process.

When used as a part of the manufacturing process, the final concentration of thimerosal in the vaccine is very small. In this case, the vaccine is labeled as containing "trace amounts" of thimerosal because anything used during vaccine manufacture might still be present in tiny amounts† (the FDA calls such chemicals "residuals"‡).[33]

---

* Thimerosal concentrations in medications are listed at *www.fda.gov/ohrms/ dockets/98fr/981109bk.pdf*.

† The thimerosal content of vaccines, either from the manufacturing process or as preservative, can be found at *www.fda.gov/Cber/vaccine/thimerosal.htm#t1*.

‡ You can find a list of vaccine components (residuals, additives, preservatives) at *www.vaccinesafety.edu/components.htm*.

Thimerosal is not the only preservative used in vaccines and other medications. For example, some vaccines contain other preservatives such as 2-phenoxyethanol or phenol; neither of these contains mercury.

WHY ARE PRESERVATIVES ADDED TO SOME VACCINES? Preservatives like thimerosal are added to multiple-dose vials of vaccines because each time a dose is to be given, a needle is pushed through the stopper to draw up the vaccine into a syringe. Each time a dose is withdrawn from the vial, there is a risk that bacteria could enter the vial and contaminate the remaining vaccine. There are tragic accounts of people who were harmed by vaccine contaminated in this fashion in the early part of the 20th century. As a consequence, the FDA requires that most vaccines in multiple dose vials contain a preservative.[33] Preservatives are not required for single-dose vaccine vials.

THIMEROSAL IN OTHER COUNTRIES

Although many developed countries have removed thimerosal preservative from their vaccines, the preservative is still used in most developing countries—a policy supported by the World Health Organization (WHO).[34] WHO's Global Advisory Committee on Vaccine Safety considers thimerosal safe based on the available evidence. Moreover, WHO says that using vaccines supplied as single doses is currently not economically feasible for the majority of countries.

For instance, a typical immunization campaign in a poor country involves thousands of health care workers going from village to village vaccinating children and adults. It would be both financially and logistically unfeasible for them to use single dose vaccines—because of the amount of space for storage at the right temperature, transport of the vaccines, and disposing of the needles and syringes.

In the absence of any evidence of harm from thimerosal-containing vaccines, the greater risks are the known diseases.

THE HISTORY OF THE THIMEROSAL SAFETY CONCERN

In 1999, the U.S. Public Health Service and the American Academy of Pediatrics issued a special statement about thimerosal-containing vaccines (see page 158). Why?

WHAT WAS KNOWN IN 1999 AND WHAT HAVE WE LEARNED SINCE THEN? Mercury exists in a number of forms. Inorganic mercury refers to the metal or its salts, and it is found in dental fillings. Organic mercury refers to compounds that are made with the mercury bound to carbon atoms. For our purposes, we will concentrate on two organic mercury compounds whose names sound similar but which have some very important differences.

METHYLMERCURY. Methylmercury is not present in vaccines or drugs but it is in some of the food we eat. Of all the environmental contaminants that we are exposed to, this form of mercury has been the most extensively studied. Methylmercury accumulates in our bodies and can affect the development of children, especially those whose mothers were exposed to methylmercury before and/or during pregnancy.[35]

Methylmercury is the most common form of mercury environmental contamination. Once methylmercury enters the food chain it concentrates in certain foods, particularly predator fish. People who eat large quantities of certain fish can be exposed to large amounts of methylmercury. Methylmercury has also been used as a fungicide to protect seed grain from spoiling and it has poisoned people who accidentally ingested it.

Methylmercury is eliminated very slowly from the body by being passed from the liver into stool. Because it is so slowly eliminated it is present for a very long time and accumulates in the body as more food containing this substance is consumed.

Methylmercury is well known to be a neurotoxin—that

is, it can damage the brain and cause developmental disabilities. It can cause developmental problems in infants born to mothers who have been eating contaminated foods; the greatest risk for brain injury is exposure to methylmercury before birth. Although it would seem that methylmercury exposure during the first few months after birth might also be associated with developmental problems, the data on this are limited. For example, one study found that children who had higher levels of methylmercury in their hair actually had better developmental measures at 12 months of age; but these children were also breastfed longer, so it may have been that the benefits of breastfeeding outweighed the risks of methylmercury exposure.[35]

After too much exposure over time, methylmercury can cause a number of neurologic symptoms including tremors, emotional lability (emotionally unstable), memory loss, weakness, sleeplessness, odd sensations, changes in the tendon reflexes, performance deficits (poor performance on cognitive and motor function testing), sensitivity to light, hearing and visual problems, and other problems. However, exposure to methylmercury has never been associated with a constellation of signs and symptoms similar to autism. The theory that children with autism had symptoms similar to methylmercury poisoning[36] did not stand up to the scrutiny by the Institute of Medicine[37] nor to side-by-side comparisons by neuroscientists.[38] In their 2004 report[23] the IOM said "... autism has never been documented as a consequence of high-dose mercury exposure ..."

Much is known about the effects of methylmercury, including how much can safely be consumed.[34] Data about the toxicity of methylmercury are based on experimental animal studies, accidental environmental exposures, and studies of island populations who have consumed large amounts of fish containing high concentrations of methylmercury. Although methylmercury is broken down to inorganic mercury in the brain, brain injury is caused by the methylmercury not the inorganic mercury.[35] After exposure, methylmercury accumulates in the body over time because it is so slowly eliminated. Because it can cause neurologic and developmental problems, researchers have calculated how much exposure to methylmercury would be safe—that is, when children, for example, have been accidentally exposed to various levels of methylmercury, researchers can calculate how much was safe because no harm was measurable at that level. These calculations then can be expressed as "safe intake levels"[§]—in other words, the amount of exposure that would be expected to be safe if it occurred daily over time. There are some differences between the safe intake levels developed by the different government regulatory agencies, since they were created for different purposes—although the values are actually very similar. All of the safe intake levels incorporate a wide margin of safety factor (usually 3–10 times) to account for unknown factors and to be sure that they really are safe estimates.

ETHYLMERCURY. Thimerosal does not contain methylmercury, it contains ethylmercury. When all the discussion about thimerosal began in 1999, there was not much information about ethylmercury toxicity or its metabolism. No estimates of safe intake levels for ethylmercury, either after being eaten or injected, have been published.

Before penicillin, a form of ethylmercury given by injection was used to treat syphilis. Ethylmercury has also been used to protect seed grain from fungal spoilage; it has caused poisoning by the accidental ingestion of the grain.

From studies of people who were poisoned by eating large

---

§ Each of the regulatory agencies calls the safe levels of exposure to various substances by different names. For simplicity, we will use the term "safe intake level" to describe these values even though the various agencies use somewhat different terms.

amounts, we know that ethylmercury can cause neurotoxicity similar to methylmercury and can cause kidney damage.[34] In other studies, at very high doses, however, ethylmercury did not do as much damage to rat brains as did methylmercury. Although both compounds are partially converted to inorganic mercury in the brain, it appears that it is the organic forms that cause the brain injury.[35]

We now know from a study in monkeys[39] that the absorption is rapid and the distribution of mercury is widespread after injection of thimerosal-containing vaccines or after the feeding of methylmercury. However, the elimination of ethylmercury from the body was much faster, and the amount of mercury in the brain was significantly lower, in the animals that received the thimerosal-containing vaccines than in those that were fed methylmercury—methylmercury levels were about 10 times higher in the brain after methylmercury exposure.

Although both methyl- and ethylmercury are distributed widely in the body, they go to different places:

- Methylmercury levels in the brain have been shown to be many times higher than ethylmercury after the same dose—this has been observed in many animal species.[35]
- Recent studies in neonatal mice[40] also showed widespread distribution of both compounds, but the methylmercury levels in the brains were 3 to 4 times higher than after the same dose of ethylmercury.
- Ethylmercury was much higher in the liver—the pathway for elimination to the stool for both compounds—and the kidney.
- Both methyl- and ethylmercury accumulated in hair in a similar fashion.

Ethylmercury—given as thimerosal-containing vaccine—is also eliminated from the bodies of children much more rapidly than ingested methylmercury.[41,42] Because it is much more rapidly eliminated it would not be expected to accumulate in the body. For this reason, blood levels of mercury cannot be used to predict brain levels of ethylmercury after intermittent vaccine administration; ethylmercury does accumulate in hair, however, so hair may prove to be a better way to demonstrate exposure to thimerosal, as it is for methylmercury.[35]

We now know that the differences between ethyl- and methylmercury are very important—just as are the differences between methyl alcohol (wood alcohol, a poison used in antifreeze) and ethyl alcohol (found in wine and beer). Thus, assessing risk for thimerosal based on methylmercury would significantly overstate any possible risk. However, in 1999, and for the next several years, much of what we now know was "missing information" about these critically important issues.

So, what happened in 1999? In 1999, the Food and Drug Administration (FDA) determined in a review[43] that, depending on which combination of vaccines an infant received for each of his or her recommended vaccines, an infant could potentially be exposed on one day to total levels of *ethylmercury* that would exceed the Environmental Protection Agency (EPA) safe intake level of 0.1 micrograms for *methylmercury* per kilogram of infant body weight per day. We now recognize that this was comparing apples to oranges.

The only known toxicities to thimerosal were allergic reactions and deaths associated with massive exposures; there was no evidence that thimerosal in vaccines was posing any health risks to infants. However, there were very few well-designed studies about developmental problems and thimerosal exposure. The information not available in 1999 was:
- The neurodevelopmental toxicity potential of ethylmercury.

- The metabolism of ethylmercury (where it goes and how it is eliminated from the body).
- Safe intake levels for ethylmercury given by injection.

Because in 1999 it was not known if ethylmercury was as toxic, or less toxic, than methylmercury, public health authorities "assumed a worst case scenario." Although most vaccine experts at the time did not believe that there was any problem, they decided to assume that the two compounds could have similar toxicities, metabolisms, and safe intake levels. Under those assumptions, they worried that some young infants, at their most vulnerable time of development, might theoretically be close to the safe intake level of mercury—even though they realized that the "safe intake level" was established to be well below the level of any actual health risk. Then—as is often the case when not all the data are available—they needed to make recommendations, balancing what was known and what was not known, weighing the *potential* risk of thimerosal against the *actual* known risk of vaccine-preventable diseases.

According to an account of those meetings, "actions proposed by participants at the meeting ranged from immediately stopping administration of all vaccines containing thimerosal to children under 6 months of age to encouraging vaccine manufacturers to expedite the elimination of thimerosal from vaccines." [44]

Although there were no disagreements about what data were available and what data were needed, the experts' deliberations about a course of action were intense, involving national leaders in public health and vaccinology as they tried to develop recommendations that would provide the greatest protection for children. They also decided to inform the public about the reasons for their decisions and about the scientific uncertainties that they had because of the lack of some information. The decision of the experts was to err on the side of caution. The U.S. Public Health Service and the American Academy of Pediatrics issued a joint statement in July 1999.[45, 46] The statement (see page 158) outlined the lack of evidence but stressed the need to take a prudent course of action. It requested that thimerosal be removed as a preservative from U.S. vaccines intended for infants less than 6 months of age and that the birth dose of hepatitis B vaccine be temporarily withheld from infants whose mothers were not infected with hepatitis B virus until formulations of the vaccine became available that did not contain thimerosal as a preservative.

How these decisions were made, how they were communicated and then implemented, was then—and continues to be—the subject of debate, but the intent to describe the uncertainty and the need to act in the best interests of children have never been an issue.

Some people didn't understand the joint statement, and some of them assumed there was something being hidden. Misinformers followed quickly and some journalists helped them. For example, here's how David Kirby (see Chapter 5) described it:

> In their far-flung corners of the country, parents like Liz [Birt], Lyn [Redwood], and Sallie [Bernard] read the statement and arrived at similar conclusions. The government and the AAP were posing an extraordinary contradiction. If thimerosal exposure had been so minimal, and if there was no evidence of harm, then why call for its removal as 'soon as possible'? (*Evidence of Harm*, p. 47)

One year after the joint statement, Bernard and Redwood (both mothers of autistic children) published their hypothesis based on a faulty understanding of what was known about organic mercury poisoning. They formed an advocacy group Sensible Action For Ending Mercury-Induced Neurological

Disorders (SafeMinds) as they were certain that mercury from thimerosal-containing vaccines caused autism.

By February 20, 2002, health departments' visits to 447 sites revealed that only 1.9% of 149,197 doses contained thimerosal.[47]

By 2003, no vaccines in the routine immunization schedule for infants under six months of age contained thimerosal as a preservative. Indeed, if any had remained, all the lots of vaccines containing thimerosal as a preservative would have expired and would have been replaced by vaccines without the preservative no later than January 14, 2003.

However, some vaccines may still contain "trace amounts" of thimerosal from the manufacturing process, as described on page 148.

Other vaccines (for example, inactivated influenza vaccine and tetanus and diphtheria vaccines for use in older children, adults, and infants who cannot receive pertussis vaccine) continue to be manufactured with thimerosal as a preservative—although influenza vaccine without thimerosal preservative is available as an option.

Since influenza vaccine has more recently been recommended for children over the age of six months, why do public health authorities not express a preference for the formulation without thimerosal preservative? Because:

- In 1999 it was known that doses of trivalent inactivated influenza vaccine contained sufficiently low amounts of thimerosal as to not be a concern—being well below the safe intake level for methylmercury in children over 6 months of age. Similarly, a dose for a pregnant woman, because of her size, was not of concern.

- We now know that methylmercury elimination is quite different than ethylmercury, which is excreted much more rapidly.

THIS IS THE JOINT STATEMENT PUBLISHED ON JULY **9, 1999**[45,46]

Notice to Readers: Thimerosal in Vaccines: A Joint Statement of the American Academy of Pediatrics and the Public Health Service

The Food and Drug Administration (FDA) Modernization Act of 1997 called for FDA to review and assess the risk of all mercury-containing food and drugs. In line with this review, U.S. vaccine manufacturers responded to a December 1998 and April 1999 FDA request to provide more detailed information about the thimerosal content of their preparations that include this compound as a preservative. Thimerosal has been used as an additive to biologics and vaccines since the 1930s because it is very effective in killing bacteria used in several vaccines and in preventing bacterial contamination, particularly in opened multidose containers. Some but not all of the vaccines recommended routinely for children in the United States contain thimerosal.

There is a significant safety margin incorporated into all the acceptable mercury exposure limits. Furthermore, there are no data or evidence of any harm caused by the level of exposure that some children may have encountered in following the existing immunization schedule. Infants and children who have received thimerosal-containing vaccines do not need to be tested for mercury exposure.

The recognition that some children could be exposed to a cumulative level of mercury over the first 6 months of life that exceeds one of the federal guidelines on methyl mercury now requires a weighing of two different types of risks when vaccinating infants. On the one hand, there is the known serious risk of diseases and deaths caused by failure to immunize our infants against vaccine-preventable infectious diseases; on the other, there is the unknown and probably much smaller risk, if any, of neurodevelopmental effects posed by exposure to thimerosal. The large risks of not vaccinating children far outweigh the unknown and probably much smaller risk, if any, of cumulative exposure to thimerosal-containing vaccines over the first 6 months of life.

Nevertheless, because any potential risk is of concern, the Public Health Service (PHS), the American Academy of Pediatrics (AAP), and vaccine manufacturers agree that thimerosal-containing vaccines should be removed as soon as possible. Similar conclusions were reached this year in a meeting attended by European regulatory agencies, European vaccine manufacturers, and FDA, which examined the use of thimerosal-containing vaccines produced or sold in European countries.

PHS and AAP are working collaboratively to assure that the replacement of thimerosal-containing vaccines takes place as expeditiously as possible while at the same time ensuring that our high vaccination coverage levels and their associated low disease levels throughout our entire childhood population are maintained.

The key actions being taken are

1. A formal request to manufacturers for a clear commitment and a plan to eliminate or reduce as expeditiously as possible the mercury content of their vaccines.

2. A review of pertinent data in a public workshop.

3. Expedited FDA review of manufacturers' supplements to their product license applications to eliminate or reduce the mercury content of a vaccine.

4. Provide information to clinicians and public health professionals to enable them to communicate effectively with parents and consumer groups.

5. Monitoring immunization practices, future immunization coverage, and vaccine-preventable disease levels.

6. Studies to better understand the risks and benefits of this safety assessment.

PHS and AAP continue to recommend that all children should be immunized against the diseases indicated in the recommended immunization schedule. Given that the risks of not vaccinating children far outweigh the unknown and much smaller risk, if any, of exposure to thimerosal-containing vaccines over the first 6 months of life, clinicians and parents are encouraged to immunize all infants even if the choice of individual vaccine products is limited for any reason.

While there is a margin of safety with existing vaccines containing thimerosal, there are steps that can be taken to increase that margin even further. Clinicians and parents can take advantage of the flexibility

within the existing schedule for infants born to hepatitis B surface antigen (HBsAg)-negative women to postpone the first dose of hepatitis B
vaccine from birth until 2 to 6 months of age when the infant is considerably larger. Preterm infants born to HBsAg-negative mothers should
similarly receive hepatitis B vaccine, but ideally not until they reach
term gestational age and a weight of at least 5.5 lbs (2.5 kg). Because of
the substantial risk of disease, there is no change in the recommendations for infants of HBsAg-positive mothers or of mothers whose status
is not known. Also, in populations where HBsAg screening of pregnant
women is not routinely performed, vaccination of all infants at birth
should be maintained, as is currently recommended. In addition to the
key actions mentioned above, the PHS Advisory Committee on Immunization Practices and the AAP Committee on Infectious Diseases will
be reviewing these issues and may make additional statements.

*Reported by: Public Health Service, U.S. Dept of Health and Human Services.
American Academy of Pediatrics, Elk Grove Village, Illinois.*

- The large body of published studies now available
  has not shown any indication of an association with
  autism and only a weak, at best, suggestion of any
  effect on other neurodevelopmental effects (such as
  tics; see next page).
- The vaccine without thimerosal preservative is
  much more expensive than the vaccine with preservative.

THE UNCERTAINTY OF MISSING INFORMATION

Following the release of the new recommendations in 1999,
researchers in many institutions and countries began looking for any evidence that thimerosal-containing vaccines had
caused any neurodevelopmental disorders. These studies took
time to complete. Most credible scientists believe that the data

are now robust that thimerosal-containing vaccines did not and do not cause autism.

On the other hand, there are some parents of autistic children who honestly believe that their children have been harmed by vaccines. Some have formed anti-thimerosal movements attracting the attention of the media, politicians, and other parents. Unfortunately, there are some parents who are so convinced that thimerosal caused their child to develop autism, that they have subjected their child to dangerous chelation therapy—administering a chemical that binds heavy metals such as lead, iron, mercury, or calcium. This treatment has never been tested for its effectiveness in children with autism and at least one child has died because of it.

COULD THIMEROSAL CAUSE NEURODEVELOPMENTAL DISORDERS? THAT IS, IS IT PLAUSIBLE?

Because methylmercury has been shown to kill brain cells in rats when given at almost lethal doses, and similar findings have been found in post-mortem studies in poisoned humans, many were concerned that ethylmercury might do the same.

One study examined the capacity of various substances—including thimerosal—to affect nerve cells in culture.[48] The researchers exposed neuroblastoma cells—nerve tumor cells—to various concentrations of lead, ethylmercury (thimerosal), aluminum, ethanol, and copper and then measured growth factor signaling by these cell. Growth factor signaling is thought to be important for cell growth. All the substances interrupted growth factor signaling. This study demonstrated a way by which these substances might affect brain development—which is not the same thing as showing that they do affect brain development. It is important to note that the concentrations of thimerosal that the researchers used were far higher than would be expected to be found in the brain after vaccinations.

In one mouse study, one group of researchers reported that a specific strain of neonatal mice had altered developmental behavior and suffered changes in the brain after exposure to thimerosal.[49] However, that study could not be duplicated even when 10 times greater amounts of thimerosal and the same strain of mice were used.[50] Indeed, in the second study, there were no differences in the brains, development, or behaviors between animals exposed to varying levels of thimerosal except for some slowness in movement that disappeared as the mice got older. These researchers also assessed social interactions, social recognition, and anxiety in the mice—behaviors relevant to the thimerosal and autism hypothesis—and found no differences.[50] The differences in results are likely explained by the greater sophistication of the brain studies and the outcome measures used in the second study.

Another hypothesis was that children with autism might have abnormal mercury metabolism. That is, perhaps some children cannot excrete mercury from their bodies as other children do, so the mercury accumulates in the body leading to adverse health effects, including autism. The two studies cited to support this hypothesis measured mercury levels in "first baby haircuts"[51] and the urinary excretion of mercury after administration of chelating agents to autistic children.[52] Both studies were so seriously flawed that they were dismissed by the IOM.[23] The data that are now available[35] would indicate that low hair values reflect lower exposure to thimerosal among children with autism rather than some alteration in metabolism. In another study, the blood and hair mercury levels among children with autism did not differ from those in control children.[53]

The 2004 IOM report *Vaccines and Autism* stated that "in the absence of experimental or human evidence that vaccination (either the MMR vaccine or the preservative thimerosal) affects metabolic, developmental, immune, or other physiological or molecular mechanisms that are causally related to the development of autism, the committee concludes that the hypotheses generated to date are theoretical only."[24] In other words, the IOM could find *no compelling mechanism* by which thimerosal could cause autism.

THIMEROSAL-CONTAINING VACCINES DO NOT CAUSE AUTISM

We can now say this with confidence. Peter Hotez, a microbiologist working to develop vaccines for neglected diseases, and the father of an autistic child, said:

> The claims of anti-vaccine groups fly in the face of overwhelming scientific evidence ... It's like religious fanaticism believing that mercury causes autism, and it's very frustrating for me because it distracts away from our genetic research efforts and services for our kids.[54]

Let's examine the evidence. Eight large studies in Sweden, Denmark, the United States, Great Britain, and Canada—conducted by different investigators, employing different techniques, looking at different populations—**consistently found no evidence** of an association between thimerosal and autism. Indeed, rates of autism continued to increase in Denmark,[55] Sweden,[56] and the United States[3] even after thimerosal was removed from vaccines.

- A population cohort study, including all children born in Denmark from January 1, 1990, to December 31, 1996, linked immunization records with diagnoses of autism.[57] In January 1993, the whole-cell DPT vaccine with thimerosal was replaced by thimerosal-preservative-free acellular pertussis vaccine (DTaP) for the entire country. Among the 467,450 children born in the time period, there were 1,227 cases of autism. The researchers did not find evidence of an association between thimerosal-containing vaccines and autism and there was no evidence that children who received a greater amount of thimerosal were more likely to develop autism.

• Retrospective cohort studies sought associations between thimerosal-containing vaccines and neurodevelopmental disorders employing the Vaccine Safety Datalink (VSD) (see page 62) at three large HMOs in the United States.[58] For analysis of autism, there were only sufficient numbers of cases at one HMO. In that HMO, there was no association between thimerosal exposure and autism and there were no differences among children exposed to different doses of thimerosal.

• An ecological study from Denmark[57] looked at the incidence of autism identified by the Danish Psychiatric Central Register. There were increasing numbers of cases diagnosed despite the removal of thimerosal-containing vaccines after 1992.

• An apparent temporal association between increasing thimerosal exposure in vaccines and increasing prevalence of cases of autism coded by the California Department of Developmental Services was reported to the IOM Vaccine Safety Review Committee.[58] However, two ecological studies compared the rates of autism in Sweden and Denmark[57]—where thimerosal-containing vaccines were discontinued in 1993 and 1992, respectively—to those findings, showing that the incidence and prevalence of autism increased with time irrespective of whether or not there was thimerosal in vaccines in Sweden, Denmark, and the United States.

- If thimerosal caused autism, it was predicted that the rates of autism would decline when thimerosal preservative was removed from vaccines given to infants.[59] An ecologic study by the California Department of Health[3] examined the prevalence of children with autism born from 1989 through 2003 that were reported to the California Department of Developmental Services using client reports for the years 1989 through March 2007. Autism increased each year (and for each age up to 10 years of age). This was true whether the data were examined by year of birth or age group. Specifically, the prevalence at ages 3 to 5 years increased for each birth year since 1999, during the period when exposure to thimerosal preservative in vaccines was reduced.
- A retrospective cohort study examined the General Practice Research Database—consisting of 152,898 children in approximately 500 general practices in Great Britain.[60] There was no evidence of an increased risk for developing autism with increasing thimerosal-containing vaccines exposure.
- An ecologic prevalence study of autism in a school system with 27,749 children in Canada found no association between autism and exposure to—and then the elimination of—thimerosal preservative-containing vaccines.[61]

DOES THIMEROSAL CAUSE OTHER TYPES OF NEURODEVELOPMENTAL DISORDERS?

Given the robust data that have now been amassed, it seems reasonable to conclude that thimerosal (ethylmercury) does not cause autism.[62] But in 1999, public health officials were more concerned about developmental problems of the type that has been associated with exposure to methylmercury. They really weren't worrying about autism at that point because autism-like symptoms had never been associated with organomercury poisoning; that all started with a hypothesis that was based on the mistaken impression that the symptoms of methylmercury poisoning were similar to the symptoms of autism;[36] as we have seen, they are quite different.

What did concern public health and policy makers was whether or not thimerosal might have caused the types of developmental disabilities that methylmercury was known to cause.[63] Rather than autism, it was critical to collect the missing information about that. And it was essential to obtain information about the toxicities and speed of elimination of ethylmercury compared to methylmercury.

The available data now are reassuring that thimerosal-containing vaccines probably do not cause these other types of neurodevelopmental problems, although the data are not yet as robust as those that show that it does not cause autism. Here is the evidence:

- The Vaccine Safety Datalink was used to screen the computer records of two HMOs from 1992 to 1998 for possible signals that might suggest associations between the amounts of thimerosal children had received from vaccines and a large number of neurodevelopmental and kidney disorders of the types that methylmercury might be expected to cause.[58] Because some signals were detected among the preliminary analyses, CDC brought together a group of 11 experts to evaluate the findings and recommend next steps before conducting the planned second phase of this study (see page 169). In the second phase of the study, the screening study findings were tested at a third HMO: cumulative exposures to thimerosal-containing vaccines were not associated with the conditions—tics, speech or language disorders, sleep disorders, or attention deficit disorders—found on the original screening.[57] Thus, in the final analysis, this study showed that none of the conditions were associated with thimerosal exposure. It also was the first study to report no association between thimerosal exposure and autism in the one HMO that had sufficient children with autism to analyze.

◆ A retrospective cohort study examined the General Practice Research Database—consisting of 152,898 children in approximately 500 general practices in Britain.[59] There was no evidence of an increased risk of most neurodevelopmental disorders associated with increasing thimerosal exposure; in fact, for some disorders, thimerosal appeared to have a "protective" effect—although there was once again some evidence that a later diagnosis of tics was associated with increasing thimerosal exposure.

◆ Between 1991 and 1992 researchers prospectively enrolled pregnant women in Avon, Great Britain.[64] The study looked at the neurodevelopment of 13,617 infants who were single born (that is, twins were excluded) and who lived at least 12 months. Once again increasing exposure to thimerosal-containing vaccines appeared to have no association with most neurodevelopmental problems—including tics and speech and language problems. However, this study did find that increased exposure to thimerosal at 3 months of age might be associated with poor "prosocial behavior" (helping, sharing types of behavior) at 47 months of age; whereas for 8 other behavioral measures increasing exposure to thimerosal appeared to be beneficial.

◆ A cohort study of 1,047 children born between 1993 and 1998 was conducted using the databases of 4 HMOs.[65] Children were enrolled in the study on the basis of their exposures to thimerosal before birth, as newborns, and during their first 7 months of life. The researchers looked at exposures to both vaccines and immune globulins (which also contain thimerosal) and estimated the amount of thimerosal the infants received from each specific product, and then summed the total exposure to thimerosal for the different time periods. Trained evaluators assessed 42 possible neuropsychological outcomes at 7 to 10 years of age. The evaluators were unaware of the children's exposure to thimerosal or their medical history. The developmental outcomes of all these children—irrespective of their exposure to thimerosal—were very similar. The associations between thimerosal and behavioral outcomes that were observed were almost equally divided between better and poorer performances in the tests. An increased frequency of tics and language delay in some subsets of children was observed, however.

The accumulating evidence does not suggest a causal association between thimerosal exposure in infancy and the subsequent development of non-autistic neuropsychological abnormalities. Because many of these studies looked at a large number of outcomes, the finding of some statistically significant outcomes—both positive and negative—were likely due to chance. However, because an increased risk of developing tics and language delay was associated with increasing thimerosal exposure in more than one study, additional studies will be needed to test these specific outcomes to assure that these findings were actually statistical flukes.

MISINFORMATION ABOUT AUTISM AND VACCINES

In 2004, a panel of respected scientists—none of whom had worked with vaccines—was convened by the Institute of Medicine of the National Academy of Sciences to review all of the available data. They concluded that there was no evidence that vaccines were associated with the development of autism.[23] Since that time, the evidence has become even more robust that there is no link between measles vaccines or thimerosal-containing vaccines and autism.

The continuing public "controversy" in the face of the scientific evidence is now considered to be misinformation. And what pervasive misinformation it has been and continues to be.

Aggressive misinformation about vaccines causing autism—presented as fact by prominent individuals—has been featured in publications and by the news media, discussed on popular TV and radio talk shows, and been the subject of TV dramas and docudramas. Because these articles feature compelling stories often by prominent people, it is little wonder that parents have become confused.

In general, misinformation about vaccines and autism follows the same pattern discussed in Chapter 5—logical fallacies, invalid assumptions, and pseudoscience.

WHAT REALLY HAPPENED AT THE SIMPSONWOOD CONSULTATION?

David Kirby in his book *Evidence of Harm*[66] and Robert Kennedy Jr. in his article *Deadly Immunity*[5] took quotes out of context from the unedited transcript of an important public health meeting in 2000 known as "Simpsonwood."[65] Kirby and Kennedy created sensational accounts about a conspiracy or cover-up that supposedly took place. What really happened at Simpsonwood?

Another important meeting came before Simpsonwood. In August 1999, the National Vaccine Advisory Committee (NVAC) of the U.S. Department of Health and Human Services convened a workshop of experts—in vaccinology, organomercury toxicology, child development, pharmacology, epidemiology, and others—in a public meeting held at the National Institutes of Health campus to examine what was known about the toxicities and elimination of methyl- and ethylmercury.[67] The scientists at the meeting had to learn about each others' areas of expertise, none of them being experts in all areas. This was not an easy task. One speaker summarized the difficulties of explaining his discipline to the rest of the group:

> So there seems to be a tremendous misunderstanding as to what these [safe intake level] guidelines mean. ... I mean, in this learned audience, it worries me that there's such a misunderstanding of the guidelines. Lord only knows what the general public views these as.[69]

At that first meeting it was agreed that there was *no evidence* that thimerosal-containing vaccines posed a risk for neurodevelopmental disorders. However, because there were no controlled studies to measure the risk, the experts discussed a research agenda. Indeed, many of the studies described elsewhere in this chapter were outlined at that conference. At the end of that meeting the question was asked to the group as to whether a study utilizing the Vaccine Safety Datalink should be undertaken to seek signals between thimerosal and neurodevelopmental outcomes. There were strong reservations voiced by many in the room because of the concern that such a study could identify associations that might not be real. In other words, there would likely be biases in how the study was set up (see Chapter 4) that could lead to finding erroneous signals.

Despite those reservations, CDC decided to go ahead and do a "two phase study" because data were needed so urgently. The Simpsonwood meeting was to consider the findings from the first *screening phase* "to see if there was any hint of association with any conditions, [and] if anything came out [they] would go to the next step and do a confirmatory study or hypothesis-testing study."[70] The screening study used computerized data collected at two HMOs. In the analyses of those screening data, CDC identified differing but statistically significant associations at the HMOs. Within weeks of recognizing this, on June 7–8, 2000, the CDC convened a group of 11 expert consultants—epidemiologists, toxicologists, heavy metal toxicologists, biostatisticians, and child development experts—at the Simpsonwood Retreat Center near Atlanta to review the data. The timing was critical because CDC wanted to present the data and the consultants' opinions later that month to the Advisory Committee on Immunization Practices (ACIP)—which advises CDC on immunization policy.

The Simpsonwood meeting[67] was characterized by lots of technical jargon (as evidenced in the transcripts), hard questions, and a great deal of give and take as the consultants dug into the data and the CDC analyses. Besides the 11 consultants, 49 specialists and observers attended and participated at Simpsonwood (one of the authors of *this* book gave the opening summary of the preceding NVAC meeting, for example), to provide additional information. This meeting was closed to the public, as are most scientific consultations; a transcript was kept, ironically, so that there would not be charges of a cover-up about a topic about which there was great public interest (the transcript was not needed for any other purpose).

At the outset, the 11 consultants were told that "... this is a scientific review to evaluate the quality of the scientific data" in advance of the ACIP meeting to be held two weeks later, where the data would be presented in that public forum.[71] In addition they were told that they were to discuss and each formally express their opinions, and then vote on three specific questions at the end of the meeting: Do the observations constitute a signal? Do they warrant further investigation? What next steps should be taken to further investigate a relationship?

The researchers had analyzed 124,170 children who were born from 1991 through 1999 at the two HMOs for many aspects of child development. Data from these HMOs suggested that thimerosal might be associated with tics and speech and language disorders (but specifically no association was found with autism). These "signals" could not be explained by reanalysis of the data. While most agreed that these findings were probably the consequence of how the dataset was collected, the consultants also agreed that:

- a signal had been found
- the observations were statistically significant, but
- the associations were "weak"; that is, they could not conclude that the associations were or were not caused by thimerosal.

The experts asked that errors in the dataset be corrected, the methods refined, additional analyses be performed, and continued follow-up of the children be performed as they became older They also agreed that the second phase of the study should be performed quickly at a third HMO to ask the questions raised by the first phase—whether or not these associations could be substantiated.

The results of these deliberations were subsequently presented to the ACIP—as was the preliminary data from the second phase of the study, which showed that none of the associations could be confirmed at the third HMO.[72]

The unedited transcripts of the Simpsonwood meeting

have a number of uncorrected transcriptional errors. The bigger problem, however, has been the dissemination of quotations taken out of context by misinformers in an attempt to describe the meeting as something that it wasn't. Some have even called it "a cover up," which it was not—the results were reported at the ACIP meeting 2 weeks later. Some have said that because the results reported in the final publication[57] differed, there must have been something done to hide the results. As is typical with scientific publications, the data analyses evolved after the preliminary results were subjected to this intense scientific peer review.

The Simpsonwood meeting was simply a gathering of scientists examining preliminary—albeit disturbing—data, speaking candidly about a difficult topic, and concluding that these were real signals but that more studies were urgently needed to either confirm or reject them.

THE BOTTOM LINE: DO VACCINES CAUSE AUTISM?!

Based on the fact that there is no evidence that MMR or thimerosal-containing vaccines increase the risk of developing autism, we conclude that vaccines do not cause autism.

Do thimerosal-containing vaccines cause other neurodevelopmental disorders? The best available data imply that thimerosal-containing vaccines do not cause other neurodevelopmental problems, but more data are needed before we can say that thimerosal-containing vaccines do not cause tics or language delay.

Note that we are not saying that thimerosal is 100% safe or that it is okay to expose children to high doses of it. We also believe that children should have their exposure to all organic mercury compounds minimized. We are pleased that we live in a wealthy country where we had the option of removing thimerosal preservative from vaccines routinely administered to young children. Nevertheless, we would not—and we did not—hesitate to give our children and grandchildren MMR and thimerosal-containing vaccines.

"WHAT IT COMES DOWN TO IS YOU HAVE TO FIND OUT WHAT REACTION THEY'RE LOOKING FOR, AND YOU GIVE THEM THAT REACTION."

Do Vaccines Cause Damage to the Immune System?!

The vaccines given in the first two years of life are literally a raindrop in the ocean of what infants' immune systems successfully encounter in their environment every day.
Paul Offit, Vaccines: What you Should Know, 2003

L ooking at the number of shots given at pediatric visits, many parents wonder whether a baby's immune system can withstand so many immunizations—almost half of the parents in a survey expressed this concern as a reason for not vaccinating their children.[1] So, they ask questions like: Do vaccines overwhelm the immune system? Do vaccines weaken a child's immune system, causing them to experience serious infections? Do vaccines cause autoimmune problems, such as type 1 (juvenile) diabetes, Guillain-Barré syndrome (GBS), or multiple sclerosis?

We will discuss those concerns in this chapter.

DEVELOPMENT OF THE IMMUNE SYSTEM

The immune system starts developing very early in pregnancy. By birth, the infant's immune system is capable of making many antibodies and immune cells that attack foreign invaders.

This is a good thing because the immune system must be prepared to face billions of bacteria and other antigens just as soon as the mother's water breaks. Within minutes of birth the child has acquired the bacteria naturally present in the mother's birth canal.

Breast milk contains billions of bacteria too. Very rapidly, the newborn's intestinal tract is full of an extraordinary number of bacteria. Many of these bacteria stay there and help digestion. But without a vigorous newborn immune system, these environmental bacteria would be very dangerous. In fact, these environmental bacteria induce components of the immune system to develop. In addition to bacteria and other microbes, newborns are exposed to other things in their natural environment that also stimulate the immune system, such as dust, tobacco smoke, pollen, pets, and many, many more.

Part of the newborn's immunity is temporary: antibodies from the mother pass across the placenta and in breast milk into the newborn. These antibodies protect the infant for several months against a number of infections.

For example, to prevent newborns from developing tetanus, it is critical that the mother pass anti-tetanus antibodies to the baby. Tetanus antibodies develop *only after* tetanus immunization, so to prevent the often fatal disease of neonatal tetanus, mothers need to be immunized before the baby is born so that the anti-tetanus antibodies can flow naturally from mother to baby.

The newborn's immune system is still developing, so there are some dangerous organisms that newborns are especially vulnerable to. Examples include chickenpox, measles, pertussis, and influenza, to name a few.

Chickenpox virus can cause very serious—even fatal if untreated—infection in the first few weeks of life; measles virus can cause a very rare but serious progressive form of encephalitis in young infants; whooping cough (pertussis) deaths and brain damage occur mostly in young infants; and influenza virus can make young infants have high fevers and irritability leading to hospitalization.

Chickenpox, measles, whooping cough, and influenza infections in young infants are best prevented by community immunity (see page 28)—that is, by those around them having been vaccinated.

There are important differences between an infant's immune system and that of older children and adults. One type of antibody inherited from the mother is targeted against *Haemophilus influenzae* type b (Hib), the bacterium that caused about 20,000 cases per year of serious infection and meningitis in young children until 1988—the year when the Hib vaccine started to be given routinely at two months of age. The story of Hib vaccine taught us a lot about the child's developing immune system and infections in children.

Before Hib vaccine became available it was known that infants were protected by the mother's antibody against Hib for about three months. After three months of age, the frequency of Hib disease would increase, but by five years of age, children had their own antibodies against Hib, so the number of infections fell dramatically after that age.

An early form of Hib vaccine didn't work in very young infants because one part of the immune system—making antibodies against the capsule that surrounds the Hib bacterium and other similar bacteria—doesn't work very well until the child is over 18 to 24 months of age. Actually that part of the immune system was discovered because the original Hib vaccine did not work very well at the younger ages.

The modern Hib vaccines used now are hooked to a carrier protein that engages the part of the immune system that is already developed in young infants so that it makes the right kind of antibodies and the child is protected early in life.

ARE CHILDREN'S IMMUNE SYSTEMS MATURE ENOUGH TO COPE WITH ALL THOSE VACCINES? WILL SO MANY VACCINES DAMAGE THE YOUNG CHILD'S DEVELOPING IMMUNE SYSTEM?

We give many more vaccines now than we used to:

- In the early 1940s only smallpox vaccine was given routinely to children.
- Later in the 1940s, the diphtheria, pertussis, and

tetanus vaccine was routinely given to children. Poliovirus vaccine was added in the late 1950s and measles in the mid 1960s.

- ♦ Nowadays, by the time a newborn is 12 years of age she will have received 30–35 doses of vaccine to protect her against 34 diseases. She can have fewer injections when vaccines containing multiple components are used.

- ♦ In addition to the vaccines that are presently available, new vaccines are being developed to protect against other important diseases.

- ♦ Because most vaccines are given by injection, the child can have multiple injections at one visit—at the very least, that is painful.

So, can a child's immune system handle all those vaccines?[2-5] The answer seems to be simple: yes it can.

- ♦ Even though an infant's immune system cannot respond to all the different types of foreign materials (called antigens) in the same way an adult can, infants do have an amazing ability to respond to an extremely large number and numerous types of antigens. The number a child can respond to is many more than the number of vaccine antigens given in the early years of life.

- ♦ Because of newer ways of making vaccines, the number of antigens (substances that induce immune responses) in vaccines has actually decreased since 1980, even though there are many more vaccines given.[2] For example, the old whole-cell pertussis vaccine contained about 3,000 antigens whereas the newer acellular pertussis vaccine contains only a few. **So while we give more shots, the number of antigens that the immune system must respond to is actually many fewer than before.**

- Before any vaccine for human use can be licensed in the United States, it has to be shown to effectively stimulate the immune system. If a vaccine contains multiple components, each of the components has to effectively stimulate the immune system (for example, measles, mumps, and rubella). If a vaccine is likely to be given at the same time as another vaccine, both vaccines must be shown to effectively stimulate the immune system.

- A number of studies have looked for but did not find any increased risk of other types of infections after vaccines and some have even shown fewer infections in immunized children.[4,6,7] One study, which looked at all the children born in Denmark from 1990 through 2001, could find no effect on hospital admissions for other types of infections regardless of how many and which vaccines a child had received.[6]

- Many vaccine researchers in the 1960s worried that there might be a temporary decrease in immunity after measles vaccine—because of reports that measles infection might activate dormant tuberculosis (TB) or make active TB worse. Because measles infection can make a TB skin test turn negative for about two weeks, sometimes physicians place a TB skin test on people before giving them a measles vaccine. Importantly, studies have found no relationship between either measles and TB[8] or an increased risk for blood-borne infections after measles, mumps, and rubella vaccine (MMR).[4]

The fact is that vaccines strengthen, not weaken, the immune system. This is true even for newborn infants. On the other hand, a natural infection clearly can weaken a child's immune system. For example, a previously healthy child who develops the usual skin rash of chickenpox (varicella) may become infected with dangerous bacteria in those breaks in the skin. In that case, an infection severe enough to require hospitalization or even cause death can develop. Similarly, a child with measles infection is more likely to develop middle ear infections.

The vaccines routinely recommended for children use only a small portion of the immune system's "memory." Scientists estimate that based on the immune system's capacity to respond, a child could theoretically get 10,000 vaccines in one day and still not "use up" his or her immune response or ability to respond.[2]

WHAT ABOUT COMBINATION VACCINES? Parents don't like to watch their children getting multiple shots—up to five at one visit—but they also worry about whether the new combination vaccines might be inferior to the individual vaccines. This is an important issue for vaccine researchers.

For example, in Great Britain, the introduction of a new DTaP-Hib combination vaccine in 2000 resulted in increased numbers of cases of Hib disease, because the combination vaccine wasn't as effective against Hib infection as prior Hib vaccines.[9] To prevent that type of problem, in the United States, the FDA requires that combinations of vaccines "not decrease the purity, potency, safety or effectiveness of any of the individual active components."[10]

This "noninferiority principle" requires additional testing of combination vaccines for both safety and immunity, as well as careful studies after the vaccine has been licensed. However, in theory, a combination vaccine could be less effective because "noninferiority" is defined as not more than 10% inferior.[11]

This is another reason why studies after licensure need to monitor vaccine effectiveness after changes to the immunization schedule.

During the confusion in Great Britain and Europe about the MMR vaccine (see Chapter 8), the media widely reported that somehow measles, mumps, and rubella vaccines given individually were safer than the MMR shot. There is no evidence to support that contention.

NOT ENOUGH SHOTS: MIKEY'S STORY

No one enjoys giving children shots, much less multiple shots on the same day. When seen by a physician at 19 months of age, Mikey had not had any immunizations since the hepatitis B vaccine at 12 months of age. His parents said "no more than four shots" at one time.

Using combination vaccines, he got "caught up" for everything except chickenpox (at that time there wasn't a chickenpox combination vaccine available, so that would have been the fifth shot). Unfortunately, three weeks later, he caught chickenpox from a playmate. Mikey's chickenpox was complicated by serious bacterial infection of skin lesions on his shoulder, which required hospitalization so he could receive intravenous antibiotics and surgery to drain the infection. He was able to go home after a week in the hospital but he will always have scars on his shoulder.

Bacterial infection of chickenpox lesions occurs in up to 5% of children who develop chickenpox. Some of these infections can be serious—sometimes fatal.

DO VACCINES CAUSE AUTOIMMUNE DISEASES?

A healthy immune system can tell the difference between the body's own cells and proteins (self) and those that are foreign (nonself). It will attack nonself, but it will not attack self. In autoimmune conditions, however, the immune system attacks self cells or proteins too.

A number of infections are known to cause autoimmune diseases. For example, acute rheumatic fever is an autoimmune disease that occurs after streptococcal throat infection; the immune response targets a protein in the bacterium that is similar to one in heart cells. This is called "molecular mimicry"—when a foreign protein is similar to a self protein.

Other examples of auto immune conditions after infection are:

- Measles infection can lead to an immune response that lowers the level of platelets in the blood[12] (which can then be associated with bleeding).
- Twenty percent of children who have congenital rubella infection will ultimately develop type 1 (juvenile) diabetes.[7]

Theoretically, if infections can trigger an autoimmune disease, then vaccines might also do it.

Illnesses can occur at about the same time as vaccines are given—just by coincidence. For example, because a number of new vaccines have recently been introduced for teenagers and young adult women, one group of researchers asked what the *background rate* of some autoimmune conditions might be just by coincidence among preadolescent girls and young women who had not been given any vaccine.

First, they determined the number of emergency consultations, hospitalizations, and outpatient consultations for some autoimmune diagnoses at an HMO during 2005. Then they calculated the number of these conditions that would have occurred by chance after any randomly selected day in the year.[13] What they determined was startling (see table on next page).

Remember that none of the women represented in the table got any vaccinations. These counts are simply the number of health problems that would have occurred within various intervals of time, in the absence of any vaccination. If a vaccine had been given these numbers show what the expected rates of coincidental findings might have been.

CONDITIONS OCCURRING BY CHANCE AMONG FEMALES (PER 100,000 PERSONS) FOLLOWING A RANDOMLY SELECTED DAY.

	9-18 Year-Old Females Time after a random day			19-30 Year-Old Females Time after a random day		
	1 day	1 week	6 weeks	1 day	1 week	6 weeks
Asthma	2.7	18.8	81.3	3.0	21.2	91.5
Allergy	1.5	10.6	45.8	2.5	17.4	75.3
Diabetes	0.4	2.9	12.8	0.6	3.9	17.0
Inflamatory Bowel Disease	0.2	1.0	4.5	0.3	2.0	8.8
Thyroid disease	0.1	0.9	4.0	2.4	16.6	71.8
Lupus	0.1	0.5	2.0	0.3	1.8	7.8
Multiple Sclerosis or Optic Neuritis	0.0	0.2	1.0	0.1	0.7	3.0

Adapted from Siegrist CA et al. 2007. Human papilloma virus immunization in adolescent and young adults: A cohort study to illustrate what events might be mistaken for adverse reactions. *Pediatrics Infectious Diseases Journal* 26:979-84. With permission of the publisher.

DO VACCINES CAUSE TYPE 1 (JUVENILE) DIABETES?

Type 1 diabetes—commonly called juvenile diabetes—is an autoimmune disease in which the beta cells in the pancreas are attacked as nonself.

Environmental factors are thought to trigger the autoimmune attack on beta cells in genetically susceptible individuals. Genetic susceptibility appears to be a necessary but not a sufficient factor (see page 50) for developing type 1 diabetes. In other words, genes play an important role (several genes are known to be particularly important), but genes are not enough by themselves.

Many possible environmental triggers have been suggested, but except for congenital rubella infection, none have been shown to trigger the onset of type 1 diabetes.

Very early in type 1 diabetes, there are antibodies against one or more proteins in the pancreas (antibodies against self proteins). In addition, first-degree relatives who have these types of antibodies are at very high risk of developing diabetes, although the disease may not appear for quite some time—that is, they are considered to have pre-diabetes. The delay in the onset of disease is thought to be because clinical signs of diabetes do not occur until 80% of the beta cells in the pancreas have been destroyed by the autoimmune process.

The incidence of type 1 diabetes varies greatly between countries and within regions of the United States. In North America, it is most common in children of European descent.

It is also clear that type 1 diabetes is increasing in incidence in the United States as well as globally.

Because some viral and bacterial infections can cause autoimmune diseases, it has been suggested that vaccines (which are made from viruses or bacteria) might also cause type 1 diabetes. Another suggestion was that the time when vaccines are given might have something to do with the development of type 1 diabetes.

Vaccines Do Not Cause Type 1 Diabetes

In 2002, the IOM Immunization Safety Review Committee concluded that the "epidemiologic and clinical evidence favors rejection of a causal relationship between multiple immunizations and an increased risk of type 1 diabetes."[7]

Subsequent studies have made the evidence even more robust.

Multiple studies—conducted by different investigators, employing different techniques, looking at different populations—consistently have found no evidence of a link between vaccines and the development of type 1 diabetes.

Here is the evidence:

- In 1997, a study suggested that if children received the Hib vaccine at certain times during their infancy, they were more likely to develop type 1 diabetes than children who received the vaccine at different ages.[14] However, later studies found no effect of the timing of Hib vaccine with the development of type 1 diabetes.[15]

- A case-control study conducted between 1985 and 1986 compared 339 children with type 1 diabetes to 528 children without diabetes who were of the same age, sex, and county of residence within Sweden. Measles and MMR vaccines appeared to have a protective effect against type 1 diabetes. There were no other significant risks relating to BCG (tuberculosis), smallpox, tetanus, pertussis, mumps, or rubella vaccines.[16]

- In September 1979, Sweden discontinued the use of pertussis vaccine because of vaccine safety concerns (see page 81), substituting DT vaccine instead. The percentage of children immunized for pertussis rapidly declined from 83% to less than 2%, while the coverage for DT after that point was 96–97%. Scientists studied children born in 1977 and 1978, who had high exposure to whole-cell pertussis vaccine, and children born in 1980 and 1981 who had low exposure to pertussis vaccine. There was no difference in the children's likelihood of developing type 1 diabetes regardless of their exposure to the vaccine.[17]

- The incidence of type 1 diabetes was examined in three groups of children born in Finland. Children born between October 1983 and September 1985 did not receive Hib vaccine. Those children were compared with children who were born between October 1985 and August 1987. During this later time period, children born on even numbered days were eligible to receive Hib vaccine at 24 months of age whereas those born on odd numbered days received the Hib vaccine at 3, 4, 6, and 14-18 months of age. There was no difference between the cumulative risk for type 1 diabetes among the groups of children.[18]

♦ A study of children who had a sibling or a parent with type 1 diabetes evaluated whether vaccines—and the ages when the vaccines were given—contributed to the development of autoantibodies (prediabetes cases) or not (controls). There were no differences in the proportion developing prediabetes among groups of children receiving hepatitis B, Hib, polio, or DTP vaccines. There were also no differences found based upon the age when the first immunizations were given or whether the hepatitis B vaccine was given at birth or later.[19]

♦ In a prospective study of 823 German children who had one or both parents with type 1 diabetes, none of the childhood vaccines (BCG, DTP, Hib, polio, tick-borne encephalitis, or MMR) was associated with the development of pre-diabetes.[20]

♦ A European population-based registry was used to identify 1,028 children who developed type 1 diabetes before 15 years of age. They were compared to a control group of children who were the same age and from the same population. There was no link between BCG, polio, DTP, MMR, or Hib vaccinations and development of type 1 diabetes.[21]

♦ A Vaccine Safety Datalink case-control study evaluated children born in 1988 through 1997 who were continuously enrolled at four HMOs. They compared 252 children who developed type 1 diabetes with 768 non-diabetic children who were matched for the same HMO, sex, birth within seven days, and length of time at the HMO. Vaccination history and other factors were obtained from the medical records. There was no link between any of the vaccines (hepatitis B, Hib, whole-cell or acellular pertussis, MMR, or varicella) and an increased risk of type 1 diabetes. Also, the timing of the first dose of hepatitis B vaccine was not related to development of type 1 diabetes.[22]

• In a 10-year follow-up of a large clinical trial of Hib vaccine in 1988–1990, children who participated were evaluated for whether or not they had developed type 1 diabetes. The follow-up included those who remained in the HMO (21,421) and those who did not choose to participate in the trial (and therefore did not get the Hib vaccine). A third group of children were those who had been randomly excluded from the study (who also did not get the Hib vaccine) as a means to control for selection bias (see page 54). The prevalence of type 1 diabetes did not differ between the groups.[23]

• In Denmark, scientists studied all 739,694 children born between January 1, 1990, and January 1, 2000. Because Denmark registers all people living in that country, the investigators were able to link specific information about vaccines, type 1 diabetes (681 cases), and whether or not the child had a sibling with type 1 diabetes (26 of the 681). There were no associations between the vaccines, the dose or time since vaccination, or the total number of vaccinations with type 1 diabetes.[24]

DO VACCINES CAUSE GUILLAIN-BARRÉ SYNDROME?

Guillain-Barré syndrome (GBS) is an autoimmune disorder of the peripheral nerves—that is, outside the brain and spinal cord—characterized by paralysis. The paralysis usually starts in the legs but can "ascend" to the arms and even to the respiratory muscles, occasionally requiring ventilator support in an intensive care unit. GBS is caused by an immune response to the myelin sheath* covering the nerves. It is usually triggered by a gastrointestinal or respiratory infection. Eventually, most patients recover nearly completely, although about 10% of patients die and as many as 20% will have some permanent disabilities.

In addition to a number of specific infections, a number of vaccines have been suggested as causes of GBS. In 2004, 38 cases of GBS with onset within 6 weeks of vaccination were reported to VAERS; 31 of these were following influenza vaccine.[25]

GBS AND INFLUENZA VACCINES. During the national "swine flu" immunization campaign in 1976-1977, people who were vaccinated had an increased risk of GBS within 6-8 weeks after vaccination. The risk was especially great in those over the age of 25 years. This association was judged to be cause-and-effect—that is, the swine flu vaccine caused GBS at a rate of about 1 per 100,000 above the estimated background rate of 0.87 cases per million persons in a six-week time period.[26,27]

The evidence as to whether GBS has been associated with other years' influenza vaccines is not clear. The Institute of Medicine was unable to conclude whether there is a causal relationship,[26] although there could be a slightly increased risk for GBS after influenza vaccine at a rate of about 1 per

---

* The myelin sheath is the envelope that surrounds nerves and nerve fibers. It provides insulation and helps transmit nerve impulses.

million.[27] No increased risk for GBS was found among British adults receiving influenza vaccine.[28]

The background rate—that is, the expected rate that would occur by chance—of GBS is low but people who have experienced GBS in the past have a much greater risk of developing GBS again than people who have never had GBS. As a consequence, these people have an increased risk of having GBS within six weeks after an influenza immunization by coincidence. Whether influenza vaccine might increase the risk of a recurrence of GBS is unknown. However, because someone who had GBS is also at increased risk from influenza infection, it would seem that the small (if any) increased risk of GBS from influenza immunization would be less than the risk of influenza infection.[29]

GBS AND TETANUS TOXOID-CONTAINING VACCINES. Because of a remarkable case report of a man who had three episodes of GBS following receipt of repeated doses of tetanus toxoid, the Institute of Medicine concluded that "the evidence favored acceptance of a causal relation between ... tetanus toxoid-containing vaccines" and GBS.[30] Other than this one man, however, analyses of cases of GBS found by active surveillance found no increased risk of GBS within six weeks following immunizations with tetanus toxoid-containing vaccines among children less than two years of age, children two to five years of age, or adults.[31]

GBS AND HEPATITIS B VACCINE. In the first few years after licensure of the first hepatitis B vaccine—which was derived from human blood—the possibility of an association between GBS and the first dose of this vaccine was suggested. That vaccine is no longer used in the United States. The hepatitis B vaccine used for the past 20 years has been manufactured by modern molecular methods utilizing yeast grown in a fermenter, similar to what is done to brew beer. In analyses of GBS cases among about 2.5 million adults who received the present hepatitis B vaccine, the number of people who had GBS was about the same as would have been expected if none of them had been vaccinated.[32]

GBS AND MENINGOCOCCAL CONJUGATE VACCINE. In January 2005, a new meningococcal conjugate vaccine (known as MCV4) was licensed and in February it was recommended for routine immunization of 11–12-year-old children with "catch-up" vaccination for older teenagers. In October 2005—when about 2.5 million doses of vaccine had been distributed—CDC informed the public that five cases of GBS had been reported 14–31 days after meningococcal vaccination of 17–18-year-olds.[33] By the end of September 2006, 15 cases had been reported in 11–19-year-olds within 6 weeks of MCV4 vaccination.

Initially this appeared to be higher than expected,[34] but then a case-control study using the Vaccine Safety Datalink (see page 62) found no association between MCV4 vaccination and GBS. There was also no association between MCV4 and facial paralysis or seizures.[35]

DO VACCINES CAUSE MULTIPLE SCLEROSIS?

Multiple sclerosis (MS) is an autoimmune disorder of the central nervous system in which the myelin sheath that surrounds the nerve cells in the brain is destroyed. In the United States, about 400,000 people are affected. Women are affected more commonly than men. New cases are most commonly recognized between the ages of 20 and 40 years but it is also recognized in children and older persons.

Clinically, MS presents many different types of neurological symptoms depending on where in the nervous system it is occurring. Optic neuritis—visual disturbances—may occur as part of MS or individually. The severity of the disease varies from person to person, and most people experience a relapsing course. The causes are unknown, but likely involve both genetic and environmental factors.

MS AND HEPATITIS B VACCINE. Hepatitis B virus (HBV) infection causes both an acute infection and a long-lasting (or chronic) infection. More than half of the people infected with the virus show no signs or symptoms at the time of infection, although they may become chronically infected, developing liver disease or liver cancer later in life.

In 1996, after a mass immunization campaign in France, there were reports of cases of multiple sclerosis (MS) following hepatitis B immunization. Because of concerns that the vaccine was causing MS, hepatitis B immunization in French schools was discontinued in 1998.

In 2002, the IOM found that the plausibility—the possible mechanisms by which HBV vaccine could cause MS— was weak. They agreed that the published studies consistently showed no link between the hepatitis B vaccination of adults and MS. They concluded that the evidence favored rejection of a cause-and-effect relationship between the hepatitis B vaccination and new cases of MS or MS relapse.[36] Subsequent studies found no increased risk of MS or optic neuritis in adults following HBV, influenza, tetanus, measles, or rubella immunizations[37] and no association of optic neuritis with anthrax, smallpox, HBV, or influenza vaccines.[38]

The overwhelming body of evidence continues to show that HBV vaccine (and other vaccines) does not cause MS or optic neuritis in adults.[39] There has been only a single study suggesting that HBV vaccine could have increased the risk of developing MS among a small proportion of the adults who subsequently developed MS.[40] Because of how the study was conducted and the fact that this study differs from so many other studies, most consider that the findings do not provide evidence of an association.

There is less evidence for a link between HBV vaccine and

MS in children. A French study compared 143 children with MS with 1,122 healthy children who were matched for age, sex, and area of residence. Immunization with HBV vaccine within six months or at any time since birth or the number of doses of vaccine did not elevate the risk of a first MS episode.[41] Similarly, hepatitis B or tetanus immunization after a first episode of illness did not increase the risk of a second episode (two episodes are required for someone to receive the diagnosis of MS).[42]

MS AND INFLUENZA VACCINE. In 2004, the IOM concluded that the data consistently demonstrated that influenza immunization did not cause MS relapses, but that there were insufficient data regarding the hypothesis that influenza immunization might trigger new cases of MS. There was only one study but it showed no increased risk for MS or optic neuritis after influenza immunization.[37] According to the IOM's report, they agreed that there was "no reason to suspect that a causal relationship might exist between influenza vaccines and onset of MS."[43]

DOES MMR VACCINE CAUSE THROMBOCYTOPENIA (LOW LEVELS OF BLOOD PLATELETS)?

Yes, but low levels of blood platelets occur more commonly from the natural measles or rubella infections than after the vaccine.[44] Both measles and rubella infections can cause reduced numbers of platelets circulating in the blood—which are an important part of the clotting process—by an autoimmune mechanism. MMR vaccine can also cause reduced numbers of platelets in blood. The course is usually short and mild and occurs in about 1 in 40,000 children aged 12-23 months of age. This condition, known as thrombocytopenia, is more common in boys than in girls.[12] The risk for this complication may be greater for someone who has had immune thrombocytopenia previously, although in one study none of 31 children who had thrombocytopenia after the first dose of MMR vaccine developed thrombocytopenia after a second MMR immunization later on.[12]

DO MEASLES VACCINES CAUSE INFLAMMATORY BOWEL DISEASE?

Concerns that measles vaccines might cause inflammatory bowel disease (IBD) (Crohn's disease and ulcerative colitis) originated with a report from Great Britain in 1995. Subsequent studies, however, have not found any link between MMR or other measles vaccines with the development of IBD. In a review of 31 studies in the literature, there was no association between MMR vaccine and IBD,[45] including these:

* A study compared 155 U.S. children with IBD who had been born between 1958 and 1989 with control children without IBD who were matched for sex, year of birth, and HMO. Vaccination with measles vaccine, given either before 12 months of age or between the ages of 12 and 18 months, was not linked to a risk for IBD.[46]
* An ecologic study in England found little change in the frequency of hospitalized cases of IBD over a 20-year period, and specifically no differences among children born before or after the introduction of measles vaccines.[47]
* In one study of 372 adults with IBD and 310 controls matched for age, sex, and residence, there were no differences in the proportions who were immune to measles (whether from infection or vaccine). Interestingly, more of those who did not have IBD were immune to rubella,[48] implying that rubella immunity might somehow protect against IBD.

Do Vaccines Cause Arthritis?

ARTHRITIS AND RUBELLA VACCINE. Joint pain and arthritis occur during natural rubella infection, much more commonly in women than in children and men. Chronic joint complaints occur after rubella infection as well.

Joint pain and arthritis also can occur after rubella vaccination, but less frequently than when associated with natural infection. After rubella vaccination, joint pain occurs in about 8 out of 1,000 young children. Joint pain and arthritis are more common in adult women, in whom arthritis occurs about 11% of the time 7 to 21 days after immunization. Joint symptoms usually go away quickly.[48]

Acute joint symptoms after infection with rubella virus or vaccine virus appear to be caused by virus infection of the joint. However, a number of studies suggested that natural rubella virus might persist and/or cause autoimmunity leading to chronic arthritis. Other studies were unable to find rubella virus in the blood of people with chronic arthritis after immunization. Virus genetic material could not be detected in blood or in joints of people with rheumatoid arthritis.[49]

Some of the early rubella vaccines were associated with higher rates of acute and chronic joint complaints, but the current vaccine does not appear to cause those adverse events. Here's the evidence:

- In one study, 485 mothers who were immunized between 1985 and 1990 with rubella vaccine after giving birth were matched to 493 control mothers who were already rubella immune for age, residence, and date of delivery. All the mothers were interviewed in 1992–1993 about joint pain and arthritis. No difference was found.[50]
- Another large study looked at three groups of women who were 15 to 59 years of age and who had been

tested for rubella immunity. One group of susceptible women was immunized (971). They were compared to an unimmunized susceptible group of
women (924) and a group of women who were unimmunized but tested immune to rubella (2,421,
matched for blood testing date and age). Over the
12 months after immunization, there was no evidence of any increased risk of new onset chronic
joint complaints.[51]

+ In a study conducted between 1989 and 1992, 546
rubella susceptible women 18–41 years of age were
randomized to receive rubella vaccine or placebo.
Acute joint reactions occurred more frequently
in the women who were vaccinated than in those
who received placebo, but there was no difference
in the frequency of persistent joint complaints after a year.[52]

ARTHRITIS AND ALUMINUM-CONTAINING VACCINES. Some vaccines contain chemicals called adjuvants to help increase the
production of antibodies against the vaccine antigens, making the vaccine more effective. The most common adjuvants
used in vaccines are aluminum salts, which can cause higher
and more prolonged antibody responses than comparable
vaccines without the adjuvant.[53] The U.S. licensed vaccines
that contain aluminum adjuvants are:

+ DTP (diphtheria-tetanus-pertussis vaccine)
+ DTaP (diphtheria-tetanus-acellular pertussis vac-
cine)
+ Some, but not all Hib (*Haemophilus influenzae* type
b) conjugate vaccines
+ Pneumococcal conjugate vaccine
+ Hepatitis B vaccines
+ All combination DTaP, Tdap, Hib, or hepatitis B
vaccines

+ Hepatitis A vaccines
+ Human papillomavirus vaccine
+ Anthrax vaccine
+ Rabies vaccine

Inactivated poliovirus vaccine (IPV), MMR, varicella vaccine, MCV4 vaccine, and influenza vaccines do not contain aluminum salts.[54]

Aluminum is a very abundant element in our environment. It is in many foods we eat, many personal hygiene products we apply to our skin (such as deodorants), and many medicines we ingest. All infants are exposed to aluminum in the environment. Breast milk, for example, contains about 40 micrograms of aluminum per liter, and infant formulas contain an average of approximately 225 micrograms of aluminum per liter.[55] Historically, however, some individuals with kidney failure—who were exposed to very large quantities of aluminum while undergoing dialysis—developed serious neurological effects. The U.S. Agency for Toxic Substances and Disease Registry has estimated safe intake levels (see page 152) for aluminum from food as well as by injection of vaccines, demonstrating an expected wide margin of safety.[53,56]

Aluminum-containing vaccines have a record of more than 75 years of safety around the world. Serious adverse effects attributable to the aluminum adjuvants are rare. On the other hand, localized reactions such as redness, swelling, and/or tenderness at the injection site occur commonly following injection of vaccines containing aluminum adjuvant. More severe local reactions such as large areas of swelling, sterile abscesses, subcutaneous nodules (small lumps under the skin, some of which have inflammation in the tissue), and allergic responses also can occur but are much less common.

+ **Aluminum in childhood vaccines.** A systematic review of studies of aluminum-containing vaccines against diphtheria, tetanus, and pertussis (DTP), found that aluminum-containing vaccines caused more localized reactions—such as pain, redness, and swelling at the injection site—but there was no evidence that aluminum salts caused any serious or long-lasting adverse events.[57] Other reviews of large numbers of studies that included hundreds of thousands of people who were given whole-cell pertussis-containing vaccines, acellular pertussis-containing vaccines, and hepatitis B vaccines—almost all of which contained aluminum salts—have also shown no evidence of long-term effects.[39,58]

• **Gulf War Illnesses.** Military personnel returning from the 1990–1991 Persian Gulf War reported numerous health problems that some believed were related to their service in the Persian Gulf. In 1998, Congress directed the Institute of Medicine to evaluate possible associations between illness and a variety of potential exposures, including anthrax, botulism, and other vaccines. The IOM Committee found that "although veterans ... report significantly more symptoms of illness than soldiers of the same period who were not deployed, studies have found no cluster of symptoms that constitute a syndrome unique to Gulf War veterans."[59] There was insufficient evidence to establish an association with most exposures, including vaccines.

• **Macrophagic myofascitis.** A group of adult French patients who had muscle and joint aches and pains and fatigue had muscle biopsies that revealed clusters of cells around aluminum crystals—a finding called macrophagic myofascitis (MMF). While the physician who first described the biopsy findings proposed that aluminum-containing vaccines caused the symptoms in his patients,[60] most scientists believe that the tissue findings showed the normal immune response to the aluminum adjuvant in some vaccines.[61,62] More recently, MMF has also been observed in muscle biopsies taken from the site of injection in the thighs of children who were being evaluated for other diseases. In those children, there was no correlation between the finding of MMF on biopsy and the clinical symptoms.[63] In other words, MMF is simply the immune response to a prior immunization with an aluminum-containing vaccine, it is not an illness.

MISINFORMATION ABOUT VACCINES AND THE IMMUNE SYSTEM

Many books and Web sites claim that immunizations overload the immune system. As we have seen in this chapter, the medical evidence does not support such a claim—it is misinformation. Some sources also claim that the rise of many chronic conditions is caused by vaccines—particularly those chronic conditions that are incompletely understood, like autoimmune diseases.

While vaccines do have some specific risks, there is no evidence to support the claims that vaccines cause asthma (Chapter 7), autism (Chapter 8), type 1 diabetes, multiple sclerosis, chronic arthritis, or inflammatory bowel disease. There is also no evidence to support claims that delaying immunizations—or spreading them out—would make vaccines safer. Delaying vaccines may place a child at risk of vaccine-preventable infections.

Many Web sites claim that vaccines "have been proven to cause" all of these autoimmune conditions. They often cite pseudoscience as providing the proof and then they either misquote valid studies or dismiss them altogether. In his online article, *Distinguishing Science and Pseudoscience*, Dr. Rory Coker from the University of Texas at Austin says that "pseudoscience appeals to the truth-criteria of scientific methodology while simultaneously denying their validity."[64] In other words, misinformers often cite invalid studies as "scientific proof" of their theories while ignoring or dismissing valid studies that contradict their views.

THE BOTTOM LINE: DO VACCINES CAUSE DAMAGE TO THE IMMUNE SYSTEM?!

Infants and children are bombarded with germs every day in the air they breathe and the food they eat, but their immune systems are designed to handle these exposures. Vaccination does not overburden a child's immune system; rather, it strengthens even the young infant's developing immune responses by preparing it to ward off specific infections that can injure the child.

Numerous studies have evaluated whether vaccines cause a variety of autoimmune diseases:

- There is no association between vaccines and type 1 diabetes or multiple sclerosis.
- Influenza vaccine in 1976 caused Guillain-Barré syndrome at a rate of about 1 per 100,000 people who were vaccinated. It may have resulted in 1 extra case per million people who have had influenza immunization since then. GBS is very rare after tetanus vaccine—there has only been one person reported who developed GBS that was caused by repeated tetanus vaccination. The first hepatitis B vaccine may have had associated cases of GBS but the vaccine we use now in the United States does not appear to cause GBS. GBS is probably not caused by the quadravalent meningococcal vaccine (MCV4)

but more studies are needed to confirm this.
- Measles vaccine does not cause inflammatory bowel disease.
- Measles vaccine does occasionally cause a temporary drop in blood platelets.
- Rubella vaccine causes joint aches in a small number of children. More frequently, it causes temporary joint aches and sometimes arthritis in adult women— but it does not cause chronic arthritis.

"... AND IT'S LOADED WITH ADDITIVES BANNED BY THE F.D.A."

Chapter 10

Other Vaccine Safety Concerns

I normally don't quote Latin before noon, but post hoc ergo propter hoc! Correlation is not causation. Just because two things happen in tandem or soon after one another doesn't prove one caused the other.
David Benzion, Lonestar Times, June 25, 2007

DO VACCINES CAUSE FEBRILE SEIZURES?

Febrile seizures are common among children but they generally have an uneventful outcome. Febrile seizures do not lead to a seizure disorder and the risk of epilepsy is not increased among children who have had a febrile seizure. But—no question about it—febrile seizures are very frightening to parents.

These seizures can occur (and re-occur) between 6 months and 5 years of age when children run a fever. A number of the vaccines routinely given to children of this age group can cause fever, so they have a chance of causing a febrile seizure. Susceptibility to febrile seizures probably is hereditary, because there is a tendency within a family to develop them.

Measles-mumps-rubella (MMR) vaccine is well tolerated and is rarely associated with severe adverse events. However, about 10% of children who receive MMR vaccine for the first time will develop a fever between 5 and 12 days later. A small proportion of these children may experience a febrile seizure.

After the first MMR, immunized children have an increased risk of a febrile seizure during the 8–14 days following vaccination than at other times. The overall increase is small: for each 1,000–3,000 children vaccinated, one child more than usual will have a febrile seizure.[1,2] Following introduction of a new vaccine that combines MMR with chickenpox vaccine (MMRV), the risk of a febrile seizure after the first immunization is increased by an additional child per 1,000 (compared to children who got MMR and varicella vaccine at different sites on the same day).[3]

Children who have previously had a febrile seizure are at increased risk of having a febrile seizure after receiving MMR vaccination. Children who had a febrile seizure after MMR vaccination are also at increased risk of seizures with other illnesses when they have fever.

Do Vaccines Cause Encephalopathy or Encephalitis?

ENCEPHALOPATHY AND PERTUSSIS VACCINES. Encephalopathy (brain injury) is a well known complication of whooping cough, particularly in young infants. Concerns about encephalopathy after pertussis (whooping cough) vaccine led to lower immunization levels and outbreaks of whooping cough in a number of countries 20 years ago (see page 77).

Although the Institute of Medicine (IOM) concluded that there was likely a link between the whole cell pertussis vaccine and encephalopathy within seven days of vaccination, it was considered a rare occurrence. It was unclear whether the number of cases of encephalopathy was increased by the vaccine or that it was a result of a pre-existing brain or metabolic disorder.[4] Many studies since then have been unable to demonstrate such an association. For example, in a study looking back at immunizations given to 2,197,000 children from 1981 through 1995—when whole-cell pertussis vaccine was used in the United States—the risk of encephalopathy wasn't greater in vaccinated children compared to unvaccinated control patients.[5]

Acellular pertussis-containing vaccines have many fewer reactions of all types than the whole-cell pertussis vaccine. Japan reported a rate of 0.5 per 10 million children for any encephalopathy or encephalitis within seven days of DTaP vaccination.[6] In Canada, between 1993 and 2002, seven cases of encephalopathy were detected within seven days of DTaP vaccination, but all had other explanations for their encephalopathy.[7]

In 2006, Australian researchers re-examined 14 cases of alleged whole-cell pertussis "vaccine encephalopathy" using new molecular tools. They showed that 11 of these cases had an alternative explanation: a genetic defect in nerve cells.[8] This defect is a common genetic cause of a number of epileptic encephalopathies—and the onset of symptoms are often preceded by fever.[9] Similarly, children with genetic defects in energy production (in the genetic material of mitochondria) may develop encephalopathy after stress (see page 141).

Encephalopathy occurring after acellular pertussis-containing vaccines is rare and usually there are alternative explanations for the brain injury. Children with certain genetic diseases may begin showing symptoms of their underlying conditions after fever, stress, or (coincidentally) immunizations.

ENCEPHALITIS AND MEASLES-CONTAINING VACCINES. Encephalitis (inflammation of the brain) occurs in about 1 in 1,000 children with measles; many die and many others have severe brain damage. It is not clear whether encephalitis occurs after measles vaccination in children with normal immune systems. In 1994, the IOM felt that the data were insufficient to decide.[10] Since then, one study could find no cases of encephalitis within 30 days after the receipt of MMR—or any other vaccine—in about 300,000 children 12–23 months old;[11] another study found no excess encephalitis among 561,000 children who received MMR;[12] and two case-control studies found no differences between those who received MMR vaccine and controls.[5,13]

SUBACUTE SCLEROSING PANENCEPHALITIS AND MEASLES VACCINE. About 1 in 100,000 children with measles develops a

degenerative brain illness called subacute sclerosing panencephalitis (SSPE). SSPE is persistent measles virus infection
of the brain that leads to severe physical and mental impair-
ment; it is ultimately fatal. Symptoms of SSPE usually develop
years after the initial measles infection. Analysis of measles
viruses from the brains of patients with SSPE have never
demonstrated vaccine virus. Indeed, after measles vaccination
was introduced, the number of cases of SSPE in the United
States declined from 40–50 cases per year to 1 or 2. Between
1989 and 1991, the country experienced a resurgence of more
than 55,000 cases of measles, with a corresponding increase
in cases of SSPE. The measles virus types recovered from the
brains of those SSPE cases were the same type associated with
the measles outbreak, but not the vaccine virus.[14]

MENINGOENCEPHALITIS AND MUMPS VACCINE. Aseptic meningitis (inflammation of the covering of the brain) occurs in
about 4–6% of children with mumps (typically it is mild).
However, this occurs more frequently in adults who may also
have encephalitis as well (or "meningoencephalitis"), sometimes with permanent damage that includes hearing loss, paralysis, and more. Some mumps vaccine strains used in other
countries caused aseptic meningitis in a few children, but the
mumps vaccine strain used in the United States has not been
associated with an increased risk of aseptic meningitis.[11,12]

DO VACCINES CAUSE SIDS?!

Sudden Infant Death Syndrome (SIDS) is the unexpected and
sudden death of a child younger than one, for which there
is no apparent cause. SIDS is not a medical condition with a
single cause. Many babies who die unexpectedly are found to
have certain other medical conditions, but there are also some
for which no cause of death is found. Some factors are known
to increase the risk of SIDS, such as tobacco smoke exposure

(before the baby is born and afterwards) and sleeping on the tummy or side or on soft materials. Most SIDS deaths occur between two and four months of age, at the time babies are beginning their immunizations. Not surprisingly, because of the timing of vaccine administration, concerns have been expressed that vaccines may be associated with SIDS.

In 2003, the IOM conducted a review of all available evidence regarding this concern. They concurred with a prior IOM report: there was not an association between the DTP vaccine nor multiple vaccines and the development of SIDS—but they could not draw that conclusion with the DTaP (the vaccine used now in the United States), Hib, hepatitis B, or polio vaccine because there were too few studies.[15] Since then a number of studies have been published that support the conclusion that vaccines are not associated with SIDS or sudden unexpected infant deaths—the more general term used to describe all infant deaths whether or not a reason for the child's death is ultimately determined. Here's the evidence:

- Birth hepatitis B vaccination appeared to have been protective against death in the first month of life among more than 350,000 infants born in California between 1993 and 1998.[16]
- A study that included half of Germany between 1998 and 2001 found that a greater proportion of SIDS cases had not received polio, diphtheria, tetanus, pertussis, Hib, hepatitis B, or a new combination vaccine compared with controls.[17]
- In an analysis of previously published case-control studies of diphtheria, tetanus, and pertussis vaccines, immunization appeared to reduce the risk for SIDS. It is not clear whether this is a direct effect of immunization (perhaps preventing unrecognized cases of infants with whooping cough, which can present with sudden cessation of breathing) or is a conse-

quence of selection biases for healthier children (because they had had their immunizations).[18]

DO VACCINES CAUSE CANCER?!

As many as 100 million Americans may have been exposed to a virus—called simian virus 40 (SV40)—that contaminated the inactivated polio vaccine when it was first introduced. SV40 also contaminated the first oral polio vaccine, but that contaminated vaccine was only given to people in the original clinical trials. In addition, SV40 contaminated some of the adenovirus vaccines used in that period among military recruits. The virus came from the monkey kidney cell cultures used to produce the vaccine and was not discovered until 1960. Once the contamination was recognized, steps were taken to eliminate it from future vaccines. No vaccines licensed for use in the United States currently are contaminated with SV40.

WHAT WERE THE EFFECTS OF THE CONTAMINATED VACCINE ON THE PEOPLE WHO RECEIVED IT? SV40 causes tumors in rodents and can transform human cell cultures into malignant-like cells. Because of these facts, SV40 has been intensively studied, both in the laboratory and epidemiologically. Although a great deal is known about the basic biology of this virus—pieces of the virus are used in almost all basic research laboratories—the role of SV40 in human cancer has been unresolved.

In 2002, the IOM's Immunization Safety Review Committee considered that the available data was "sufficiently flawed" that they were unable to conclude whether or not the contaminated polio vaccine may have caused cancer.[19] Since then, other studies were conducted:

 ♦ Newborn babies who received SV40 in polio vaccine were followed for 35 years and had no excess risk of

cancer. This is particularly important because newborn animals are much more susceptible to SV40
tumors than older animals.[20]

* A case-control study of cancers among Army veterans found no risk of brain tumor, mesothelioma,
or non-Hodgkin's lymphoma associated with receipt
of adenovirus vaccine that contained large amounts
of SV40.[21]

* People infected with human immunodeficiency virus (HIV)—the cause of acquired immune deficiency
syndrome (AIDS)—are at increased risk of developing non-Hodgkin's lymphoma. This risk was not
increased if they had received SV40-contaminated
polio vaccine compared to those who had not received it.[22]

Recent advances in testing for antibodies and the detection
of SV40 in tumor cells have finally begun to clarify the scientific controversies about this virus and human cancers.[23]
However, there remain many conflicting pieces of evidence:

* Earlier studies reported that many people had antibodies against SV40, but those studies more likely
measured antibodies to human viruses similar to
SV40. Using new methods to test for SV40 antibody, recent studies have demonstrated a lack of
SV40 antibody response in humans—in contrast to
animals—and exposure to SV40 does not seem to
be associated with human cancers.[23]

* Molecular tools frequently used to detect SV40 in
cancerous tissues may have commonly detected
SV40 contaminants in the laboratory when, in fact,
it was not present.[24]

* If SV40 caused cancer in humans, the proteins it
produces in animal tumor cells should be measurable. So far they have not been detectable.[23]

DO VACCINES CAUSE AIDS?

Many scientists believe that human immunodeficiency virus (HIV) is derived from a closely related virus in chimpanzees and arose by infection of a hunter. In 1999, British journalist Edward Hooper theorized in a widely publicized book, *The River: A Journal to the Source of HIV and AIDS*, that field trials of an early oral poliovirus vaccine were the origin of the global acquired immunodeficiency syndrome (AIDS) epidemic.

Hooper speculated that chimpanzee cells were used in the production of the experimental vaccine lots of type 1 oral polio vaccine developed by Hilary Koprowski, which was tested in the former Belgian Congo between 1957 and 1960. Hooper wrote in *The River* that the monkey cells used to prepare the vaccine were contaminated with chimpanzee cells and the chimpanzee immunodeficiency virus—and that ingestion of the virus during oral polio vaccination led to the human infection with a virus that was to evolve into HIV-1. The theory relied heavily on the coincidental recognition of cases of AIDS in a region near some of the sites where the vaccine was tested in Central Africa.

A large collection of scientific evidence is available that rejects these allegations:[25,26]

* The same lot of vaccine tested in Africa was also tested in many people in Europe (for example, 7.2 million in Poland) without giving rise to HIV or AIDS.
* Three independent laboratories examined several old vials of vaccine and showed only evidence of monkey cells; specifically there was no evidence of chimpanzee cells. The presence of polio virus was confirmed but there was no evidence for any HIV-like virus.
* Studies of the evolution of the origin of HIV have

shown that the virus was first acquired by humans about 30 years before the vaccine trials, in an altogether different region of Africa.

• Chimpanzee immunodeficiency viruses from animals in the region of Africa where all this was supposed to have occurred are clearly different from the strain from which all strains of HIV-1 were likely to have been derived.

The theory that HIV arose from an early experimental polio vaccine has been firmly rejected.

DO VACCINES CAUSE MAD COW DISEASE?

Transmissable spongiform encephalopathies (TSE) are a group of illnesses caused by a normal protein in the brain (called "prion") that is folded incorrectly and that then accumulates in brain cells causing dementia leading to death. Examples of TSEs are Creutzfeldt-Jakob disease (CJD), which occurs in man; bovine spongiform encephalopathy (BSE)—or mad cow disease—which occurs in cattle; scrapie, which occurs in sheep; and "chronic wasting disease," which occurs in elk and deer.

There are several forms of CJD. CJD can be an inherited disease because of a mutation in the prion protein. It can also occur sporadically at a rate of 1-2 cases per million people. It can also be transmitted from person to person by transplantation of nervous tissue. We now know that BSE can be transmitted from cattle to man—this form of the disease is called variant CJD or vCJD.

In the 1990s, an outbreak of mad cow disease occurred in the United Kingdom, resulting in the slaughter of thousands of cows. Up until then, cattle were fed what was left over from slaughter houses as part of their feed. Many scientists believe that BSE is the scrapie prion that was transmitted that way from sheep to cattle, then to more cattle, and finally it appeared in man who ate the meat, probably the nervous tissues.

Cattle products have been used to prepare some vaccines, although nervous tissue has not. So there could be a risk, at least theoretically. To examine that risk, in July 2000, the FDA's Center for Biologics Evaluation and Research conducted a careful review of which vaccines had beef products, where the beef came from, and what was the theoretical possibility that a product could have come from a cow with BSE. FDA statisticians calculated that the theoretical risk of any bacterial or viral vaccine contamination by the agent of BSE was remote, ranging from 1 in 2 billion to 1 in 200 billion doses.[27]

There have been no cases of vCJD related to vaccines.[28]

DO VACCINES CAUSE BIRTH DEFECTS?

Ideally, women of child-bearing age should be immunized before becoming pregnant. For example, rubella causes serious damage to the unborn fetus and is preventable by rubella vaccine. Varicella (chickenpox) can cause birth defects in the fetus and fatal pneumonia in the mother; it is preventable by varicella vaccine. Tetanus in the newborn, almost always fatal, is prevented if the mother has been immunized, as is the case with many other vaccine-preventable diseases.

Although many medications, including some vaccines, are avoided during pregnancy because of potential harm to the mother or fetus, some vaccines are recommended for pregnant women. Thus, certain immunizations during pregnancy can enhance the mother's health, while others can protect the child by means of the mother's antibodies that remain in the child for the first 3-6 months of life.[29]

According to the Advisory Committee on Immunization

Practices (ACIP), the risk of a developing fetus being harmed by vaccination of the mother during pregnancy is only theoretical.[30] Currently, no evidence exists of risk from vaccinating pregnant women with any inactivated viral or bacterial vaccine or toxoid. Live attenuated vaccines, including MMR and varicella, are of greater theoretical concern so it is recommended that pregnancy be avoided as a precautionary measure for at least 28 days after administration of these vaccines. This 28-day rule is used even though there is no evidence of damage to the fetus in prior studies.

The Centers for Disease Control and Prevention (CDC) has published a recommended adult immunization schedule, including for pregnant women.[30]

VACCINES RECOMMENDED FOR ALL SUSCEPTIBLE PREGNANT WOMEN

Pregnant women are at a higher risk of serious medical complications from **influenza** than non-pregnant women. Because of this, CDC recommends that all women who will be pregnant during the influenza season should be immunized with the injectable inactivated vaccine. One study of influenza vaccination of more than 2,000 pregnant women demonstrated no adverse effects in the fetus from the vaccine.[31] However, the nasal influenza vaccine should not be given to pregnant women because it is a live virus vaccine.

Tetanus in newborn infants, once common throughout the Americas, is prevented if the mother has been immunized. This is because an immune mother passes antibodies to the baby across the placenta. The mother is immune if she has been immunized before becoming pregnant or during pregnancy. An expectant mother whose tetanus immunization status is uncertain or whose last immunization was more than 10 years ago should be immunized against tetanus. This is usually given combined with diphtheria toxoid vaccine (a product called Td). Recently a new vaccine containing pertussis, Tdap, has been licensed for use for women in the child-bearing age group. Pregnancy is not a contraindication to Tdap immunization. At this time, CDC recommends that pregnant women who received the last tetanus toxoid-containing vaccine less than 10 years ago receive Tdap in the post-partum period according to the routine vaccination recommendations, and if the last dose of tetanus toxoid-containing vaccine was more than 10 years previously, that they would give preference to her being immunized with Td in preference to Tdap during the second and third trimester.[32]

VACCINES THAT ARE CONTRAINDICATED FOR PREGNANT WOMEN

Generally, live-attenuated vaccines are contraindicated for pregnant women because of the theoretical risk of transmission of the vaccine virus to the fetus. The following live, attenuated vaccines should NOT be administered during pregnancy except in unusual circumstances:[29]

- Influenza virus vaccine (nasal spray)
- Oral poliovirus vaccine (no longer distributed in the United States)
- Measles-containing vaccines
- Mumps-containing vaccines
- Rubella-containing vaccines
- Smallpox (vaccinia) vaccine
- Typhoid vaccine (Ty21a)
- Varicella (chickenpox) live virus vaccine
- Yellow fever vaccine

Varicella vaccine is universally recommended for all children and nonpregnant adults who are susceptible, but it is not given to pregnant women. Pregnant women who develop chickenpox (varicella) are at increased risk of having severe illness and a small proportion of their newborns may be born with congenital varicella syndrome. Susceptible women who are exposed to varicella (or shingles, which is caused by the same virus) should receive varicella-zoster immune globulin (VariZIG) within 96 hours, which may prevent or modify infection. Antiviral drugs usually are reserved for pregnant women with severe chickenpox illness. Infants born to mothers who had chickenpox within 5 days of delivery are also given VariZIG within 48 hours of delivery to prevent them from having serious illness. Vaccination with varicella live virus vaccine during pregnancy is not recommended, although inadvertent vaccinations have not been associated with adverse outcomes.[29,33] A pregnant household member is not a contraindication for varicella immunization of a child within that household.[34]

The varicella vaccine virus rarely spreads from a vaccinated person who develops rash to susceptible persons within households. The risk for a susceptible pregnant woman and her fetus should be very low after this type of exposure. However, the pregnant woman who believes that she is susceptible to chickenpox and who has a household exposure to someone who develops rash after varicella immunization should inform her physician.

Ideally women should be immune to varicella before pregnancy, either from vaccine or chickenpox. At the completion of pregnancy, susceptible women should receive the first dose of varicella vaccine before discharge from the healthcare facility. A second dose should be administered four to eight weeks later.

Measles, mumps, and rubella live virus vaccines—usually given together as MMR—should not be administered during pregnancy. However, because measles increases the risk for spontaneous abortion or premature delivery, pregnant susceptible women are given immune globulin within six days of exposure. The mumps virus has not been associated with problems during pregnancy. Wild rubella virus infection in early pregnancy has a high risk of causing congenital rubella syndrome (CRS) in fetuses. This is a devastating disease that is preventable by the use of vaccine prior to pregnancy. Pregnant women are screened early in pregnancy to be certain that they are immune. If susceptible and exposed, the pregnant woman and her physician together will need to consider her options. The rubella-susceptible woman should be immunized with MMR in the immediate post-partum period. CDC has followed the outcomes of inadvertent rubella vaccination of pregnant women and no cases of CRS have been detected.[35]

Transmission of MMR vaccine viruses within households has not been demonstrated (except rubella virus from nursing mothers to their infants). Thus, susceptible children should be immunized whether or not there is a pregnant household contact.[36]

Live attenuated **yellow fever** vaccine is not known to cause developmental malformations. It is only administered to pregnant women if travel to an endemic area is unavoidable where she is going to be at risk of exposure to yellow fever.

Neither the live attenuated Ty21a nor the Vi polysaccharide **typhoid fever** vaccines have been tested in pregnant or breastfeeding women. Some experts might consider the polysaccharide vaccine for pregnant or lactating women if travel to an endemic area is unavoidable and she is likely to be at risk of exposure to *Salmonella typhi* (the cause of typhoid fever).

VACCINES FOR PREGNANT WOMEN WHO ARE AT RISK

The following vaccines should be considered for pregnant women who are at risk for acquiring or being exposed to these diseases. Because spontaneous abortion occurs more commonly in the first trimester of pregnancy, some obstetricians prefer to avoid administering vaccines during this time, if possible, to avoid any temporal associations that might oc-cur.[29] Specific recommendations for travel by pregnant women (and others) can be obtained at *www.cdc.gov/travel.*

- **Hepatitis B virus (HBV)** infection during pregnan-cy can result in severe disease for both the mother, the fetus, and ultimately for the neonate. Immuni-zation is recommended universally in the United States for everyone under the age of 18 years and those older than that who have increased risk of exposure. Pregnancy is not a contraindication for HBV immunization and vaccine should be given to persons with occupational or lifestyle risks, special patients risk groups (such as those undergoing hemo-dialysis), those who have another sexually transmit-ted disease, household and sexual contacts of HBV carriers, prison inmates, and for international trav-elers to endemic areas. All pregnant women should have early prenatal screening for immunity and, if susceptible and if they have a risk factor, should be immunized. Screening for active hepatitis B infec-tion is a "standard of care" because it permits a new-born infant to receive birth doses of both vaccine and hepatitis B immune globulin.[37]

- **Pneumococcal polysaccharide vaccine (PPV23)** is indicated for specific medical conditions (such as asplenia [absence of the spleen], metabolic, renal, cardiac, and pulmonary diseases, and immunosup-pression). Pregnant women with those conditions should also receive the vaccine, preferably prior to pregnancy—but it can be given to a pregnant woman if she has not previously been immunized.[38]

- The risk of **rabies** far exceeds the theoretical risk from the vaccine if the expectant mother has been exposed to the disease.[38]

- Studies of pregnant women immunized with menin-gococcal polysaccharide vaccine and their newborns have not demonstrated any adverse effects. This means that that vaccine would likely be safe for a pregnant woman at high risk for **meningococcal infection**.[38,39] Because the new meningococcal conjugate vaccine (MCV4) is the preferred vaccine for people 11-55 years of age, many experts would prefer to give MCV4 in this setting, although there are no data on the safety of MCV4 during pregnancy.

- Pregnant women are at risk of acquiring **hepatitis A** virus infection if there is someone infected in the household, if they have occupational exposure, or by traveling to areas where hepatitis A is endemic. Although formal studies of hepatitis A vaccine in pregnant women have not been performed, the vaccine is produced from inactivated virus so the theoretical risk for the fetus should be low.[40] The vaccine has been used in pregnant women without adverse events having been reported.[29] Because international travel is now the most frequent source of exposure for Americans to hepatitis A, vaccination prior to travel to endemic areas is particularly important. For pregnant women who have been exposed to hepatitis A virus, testing for susceptibility may be warranted but should not delay the administration of immune globulin ("gamma globulin").

- **Polio** viruses have been eliminated in the United States and thus there is not usually an indication for immunization of the pregnant woman except for those women traveling to endemic areas. If polio vaccine is indicated, only the inactivated vaccine should be given to a pregnant woman and not the oral live virus vaccine.[38]

- Women vaccinated against **anthrax** earlier in life
  have had no problems with their pregnancies or
  babies.[41] No studies have been published regarding
  use of anthrax vaccine among pregnant women, although an ongoing study by the Naval Health Research Center and the National Center for Birth
  Defects and Developmental Disabilities suggest that
  children born to women who were immunized with
  anthrax vaccine in the first trimester of pregnancy
  could have an increased risk of birth defects.[42] The
  Advisory Committee for Immunization Practices
  recommends that pregnant women not be vaccinated against anthrax.[43] However, in the circumstances of an exposure to aerosolized anthrax, the
  theoretical risks of the vaccine would likely be far
  less than the risk of disease; pregnant women should
  be vaccinated against anthrax only if the potential
  benefits of vaccination outweigh the potential risks
  to the fetus.[44]
- Although the initial clinical trials of **human papillomavirus** (HPV) vaccine specifically excluded
  pregnant women, 1,244 pregnancies occurred in
  the vaccine group and 1,272 occurred among the
  women who received placebo. There were no differences in the rates of miscarriage, late pregnancy fetal
  deaths, or birth defects among their babies.[45] Infants
  of 500 women who were breast feeding when they
  received vaccine had no more adverse events than
  did those who got placebo and none of the events
  was considered related to vaccine. The FDA has established a registry to record the outcomes of pregnancy among women who are inadvertently given
  vaccine while pregnant.

Pregnant women and health care providers should always

consider the risks and benefits of the vaccine as well as the risks of the disease before administering or receiving the vaccine. Immunization before conception is always preferred to immunization during pregnancy to prevent disease in the child. After delivery, women susceptible to rubella or varicella should be immunized with MMR or varicella vaccine before discharge from the hospital.[38]

Breast-feeding does not interfere with the response to the vaccines recommended for adults. Although rubella vaccine virus has been found in human milk, this and other vaccines provided to the mother during pregnancy or immediately post partum have not been shown to interfere with the immune response of children to vaccine and no child has developed disease secondary to vaccine administered to their mother.[29] Human milk contains antibodies and other factors that may help protect infants against many infectious diseases.

Vaccine Safety Terms: A Glossary

Vaccine research concerns various scientific disciplines, such as epidemiology, genetics, immunology, and statistics. The terms used in vaccine research are sometimes technical and hard to understand for the lay reader. Sometimes words used in vaccine research have very different meanings when used in ordinary conversation (see also page 45). Below is a list of common terms used in the scientific literature related to vaccines and vaccine safety.

Absolute risk: The incidence of a disease in a population. It indicates the magnitude of the risk in a group of people with a certain exposure to a disease. For example, more than 95% of susceptible household contacts to a case of chickenpox will develop chickenpox.

Acellular vaccine: Vaccines composed of antigens (fragments) of a pathogen such as the acellular pertussis vaccine.

Adjuvant: Substances that, when mixed with an antigen, increase the immune response, such as aluminum salts.

Adverse event: Something untoward that occurs at about the same time as a vaccination, which may *or may not* be caused by the vaccine.

Antibody: A molecule produced by some cells in the body that binds to a specific antigen during an immune response. An antibody can bind to a toxin, a virus, or a bacterium, preventing them from doing harm.

Antigen: A chemical substance that induces an immune response after a period of time (days to weeks). For example, there is a protein antigen called hemagglutinin on the surface of the influenza virus that induces protective antibody to be made after infection or vaccination.

Attack rate (or case rate): The number of new cases—usually expressed as a percentage or the number of cases per a group of people, such as 10/100,000.

Attributable risk: The amount or proportion of disease incidence (or disease risk) that can be attributed to a specific exposure.

Bias: A systematic error in the design, conduct, or analysis of a study that could lead to the wrong conclusion. For example, selection bias means the manner by which subjects were selected could have influenced the results. This research use of this word is in contrast to the conversational use of the word, which implies not having an open mind or a conscious attempt to distort findings.

Case-control study: A study that compares individuals affected by a disease with a comparable group of people who do not have that disease, to seek possible causes or associations.

Case-fatality rate: The proportion of persons diagnosed as having a disease who die as a result of that disease within a particular period of time.

Clinical trial: A research study to determine whether a vaccine works and whether it causes reactions. Clinical trials answer questions about the safety and effectiveness of vaccines (and other type of drugs and treatments).

Cohort study: A study of groups of people, or cohorts, followed over time to see an outcome.

Combination vaccine: A vaccine against more than one pathogen, which is given in a single dose, such as the measles, mumps, and rubella vaccine.

Community immunity (or herd immunity): The indirect protection against a disease or infectious agent that nonimmune persons obtain by being surrounded by immune persons.

Confidence interval: This is a measure of precision around a given risk or value. In a measurement of a result in a sample of a large population, the confidence interval estimates the range within which the real value probably lies. Vaccine researchers often use something called the 95% confidence interval, which means the risk that was measured has a margin of error within this interval—the estimate of risk value could be different than was found but would likely lie within the 95% confidence limits.

Confounders: Other factors or explanations that may affect a result or conclusion.

Conjugate vaccine: A vaccine where the antigen(s) is linked to another molecule, enhancing the immune response. Conjugation of a fragment of the *Haemophilus influenzae* type b capsule to a protein makes it possible to immunize young children who cannot respond to the fragment of the capsule alone.

Control group: A group of animals or people used in research as an untreated standard for comparison, to see how they differ from an experimental group—such as people receiving a vaccine.

Controversy: There are different but plausible interpretations of the same data within the scientific community. This technical use of the word is in contrast to the conversational use of the word meaning there is a difference of opinion.

Correlation: The extent to which two or more variables in an association are related. For example, the extent by which disease incidence changes in response to immunization rates.

Cost benefit: In vaccine economics, cost-benefit analyses include all the costs and benefits that might arise from an immunization program up to a particular time.

Cost effectiveness: In vaccine economics, cost-effectiveness analyses take into account the costs and savings that result from an immunization program using a predefined unit of health outcome—for example, years of life saved or cases of the disease avoided.

Cost saving: When the cost benefit analysis demonstrates that the immunization program saves more money than it costs. For example, for every dollar spent, there is a $5 saving in health care costs.

Denies: As in "the patient denies 'xyz'" means that the patient said s(he) doesn't have those symptoms or hasn't had that illness. This meaning is in contrast to the conversational use that the patient reacts defensively to an accusation.

Disease carrier: A person or animal that harbors a specific infectious agent in the absence of discernible clinical disease and serves as a potential source of infection.

Double-blinded study: In a double-blinded study, neither the person being treated, nor the person giving the treatment (and observing the outcome) know which treatment has been given. See *Placebo*.

Effectiveness: The extent to which a vaccine achieves its intended purpose—for example, a vaccine protects against a disease, such as pneumonia or influenza-like illness.

Efficacy: The extent to which a vaccine produces a specific outcome, such as the prevention of influenza virus type A infection.

Efficiency: A measure of effectiveness. Efficiency refers to the production of the desired effects or results with minimum waste of time, money, effort, or skill. For example, an efficient vaccine delivery system would allow immunizing a population without spending excess money or efforts.

Endemic: The constant presence of a disease in a community or region.

Endotoxin: Part of the cell wall of certain bacteria. It is a poisonous substance that may be released when the bacterium is destroyed.

Environmental factors: External factors such as overcrowding or poor sanitation that contribute to the development of disease. These interact often with genetic factors.

Epidemic: The occurrence in a community or region of cases of an illness in excess of what is expected. A smaller number of cases, such as polio in countries that had not seen a case in decades, is often referred to as an outbreak.

Epidemiology: The study of how disease is distributed in a population and of the factors that influence or determine this distribution. Epidemiology helps to identify the causes and risk factors of a disease in a community.

Etiology: The cause(s) of disease.

Experimental group: The treated group in a research study. For example, the group that receives the vaccine that is being tested, as opposed to the control group, which receives a placebo or no treatment.

False negative: The failure to find a result or effect when there is one.

False positive: Finding a result or effect when it does not exist.

Febrile seizures: Scary but self-limited seizures that occur in young children when they have a high fever.

First-degree relative: The parents, siblings, or children of an individual.

Formalin: The chemical formaldehyde diluted in water.

Genetics: The branch of science concerned with the biology of inheritance and its consequences.

Genetic factors: Inherited characteristics that contribute to the development of disease (or immunity to the disease).

Genetic predisposition: An inherited susceptibility to disease, which may be activated under certain conditions.

Health outcome: A measure of whether or not a patient benefits from a vaccination—for example, a health outcome may be expressed in the number of cases of measles prevented or years of life saved through measles immunizations.

Immunity: Resistance against a disease, often measured by the presence of antibodies against the pathogen that causes the disease.

Inactivated vaccine: A vaccine made from pathogens that have been killed, such as the inactivated polio vaccine.

Incidence: The number of *new* cases of a disease during a specified period in a specified population. Incidence is usually expressed as cases per 1,000 or per 100,000 of the population per year. For example, between 1990 and 2002, the incidence of acute hepatitis B declined 67%, from 8.5 per 100,000 population (21,102 total cases reported) to 2.8 per 100,000 population (8,064 total cases reported).

Incubation period: The time interval between exposure to a pathogen and the first symptoms of the disease.

Intussusception: A serious and potentially life-threatening condition that occurs when one portion of the intestine telescopes into another portion, causing intestinal obstruction and, if untreated, a portion of the intestine can die. The most common site is where the small intestine joins the large intestine. The disease is most common among young infants. While at times the cause is a tumor or enlarged lymph nodes, it mostly occurs spontaneously. It has only rarely been associated with rotavirus infections but one rotavirus vaccine, Rotashield, was shown to cause intussusception at a rate of about one in 10,000 infants, usually within 3–14 days after reciept of the first dose.

Live attenuated vaccine: The virulence of the pathogen has been reduced but the pathogen retains the ability to infect and to induce immunity. For example, live attenuated measles virus vaccines.

Log$_{10}$: The logarithm to the base 10 is a mathematical expression of the power to which 10 must be raised to equal a given number. A logarithm scale on a figure shows the distance from 1 to 10 and from 10 to 100 as the same.

Meta-analysis: An analysis that looks at results combining several studies.

Molecular mimicry: When a foreign protein is similar to the body's own cells or proteins.

Morbidity: The proportion of the population that becomes sick.

Mortality: The proportion of the population that dies.

Myelin sheath: The envelope that surrounds nerves and nerve fibers. It provides insulation and helps transmit nerve impulses.

Naïve: The person or animal that has not previously been exposed to a particular infection, drug, or vaccine. This meaning of the word is in contrast to its conversational use meaning unsophisticated or lacking in experience or training.

Observational study: A study that simply observes and describes, offering clues but not a positive determination of cause and effect.

Odds ratio: A way of comparing whether the probability of a certain event is the same for two groups—for example, is the probability of developing a disease the same for vaccinated children as for unvaccinated children? The odds of acquiring a disease are calculated as the number of cases divided by the number of non-cases. An odds ratio of 1 implies that both groups are equally likely to develop the disease; an odds ratio greater than one implies that the vaccinated group is more likely to develop the disease; an odds ratio less than one implies that the vaccinated group is less likely to develop the disease. Odds ratios are usually expressed as a range. For example an odds ratio that goes from less than one to more than one implies no association but a ratio that goes from more than one to a higher number implies an association.

Outbreak: A cluster of cases of a disease.

Pandemic: A disease affecting the population of an extensive region, such as a world-wide outbreak.

Pathogen: An infectious agent, such as a bacterium or a virus that causes an infection.

Paralysis: Loss of the ability to move a body part usually as a result of nerve damage. This use of the word is in contrast to the conversational use of the word meaning the inability to act or helpless inactivity.

Person-years: The product of the number of years times the number of members of a population who have been affected by a certain condition. For example, the number of years of paralysis a group of polio survivors might experience.

Phase I, II, III, and IV: Clinical trials are conducted in phases. Phases I, II, and III are the regulatory steps in vaccine development before the vaccine is licensed. Phase IV refers to studies after the vaccine is licensed by the FDA.

Placebo: An inert compound identical in appearance to material being tested in experimental research, which may or may not be known to the investigator and/or patient, administered to distinguish between drug action and suggestive effect of the material under study. For example, in a case-control study, a control group might receive saltwater—the placebo—instead of the actual vaccine. If neither the person giving the vaccine nor the person receiving the vaccine knows whether it is vaccine or placebo the study is said to be "double blinded."

Plausible: Theoretically possible. This use of the word is in contrast to how this word is often used in conversation, where it is often used to mean "worthy of belief" or "factual."

Positive: The results of the study agree with the hypothesis; having a value greater than one. This use of the word is in contrast to its conversational use meaning "good."

Power: The likelihood of a study finding an effect, if there was one. This is in contrast to the conversational use of this word which means "energy," "strength," "control." Another use of the word power is by mathematicians who use it to mean the number of times a number is multiplied by itself.

Prevalence: The total number of cases of a disease existing in a given population at a specific period of time (period prevalence) or at a particular moment in time (point prevalence). For example, the prevalence of chronic hepatitis B infection is higher among Asian Americans than among other ethnic groups in the United States.

P value: The probability that an observed result or effect could have occurred by chance if there had actually been no real effect. See *Statistical Significance.*

Randomized trials: In clinical trials, when the selection of individuals into the experimental and control groups is done by some random method that reduces the chances of selection bias.

Range: A measure of spread—for example, the spread between the youngest and oldest child in a study.

Rate: The proportion of a disease in a group during a particular time period, with a numerator and a denominator. For example, the rate of cases of a disease is 12 cases per 100,000 population per year.

Recombinant vaccine: Vaccine produced by the introduction of a piece of genetic material into another cell, which then produces the antigen. For example the hepatitis B surface antigen is manufactured in yeast cells for preparation of hepatitis B vaccine.

Relative risk (or risk ratio): A comparison of two morbidity or mortality rates by calculating the ratio of one to the other. Relative risk (RR) is equal to the risk in those exposed divided by the risk in those not exposed. If RR is equal to 1, then the risk in exposed persons is the same in non-exposed persons (therefore, the disease is not related to the alleged exposure); if RR is greater than 1, then the risk is greater in the exposed person (thus a causal association may exist); if RR is less than 1, then the risk is less in the exposed person (that means a "protective effect" exists). Risk ratios are usually expressed as a range. For example, a risk ratio that goes from less than 1 to more than 1 implies the risks are the same; a ratio that goes from more than 1 to a higher number implies a higher risk. When the range is below 1, it implies no risk, but protection.

Resistance: The natural or acquired ability to resist the effects of an antagonistic agent, such as being immune against infection by measles virus or to the toxin (poison) produced by the tetanus bacterium.

Safe: The risk is very small.

Sample: A part of a population that is used to represent the whole population.

Selection bias: A non-random selection of study subjects that could have influenced the results (see bias).

Sign: A change in condition perceived by someone other than the patient such as rash.

Significant: The finding may not be a chance difference. "Not significant" means that the differences were likely due to chance. By convention, a finding is said to be significant when p is less than 0.05. These uses of the word are different from the manner it is usually used in ordinary conversation where it often is intended to mean "important."

Statistical significance: In an experiment or a clinical trial, statistical significance means that there is only a small probability that the same result could have been found by chance alone. For example, $p<0.05$ means that the chance of the outcome having occurred by chance was less than 5% (but it also means that the outcome could have been found by chance 5% of the time).

Surrogate measures: These are outcomes—other than the number of cases of disease prevented—that are sometimes used to estimate vaccine effectiveness. For example, a rise in antibody after immunization to a level expected to protect against disease might be used as a surrogate measure.

Susceptible: The lack of resistance against a particular infection or disease; the individual is capable of contracting the disease when exposed to the pathogen (such as a virus or bacterium).

Symptom: A change in condition that is perceived by the patient such as headache.

Toxoid vaccine: *Clostridium tetani* and *Corynebacterium diphtheriae* are bacteria that cause disease because they make very potent toxins. Tetanus and diphtheria vaccines contain inactivated toxins. These toxoids are no longer toxic but they induce antibodies that inactivate the toxin.

Uncertainty: When the available scientific information is not sufficient to prove a relationship or is not sufficient to favor rejection of a rela-tionship. Statistical uncertainty is a term used to express the estimated amount by which an observed value may differ from the actual value. This use of the word is in contrast to its conversational use meaning "I don't know."

Virulence: The ability of a virus or bacterium to invade and cause ill-ness; the degree of disease severity the pathogen is able to cause—usually expressed in case-fatality rates.

Wild type: As it occurs in nature (as opposed to vaccine-type vi-rus—the weakened or attenuated type in a vaccine).

SOURCES

Chin J, ed. 2000. *Control of communicable diseases manual*, 17th ed. Wash-ington, DC: American Public Health Association.

Cohen V, Cope L. 2001. *News & Numbers*. 2nd ed. Ames, IA: Iowa State University Press.

Gordis L. 2000. *Epidemiology*. 2nd ed. Philadelphia, PA: W.B. Saunders Company.

Jefferson T. 2001. A basic glossary of vaccinology. *Journal of Epidemiology and Community Health* 55:294-5.

Stedman's Online Medical Dictionary.

Dictionary.com

Thanks

The National Network for Immunization Information (NNii) is 'what we do'. It's mission is to provide up-to-date, science-based information to healthcare professionals, the media, and the public: everyone who needs to know the facts about vaccines and immunization. One of the important things we do is run our Web site *www.immunizationinfo.org*. In addition to providing information about the different vaccines, we quickly learned that our readers would tell us what they wanted us to write about. When we write about topics that we are interested in but they aren't, it is obvious! Thank you to our readers who have asked the questions and expressed the interest that form the basis of this book. Also, thanks to our steering committee, who represent the affiliate organizations, for all your support over the 10 years that NNii has existed and for encouraging us to write this book.

Drs. Samuel Katz and Louis Cooper are well known in the vaccinology community because of their leadership roles in vaccine development and vaccine education. They critiqued our book and they make NNii what it is. Several generations of children are healthier because of their efforts in many areas surrounding vaccine development, immunization policy, vaccine financing, and public education.

Dr. Paul Offit, vaccine spokesperson extraordinaire, deserves special thanks for encouragement and advice on how to write a book such as this.

A very special thanks to our wives, Diana Pineda and Beverly Myers, for their reviews and suggestions through the earlier drafts. There is no greater motivator to rewriting a chapter than the words "This is important and I understand it but a busy mother won't have the time to spend trying to understand it as I did"! The encouragement and advice of

Diana Olson who is both a wonderful writer as well as critic at IDSA was invaluable.

This book encompasses a wide range of topics in which we were fortunate to have the aid of experts like Drs. Patricia Beach, Thomas Clarkson, Randall Goldblum, John Grabenstein, Frederick Huang, Samuel Katz, Edgar Marcuse, Martin Myers Jr., Dennis Murray, Walter Orenstein, Janak Patel, John Shanley, Andy Shih, and Lawrence Stanberry.

We are deeply grateful to the many reviewers who helped us so generously in our efforts to be both clear and accurate.

Finally, we thank our copyeditor, Sarah Enticknap, for her hard work on the manuscript.

Notes

CHAPTER 1

1. Mills E, Jadad AR, Ross C, Wilson K. 2005. Systematic review of qualitative studies exploring parental beliefs and attitudes toward childhood vaccination identifies common barriers to vaccination. *Vaccine* 58:1081-8.

2. Centers for Disease Control and Prevention. 1999. Achievements in public health, 1900-1999. Impact of vaccine universally recommended for children—United States, 1900-1998. *Morbidity & Mortality Weekly Report* 48:243-8. (Accessed November 2, 2007, at *www.cdc.gov/mmwR/preview/mmwrhtml/00056803.htm*). Invasive S. pneumoniae cases were projected for 1998-9 of which 82.9% were vaccine serotypes (CDC. 2005. Direct and indirect effects of routine vaccination of children with 7-valent pneumococcal conjugate vaccine on incidence of invasive pneumoccal diseases—United States—1998-2003. *Morbidity & Mortality Weekly Report* 54(36): 893-7). This same study projected 4,454 cases (of which 876, or 19.7%, would be vaccine serotypes in 2003. Pre-vaccine numbers of cases of hepatitis A and hepatitis B were estimates for acute hepatitis in 1994 and 1986, respectively (Wesley A, Miller J, Finelli L. 2007. Surveillance for acute viral hepatitis—United States, 2005. *Morbidity & Mortality Weekly Report* 56(SS03): 1-24. Varicella cases and deaths prior to vaccine introduction were estimated retrospectively because it was not a nationally notifiable disease at that time (Marin M, Guris D, Chaves SS, et al. 2007. Prevention of varicella: Recommendations of the Advisory Committee on Immunization Practices. *Morbidity & Mortality Weekly Report* 56 (RR04): 1-40.

3. Centers for Disease Control and Prevention. 2005. Summary of notifiable diseases—United States, 2003. *Morbidity & Mortality Weekly Report* 52:1-85. (Accessed November 2, 2007, at *iier.isciii.es/mmwr/preview/mmwrhtml/mm5254a1.htm*.)

4. Centers for Disease Control and Prevention. 2006. Summary of notifiable diseases—United States, 2004. *Morbidity & Mortality Weekly*

Report 53:1-79. (Accessed November 2, 2007, at *www.cdc.gov/mmwR/ preview/mmwrhtml/mm5353a1.htm.*)

5.   Centers for Disease Control and Prevention. 2007. Summary of no-tifiable diseases—United States, 2005. *Morbidity & Mortality Weekly Report* 54:2-92. (Accessed November 2, 2007, *www.cdc.gov/mmwr/ preview/mmwrhtml/mm5453a1.htm.*)

6.   Centers for Disease Control and Prevention. 2008. Summary of no-tifiable diseases—United States, 2006. *Morbidity & Mortality Weekly Report* 55:1-94. (Accessed April 7, 2008, at *www.cdc.gov/mmwR/pre-view/mmwrhtml/mm5553a1.htm.*)

CHAPTER 2

1.   Paulos JA. 1988. *Innumeracy: Mathematical illiteracy and its consequenc-es.* New York, NY: Hill and Wang.

2.   Lasky T, Terracciano GJ, Magder L, et al. 1998. The Guillain-Barre syndrome and the 1992-1993 and 1993-1994 influenza vaccines. *New England Journal of Medicine* 339:1797-802.

3.   Plotkin SA, Orenstein WA, eds. 2004. *Vaccines.* 4th ed. Philadel-phia, PA: W.B. Saunders Company.

4.   Dannetun E, Tegnell A, Hermansson G, et al. 2005. Parents' re-ported reasons for avoiding MMR vaccination. *Scandinavian Journal of Primary Health Care* 23:149-53.

5.   Reynolds, B. 2002. *Crisis and emergency risk communication.* Atlanta, GA: Centers for Disease Control and Prevention.

6.   Bennett P. 1999. Understanding responses to risk: Some basic find-ings. In: Bennett P, Calman K, eds. *Risk communication and public health.* New York: Oxford University Press.

7.   Sutter RW, Kew OM, Cochi SL. 2004. Poliovirus vaccine—Live. In: Plotkin SA, Orenstein WA, eds. *Vaccines.* 4th ed. Philadelphia, PA: W.B. Saunders Company, Chapter 25.

8.   Smith PJ, Chu SY, Barker LE. 2004. Children who have received no vaccines: Who are they and where do they live? *Pediatrics* 114:187-95.

9.   Salmon DA, Haber M, Gangarosa EJ, et al. 1999. Health conse-

quences of religious and philosophical exemptions from immunization laws: Individual and societal risk of measles. *Journal of the American Medical Association* 282:47-53.

Chapter 3

1. Edwards KM, Decker MD. 2004. Pertussis vaccine. In: Plotkin SA, Orenstein WA, eds. *Vaccines.* 4th ed. Philadelphia, PA: W.B. Saunders Company, Chapter 21.

2. Gangarosa EJ, Galazka AM, Wolfe CR, Phillips LM, Gangarosa RE, Miller E, Chen RT. 1998. Impact of anti-vaccine movements on pertussis control: The untold story. *The Lancet* 351:356-61.

3. Howson CP, Howe CJ, Fineberg HV, eds. 1991. Committee to Review the Adverse Consequences of Pertussis and Rubella Vaccines, Institute of Medicine. *Adverse effects of pertussis and rubella vaccines.* Washington, DC: National Academies Press.

4. Based on a story first published in the Winter 1999 issue of the "Immunize Georgia's Little Guys" newsletter of Children's Healthcare of Atlanta.

5. Jacobson RM, Adegbenro A, Pankratz VS, Poland GA. 2001. Adverse events and vaccination—The lack of power and predictability of infrequent events in pre-licensure study. *Vaccine* 19:2428-33.

6. Chen RT, Davis RL, Sheedy KM. 2004. Safety of immunizations. In: Plotkin SA, Orenstein WA, eds. *Vaccines.* 4th ed. Philadelphia, PA: W.B. Saunders Company, Chapter 61.

7. Karron RA. 2004. Respiratory syncytial virus vaccine. In: Plotkin SA, Orenstein WA, eds. *Vaccines.* 4th ed. Philadelphia, PA: W.B. Saunders Company, 1317-26.

Chapter 4

1. Walboomers JM, Jacobs MV, Manos MM, et al. 1999. Human papillomavirus is a necessary cause of invasive cervical cancer worldwide. *Journal of Pathology* 189:12-19.

2. National Cancer Institute. 2005. Human papillomaviruses and cancer: Questions and answers. (Accessed November 2, 2007, at

www.cancer.gov/cancertopics/factsheet/Risk/HPV.)

3. Rothman KJ, Greenland S. 2005. Causation and causal inference in epidemiology. *American Journal of Public Health* 95:S144-S150.

4. Global Advisory Committee on Vaccine Safety, WHO. 2001. Causality assessment of adverse events following immunization. *Weekly Epidemiological Record* 12:85-92.

5. Institute of Medicine. 2004. *Immunization safety review: Vaccines and autism*. Washington, DC: National Academies Press.

6. Peter G, Myers MG. 2002. National Vaccine Advisory Committee; National Vaccine Program Office. Intussusception, rotavirus, and oral vaccines: Summary of a workshop. *Pediatrics* 110:e67.

7. Centers for Disease Control and Prevention. 1999. Rotavirus vaccine for the prevention of rotavirus gastroenteritis among children. *Morbidity & Mortality Weekly Report* 48:1-20.

8. Parashar UD, Alexander JP, Glass RI. 2006. Prevention of rotavirus gastroenteritis among infants and children: Recommendations of the Advisory Committee on Immunization Practices (ACIP). *Morbidity & Mortality Weekly Report* 55:1-13, and FDA. 2008. FDA Approves new vaccine to prevent gastroenteritis caused by rotavirus. FDA News. (Accessed April 23, 2008, at *www.fda.gov/bbs/topics/ NEWS/2008/NEW01814.html*.)

9. Murphy TV, Gargiullo PM, Massoudi MS, et al. 2001. Intussusception among infants given an oral rotavirus vaccine. *New England Journal of Medicine* 344:564-72.

10. Kramarz P, France EK, Destefano F, et al. 2001. Population-based study of rotavirus vaccination and intussusception. *The Pediatric Infectious Disease Journal* 20:410-6.

11. Murphy BR, Morens DM, Simonsen L, et al. 2003. Reappraisal of the association of intussusception with the licensed live rotavirus vaccine challenges initial conclusions. *Journal of Infectious Diseases* 187:1301-8.

12. Varricchio F, Iskander J, Destefano F, Ball R, Pless R, Braun MM, Chen RT. 2004. Understanding vaccine safety information from the Vaccine Adverse Event Reporting System. *The Pediatric Infectious Disease Journal* 23:287-94.

13. Offit, Paul. 2005. *The Cutter incident.* New Haven, CT: Yale University Press.

14. Chen RT, Glasser J, Rhodes P, et al. 1997. The vaccine safety datalink project: A new tool for improving vaccine safety monitoring in the United States. *Pediatrics* 99:765-73.

15. Institute of Medicine. 2003. Immunization Safety Review: Vaccinations and sudden unexpected death in infancy. Washington, DC: National Academies Press.

16. Lieu T, Kulldorff M, Davis RL, et al. 2007. Real-time vaccine safety surveillance for the early detection of adverse events. *Medical Care* 45:S89-95.

17. Lieu T. 2008. Rapid cycle analysis for early detection of vaccine adverse events. Presentation to the Advisory Committee on Immunization Practices, February 27, 2008.

18. DeStefano F, Gu D, Kramarz P, et al. 2002. Childhood vaccinations and risk of asthma. *Pediatric Infectious Diseases Journal* 21:498-504.

19. Eriksen EM, Perlman JA, Miller A, et al. 2004. Lack of association between hepatitis B birth immunization and neonatal death: A population-based study from the Vaccine Safety Datalink Project. *The Pediatric Infectious Disease Journal* 23:656-62.

20. Institute of Medicine. 2005. *Vaccine safety research, data access, and public trust.* Washington, DC: National Academies Press.

21. Harry GJ, Billingsley M, Bruinink A, et al. 1998. In vitro techniques for the assessment of neurotoxicity. *Environmental Health Perspectives* 106:131-58.

22. Cohn V, Cope L. 2001. *News & numbers: A guide to reporting statistical claims and controversies in health and other fields.* 2nd ed. Ames, IA: Iowa State University Press.

CHAPTER 5

1. Edwards KM, Decker MD. 2004. Pertussis vaccine. In: Plotkin SA, Orenstein WA, eds. *Vaccines.* 4th ed. Philadelphia, PA: W.B. Saunders Company, Chapter 21.

2. Evans G, Harris D, Levine EM. 2004. Legal issues. In: Plotkin SA,

Orenstein WA, eds. *Vaccines.* 4th ed. Philadelphia, PA: W.B. Saunders Company, Chapter 63.

3.   Kulenkampff M, Schwartzman JS, Wilson J. 1974. Neurological complications of pertussis inoculation. *Archives of Disease in Childhood* 49:46-49.

4.   Cherry JD, Brunell PA, Golden GS, et al. 1988. Report of the task force on pertussis and pertussis immunization—1988. *Pediatrics* 81:933-84.

5.   Alderslade R, Bellman MH, Rawson NSB, Ross EM, Miller DL. 1981. The National Childhood Encephalopathy Study: A report on 1000 cases of serious neurological disorders in infants and young children from the NCES research team. In: *Whooping cough: Reports from the Committee on the Safety of Medicines and the Joint Committee on Vaccination and Immunisation.* London: Her Majesty's Stationery Office.

6.   Ray P, Hayward J, Michelson D, et al. 2006. Encephalopathy after whole-cell pertussis or measles vaccination: Lack of evidence for a causal association in a retrospective case-control study. *The Pediatric Infectious Disease Journal* 25:768-73.

7.   Berkovic SF, Harkin L, McMahon JM, et al. 2006. De-novo mutations of the sodium channel gene SCN1A in alleged vaccine encephalopathy: A retrospective study, *The Lancet Neurology* 5:488-92.

8.   Gangarosa EJ, Galazka AM, Wolfe CR, Phillips LM, Gangarosa RE, Miller E, Chen RT. 1998. Impact of anti-vaccine movements on pertussis control: The untold story. *The Lancet* 351:356-61.

9.   D'Souza YD, Fombonne E, Ward BJ. 2006. No evidence of persisting measles virus in peripheral blood mononuclear cells from children with autism spectrum disorder. *Pediatrics* 118:1664-75.

10. Jansen VAA, Stollenwerk N, Jensen HJ, et al. 2003. Measles outbreaks in a population with declining vaccine uptake. *Science* 301:804.

11. Centers for Disease Control and Prevention. 2006. Mumps epidemic—United Kingdom, 2004–2005. *Morbidity & Mortality Weekly Report* 55:173-5.

12. Health Protection Agency. Measles cases so far in 2006. Press State-

ment, 15 June 2006. (Accessed September 28, 2006, at *www.hpa.org. uk/hpa/news/articles/press_releases/2006/060615_measles.htm.*)

13. Doja A, Roberts W. 2006. Immunizations and autism: A review of the literature. *Canadian Journal of Neurological Science* 33:341-6.

14. Murch SH, Anthony A, Cassen DH, et al. 2004. Retraction of an interpretation. *The Lancet* 363:750.

15. Horton R. 2004. A statement by the editors of *The Lancet*. *The Lancet* 363:820-1.

16. Snyder B. Vaccine safety morality hit home for girl's parents. *The Tennessean*, September 17, 2000.

17. Shapiro CN, McCaig LF, Gensheimer KF, et al. 1989. Hepatitis B virus transmission between children in day care. *Pediatric Infectious Diseases Journal* 8:870-5.

18. Oleske J, Minnefor A, Cooper R Jr, et al. 1980. Transmission of hepatitis B in a classroom setting. *Journal of Pediatrics* 97:770-2.

19. Daseda CC, Shapiro CN, Carroll K, et al. 1994. Hepatitis B virus transmission between a child and staff member at a day-care center. *The Pediatric Infectious Diseases Journal* 13: 828-30.

20. Enzi MB. 2007. Thimerosal and autism spectrum disorders: Alleged misconduct by government agencies and private entities. Report of the Ranking Member, United States Senate Committee on Health, Education, Labor and Pensions, September 28, 2007.

21. Davies P, Chapman S, Leask J. 2002. Antivaccination activists on the World Wide Web. *Archives of Disease in Childhood* 87:22-25.

22. Wolfe RM, Sharp LK, Lipsky MS. 2002. Content and design attributes of antivaccination web sites. *Journal of the American Medical Association* 287:3245-8.

23. Generation Rescue. 2005. Mercury Poisoning: 25 Mercury Myths. (Accessed August 20, 2006, at *www.generationrescue.org.*)

24. Kirby D. 2005. *Evidence of harm: Mercury in vaccines and the autism epidemic: A medical controversy.* New York: St. Martin's Press.

25. Office of Special Masters. 2007. Autism update—September 28, 2007. U.S. Court of Federal Claims, Washington, DC.

26. American Medical Association. 2004. H-265.994 Expert Witness

Testimony. In: AMA *code of medical ethics: Current opinions with annotations 2004-2005*. AMA Council on Ethical and Judicial Affairs and American Medical Association.

27. U.S. Court of Federal Claims. Office of Special Masters. October 9, 2003. (Accessed April 30, 2008, at *www.immunizationinfo.org/assets/files/pdfs/geier_in_court_03-1009.pdf*.)

28. Burton D. Refuting the IOM's latest vaccines and autism report. Press release, June, 2, 2004. (Accessed May 2, 2006, at *www.house.gov/burton/pr/2004/pr060204.htm*.)

29. Centers for Disease Control and Prevention. 2006. Diabetes and Vaccines Q&A. (Accessed August 10, 2006, at *www.cdc.gov/nip/vacsafe/concerns/diabetes/q&a.htm*).

30. Laidler JR. Chelation & autism. Neurodiversity weblog. (Accessed May 2, 2006, at *neurodiversity.com/weblog/article/14/chelation-autism*.)

31. Parker SK, Schwartz B, Todd J, Pickering LK. 2004. Thimerosal-containing vaccines and autistic spectrum disorder: A critical review of published original data. *Pediatrics* 114:793-804.

32. Generation Rescue's ad in the *New York Times*. (Accessed May 2, 2006, at *www.generationrescue.org/pdf/051114.pdf*.)

33. General confusion and the *New York Times*, November 25, 2005. (Accessed April 30, 2008, at *autismdiva.blogspot.com/2005/11/general-confusion-and-nyt.html*.)

34. Deer B. MMR doctor given legal aid thousands. *The Sunday Times*, December 31, 2006.

35. Kennedy RF Jr. Deadly immunity. *Rolling Stone*, June 20, 2005. (Accessed April 30, 2008, at *www.rollingstone.com/politics/story/7395411/deadly_immunity/*.)

36. Simpsonwood transcripts are available online at *www.safeminds.org/legislation/foia/Simpsonwood_Transcript.pdf*. (Accessed April 30, 2008.)

37. The Institute of Medicine Transcripts are available at *www.nomercury.org/iom/iom.pdf*. (Accessed April 30, 2008.)

CHAPTER 6

1. Gellin BG, Maibach EW, Marcuse EK. 2000. Do parents understand immunizations? A national telephone survey. *Pediatrics* 106:1097-1102.
2. Patel J. 2006 Personal communication.
3. Pribble JM, Goldstein KM, Fowler EF, Greenberg MJ, Noel SK, Howell JD. 2006. Medical news for the public to use? What's on local TV news. *American Journal of Managed Care* 12:170-6.

CHAPTER 7

1. American Lung Association. 2005. Trends in asthma morbidity and mortality (Accessed January 2, 2008, at *www.lungusa.org.*)
2. Ober C, Hoffjan S. 2006. Asthma genetics 2006: The long and winding road to gene discovery. *Genes and Immunity* 7:95-100.
3. Selgrade MK, Lemanske RF, Gilmour MI, et al. 2006. Induction of asthma and the environment: What we know and need to know. *Environmental Health Perspectives* 114:615-9.
4. Akinbami LJ, Schoendorf KC. 2002. Trends in childhood asthma: Prevalence, health care utilization, and mortality. *Pediatrics* 110:315-22.
5. Eder W, Ege MJ, Von Mutius E. 2006. The asthma epidemic. *New England Journal of Medicine* 355:2226-35.
6. O'Connor G, Neas L, Vaughn B, et al. 2008. Acute respiratory health effects of air pollution on asthmatic children in US inner cities. *Journal of Allergy and Clinical Immunology.* In Press. Available online April 11, 2008.
7. Yeatts K, Sly P, Shore S, et al. 2006. A brief targeted review of susceptibility factors, environmental exposures, asthma incidence, and recommendations for future asthma incidence research. *Environmental Health Perspectives,* 114:634-40.
8. WHO. 2006. Asthma. (Accessed November 27, 2007, at *www.who. int/mediacentre/factsheets/fs307/en/index.html.*)
9. Thomson CC, Clark S, Camargo CA Jr. 2003. Body mass index

and asthma severity among adults presenting to the emergency department. *Chest* 124:795-802.

10. Castro-Rodríguez JA, Holberg CJ, Morgan WJ, et al. 2001. Increased incidence of asthmalike symptoms in girls who become overweight or obese during the school years. *American Journal of Respiratory and Critical Care Medicine* 163:1344-9.

11. Gold DR, Damokosh AI, Dockery DW, et al. 2003. Body-mass index as a predictor of incident asthma in a prospective cohort of children. *Pediatric Pulmonology* 36:514-21.

12. Aaron SD, Fergusson D, Dent R, et al. 2004. Effect of weight reduction on respiratory function and airway reactivity in obese women. *Chest* 125:2046-52.

13. Strachan DP. 1989. Hay fever, hygiene, and household size. *British Medical Journal* 299:1259-60.

14. Ramsey CD, Celedon JC. 2005. The hygiene hypothesis and asthma. *Current Opinion in Pulmonary Medicine* 11:14-20.

15. Martinez FD. 2001. The coming-of-age of the hygiene hypothesis. *Respiratory Research* 2:129-32.

16. Gereda JE, Leung DYM, Thatayatikom A, et al. 2000. Relation between house-dust endotoxin exposure, type 1 T-cell development, and allergen sensitisation in infants at high risk of asthma. *The Lancet* 355:1680-3.

17. von Mutius E, Martinez FD, Fritzsch C, et al. 1994. Prevalence of asthma and atopy in two areas of West and East Germany. *American Journal of Respiratory and Critical Care Medicine* 149:358-64.

18. Institute of Medicine. 2002. *Immunization safety review: Multiple immunizations and immune dysfunction.* Washington, DC: National Academies Press.

19. Rottem M, Shoenfeld Y. 2004. Vaccination and allergy. *Current Opinion in Otolaryngology and Head and Neck Surgery* 12:223-31.

20. Wickens K, Crane J, Kemp T, et al. 2001. A case-control study of risk factors for asthma in New Zealand children. *Australian and New Zealand Journal of Public Health.* 25:44-9.

21. Hurwitz EL, Morgenstern H. 2000. Effects of diphtheria-tetanus-per-

tussis or tetanus vaccination on allergies and allergy-related respiratory symptoms among children and adolescents in the United States. *Journal of Manipulative and Physiological Therapeutics*, 23:81-90.

22. Farooqi IS, Hopkin JM. 1998. Early childhood infection and atopic disorder. *Thorax* 53:927-32.

23. Nilsson L, Gruber C, Granstrom M, et al. 1998. Pertussis IgE and atopic disease. *Allergy.* 53:1195–201.

24. Kemp T, Pearce N, Fitzharris P, et al. 1997. Is infant immunization a risk factor for childhood asthma or allergy? *Epidemiology* 8:678-80.

25. DeStefano F, Gu D, Kramarz P, et al. 2002. Childhood vaccinations and risk of asthma. *Pediatric Infectious Disease Journal* 21:498-504.

26. Maher JE, Mullooly JP, Drew L, et al. 2004. Infant vaccinations and childhood asthma among full-term infants. *Pharmacoepidemiology and Drug Safety* 13:1-9.

27. Maitra A, Sherriff A, Griffiths M, et al. 2004. Pertussis vaccination in infancy and asthma or allergy in later childhood: Birth cohort study. *British Medical Journal* 328:925-6.

28. Bernsen RM, Koes BW, de Jongste JC, et al. 2006. Haemophilus influenzae type b vaccination and reported atopic disorders in 8–12-year-old children. *Pediatric Pulmonology* 41:463-9.

29. Bernsen RM, de Jongste JC, Koes BW, et al. 2006. Diphtheria tetanus pertussis poliomyelitis vaccination and reported atopic disorders in 8–12-year-old children. *Vaccine* 24:2035-42.

30. Balicer RD, Grotto I, Mimouni M, et al. 2007. Is childhood vaccination associated with asthma? A meta-analysis of observational studies. *Pediatrics* 120:e1269-77.

31. Poehling KA, Edwards KM, Weinberg GA, et al. 2006. The unrecognized burden of influenza in young children. *New England Journal of Medicine* 355:31-40.

32. Miller EK, Griffin MR, Edwards KM, et al. 2008. Influenza burden for children with asthma. *Pediatrics* 121:1-8.

33. Prosser LA, Bridges CB, Uyeki TM, et al. 2006. Health benefits, risks, and cost-effectiveness of influenza vaccination of children. *Emerging Infectious Diseases* 12:1548-58.

34. Bohlke K, Davis RL, Marcy SM, et al. 2003. Risk of anaphylaxis after vaccination of children and adolescents. *Pediatrics* 112:815-20.

35. Fisher BL. *NVIC News*, April 14, 2004.

36. Fisher BL. *NVIC News*, July 5, 2005.

37. Neustaedter R. Do vaccines disable the immune system? (Accessed July 25, 2006, at *www.healthychild.com/database/do_vaccines_disable_the_immune_system.htm.*)

38. Stanley SK, Ostrowski MA, Justement JS, et al. 1996. Effect of immunization with a common recall antigen on viral expression in patients infected with human immunodeficiency virus type 1. *New England Journal of Medicine* 334:1222-9.

CHAPTER 8

1. Centers for Disease Control and Prevention. 2007. Prevalence of autism spectrum disorders—autism and developmental disabilities monitoring network, 14 sites, United States, 2002. *Morbidity & Mortality Weekly Report* 56 (SS-1):12-28.

2. Centers for Disease Control and Prevention. 2007. Autism Information Center. Available on line at *www.cdc.gov/ncbddd/autism/overview.htm.*

3. Schecter R, Grether JK. 2008. Continuing increases in autism reported to California's Developmental Services System. *Archives of General Psychiatry* 63:19-24.

4. AAP Committee on Children with Disabilities. 2001. The pediatrician's role in the diagnosis and management of autistic spectrum disorder in children. *Pediatrics* 107:1221-6.

5. Kennedy RF Jr. Deadly immunity. *Rolling Stone*, June 20, 2005. (Accessed April 30, 2008, at *www.rollingstone.com/politics/story/7395411/deadly_immunity/.*)

6. Nylander L, Gillberg C. 2001. Screening for autism spectrum disorders in adult psychiatric out-patients: A preliminary report. *Acta Psychiatrica Scandinavica* 103:428-34. See also La Malfa G, Lassi S, Bertelli M, Salvini R, Placidi GF. 2004. Autism and intellectual disability: A study of prevalence on a sample of the Italian population.

Journal of Intellectual Disability Research 48:262-67.

7. Baron-Cohen S, Wheelwright S, Skinner R, Martin J, Clubley E. 2001. The Autism-Spectrum Quotient (AQ): Evidence from Asperger syndrome/high-functioning autism, males and females, scientists and mathematicians. *Journal of Autism and Developmental Disorders* 31:5-17.

8. Bailey A, Le Couteur A, Gottesman I, et al. 1995. Autism as a strongly genetic disorder: Evidence from a British twin study. *Psychological Medicine* 25:63-77.

9. Muhle R, Trentacoste SV, Rapin I. 2004. The genetics of autism. *Pediatrics* 113:e472-86.

10. Pons R, Andreu AL, Checcarelli N, et al. 2003. Mitochondrial DNA abnormalities and autistic spectrum disorders. *Journal of Pediatrics* 144:81-5.

11. Poling JS, Frye RE, Shoffner J, et al. 2006. Developmental regression and mitochondrial dysfunction in a child with autism. *Journal of Child Neurology* 21:170-72.

12. United States Court of Federal Claims. November 9, 2007, Respondent's Rule 4(c) Report. These reports are protected under the confidentiality provisions of the National Vaccine Injury Act. However, this particular report has been widely distributed on the Internet and reported in the media. (Accessed April 30, 2008, at *www.huffingtonpost.com/david-kirby/the-vaccineautism-court-_b_88558.html.*)

13. National Vaccine Injury Compensation Program (VICP). (Accessed April 22, 2008, at *www.hrsa.gov/vaccinecompensation.*)

14. Plotkin SA, Reef S. 2004. Rubella vaccine. In Plotkin SA, Orenstein WA, eds., *Vaccines*, 4th ed. Philadelphia, PA: W.B. Saunders Company.

15. Stephan DA. 2008. Unraveling autism. *American Journal of Human Genetics* 82:7-9.

16. Weiss LA, Shen Y, Korn JM, et al. 2008. Association between microdeletion and microduplication at 6p11.2 and autism. *New England Journal of Medicine* 358:1-9.

17. U.S. Department of Education, Office of Special Education and

Rehabilitative Services, Annual Report to Congress on the Implementation of The Individuals with Disabilities Education Act, various years, and unpublished tabulations; and National Center for Education Statistics, Common Core of Data survey. Table 52. Children 3 to 21 years old served in federally supported programs for the disabled, by type of disability: 1976-77 to 2000-01. (This table was prepared March 2002.) Available on line at *nces.ed.gov/programs/digest/d02/dt052.asp.*

18. Chakrabarti S, Fombonne E. 2001. Pervasive developmental disorders in preschool children. *Journal of the American Medical Association* 285:3093-9.

19. Bishop DVM, Whitehouse AJO, Watt HJ, et al. 2008. Autism and diagnostic substitution: Evidence from a study of adults with a history of developmental language disorder. *Developmental Medicine and Child Neurology* 50:341-5.

20. Newschaffer CJ. 2006. Investigating diagnostic substitution and autism prevalence trends. *Pediatrics* 117:1436-7.

21. Wakefield AJ, Murch SH, Anthony A, Linnell J, Casson DM, Malik M, et al. 1998. Ileal-lymphoid-modular hyperplasia, non-specific colitis, and pervasive developmental disorder in children. *The Lancet* 351:637-41.

22. Hall C, Medical Editor. *Daily Telegraph*, 27 February, 1998.

23. Murch SH, Anthony A, Cassen DH, et al. 2004. Retraction of an interpretation. *The Lancet* 363:750.

24. Institute of Medicine. 2004. *Immunization Safety Review: Vaccines and Autism*. Washington, DC: National Academies Press.

25. D'Souza Y, Fombonne E, Ward BJ. 2006. No evidence of persisting measles virus in peripheral blood mononuclear cells from children with autism spectrum disorder. *Pediatrics* 118:664-75.

26. Afzal MA, Ozoemena LC, O'Hare A, et al. 2006. Absence of detectable measles virus genome sequence in blood of autistic children who have had their MMR vaccination during the routine childhood immunization schedule of UK. *Journal of Medical Virology* 78:623-30.

27. Katz S. 2006. Has the measles-mumps-rubella vaccine been fully

exonerated? *Pediatrics* 118:1744-5.

28. Baird G, Pickles A, Simonoff E, et al. 2008. Measles vaccination and antibody response in autism spectrum disorders. *Archives of Disease in Childhood* [Epub ahead of print].

29. Deer B. 2006. MMR doctor given legal aid thousands. *The Sunday Times.* December 31, 2006.

30. Demichelli V, Jefferson T, Rivetti A, Price D. 2005. Vaccines for measles, mumps and rubella in children. *The Cochrane Database of Systematic Reviews*, 4.

31. Myers MG, Pineda D. 2008. Misinformation about vaccines. In Stanberry LR, Barrett A., eds., *Vaccines for Biodefense and Emerging and Neglected Diseases.* Oxford: Academic Press.

32. Deer B. 2007. Andrew Wakefield & MMR. The MMR-autism scare – our story so far. (Accessed January 24, 2008, at *briandeer.com/mmr/lancet-summary.htm.*)

33. Finn TM, Egan W. 2004. Vaccine additives and manufacturing residuals in United States-licensed vaccines. In Plotkin SA, Orenstein WA, eds., *Vaccines*, 4th ed. Philadelphia, PA: W.B. Saunders.

34. WHO. 2002. Recommendations from the Strategic Advisory Group of Experts. *Weekly Epidemiological Record FDI World* 6:9.

35. Clarkson TW, Magos L. 2006. The toxicology of mercury and its chemical compounds. *Critical Reviews in Toxicology* 30:609-62.

36. Bernard S, Enayati A, Redwood L, Roger H, Binstock T. 2001. Autism: A novel form of mercury poisoning. *Medical Hypotheses* 56:462-71.

37. IOM. 2001. *Thimerosal-containing vaccines and neurodevelopmental disorders.* Washington, DC: National Academic Press.

38. Nelson KB, Bauman ML. 2003. Thimerosal and autism? *Pediatrics* 111:674-9.

39. Burbacher TM, Shen DD, Liberato N, Grant KS, Cernichiari E, Clarkson T. 2005. Comparison of blood and brain mercury levels in infant monkeys exposed to methylmercury or vaccines containing thimerosal. *Environmental Health Perspectives* 113:1015-21.

40. Zareba G, Cernichiari E, Hojo R, et al. 2007. Thimerosal distribu-

tion and metabolism in neonatal mice: Comparison with methyl mercury. *Journal of Applied Toxicology* 27:511-8.

41. Pichichero ME, Cernichiari E, Lopreiato J, Treanor J. 2002. Mercury concentrations and metabolism in infants receiving vaccines containing thiomersal: A descriptive study. *The Lancet* 360:1737-41.

42. Pichichero ME, Gentile A, Giglio N, et al. 2008. Mercury levels in newborns and infants after receipt of thimerosal-containing vaccines. *Pediatrics* 121:e208-14.

43. Ball LK, Ball R, Pratt RD. 2001. An assessment of thimerosal use in childhood vaccines. *Pediatrics* 107:1147-54.

44. Freed GL, Andreae MC, Cowan AE, Katz SL. 2002. The process of public policy formulation: The case of thimerosal in vaccines. *Pediatrics* 109:1153-9.

45. American Academy of Pediatrics. 1999. Joint Statement of the American Academy of Pediatrics (AAP) and the United States Public Health Service (USPHS). *Pediatrics* 104:568-9.

46. Centers for Disease Control. 1999. Notice to readers: Thimerosal in vaccines: A joint statement of the American Academy of Pediatrics and the Public Health Service. *Morbidity & Mortality Weekly Report* 48:563-5.

47. Mason D. Presentation to Advisory Committee on Immunization Practices. February 21, 2002. Atlanta, GA: Centers for Disease Control and Prevention.

48. Waly M, Olteanu H, Banerjee R, Choi SW, Mason JB, Parker BS, et al. 2004. Activation of methionine synthase by insulin-like growth factor-1 and dopamine: A target for neurodevelopmental toxins and thimerosal. *Molecular Psychiatry* 9:358-70.

49. Hornig M, Chian D, Lipkin WI. 2004. Neurotoxic effects of postnatal thimerosal are mouse strain-dependent. *Molecular Psychiatry* 9:833-45.

50. Berman RF, Pessah IN, Mouton PR, et al. 2008. Low-level neonatal thimerosal exposure: Further evaluation of altered neurotoxic potential in SJL mice. *Toxicological Sciences* 101:294-309.

51. Holmes AS, Blaxill MF, Haley BE. 2003. Reduced levels of mercu-

ry in first baby haircuts of autistic children. *International Journal of Toxicology* 22:277-85.

52. Bradstreet J, Geier D, Kartzinel J, Adams J, Geier M. 2003. A case-control study of mercury burden in children with autistic spectrum disorders. *Journal of American Physicians and Surgeons* 8:76-9.

53. Ip P, Wong V, Ho M, et al. 2004. Mercury exposure in children with autistic spectrum disorder: Case-control study. *Journal of Child Neurology* 19: 431-4. See also, Wong V. 2007. Erratum. *Journal of Child Neurology* 22:1324.

54. Hotez P. quoted by James SD. Vaccine-autism debate moves to small screen. ABC News, January 31, 2008. (Accessed January 31, 2008, at *abcnews.go.com/Health/story?id=4218078&page=1.*)

55. Madsen KM, Lauritsen MB, Pedersen CB. 2003. Thimerosal and the occurrence of autism: Negative ecological evidence from Danish population-based data. *Pediatrics* 112:604-6.

56. Stehr-Green P, Tull P, Stellfeld M, Mortenson PB, Simpson D. 2003. Autism and thimerosal-containing vaccines: Lack of consistent evidence for an association. *American Journal of Preventive Medicine* 25:101-6.

57. Hviid A, Stellfeld M, Wohlfahrt J, et al. 2003. Association between thimerosal-containing vaccine and autism. *Journal of the American Medical Association* 290:1763-6.

58. Verstraeten T, Davis RL, DeStefano F, et al. 2003. Safety of thimerosal-containing vaccines: A two-phased study of computerized health maintenance organization databases. *Pediatrics* 112:1039-48.

59. Blaxill M. 2001. Presentation to Immunization Safety Review Committee. Rising Incidence of Autism: Association with Thimerosal. Washington, DC.

60. Andrews N, Miller E, Grant A, et al. 2004. Thimerosal exposure in infants and developmental disorders: A retrospective cohort study in the United Kingdom does not support a causal association. *Pediatrics* 114:584-91.

61. Fombonne E, Zakarian R, Bennett A, et al. 2006. Pervasive developmental disorders in Montreal, Quebec, Canada: Prevalence and

links with immunizations. *Pediatrics* 118:e139-50.

62. Parker SK, Schwartz B, Todd J, Pickering LK. 2004. Thimerosal-containing vaccines and autistic spectrum disorder: A critical review of published original data. *Pediatrics* 114:793-804.

63. National Vaccine Advisory Committee. 1999. Workshop on thimerosal vaccines. (Accessed April 30, 2008, at *www.fda.gov/ohrms/dockets/dailys/04/aug04/080404/04p-0349-cp00001-toc.htm.*)

64. Heron J, Golding J, ALSPAC Study Team. 2004. Thimerosal exposure in infants and developmental disorders: A prospective cohort study in the United Kingdom does not support a causal association. *Pediatrics* 114:577-83.

65. Thompson WW, Price C, Goodson B, et al. 2007. Early thimerosal exposure and neuropsychological outcomes at 7 to 10 years. *New England Journal of Medicine* 357:1281-92.

66. Kirby D. 2005. *Evidence of harm: Mercury in vaccines and the autism epidemic: A medical controversy.* New York: St. Martin's Press.

67. Centers for Disease Control and Prevention. Scientific review of Vaccine Safety Datalink information. Verbatim Transcript. Norcross, GA. June 7-8, 2000.

68. Department of Health and Human Services. National Vaccine Advisory Committee sponsored workshop on thimerosal vaccines. Verbatim Transcript. Bethesda MD. August 11-12, 1999.

69. ibid. Dr. Tom Clarkson, Day 2 page 174.

70. Dr. Frank DeStefano. Centers for Disease Control and Prevention. Scientific review of vaccine safety datalink information. Verbatim Transcript. Norcross, GA. June 7-8, 2000. Day 1, page 30.

71. Orenstein WA. Centers for Disease Control and Prevention. Scientific review of vaccine safety datalink information. Verbatim Transcript. Norcross, GA. June 7-8, 2000. Day 1, page 2.

72. Centers for Disease Control and Prevention. Advisory Committee on Immunization Practices. Verbatim Transcript. Volume I – Day One. Atlanta, Georgia. June 21, 2000, pp. 248-387.

CHAPTER 9

1. Salmon DA, Moulton LH, Omer SB, deHart MP, Stokley S, Halsey NA. 2005. Factors associated with refusal of childhood vaccines among parents of school-aged children: A case-control study. *Archives of Pediatrics and Adolescent Medicine* 159:470-6.

2. Offit PA, Quarles J, Gerber MA, et al. 2002. Addressing parents' concerns: Do multiple vaccines overwhelm the infant's immune system? *Pediatrics* 109:124-9.

3. Hilton S, Petticrew M, Hunt K. 2006. 'Combined vaccines are like a sudden onslaught to the body's immune system': Parental concerns about vaccine 'overload' and 'immune vulnerability'. *Vaccine* 24:4321-7.

4. Gregson AL, Edelman R. 2003. Does antigenic overload exist? The role of multiple immunizations in infants. *Immunology and Allergy Clinics of North America* 23:649-64.

5. Gellin BG, Maibach EW, Marcuse EK, et al. 2000. Do parents understand immunizations? A national telephone survey. *Pediatrics* 106:1097-102.

6. Hviid A, Wohlfahrt J, Stellfeld M, et al. 2005. Childhood vaccination and nontargeted infectious disease hospitalization. *Journal of the American Medical Association* 294:699-705.

7. Institute of Medicine Immunization Safety Review Committee. 2002. Multiple immunizations and immune dysfunction. Washington, DC: National Academies Press.

8. Lee C-H, Lee EG, Lee J-Y, et al. 2008. The incidence of tuberculosis after a measles outbreak. *Clinical Infectious Diseases* 46:902-4.

9. McVernon J, Andrews N, Slack MPE, et al. 2003. Risk of vaccine failure after Haemophilus influenzae type b (Hib) combination vaccines with acellular pertussis. *The Lancet* 361:1521-3.

10. Code of Federal Regulations, 1999 revision. Title 21, part 601.25 (d) (4). (Accessed March 13, 2008, at *www.access.gpo.gov/cgi-bin/cfrassemble.cgi?title=199921*.)

11. Postema AS, Myers MG, Breiman RF. 2001. Challenge for the development, licensure and utilization of combination vaccines. *Clinical Infectious Diseases* 33S4:261-6.

12. France EK, Glanz J, Xu S, et al. 2008. Risk of immune thrombocytopenic Purpura after measles-mumps-rubella immunization in children. *Pediatrics* 121:e687-92.

13. Siegrist CA, Lewis EM, Eskola J, et al. 2007. Human papilloma virus immunization in adolescent and young adults: A cohort study to illustrate what events might be mistaken for adverse reactions. *Pediatrics Infectious Diseases Journal* 26:979-84.

14. Classen DC, Classen JB. 1997. The timing of pediatric immunization and the risk of insulin-dependent diabetes mellitus. *Infectious Diseases in Clinical Practice* 6:449-54.

15. Offit PA, Hackett CJ. 2003. Addressing parents' concerns: Do vaccines cause allergic or autoimmune diseases? *Pediatrics* 111:653-9.

16. Blom L, Nystrom L, Dahlquist G. 1991. The Swedish childhood diabetes study. Vaccinations and infections as risk determinants for diabetes in childhood. *Diabetologia* 34:176-81.

17. Heijbel H, Chen RT, Dahlquist G. 1997. Cumulative incidence of childhood-onset IDDM is unaffected by pertussis immunization. *Diabetes Care* 20:173-5.

18. Karvonen M, Cepaitis Z, Tuomilehto J. 1999. Association between type 1 diabetes and Haemophilus influenzae type b vaccination: Birth cohort study. *British Medical Journal* 318:1169-72.

19. Graves PM, Yu L, Barriga KJ, et al. 1999. Lack of association between early childhood immunizations and B-cell autoimmunity. *Diabetes Care* 22:1694-7.

20. Hummel M, Schenker M, Futenbusch M, et al. 2000. No major association of breast-feeding, vaccinations, and childhood viral diseases with early islet autoimmunity in the German BABYDIAB study. *Diabetes Care* 23:969-74.

21. EURODIAB Substudy 2 Study Group. 2000. Infections and vaccinations as risk factors for childhood type 1 (insulin-dependent) diabetes mellitus: A multicentre case-control investigation. *Diabetologia* 43:47-53.

22. DeStefano F, Mullooly JP, Okoro CA, et al. 2001. Childhood vaccinations, vaccination timing, and risk of type 1 diabetes mellitus. *Pediatrics* 108:E112.

23. Black SB, Lewis E, Shinefield HR, et al. 2002. Lack of association between receipt of conjugate Haemophilus influenzae type b vaccine (HbOC) in infancy and risk of type 1 (juvenile onset) diabetes: Long term follow-up of the HbOC efficacy trial cohort. *Pediatric Infectious Diseases Journal* 21:568-9.

24. Hviid A, Stellfeld M, Wohlfahrt J, et al. 2004. Childhood vaccination and type 1 diabetes. *New England Journal of Medicine* 350:1398-404.

25. Souayah N, Nasar A, Suri MFK, et al. 2007. Guillain-Barré syndrome after vaccination in United States: A report from the CDC/FDA Vaccine Adverse Reporting System. *Vaccine* 25:5253-5.

26. Institute of Medicine. 2004. *Immunization safety review: Influenza vaccines and neurological complications.* Washington, DC: National Academies Press.

27. Lasky T, Terracciano GJ, Magder L, et al. 1998. The Guillain-Barré syndrome and the 1992–1993 and 1993–1994 influenza vaccines. *New England Journal of Medicine* 339:1797-802.

28. Hughes RA, Charlton J, Latinovic R, et al. 2006. No association between immunization and Guillain-Barré Syndrome in the United Kingdom. *Archives of Internal Medicine* 166:1301-4.

29. Centers for Disease Control and Prevention. 2006. Prevention and control of influenza. Recommendations of the Advisory Committee on Immunization Practices (ACIP). *Morbidity & Mortality Weekly Report* 55(RR-10):1-42.

30. Institute of Medicine. 1994. *Adverse events associated with childhood vaccines: Evidence bearing on causality.* Washington, DC: National Academies Press.

31. Tuttle J, Chen RT, Rantala H, et al. 1997. The risk of Guillain-Barré syndrome after tetanus-toxoid-containing vaccines in adults and children in the United States. *American Journal of Public Health* 87:2045-8.

32. Centers for Disease Control and Prevention. 2006. A comprehensive immunization strategy to eliminate transmission of hepatitis B virus infection in the United States. Recommendations of the Advisory Committee on Immunization Practices (ACIP). Part II: Immunization of adults. *Morbidity & Mortality Weekly Report* 55(RR-16):1-25.

33. Centers for Disease Control and Prevention. 2005. Guillain-Barré syndrome among recipients of Menacta meningococcal conjugate vaccine—United States, June–July 2005. *Morbidity & Mortality Weekly Report* 54:1023-5.

34. Centers for Disease Control and Prevention. 2006. Update: Guillain-Barré syndrome among recipients of Menactra® meningococcal conjugate vaccine—United States, June 2005–September 2006. *Morbidity & Mortality Weekly Report* 55:1120-4.

35. Lieu T, Kulldorff M, Davis RL, et al. 2007. Real-time vaccine safety surveillance of the early detection of adverse events. *Medical Care* 45:S89-95.

36. Institute of Medicine. 2002. *Hepatitis B vaccine and demyelinating neurological disorders*. Washington, DC: National Academies Press.

37. DeStefano F, Verstraeten T, Jackson LA, et al. 2003. Vaccinations and risk of central nervous system demyelinating diseases in adults. *Archives of Neurology* 60:504-9.

38. Payne DC, Rose CE, Kerrison J, et al. 2006. Anthrax vaccination and risk of optic neuritis in the United States military, 1998–2003. *Archives of Neurology* 63:871-5.

39. Demicheli V, Rivetti A, DiPietrantonj C, et al. 2003. Hepatitis B vaccination and multiple sclerosis: Evidence from a systematic review. *Journal of Viral Hepatitis* 10:343-4.

40. Hernan MA, Jick SS, Olek MJ et al. 2004. Recombinant hepatitis B vaccine and the risk of multiple sclerosis: A prospective study. *Neurology* 63:838-42.

41. Mikaeloff Y, Caridade G, Rossier M. 2007. Hepatitis B vaccination and the risk of childhood-onset multiple sclerosis. *Archives of Pediatrics and Adolescent Medicine* 161:1176-82.

42. Mikaeloff Y, Caridade G, Assi S, et al. 2007. Hepatitis B vaccine

and risk of relapse after a first childhood episode of CNS inflammatory demyelination. *Brain* 130:1105-10.

43. Institute of Medicine. 2004. *Immunization safety review: Influenza vaccines and neurological complications.* Washington, DC: National Academies Press.

44. Chen RT, Pless R, DeStefano F. 2001. Epidemiology of autoimmune reactions induced by vaccination. *Journal of Autoimmunity* 16:309-18.

45. Demicheli V, Jefferson T, Rivetti A, et al. 2005. *Vaccines for measles, mumps and rubella in children.* Cochrane Database Syst Rev., CD004407.

46. Davis RL, Kramarz P, Bohlke K, et al. 2001. Measles-mumps-rubella and other measles-containing vaccines do not increase the risk of inflammatory bowel disease. *Archives of Pediatrics and Adolescent Medicine* 155:354-9.

47. Seagroatt V, Goldacre MJ. 2003. Crohn's disease, ulcerative colitis, and measles vaccine in an English population, 1979–1998. *Journal of Epidemiology and Community Health* 57:883-7.

48. Bernstein CN, Rawthorne P, Blanchard JF. 2007. Population-based case-control study of measles, mumps, and rubella and inflammatory bowel disease. *Inflammatory Bowel Diseases* 13:759-62.

49. Plotkin SA, Reef S. 2004. Rubella vaccine. In: Plotkin SA, Orenstein WA, eds. 2004. *Vaccines.* 4th ed. Philadelphia, PA: W.B. Saunders.

50. Slater PE, Ben-Zvi T, Fogewl A, et al. 1995. Absence of an association between rubella vaccination and arthritis in underimmune postpartum women. *Vaccine* 13:1529-32.

51. Ray P, Shinefield H, Dillon A, et al. 1997. Risk of chronic arthropathy among women after rubella vaccination. Vaccine Safety Datalink Team. *Journal of the American Medical Association* 278:551-6.

52. Tingle AJ, Mitchell LA, Grace M, et al. 1997. Randomised double-blind placebo-controlled study on adverse effects of rubella immunisation in seronegative women. *The Lancet* 349:1277-81.

53. Eickhoff TC, Myers MG. 2002. Workshop summary: Aluminum in vaccines. *Vaccine* 20:S1-S4.

54. Hunter RL. 2002. Overview of vaccine adjuvants: Present and future. *Vaccine*, 20:S7-S12.

55. Offit PA, Jew RK. 2003. Addressing parents' concerns: Do vaccines contain harmful preservatives, adjuvants, additives, or residuals? *Pediatrics* 112:1394-1401.

56. Keith LS, Jones DE, Chou C-HSJ. 2002. Aluminum toxicokinetics regarding infant diet and vaccinations. *Vaccine* 20:S13-17.

57. Jefferson T, Rudin M, Di Pietrantonj C. 2004. Adverse events after immunisation with aluminium-containing DTP vaccines: Systematic review of the evidence. *The Lancet Infectious Diseases* 4:4-90.

58. Jefferson T, Rudin M, DiPietrantonj C. 2003. Systematic review of the effects of pertussis vaccines in children. *Vaccine* 21:2003-14.

59. Institute of Medicine. 2006. *Gulf War and health: Volume 4. Health effects of serving in the Gulf War.* Washington, DC: National Academies Press.

60. Gherardi RK, Coquet M, Chérin P, et al. 1998. Macrophagic myofasciitis: An emerging entity. *The Lancet* 352:347-52.

61. Verdier F, Burnett R, Michelet-Habchi C, et al. 2005. Aluminum assay and evaluation of the local reaction at several time points after intramuscular administration of aluminum containing vaccines in the Cynomolgus monkey. *Vaccine* 23:1359-67.

62. Brenner A. 2002. Macrophagic myofasciitis: A summary of Dr. Gherardi's presentation. *Vaccine* 20:S5-6.

63. Lach B, Cupler EJ. 2008. Macrophagic myofascitis in children is a localized reaction to vaccination. *Journal of Child Neurology* [Epub ahead of print].

64. Coker R. Distinguishing science and pseudoscience. (Accessed September 7, 2006, at *www.quackwatch.org/01QuackeryRelatedTopics/pseudo.html*.)

CHAPTER 10

1. Vestergaard M, Hviid A, Madsen KM, et al. 2004. MMR vaccination and febrile seizures: Evaluation of susceptible subgroups and long-term prognosis. *Journal of the American Medical Association* 292:351-7.

2. Barlow WE, Davis RL, Glasser JW, et al. 2001. The risk of seizures after receipt of whole-cell pertussis or measles, mumps, and rubella vaccine. *New England Journal of Medicine* 345:656-61.

3. Centers for Disease Control and Prevention. 2008. Update: Recommendation from the Advisory Committee on Immunization Practices (ACIP) regarding administration of combination MMRV vaccine. *Morbidity & Mortality Weekly Report* 57:258-60.

4. Institute of Medicine. 1994. *DPT vaccine and chronic nervous system dysfunctions: A new analysis.* Washington, DC: The National Academies Press.

5. Ray P, Hayward J, Michelson D, et al. 2006. Encephalopathy after whole-cell pertussis or measles vaccination. Lack of evidence for a causal association in a retrospective case-control study. *Pediatric Infectious Disease Journal* 25:768-73.

6. Kuno-Sakai H, Kimura M. 2004. Safety and efficacy of acellular pertussis vaccine in Japan, evaluated by 23 years of its use for routine immunization. *Pediatrics International* 46:650-5.

7. Moore DL, Le Saux N, Scheifele D, et al. 2004. Lack of evidence of encephalopathy related to pertussis vaccine: Active surveillance by IMPACT, Canada 1993-2002. *Pediatric Infectious Disease Journal* 23:568-71.

8. Berkovic SF, Harkin L, McMahon JM, et al. 2006. De-novo mutations of the sodium channel gene SCN1A in alleged vaccine encephalopathy: A retrospective study. *Lancet Neurology* 5:488-92.

9. Marini C, Mei D, Temudo T, et al. 2007. Idiopathic epilepsies with seizures precipitated by fever and SCN1A abnormalities. *Epilepsia* 48:1678-85.

10. Institute of Medicine. 1994. *Adverse events associated with childhood vaccines: Evidence bearing on causality.* Washington DC: National Academies Press.

11. Black S, Shinefield H, Pay P, et al. 1997. Risk of hospitalization because of aseptic meningitis after measles-mumps-rubella vaccination in one- to two-year-old children: An analysis of Vaccine Safety Datalink (VSD) project. *Peditatric Infectious Disease Journal* 16:500-3.

12. Mäkelä A, Nuorti JP, Peltola H. 2002. Neurologic disorders after measles-mumps-rubella vaccination. *Pediatrics* 110:957-63.

13. Miller D, Wadsworth J, Diamond J, et al. 1997. Measles vaccination and neurological events. *The Lancet* 349:730-1.

14. Bellini WJ, Rota JS, Lowe LE, et al. 2005. Subacute sclerosing panencephalitis: More cases of this fatal disease are prevented by measles immunization than was previously recognized. *Journal of Infectious Diseases* 192:1686-93.

15. Institute of Medicine. 2003. *Vaccinations and sudden unexpected death in infancy*. Washington, DC: National Academies Press.

16. Eriksen EM, Perlman JA, Miller A, et al. 2004. Lack of association between hepatitis B birth immunization and neonatal death: A population-based study from the vaccine safety datalink project. *Pediatric Infectious Disease* 23:656-62.

17. Vennemann MMT, Buterfab-Bahloul T, Jorch G, et al. 2007. Sudden infant death syndrome: No increased risk after immunization. *Vaccine* 25:336-40.

18. Vennemann MMT, Hoffgen M, Bajanowski T, et al. 2007. Do immunizations reduce the risk for SIDS? A meta analysis. *Vaccine* 25:4875-9.

19. Institute of Medicine. 2002. *Immunization safety review: SV40 contamination of polio vaccine and cancer*. Washington, DC: National Academies Press.

20. Carroll-Pankhurst C, Engels EA, Strickler HD, et al. 2001. Thirty-five year mortality following receipt of SV40-contaminated polio vaccine during the neonatal period. *British Journal of Cancer* 85:1295-7.

21. Rollison DE, Page WF, Crawford H, et al. 2004. Case-control study of cancer among US Army veterans exposed to simian virus 40-contaminated adenovirus vaccine. *American Journal of Epidemiology* 160:317-24.

22. Engels EA, Rodman LH, Frisch M, et al. 2003. Childhood exposure to simian virus 40-contaminated poliovirus vaccine and risk of AIDS-associated non-Hodgkin's lymphoma. *International Journal of Cancer* 106:283-7.

23. Poulin DL, DeCaprio JA. 2006. Is there a role for SV40 in human cancer. *Journal of Clinical Oncology* 24:4356-65.

24. López-Ríos F, Illei PB, Ladanyi M. 2004. Evidence against a role for SV40 infection in human mesotheliomas and high risk of false-positive PCR results owing to presence of SV40 sequences in common laboratory plasmids. *The Lancet* 364:1157-66.

25. Worobey M, Santiago ML, Keele BF, et al. 2004. Contaminated polio vaccine theory refuted. *Nature* 428:820.

26. Plotkin SA. 2004. Chimpanzees and journalists. *Vaccine* 22:1829-30.

27. Transcript of July 27, 2000, CBER meeting, p. 120. (Accessed April 30, 2008, at *www.fda.gov/ohrms/dockets/ac/00/transcripts/3635t1b.pdf*.)

28. Gibbons RV, Holman RC, Belay ED, Schonberger LB. 2000. Creutzfeldt-Jakob disease in the United States: 1979-1998. *Journal of the American Medical Association* 284:2322-3.

29. Gall, SA 2003. Maternal immunization. *Obstetrics and Gynecology Clinics of North America* 30:632-6.

30. Centers for Disease Control and Prevention. 1998 (updated 2007). Guidelines for vaccinating pregnant women. (Accessed March 27, 2008, at *www.cdc.gov/vaccines/pubs/preg-guide.htm*.)

31. Centers for Disease Control and Prevention. 2006. Prevention and control of influenza: Recommendations of the Advisory Committee on Immunization Practices (ACIP). *Morbidity & Mortality Weekly Report* 55 (RR-10):1-41.

32. Centers for Disease Control and Prevention. 2006. Preventing tetanus, diphtheria, and pertussis among adults: Use of tetanus toxoid, reduced diphtheria toxoid and acellular pertussis vaccine. *Morbidity & Mortality Weekly Report* 55(RR-17):1-37.

33. Wison E, Goss MA, Marin M, et al. 2008. Varicella vaccine exposure during pregnancy: Data from 10 years of the pregnancy registry. *Journal of Infectious Diseases* 197:S178-84.

34. AAP, Committee on Infectious Diseases. 2006. Varicella-Zoster infections. In: Pickering LK, ed. *Red Book: 2006 Report of the Commit-*

tee on Infectious Diseases. 27th ed. Elk Grove Village, IL: American Academy of Pediatrics, pp. 711-25.

35. Centers for Disease Control and Prevention. 2008. Rubella. In: Atkinson W, Hamborsky J, McIntyre L, Wolfe S, eds. *Epidemiology and prevention of vaccine-preventable diseases.* 10th ed. Washington, DC: Public Health Foundation.

36. AAP, Committee on Infectious Diseases. 2006. Rubella. In: Pickering LK, ed. *Red Book: 2006 Report of the Committee on Infectious Diseases.* 27th ed. Elk Grove Village, IL: American Academy of Pediatrics, pp. 574-9.

37. Centers for Disease Control and Prevention. 2008. Hepatitis B. In: Atkinson W, Hamborsky J, McIntyre L, Wolfe S, eds. *Epidemiology and prevention of vaccine-preventable diseases,* 10th ed. Washington, DC: Public Health Foundation.

38. American College of Obstetricians and Gynecologists. 2003. ACOG Committee Opinion 282: Immunization during pregnancy. *International Journal of Gynecology and Obstetrics* 81:123-8.

39. Centers for Disease Control and Prevention. 2005. Prevention and control of meningococcal disease. *Morbidity & Mortality Weekly Report* 55(RR07):1-21.

40. Centers for Disease Control and Prevention. 2006. Prevention of hepatitis A through active or passive immunization. Recommendations of the Advisory Committee on Immunization Practices (ACIP). *Morbidity & Mortality Weekly Report* 55(RR-7):1-23.

41. Wiesen AR, Littell CT. 2002. Relationship between prepregnancy anthrax vaccination and pregnancy and birth outcomes among US Army women. *Journal of the American Medical Association,* 287:1556-60.

42. Department of Defense. (Accessed March 27, 2008, at *www.anthrax. osd.mil/resource/qna/qaAll.asp?cID=312.*)

43. Centers for Disease Control and Prevention. 2000. Use of anthrax vaccine in the United States: Recommendations of the Advisory Committee on Immunization Practices. *Morbidity & Mortality Weekly Report* 49(RR15):1-20.

44. Centers for Disease Control and Prevention. 2002. Notice to readers: Status of U.S. Department of Defense preliminary evaluation of the association of anthrax vaccination and congenital anomalies. *Morbidity & Mortality Weekly Report* 51:127.

45. Centers for Disease Control and Prevention. 2007. Quadrivalent human papillomavirus vaccine. Recommendations of the Advisory Committee on Immunization Practices (ACIP). *Morbidity & Mortality Weekly Report* 56(RR-2):1-23.

Index

A

D

E

F

J

K

L

M

R

S

T

U

uncertainty, scientific— *38*
United Kingdom— *37, 80-84, 209*

V

Vaccine Adverse Event Reporting System (VAERS)— *42, 60-63, 86, 99, 100, 105, 188*
vaccine-associated paralytic polio (VAPP)— *26*
Vaccine Injury Compensation Program— *37, 38, 94, 141, 142*
Vaccine Safety Datalink (VSD)— *42, 62-66, 134, 164, 166, 170, 186, 190*
varicella. SEE *chickenpox*

W

Wakefield— *82, 84, 100, 103, 104, 146, 147*
whooping cough. SEE *pertussis*
World Health Organization— *115, 125, 149*

Y

yellow fever— *134, 214*

About the Authors

Martin G. Myers, MD and Diego Pineda, MS are, respectively, the editor and the science writer for the National Network for Immunization Information (NNii). They have co-authored more than 80 peer-reviewed articles on immunization issues and the best-selling booklet *Are Vaccines Safe? Evaluating Information About Immunizations on the Internet.*

Dr. Myers is an internationally recognized vaccine expert and former director for the Department of Health and Human Service's National Vaccine Program Office. He is presently a professor in the Departments of Pediatrics at the University of Texas Medical Branch at Galveston (UTMB). He is a pediatrician who received his AB (Magna Cum Laude) from Princeton University and his MD from The John Hopkins University.

Mr. Pineda is an officer in the southwest chapter of the American Medical Writers Association (AMWA) and is actively involved in the medical writing community. He often presents at conferences on the topics of risk communication and medical writing. He holds a masters degree in science and technology journalism from Texas A&M University.

Quick Order Form
Immunizations for Public Health (i4ph)

FAX ORDERS: 409-772-5208. Send this form.
TELEPHONE ORDERS: Call 409-772-0199. Have your credit card ready.
EMAIL ORDERS: nnii@i4ph.org
INTERNET ORDERS: **www.DoVaccinesCauseThat.com**
POSTAL ORDERS: Immunizations for Public Health
301 University Blvd., Galveston, TX 77555-0351, USA.

Do Vaccines Cause That?!
A Guide for Evaluating Vaccine Safety Concerns

NAME: _____

ADDRESS: _____

CITY, STATE, & ZIP: _____

PHONE: _____

EMAIL: _____

COST: $14.95 X _____ (number of copies) = $ _____

SALES TAX: _____ Please add 8.25% for books shipped to Texas addresses.

SHIPPING:

US: $5.00 for first book and $3.00 for each additional book (3–5 days).

International: $10.00 for first book to Canada and Mexico and $6.00 for each additional book (6–10 days). Other countries, $12.00 for first book and $8.00 for each additional book.

ORDER TOTAL: _____

For other related products, visit:
www.immunizationinfo.org/bookstore.cfm

events. . . . That he is also a novelist is evident in his prose; he's skillful in making characters come alive and keeping readers engaged." —Sandee Brawarsky, *Jewish Week*

"As a comprehensive examination of the Unites States' association with the Middle East, his much-needed book fills a gap in the literature. . . . This is a wonderfully rich and thought-provoking history. . . . Highly recommended for all public and academic libraries."
—*Library Journal*

"Even at more than 700 pages, the book leaves a reader wanting more. And because the detailed text reads so fluidly, all of that information is palatable, and much of it is downright gripping. . . . With Oren's survey as a guide, any reader can become grounded in the realities of the vast Middle East."
—Steve Weinberg, *St. Louis Post-Dispatch*

"*Power, Faith, and Fantasy* provides a rich and complex context for assessing America's embattled role in the Middle East today."
—Lawrence Grossman, *The New Leader*

"Oren knows how to tell a story, turn a phrase and tweak a delightful detail." —Glenn Altschuler, *Baltimore Sun*

"There is no better introduction to the history of U.S. involvement in the Middle East than this highly readable book."
—Paul Collins, *Sydney Morning Herald*

"Oren provides not an exhaustive study of recent Middle East history but rather an indispensable overview of its crucial turning points and trends." —Jack Fischel, *Courier Mail*

"Because there is no other book with such a sweeping view of the subject, the vast cast of characters Oren presents and the exhaustively researched tales of the way they played on each other will shape our thinking about America and the Middle East for years. . . . For now *Power, Faith, and Fantasy* is the best history we have of the history we've had, and an indispensable guide from point A to point Z."　　　　　　　　　　—Christopher Dickey, *Newsweek*

"*Power, Faith, and Fantasy: America in the Middle East, 1776 to the Present*, Michael B. Oren's brilliant, sweeping account of America's considerably longer, vastly more complex entanglement in the region is a much-needed antidote, a fuller picture of the motivations behind an engagement that began in the very infancy of the republic, when Israel was a mere dream and the combustion engine not even a blueprint. . . . This is a majestically told story, its grand themes brought to life by a succession of riveting characters."
　　　　　　　　　—Gerard Baker, *The Times* (London)

"Mr. Oren goes on to list almost a dozen titles, some very highly regarded, on America and the Middle East that have fallen short of providing 'the full sweep of America's centuries-old engagement with the Middle East in all of its military, economic, and cultural aspects.' This is exactly what he provides, and much of the pleasure of working through the book is realizing how well he does it. . . . An abundance of little stories and vignettes, persons and personalities, touching on all these themes make up Mr. Oren's narrative. . . . To say this book is timely is only to say that all well-written history is timely. . . . As captivating as many of these stories are, the real worth of the book comes only when the reader takes it as a whole. A subtle and refreshing assumption about the importance of history and its relationship to the present underlies every page. . . . Mr. Oren has made a significant and readable contribution to the understanding of the historic relationship of America with the Middle East. It is a book worth seeking out."　　　—David A. Smith, *Washington Times*

"One of the most important books on the subject to be published in this or any other year. . . . *Power, Faith, and Fantasy: America in the Middle East, 1776 to the Present* by Israeli historian Michael Oren fills a void that has long existed in the historiography of the Middle East. Until the release of this beautifully written and meticulously researched volume this month, there simply was no comprehensive history of American involvement in the region. . . . Oren's achievement is must-reading for policymakers and the general public alike. In an era in which global terror based in the Middle East is the primary challenge to the survival of democracy, *Power, Faith, and Fantasy* ought to be read and understood by as many Americans as possible." —Jonathan S. Tobin, *Jerusalem Post*

"In his magisterial history of the relationship between the United States and the Middle East, Michael Oren provides an exhaustively researched and compellingly told exercise in déjà vu. . . . Oren's engrossing narrative reads like a who's who of American history. . . . Even the historical footnotes are fascinating. . . . Oren is a wonderful storyteller. The ability to move from minute-by-minute chronicling to sketching the grand sweep of history is no easy feat, but he does so with elegance and a flair for the dramatic." —Robert Satloff, *New York Post*

"What Oren does is cull the history and put together a single, easy-to-read package. He's thorough without sounding academic, which is a definite plus when you sit down with more than 700 pages of history. . . . Possess even the scantest level of curiosity, and this is the kind of book that'll lead you into an adventure of discovery." —Zachary Reid, *Richmond Times-Dispatch*

"Oren effectively traces and harnesses the many threads of America's connectedness to the Middle East, from its evangelical missions to its consuming thirst for oil. It is a panoramic view, ranging from the adventures of early visitors like John Ledyard, who fell in love with the Oregon territory when he sailed with Captain Cook but became the first American to explore the Middle East, to the cynical observations of Mark Twain, who wrote that the holy city of Jerusalem was 'grimy and impoverished,' full of lepers, idiots and Western pilgrims. Oren's book is a rare hybrid: It is appealing as entertainment and useful as a reference work on America's long and volatile engagement with the Middle East." —Mike Francis, *The Oregonian*

"Compelling. . . . Mr. Oren's sweeping, highly textured history of the 230-year interaction between America and the Middle East told me much I did not know. . . . Mr. Oren's work is prodigious, drawing upon hundreds of original and archival sources—letters, memoirs, books, and government documents, which he skillfully weaves into a finely drawn narrative that alternates among cultural, political, and economic interactions."   —Judith Miller, *New York Sun*

POWER, FAITH, AND FANTASY

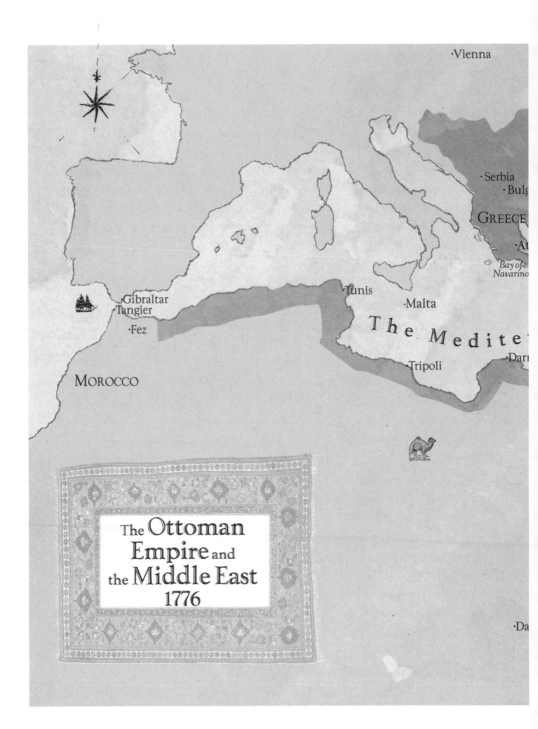

·Vienna

·Serbia
·Bulg

GREECE

At

Bay of
Navarino

Gibraltar
·Tangier

·Fez

·Tunis

·Malta

The Mediter

·Tripoli

·Dar

MOROCCO

The Ottoman
Empire and
the Middle East
1776

·Da

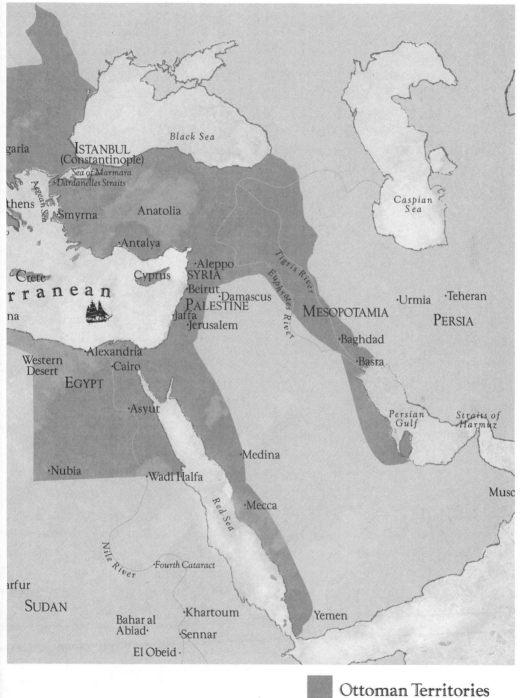

ISTANBUL
(Constantinople)

Sea of Marmara
Dardanelles Straits

garia

Black Sea

Caspian
Sea

thens

Aegean Sea

·Smyrna

Anatolia

Crete

·Antalya

Cyprus

·Aleppo
SYRIA
·Beirut
·Damascus

·Urmia   ·Teheran

PERSIA

rranean

PALESTINE
·Jaffa
·Jerusalem

Tigris River
Euphrates River

MESOPOTAMIA

·Baghdad

·Basra

na

·Alexandria
·Cairo

Western
Desert

EGYPT

Persian
Gulf

Straits of
Harmuz

·Asyut

·Nubia

·Wadi Halfa

·Medina

Musc

Red Sea

·Mecca

Nile River

arfur

SUDAN

·Fourth Cataract

·Khartoum

Bahar al
Abiad·

·Sennar

El Obeid ·

Yemen

Ottoman Territories

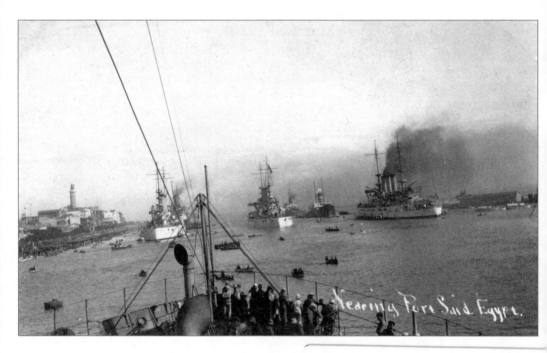

Warships of America's Great White Fleet preparing to enter the
Suez Canal in January 1909.

POWER, FAITH, AND FANTASY

America in the Middle East,
1776 to the Present

Michael B. Oren

W. W. NORTON & COMPANY
NEW YORK   LONDON

For information about permission to reproduce selections from this book,
write to Permissions, W. W. Norton & Company, Inc.,
500 Fifth Avenue, New York, NY 10110

Manufacturing by RR Donnelley, Harrisonburg
Book design by Lovedog Studio
Production manager: Devon Zahn

Library of Congress Cataloging-in-Publication Data

Oren, Michael B., 1955–
Power, faith, and fantasy : America in the Middle East, 1776 to the present /
Michael B. Oren.
p.   cm.
Includes bibliographical references and index.
ISBN-13: 978-0-393-05826-0 (hardcover)
ISBN-10: 0-393-05826-3 (hardcover)
1. Middle East—Foreign relations—United States. 2. United States—
Foreign relations—Middle East. I. Title.
DS63.2.U5054 2007
327.73056—dc22
2006036571

ISBN 978-0-393-33030-4 pbk.

W. W. Norton & Company, Inc.
500 Fifth Avenue, New York, N.Y. 10110
www.wwnorton.com

W. W. Norton & Company Ltd.
Castle House, 75/76 Wells Street, London W1T 3QT

3 4 5 6 7 8 9 0

To Yossi Klein Halevi, my colleague and friend,
who helped make this book possible,
and for my wife, Sally,
who makes everything possible.

CONTENTS

Part Six
OIL, WAR, AND ASCENDANCY

Part Seven
IN SEARCH OF PAX AMERICANA

Black Sea

Russia

Caspian Sea

• Ankara

Turkey

Mersin •

Lake Van

Lake Urmia

• Urfa

Alexandretta

Mosul •

Persia

Cyprus

Latakia

Syria

French

• Hamdan

Lebanon

• Beirut

• Damascus

Tigris

• Kermanshah

Iraq

British

• Baghdad

Mediterranean Sea

Palestine

• Amman

Jerusalem •

Euphrates

Trans-Jordan

Egypt

Aqaba •

• Jauf

Basra •

Persian Gulf

Hejaz

• Kuweit

Arabia

Red Sea

Postwar Middle East Mandates

.... Railways   Border

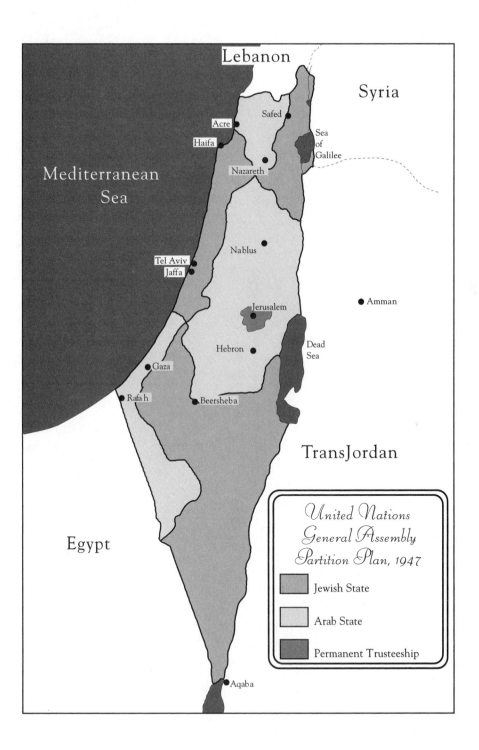

Lebanon

Syria

Mediterranean
Sea

Safed

Acre

Haifa

Sea
of
Galilee

Nazareth

Nablus

Tel Aviv
Jaffa

Jerusalem

Amman

Hebron

Dead
Sea

Gaza

Rafah

Beersheba

TransJordan

Egypt

United Nations
General Assembly
Partition Plan, 1947

Jewish State

Arab State

Permanent Trusteeship

Aqaba

CHRONOLOGY

1776–1800

1776 By declaring its independence, the United States forfeits the protection of Britain's navy and faces the Barbary pirates alone.

1777 Morocco recognizes American independence.

1784 The Boston brig *Betsy* is seized by Moroccan pirates.

1785 John Lamb conducts the first American diplomatic mission to the Middle East.

1785 Thomas Jefferson and John Adams meet with the emissary of Tripoli.

1787 Spurred in part by the need to confront North Africa, delegates meet in Philadelphia to draft a constitution.

1788 John Ledyard, the first American to explore the Middle East, arrives in Egypt.

1794 Congress votes to create a navy "adequate for the protection of the commerce of the United States against Algerian corsairs."

1801–1900

1801 Tripoli declares war on the United States.

1803 Tripoli captures the USS *Philadelphia* and its 305-man crew.

1804 American forces burn the *Philadelphia* in Tripoli's harbor.

1805 William Eaton and U.S. Marines and mercenaries attack Darna, on the North African coast. Jefferson makes a separate peace arrangement with Tripoli.

1815 James Madison dispatches an American fleet to force Algiers, Tripoli, and Tunis to cease attacks against American ships.

1819 The first American missionaries to the Middle East, Levi Parsons and Pliny Fisk, depart Boston.

1821 The Greek war of independence begins, forcing the United States to choose between its democratic ideals and its economic interests in the Ottoman Empire.

1823 Pliny Fisk establishes the first American school in the Middle East.

1830 President Andrew Jackson secures a treaty between the United States and the Ottoman Empire.

1831 David Porter, America's first ambassador in the Middle East, arrives in Istanbul.

1832 Washington Irving publishes *Alhambra*, an anthology of Arabian tales. The United States signs a commercial treaty with Muscat, today's Oman.

1835 The American traveler John Lloyd Stephens lands in Alexandria.

1837 Edward Robinson establishes the field of biblical archaeology.

1837 The American evangelist Harriet Livermore sets out for Palestine.

1840 The *Sultanah* becomes the first Middle Eastern vessel to dock in the United States.

1842 Cyrus Hamlin opens a school on the outskirts of Istanbul, laying the foundation for Robert College.

1844 Warder Cresson, restorationist and U.S. consul, sets sail for Palestine.

1848 William Francis Lynch becomes the first explorer to navigate the Jordan River from the Sea of Galilee to the Dead Sea.

1851 Clorinda Minor arrives in Palestine with the goal of establishing an agricultural school to furnish the Jews with the skills necessary for statehood.

1856 Herman Melville tours the Middle East.

1858 Washington dispatches the diplomat Edwin De Leon to Jaffa to demand justice for the victims of an Arab assault on the Dickson colony. The former slave David F. Dorr publishes an account of his Middle Eastern travels.

1862 Daniel Bliss formally proposes the opening of the Arab world's first modern university—the Syrian Protestant College, later renamed the American University at Beirut.

1863 President Lincoln protests the presence of Egyptian troops in Mexico.

1865 John Surrat, a conspirator in the Lincoln assassination, is arrested in Egypt.

1866 George Adams recruits 156 Americans to form a colony in Palestine.

1867 Mark Twain tours the Middle East and publishes his impressions in *The Innocents Abroad.*

1868 The Egyptian leader Isma'il enlists Civil War veterans to modernize his army and strengthen U.S.-Egyptian ties.

1872 General William Tecumseh Sherman and Ralph Waldo Emerson tour the Middle East.

1878 The former president Ulysses S. Grant tours the Middle East.

1880 An ancient Egyptian obelisk, popularly known as Cleopatra's Needle, is erected in New York's Central Park.

1881 Followers of the Spafford family establish the American Colony in Jerusalem.

1882 Marines land in Alexandria, Egypt, after the British bombard the city. The poet Emma Lazarus pioneers American Zionism.

1883 Samuel Benjamin heads America's first official mission to Persia.

1888 The Lebanese poet and political activist Ameen Rihani arrives in the United States.

1890 Samuel Zwemer, the first Western missionary to penetrate the Arabian Peninsula, departs for the Middle East.

1891 William Blackstone submits his memorial calling for American support for Jewish statehood in Palestine to President Benjamin Harrison.

1893 Millions of Americans partake of Middle Eastern fantasy at Chicago's World Columbian Exposition.

1896 Clara Barton travels to Turkey to aid the Armenian victims of Turkish atrocities.

1897 The First Zionist Congress is held in Basel, Switzerland; four Americans participate.

1900–1945

1901 Ellen Stone, an American missionary in Bulgaria, is kidnapped by local Christians attempting to finance their revolt against Turkey.

1902 The American naval theorist Alfred Mahan coins the term "Middle East."

1904 The expatriate businessman Ion Perdicaris is kidnapped by the Moroccan chieftain Raisuli.

1906 Theodore Roosevelt helps resolve a Franco-German conflict over imperial rights in North Africa at the Algeciras Conference.

1909 The State Department Division of Near Eastern Affairs (NEA) is created.

1909 The American missionary Howard Baskerville is killed while leading an Iranian peasant revolt.

1910 Theodore Roosevelt tours the Middle East.

1912 Henrietta Szold establishes the women's Zionist organization Hadassah.

1915 The American ambassador to Turkey Henry Morgenthau tries to aid the victims of the Armenian genocide. American cruisers evacuate Jews from Palestine and missionaries from Beirut.

1917 Louis Brandeis helps persuade Woodrow Wilson to endorse the Balfour Declaration, the British government's pledge to foster a Jewish homeland in Palestine. Ameen Rihani urges Arab Americans to volunteer for military service.

1918 President Woodrow Wilson promises self-determination for the nations of the Middle East.

1919 The Paris Peace Conference. President Woodrow Wilson vainly attempts to secure independence for the Middle East.

1921 Rudolph Valentino stars in *The Sheikh of Araby*, Hollywood's first Middle Eastern fantasy. Golda Meir leaves Wisconsin for Palestine.

1923 Khalil Gibran's *The Prophet* is published.

1924 American and European oil companies form the Iraq Petroleum Company (IPC). The journalist Lowell Thomas publishes *With Lawrence in Arabia*. The United States recognizes the British mandate over Palestine.

1928 The Red Line Agreement, specifying areas for IPC oil exploration in the Middle East, is concluded.

1931 Charles Crane meets with ibn Saud, laying the foundation for future American-Saudi cooperation.

1932 The American engineer Karl Twitchell surveys the Arabian Peninsula for water, mineral deposits, and oil.

1933 Saudi Arabia grants American oil companies the right to prospect for oil.

1938 Conservationist Walter Lowdermilk devises an irrigation system for the Jewish community of Palestine.

1938 American engineers strike oil in Damman, Saudi Arabia.

1939 American Zionists protest the issuance of Britain's White Paper that curtails Jewish immigration to Palestine.

1942 Operation Torch commences as American troops lead an invasion of North Africa. Zionist representatives meet at New York's Biltmore Hotel and declare their goal of establishing an independent Jewish state in Palestine.

1943 The United States, together with Great Britain, compels France to respect Lebanon's independence. James McCauley Landis becomes director of the Middle East Supply Center. Roosevelt's personal emissary to the Middle East, Patrick J. Hurley, recommends American support for native nationalism.

1945 FDR meets with ibn Saud on the Great Bitter Lake, cementing the American-Saudi partnership. The new Truman administration forces France to remove its troops from Syria and blocks Soviet attempts to gain control over Libya.

1946–The Present

1946 The United States, working through the United Nations, successfully pressures the Soviet Union to withdraw from Iran.

1947 President Truman declares his doctrine for defending Greece and Turkey from Soviet aggression. The United States, along with thirty-two other nations, votes in favor of UN Resolution 181, partitioning Palestine into independent Arab and Jewish states.

1948 Eleven minutes after its creation, Israel receives de facto recognition from the United States.

1952 The CIA assists a group of Free Officers, including Colonel Gamal Abdul Nasser, to seize power in Egypt.

1953 A coup facilitated by the CIA ousts Iranian nationalist leader Mossadegh from power.

1955 The Baghdad Pact, an American-backed, anticommunist coalition, is created.

1956 The Suez Crisis. The United States, together with the Soviet Union, compels Britain, France, and Israel to withdraw their forces from Egyptian territory and uphold Nasser's nationalization of the Suez Canal.

1957 President Eisenhower issues his doctrine for the defense of the Middle East against communism.

1958 American troops land in Lebanon in support of the pro-Western government of Camille Chamoun.

1961 President Kennedy initiates a correspondence with President Nasser of Egypt.

1962 The Kennedy administration approves the sale of Hawk antiaircraft missiles to Israel. The film *Lawrence of Arabia* is released to popular acclaim.

1967 The United States supports Israel in its six-day victory over Arab armies and its conquest of the West Bank, Gaza, Jerusalem, the Golan Heights, and the Sinai Peninsula. The Johnson administration initiates the Arab-Israeli peace process on the basis of the territory-for-peace formula contained in UN Resolution 242.

1969 Secretary of State William Rogers announces his plan for Arab-Israel peace based on UN Resolution 242.

1970 The PLO attempts to seize power in Jordan in a brutal internecine conflict known as Black September.

1973 The United States undertakes a massive airlift to Israel after Egypt and Syria launch a surprise attack. Saudi Arabia spearheads an oil boycott against the United States because of American support for Israel.

1974 Henry Kissinger's famous "shuttle diplomacy" produces a disengagement of Egyptian and Israeli forces in the Sinai Peninsula.

1979 President Jimmy Carter mediates a peace agreement between Egypt and Israel. Fifty-two Americans, most of them employees of the U.S. embassy, are taken hostage by Islamic revolutionary militants in Teheran.

1980 An attempt to rescue the American hostages in Iran fails. President Carter tells Congress of his commitment to defend American interests in the Persian Gulf.

1981 American jets shoot down two Libyan fighters in the Gulf of Sidra. The Reagan administration condemns Israel's attack on the Iraqi nuclear reactor at Osirk.

1983 A suicide bombing ordered by Hizbollah kills 241 American Marines sent to maintain the peace in Lebanon's civil war.

1984 The United States withdraws its forces from Lebanon. William Buckley, the American CIA chief in Beirut, is kidnapped and tortured to death.

1986 In response to a terror attack on American servicemen in a Berlin nightclub, President Reagan bombs Libya.

1986 The Iran-Contra scandal breaks, exposing illicit arms deals between the Reagan White House and Iran's revolutionary government.

1987 The Palestinian uprising, or *intifada*, begins in Gaza and the West Bank.

1987 The U.S. Navy provides escorts for Kuwaiti oil tankers in order to deter attacks from Iran.

1990 Iraq invades Kuwait.

1991 An American-led coalition expels Iraqi forces from Kuwait, but leaves Saddam Hussein in power. After the war, the United States convenes the Madrid Peace Conference, an attempt to achieve a general Arab-Israeli settlement.

1993 The Oslo Accords, the result of secret Israeli-Palestinian negotiations in Norway, are signed on the White House Lawn.

1996 Nineteen Americans troops are killed in a terror attack on the Khobar Towers housing complex in Saudi Arabia.

1998 President Clinton brokers an interim Palestinian-Israeli agreement at Wye River Plantation. Responding to al-Qaeda attacks in Africa, the United States bombs presumed terrorist targets in Sudan.

2000 A suicide bomber kills seventeen sailors aboard the USS *Cole* near the Yemen coast.

2001 Al-Qaeda attacks in New York, Virginia, and Pennsylvania kill nearly three thousand civilians.

2002 The United States declares war on and topples the Taliban regime in Afghanistan.

2003 The United States invades Iraq.

POWER, FAITH, AND FANTASY

John Ledyard

A PASSAGE
TO GLORY

IN A CANOE THAT HE HOLLOWED OUT WITH HIS OWN hands from a great white pine tree, John Ledyard paddled down the Connecticut River. A thick-chested youth, he rowed, his tawny hair streaming behind him, his aquiline nose pitched toward the prow. He descended on waters swollen by the springtime thaw, past mountains stippled with ice, several hundred miles to the Long Island Sound. Vast distances still stretched before him, though, before he reached his ultimate destination—a land of labyrinthine ruins and deserts annealed by the sun. Though he scarcely knew it then, in 1773, John Ledyard would become the first citizen of an independent United States to explore the Middle East, to record his impressions of the region, and to render it intelligible to Americans.

Ledyard's concern that spring was not to reach the Middle East but rather to escape the scrutiny of the Reverend Eleazar Wheelock, Dartmouth's domineering president. Wheelock had been convinced that Ledyard, a New Hampshire frontiersman who once lived among the Iroquois, would make a superior missionary and pressured him to attend the college. But Ledyard, at twenty-three, was far more interested in exploration than in theology. He yearned for adventure, to become, as he wrote his widowed mother, "the greatest traveler in history . . . excentric, irregular, rapid, unaccountable, curious and . . . majestic as a comet." He lasted a single semester at Dartmouth before canoeing down the Connecticut, plying toward the ocean and the world.[1]

Ledyard began his journey inauspiciously, as a simple sailor aboard a merchantman bound for the West Indies. Life aboard the rat-infested sloops of the late eighteenth century was hardly swash-buckling, though, and as the vessel turned eastward toward the Mediterranean, Ledyard again decided to flee. Disembarking at Gibraltar in July 1776, he joined the British marines. That same month, Great Britain went to war against its rebellious American colonies, now cohered as the United States, and Ledyard might well have found himself battling against his countrymen. Providentially, though, he was posted not to a gunboat but to the HMS *Resolution*, the flagship of Britain's most celebrated captain, James Cook.

The discoverer of Tahiti and the Hawaiian Islands, Cook was now embarking on his third world excursion, traversing the Pacific to the Oregon and Alaskan coasts in search of a waterway across the con-tinent—the legendary Northwest Passage. Ledyard kept a journal of the expedition, vividly describing the tattooed South Sea Islanders he encountered and the Hawaiian warriors who, on February 14, 1779, ambushed and murdered Cook. The horror of that incident could not, however, eclipse the splendor of the densely forested Oregon Territory, on the North American coast. Ledyard yearned to return to the area and to make his fortune by fur trapping. He set out to realize that dream by jumping ship off the shoreline of Long Island in 1782 and reuniting with his native land.

Though America had nearly achieved its independence by that time, the Continental Army remained on a war footing and Ledyard might still have served in its ranks. But he was far too restive to reen-list. He saw himself "dancing through life between . . . two extremes," misery and happiness, "a being indigenous to no sphere or unfit for any." He published his journal of the Cook expedition, which became the first major travel book printed in the United States and, by eighteenth-century terms, a bestseller. At age thirty-three, Ledyard had probably seen more of the world—and more of the North American continent—than perhaps any other person alive.

His mind, though, remained fixed on Oregon and his vision of establishing a fur-trading post. Failing to find backers for his scheme in the United States, however, Ledyard once more exited his homeland and in 1785 set sail for France.

Ledyard embodied the American frontier spirit that Frenchmen at that moment revered and they afforded him access to some of the most exalted personages in Paris. He also befriended Benjamin Franklin, America's first representative to France, as well as the Revolutionary firebrand Tom Paine and Continental Navy hero John Paul Jones. His warmest and most influential relationship, though, was with a worldly aristocrat who appeared to have little in common with this former backwoodsman and deckhand.

"[W]hile at Paris, I became acquainted with John Ledyard . . . a man of genius, of some science, and of fearless courage and enterprise," wrote Thomas Jefferson, who had succeeded Franklin as ambassador. Tall, lanky, and fair-skinned, Jefferson cut a contrasting figure with the brawny, weather-beaten voyager, but the two men immediately bonded. Jefferson regarded Ledyard as "a man of truth" possessed of "unrivalled intrepidity" and "roaming, restless character." Returning the commendation, Ledyard called Jefferson "my brother my father my friend."[2]

Jefferson was riveted by Ledyard's descriptions of Oregon and tantalized by the possibility of finding a water route between that territory and America's east coast. He persuaded Ledyard to return to Oregon by way of Russia and the Bering Strait and to search for this fabled Northwest Passage. Jefferson even appealed to the Russian empress Catherine the Great to permit Ledyard to cross through her lands unscathed. Catherine dismissed the project as "chimerical," but her skepticism failed to daunt Ledyard. Starting in the winter of 1787, he walked from Stockholm to St. Petersburg and then proceeded by canoe and snowsled, three thousand frozen miles, to eastern Siberia. Catherine's agents arrested him there, however, and deported him from Russia.

The ordeal left Ledyard visibly aged, but otherwise undeterred. "An American face does not wear well like an American heart," he proclaimed. He kept up a vigorous correspondence with Jefferson, positing the then groundbreaking theories that Native Americans were the descendants of prehistoric emigrants from Asia and that all human beings, irrespective of race, shared a single ancestor. But he never abandoned his ambition of exploring uncharted territories, and in search of a new sponsor, Ledyard relocated to London. There he gained the attention of the prestigious African Society and of its flamboyant secretary, Henry Beaufoy. Impressed with the "manliness of his person, the breadth of his chest, the openness of his countenance, and the inquietude of his eyes," Beaufoy proposed that Ledyard probe the length of the Nile, from Cairo to Sennar in the eastern Sudan, a journey never before undertaken by a Westerner. Ledyard volunteered to leave at once, but Beaufoy explained that the society planned its expeditions meticulously and that several months at least would pass before he could depart for Egypt.

Ledyard readied himself physically with twenty-mile hikes, and mentally by poring over maps of the Middle East, most of which were conjectural. He made contact with America's acting minister to Great Britain, William Stephens Smith, and through him agreed to "exercise his talents and Industry for the immediate service of his own country" by exploring in the name of the United States. Finally, on June 30, 1788, with the preparations for his journey completed, Ledyard left London for Marseille. "My path will be from here . . . across the Mediterranean . . . to Grand Cairo," he jotted in a final note to his mother. "Beyond is unknown, and my discoveries begin. Where they will terminate, and how, you shall know, if I survive." He also wrote Jefferson, thanking him for his friendship and trust and promising to honor them both. "I . . . do not think that mountains or oceans shall oppose my passage to glory," Ledyard predicted. "My heart is on fire."

John Ledyard was bound for the Middle East, a region steeped in myths, an area that few Westerners of his time had ever visited, much less penetrated in depth. What, beside hardship and hostility, did he expect to find there? What similarities of history, theology, and culture could possibly bind these distant, alien lands to the recently wrought democracy of the United States? And what sort of common future might these seemingly incompatible sections of the globe, America and the Middle East, forge?

Such questions were certainly pertinent in the 1780s, yet Americans have continued to raise them ever since. While Ledyard, whose journey to Egypt will be recounted in a subsequent chapter, was the first American to explore the Middle East, he was merely one of the millions of his countrymen and women who, over the course of more than two centuries, traveled and ministered to the region, studied and wrote about it, abetted and battled it. That interaction would indelibly transform the Middle East, but it would also alter, sometimes strengthen and at other times divide, the United States.

Ledyard's voyage to the Middle East was indeed a "passage to glory" for him as well as for his fellow Americans, both then and now. "Behold," the adventurer exclaimed as his ship weighed anchor for Egypt. "I afford a new character to the world, and a new subject to biography."[3] And, he might have added, a beginning to America's extraordinary involvement in the Middle East.

Introduction

RECOVERING
A PIVOTAL PAST

FEW AMERICANS TODAY WOULD RECOGNIZE THE NAME John Ledyard, much less appreciate his contribution to America's relationship with the Middle East. Nevertheless, since the Gulf War of 1991 and certainly since 9/11, familiarity with the Middle East has expanded immensely among Americans. Fifteen years ago, how many of them knew the meaning of *jihad*, or were acquainted with the words *al-Qaeda, intifada,* and *Wahhabi*? How many could distinguish between Arabs and Iranians, Ba'athists and Islamists, and Sunni and Shi'ite Muslims? Indeed, the names of Middle Eastern towns such as Faluja and Jenin are often more familiar to Americans today than those of their own midwestern cities.

The growing familiarity that Americans display toward the Middle East reflects the essential role that the region now occupies in their lives. The United States is extensively, profoundly, and perhaps even existentially involved in the Middle East. The war in Iraq, the terrorist threat, and the quest for dependable sources of fuel permeate the media and dominate the national agenda. A source of religious inspiration for millions of Americans, the Middle East has also become a fountainhead of American fears. Tellingly, the Asian greens that once camouflaged the fatigues of U.S. troops have burnished to

Arabian browns and yellows, and Arabic has supplanted Russian as the *lingua sancta* of the intelligence services. More materially than South America, Africa, or Europe, more immediately than North Korea or even China, the Middle East impacts the security of the United States and the well-being of all of its citizens.

In spite of the paramount importance of the Middle East, Americans remain largely unaware of their country's rich and multidimensional history in the area. A majority of them seem to believe that the United States became active in the Middle East shortly after the Second World War, with the advent of the Arab-Israeli conflict or the tapping of Saudi oil. Many would respond incredulously to the claim that relations with a region so physically remote—some thirty-five hundred miles separate New York from the closest Middle Eastern city, Sidi Ifni in Morocco—could have influenced the drafting of the Constitution and the creation of the U.S. Navy. Most would be surprised to learn that Americans and Middle Eastern peoples have met not only on oil fields and battlefields but also in the spheres of art, education, and philanthropy. Americans built the first modern universities in the Middle East and both the Star Spangled Banner and the Statue of Liberty originated in America's Middle Eastern experience.

The lack of knowledge about America's history in the Middle East stems, at least partially, from the absence of a comprehensive book on the subject. While British citizens interested in reading about their country's history in the region can consult Elizabeth Monroe's classic *Britain's Moment in the Middle East* or several exceptional works by William Roger Louis, Americans must wade through a daunting mass of publications. Several dozen books have been written on the Barbary Wars—America's first conflict with the Middle East—and on U.S. policy toward the post–World War I Middle East settlement, but there is no single study of American military interventions in the Middle East or of America's role in the decolonization process. The bibliography on American policy toward Israel and the Palestine dispute spans several pages, but no work exists on America's literary tradition in the Middle East or on the integration of the U.S. and the Middle Eastern economies since 1776.

Several scholars have, however, sought to investigate broader aspects of America's Middle East history. In his *Pioneers East*, issued in 1967, David Finnie offered a colorful narrative of Americans working, traveling, and preaching in the area in the late eighteenth and nineteenth centuries. Two years later, James A. Field added academic depth to Finnie's more popular survey and produced *America and the Mediterranean World, 1776–1882*. John DeNovo followed Field with his *American Interests and Policies in the Middle East, 1900–1939*, an encyclopedic work, and after DeNovo, Joseph L. Grabill authored his groundbreaking *Protestant Diplomacy and the Near East: Missionary Influence on American Policy, 1810–1927*. The last of these far-reaching studies was Thomas Bryson's *American Diplomatic Relations with the Middle East, 1784–1975*, published thirty years ago. Since then, historians have focused on the post–World War II period and on the political and strategic dimensions of America's Middle East relations. George Lenczowski's *American Presidents and the Middle East*, Steven L. Spiegel's *The Other Arab-Israeli Conflict*, and William B. Quandt's *Peace Process* are three of the genre's finer examples. Another essential book, *The Arabists* by Robert D. Kaplan, covers a wider chronological span, but primarily examines the State Department's influence on American Middle East policy.

Still missing from this list is an examination of the full sweep of America's centuries-old engagement with the Middle East in all of its military, economic, and cultural aspects. No study has attempted to identify the recurrent themes in that history or to provide a methodological framework for analyzing it. To date, no work has presented an academic, yet compelling, account of the history of American involvement in the Middle East, one that is accessible to scholars as well as to general readership. This book strives to fill that vacuum.

Writing such a book gives rise to many challenges, the first of which is answering the question, "Where is the Middle East?" Though the term "Middle East" is today almost universally accepted, there is, in fact, no consensus on the region's borders. Many scholars classify Morocco, Tunisia, and Algeria as Middle Eastern countries, while others regard all of North Africa as a separate entity. The Middle Eastern Studies departments at some universities exclude Afghanistan and Pakistan from their scope, but other programs cover the Cacusus and Southwest Asia. Disagreements over the parameters of the area deepen the further one retreats into history. Historians differ over whether a discussion of the eighteenth-century Middle East should incorporate Ottoman Bulgaria and Greece or whether these provinces belonged to a discrete and nebulous Near East. Some deny that a Middle East could have existed before 1902, when the term was first employed.

This book resolves these issues by treating "Middle East" as synonymous with the region once known to Americans—indeed to most Westerners—as "the Orient." Prior to the twentieth century, at least, "the Orient" comprised a vast area stretching from Anatolia and Western Thrace to North Africa and Egypt, and from Arabia to the Persian Gulf. Ottoman possessions in Europe and Central Asia were also included in this category, though they became less "Oriental" after achieving independence. These lands were linked in the American mind by a common civilization, by similarities of dress, architecture and art, religious beliefs, and modalities of government. Even today, the bulk of Americans place Libyans and Iranians, along with Palestinians, Tunisians, and Lebanese, within the geopolitical framework they call the Middle East.

After demarcating the Middle East, the next task is to delineate the study's structure. Here, too, fundamental questions arise. Should equal attention be given to all stages of America's history in the Middle East or only to those periods on which little has been written? What, apart from perspective, can the book contribute to previously researched subjects such as Eisenhower's policy toward the 1956 Suez crisis or Nixon's stand in the 1973 Arab-Israeli War? How can a text that relies on declassified diplomatic papers in reconstructing the first two centuries of U.S.-Middle East relations document the last thirty years of that interaction, the files for which are not yet open to the public?

The answers to all of these questions are reflected in the book's structure. Accordingly, the first six parts of the study present a detailed account of America's relations with the Middle East from the late eighteenth century to the mid-twentieth. A final part surveys the events of the last sixty years, from the Cold War to the war in Iraq. Throughout the book, emphasis will be placed on identifying the central motifs in America's involvement in the Middle East and tracing the themes that run threadlike through the text, binding and embellishing it.

The most tangible and pervasive of these themes is power. Power refers to the pursuit of America's interests in the Middle East through a variety of means—military, diplomatic, and financial. Power describes President Madison's decision to send warships against Algiers in 1815 and Lincoln's efforts in 1863 to dissuade Egypt from intervening in Mexico. But America also employed power in the Middle East to protect its citizens who were residing there and to defend imperiled minorities. When, in 1844, the USS *Independence* rescued endangered American missionaries in Lebanon or when the *Tennessee* evacuated Jewish refugees from Palestine during World War I, power was not serving political or economic interests alone. It was assisting, rather, American faith.

Faith, the second theme, refers to the impact of religion in the shaping of American attitudes and policies toward the Middle East. Though Catholics and Jews played an active role in determining the course of America's relationship with the area, especially after World War II, Protestant influence traditionally predominated. The first Protestant missionaries departed Boston for the Middle East in 1819 with the goal of restoring Palestine to Jewish sovereignty and saving the souls of Orthodox Christians, Maronites, and Druze. But faith for the United States also had a secular, civic dimension, propelling Americans to export their concepts of patriotism and democracy abroad. The missionaries failed at re-creating the Jewish state and making converts, but they succeeded in establishing the first modern universities in Turkey and the Arab world. By instilling their students with a sense of national identity and pride, these institutions unleased powerful new forces in the Middle East and changed the region's politics irrevocably.

The third theme is fantasy. The idea of the Middle East has always enchanted Americans, enthralling them with an ethereal montage of minarets and pyramids, oases, camels, and dunes. Romantic notions of the region originated in the Bible, traditionally the most widely read book in America, with its otherwordly depictions of the desert. Another popular volume, *A Thousand and One Arabian Nights*, the medieval Persian anthology, further endowed the Middle East with a sexual aura. Lured by these seductive images, great numbers of nineteenth-century Americans traveled to the Middle East and vividly portrayed its landscapes in their prose. Later, when film and sound recordings replaced books as the primary means of perpetuating myths, Middle Eastern motifs became the rage in Hollywood and the music industry. Such revelries not only influenced the public's perceptions of the area, they also impacted government policy. Fantasy, it will be shown, contributed to President Polk's decision to sponsor a naval expedition to the Jordan River, and the 1856 congressional bill creating a U.S. Camel Corps with dromedaries imported from Egypt.

None of these themes was exclusive to America's interaction with the Middle East; Europeans also incorporated elements of power, faith, and fantasy in their Middle Eastern policies. Still, the persistence of these patterns over the course of more than two hundred years of America's Middle East involvement—and the dynamic interplay between them—was unique to the United States.

By exploring these themes and reconstructing the history of America's relationship with the Middle East, this book aims to facilitate a deeper and more nuanced understanding of this pivotal part of America's past. It also provides a historical context for analyzing the country's current role in the region. America's policies in Iraq, Iran, and the Israeli-Palestinian dispute are today the focus of intense controversy both within the United States and abroad. The purpose of this book is not to advocate for any side in these disputes or to advance a specific course of action. Rather, it seeks to generate an appreciation of the common legacy of the two worlds in which I live and which I equally esteem, America and the Middle East.

—Jerusalem and New Haven, 2006

Part One

EARLY AMERICA
ENCOUNTERS THE
MIDDLE EAST

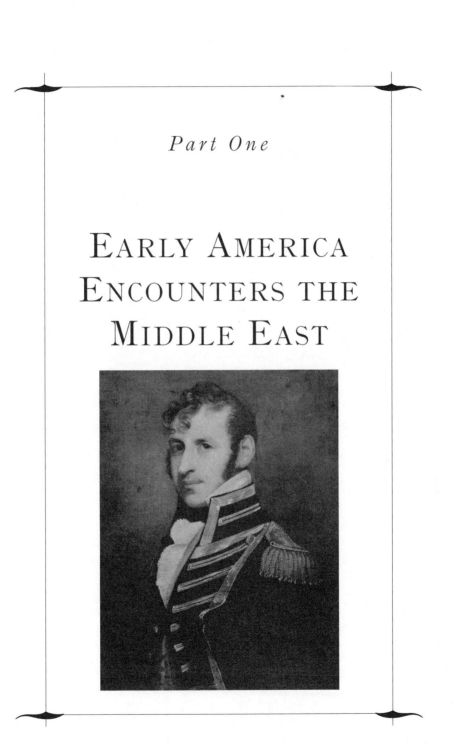

1

A MORTAL AND MORTIFYING THREAT

In 1776, suddenly, Americans were on their own. Previously, merchants from the New World blithely sailed the oceans in their brigs, sloops, and schooners, confident of the protection of history's most powerful navy. That security vanished overnight, however, with the outbreak of the Revolution. The massive British fleet that had once shielded American commerce from harm was now its lethal enemy. With no real navy of their own to defend them, American vessels were exposed to attack from the moment they left their moorings and almost helpless in the open sea.

The absence of a naval capability not only endangered American sailors but also imperiled the country's survival. Concentrated along the eastern seaboard, blessed with natural harbors and an abundance of superior shipbuilding wood, eighteenth-century America was in large part a seafaring nation, dependent on foreign trade. A blow to that commerce could pitch the fledgling United States, struggling to preserve its tenuous independence, into bankruptcy. As Continental troops battled against better-armed and trained British forces, the former colonies clung to their maritime lifeline. One of these led south to the West Indies, but another, no less critical route, extended across the Atlantic eastward to the blue-water ports of the Mediterranean.

Stretching from the Rock of Gibraltar to the Levantine and Anatolian coasts, the Mediterranean basin represented one of the world's last remaining spheres free of European domination, where enterprising Americans could still seek their fortunes unchecked. Though the trip from North America to the Mediterranean was rarely pleasant, requiring six weeks' sailing time aboard cold, cramped, and unsanitary vessels, the profits often outweighed the hardships. Local merchants were delighted to exchange capers, raisins, figs, and other Oriental delicacies for New World commodities such as timber, tobacco, and sugar. A singularly brisk business involved the export of puncheons of rum—"Boston Particular"—brewed by the descendants of New England Puritans and traded for barrels of Turkish opium, which the colonists then conveyed to Canton, China, or brought home for medicinal purposes. By the 1770s, an estimated one-fifth of the colonies' annual exports were destined for Mediterranean docks, borne in the holds of some one hundred American ships. "Go where you will," one British businessman in the area grumbled, "there is hardly a petty harbor . . . but you will find a Yankee . . . driving a hard bargain with the natives."[1]

Prior to the Revolution, the only major threat to America's vital Mediterranean trade came from the Middle East. Styling themselves as mujahideen—warriors in an Islamic holy war—Arabic-speaking pirates preyed on Western vessels, impounding their cargoes and enslaving their crews. These corsairs, as early Americans called them, sailed from the independent empire of Morocco and the semi-autonomous Ottoman regencies of Tripoli, Tunis, and Algiers, an area of the Middle East known collectively in Arabic as al-Maghrib, "the West." Westerners, though, had a different name for the region, one that evoked its Berber location but also its ferocious reputation. They called it Barbary.

Throughout the sixteenth and seventeenth centuries, Barbary was Europe's nightmare. Most of the men the pirates captured—among them Miguel de Cervantes, who based his first play on the ordeal—were sold as slaves destined for deadly toil in mines and galleys.

European women, prized for their fair complexions, fetched premium prices in the harems. Escape was virtually impossible. Mrs. Maria Martin, a British citizen purportedly seized by Algiers, told of being stripped, extensively inspected, and chained in a lightless cell for over two years, merely for refusing to serve as a concubine. In despair, some captives converted to Islam ("turned Turk") and served their rulers as advisers and physicians, or joined the pirate navy as renegades. Most, however, waited hopelessly to be ransomed by their families back home, for few could afford the exorbitant fee.[2]

Though directed principally against Europeans, North African piracy occasionally claimed victims from the New World. The earliest documented attack occurred in 1625, when Moroccan corsairs captured a merchant ship sailing from the North American colonies. Twenty years later, seamen from Cambridge, Massachusetts, repelled an assault by Algerians, but in 1678 Algiers seized another Massachusetts ship and thirteen vessels from Virginia. Of the 390 English captives ransomed from Algiers in 1680, eleven were residents of New England and New York. "We had already lost five or six of our vessels by . . . pirates," the Massachusetts governor Simon Bradstreet reported. "Many more of our inhabitants continue in miserable condition among them." One of those residents was Joshua Gee, a Boston merchant who suffered "sorrows & exarsises"—forced labor, plague and occasional beatings—throughout his seven years' captivity and who wept "tears of Joy . . . praising god . . . for his manifold merses," upon his release.[3]

Pirate attacks against New World ships nevertheless grew infrequent over the course of the eighteenth century, as American vessels came under the protection of Britain's vastly expanding and technologically superior navy. In their single-masted polaccas, xebecs, or feluccas, each with no more than twenty cannons and a few dozen armed men, the corsairs thought twice before waylaying a merchantman protected by a Royal Navy ship of the line manned by as many as 850 sailors and bristling with a hundred guns. For the British, North Africa was merely a gadfly scarcely worth a broadside, much less a war. Instead of resisting them, London mollified the Barbary States with annual installments of "tribute," a euphemism for protection money. Bribed not to attack British boats, the pirates turned their attention to those of the less muscular powers, such as Portugal, Denmark, and Spain.

The safeguards for American shipping remained in place until the issuance of the Declaration of Independence, in 1776. Yankee merchants promptly became the targets not just of North African corsairs but, more disastrously, of the British fleet that had once protected them. The patchwork Continental Navy nevertheless managed to meet those challenges with the leadership of intrepid captains like John Paul Jones and the assistance of French men-of-war, but by the time the fighting ended in 1783, most of America's warships had either been captured, sold off, or sunk. The country was scarcely capable of defending its own coastline, let alone its overseas trade. "At present we are not in a condition to be at War with any nation, especially one [Algiers] from whom we expect nothing but hard knocks," Pierse Long, a New Hampshire delegate to the Continental Congress, justifiably lamented. Algiers's flotilla—nine large battleships and fifty gunboats strong—vastly outgunned that of the United States. Britain's Lord Sheffield, a notorious opponent of American independence, affirmed, "The Americans cannot protect themselves [from Barbary]; they cannot pretend to a Navy."

America Cannot Retaliate

Sheffield had reason to gloat. A national navy could be created only by a strong central government, which the country still lacked. Loosely bound by the Articles of Confederation, the states could not even raise national taxes, much less a countrywide military force. Indeed, the articles specifically ruled out the construction of a standing peacetime navy. And while the confederation in theory permitted any state "infested by pirates" to outfit warships for self-defense, in practice no single state was capable of generating the armed power necessary to ward off Barbary. America, moreover, could make war against North Africa only with the consent of nine of the thirteen states, each of which possessed the right to exercise "its sovereignty, freedom, and independence."

The reluctance of the Americans to forfeit their state prerogatives in order to present a common front to the world was reinforced by their aversion to international affairs in general. "No nation can be trusted farther than it is bound by its own interests," George Washington warned, and no nations were deemed less trustworthy than the Europeans. Fear of foreign entanglements led many Americans to oppose creating a navy that could become embroiled with European fleets, or, worse, turn its guns on the nation's nascent democratic institutions. Having just narrowly survived a confrontation with one European navy (Britain's), many Americans were wary of any ocean-going force, even their own. There was also a financial consideration: warships were fabulously expensive to build, and, groaning under a colossal war debt, the United States treasury seemed incapable of bearing the burden.[4]

THE LACK of gunboats and the authority to construct them compelled the United States to overcome its aversion to European politics and to appeal to its Revolutionary allies, the French. According to the Franco-American Treaty of Amity and Commerce signed in 1778, France was "to use its best offices to . . . obtain . . . the immunity of the ships, citizens, and goods of the United States, against any attack, violence or depredation of . . . the States of Barbary." But when America called on France to honor that commitment, the response was negative. French leaders were keen to promote their own Mediterranean trade and feared the impact of American competition on the southern ports of Toulon, Nice, and Marseille. Concluding that "there is no advantage to us in procuring for them [the Americans] a tranquil navigation in the Mediterranean," Paris ignored the request.

Abandoned by France, Americans became easy prey for the pirates. In September 1783, Algerian xebecs reportedly harassed an American convoy sailing home from peace talks with Britain. "If there were no Algiers, it would be worth England's while to build one," quipped Benjamin Franklin, echoing the popular belief that the British were secretly paying the pirates. In fact, North Africa needed no encouragement from Britain or any other European power to attack ships of a United States that was now defenseless, friendless, and too impecunious to pay tribute.[5]

The North Africans' impunity in raiding American ships was illustrated in October 1784 by the attack on the *Betsey*. The 300-ton brig was sailing from Boston to Tenerife Island, one hundred miles from North Africa's coast, when it encountered an unidentified vessel. With the aid of a double bank of oars, the supple craft swiftly closed in and aligned its gunwales with those of the cumbrous *Betsey*. Then, with "sabers grasped between their teeth and their loaded pistols in their belts," as one American sailor remembered them, bare-chested pirates in turbans and pantaloons swarmed onto the merchantman's deck. "They made signs for us to all go forward," another eyewitness recounted, "assuring us in several languages that if we did not obey their demands, they would massacre us all." Surrendering crew members were stripped of all valuables and most of their clothing before being locked in the hold as human cargo, headed for the slave markets of Morocco.[6]

Three months after the *Betsey*'s capture, two more American ships, the *Dauphin* and the *Maria*, were abducted, this time by Algiers. Twenty-one American crewmen were fettered and paraded past jeering crowds to the court of the dynastic sovereign or dey, Hassan, who allegedly spat at them, "Now I have got you, you Christian dogs, you shall eat stones." A seventeen-year-old seaman named James Leander Cathcart recalled being cast into a dungeon, "perfectly dark . . . where the slaves sleep four tier deep . . . many nearly naked, and few with anything more than an old tattered blanket to cover them in the depth of winter." The daily ration, according to Cathcart, was a mere fifteen ounces of bread. The slightest resistance was punishable by bastinado (beatings on the feet), beheading, or impalement on iron spikes.

"Curse and doubly curse the Algerines for these pirates I fear have certainly made war on our commerce," raged the Virginia patriot Richard Henry Lee, a signer of the Declaration of Independence. Secretary of Foreign Affairs John Jay warned that the "alarming evil" of Barbary not only endangered American trade but also signaled America's weakness to the "jealous" powers of Europe. Unfounded newspaper reports of corsair attacks against American ships in the

Atlantic also compounded the panic. "The Algerians are cruising in different squads of six and eight sail, and extend themselves out as far as the western islands," fretted the usually unflappable John Paul Jones. Yet, in spite of this aggression—real and imagined—the states never once contemplated retaliating against the pirates. Apart from banishing three Virginian Jews on spurious charges of spying for North Africa, America remained passive.

The United States had just achieved independence and already encountered its first acute foreign threat—from the Middle East. The capture of the *Betsey*, the *Dauphin*, and the *Maria* was merely the first of many instances of hijacking and hostage taking that America later faced in the region. Yet, uniquely, the Barbary crisis raised fundamental questions about the nature, identity, and viability of the United States. Would the states survive if they tried to address the danger individually, or could they join in an effective defense? Would Americans imitate Europe and bribe the pirates, or would they create a revolutionary precedent and fight them? Though the answers to those questions may seem obvious today, in the late eighteenth century they were far from unequivocal. "It will not be an easy matter to bring the American States to act as a nation," Lord Sheffield taunted. "America cannot retaliate."[7]

Innocence or Independence?

Before they could prove Sheffield wrong, Americans first had to engage in protracted and often agonizing debates over the essence of their nation's constitution and character. Among the most outspoken participants in that dispute was the former governor of Virginia and principal framer of the Declaration of Independence. A provincial landowner who had never been east of Paris and had never fought in a war, Thomas Jefferson nevertheless insisted that he understood the Middle East and the need to confront it with power.

Much like his country—adverse to European politics but hungry for overseas trade, eager for national unity but protective of state prerogatives, committed to the Rights of Man while denying those rights to blacks and Native Americans—Jefferson was a ganglion of contradictions. Alternatively foppish and unkempt, garrulous and tight-lipped, he claimed to be a man of the people while cloistered in his splendorous Monticello estate. The conflicts between his effete and egalitarian sides, his republicanism and his Epicureanism, his pacifism and his ardor for France's blood-soaked revolution were just some of the many paradoxes that would baffle his biographers. Jefferson "combined great depth with great shallowness," conceded the historian Joseph Ellis, "massive learning with extraordinary naïveté, piercing insights into others with daunting powers of self-deception."

On few issues was Jefferson more inconsistent than in his attitudes toward the Barbary pirates. The owner of African American slaves, one of whom, Sally Hemmings, he almost certainly exploited sexually, he could not abide the thought of Africans possessing white people and violating American women in harems. The same Jefferson who warned against constructing warships liable "to sink us under them" could, in another breath, say, "We ought to begin a naval power, if we mean to carry our own commerce."

On one crucial point, though, Jefferson remained unswerving. Proud and parsimonious Americans, he believed, would rather "raise ships and men to fight the pirates into reason than money to bribe them." This peculiar "temper" translated naturally into the "erect and independent attitude" that Jefferson hoped would characterize American foreign policy, a posture that was inherently incompatible with payoffs. By deterring, rather than appeasing, Barbary, the United States would preserve its economy and send an unambiguous message to potentially hostile powers. "It will procure us respect in Europe," Jefferson held. "And respect is a safeguard to interest."[8]

In the fall of 1784, Jefferson was slated to serve as America's "minister" to France (the title "ambassador" sounded monarchical to Revolutionary American ears) and its representative to various European courts. He first recommended that the United States act in concert against Barbary, joining with Spain, Portugal, Naples, Denmark, Sweden, and France. The combined navies would maintain a permanent presence along the North African coast, compelling its residents to desist from piracy and to take up a peaceful profession—farming, Jefferson suggested. Unsure, however, of Europe's reaction to the initiative of an upstart United States, Jefferson sought the help of the Marquis de Lafayette, the French nobleman who had aided America's Revolution. Lafayette duly circulated the plan, but the responses were overwhelmingly negative. While several kingdoms expressed an interest in the concept, they refused to contribute ships to any alliance and continued paying tribute to Barbary. The French rejected the very idea of coalition.[9]

For Jefferson, the response of the United States to his proposal was even more disappointing. Congress staunchly refused to allocate the $2 million needed, according to Jefferson's math, to build a fleet of 150 guns. Instead, representatives allotted $70,000 for purchasing what Secretary Jay called "the Influence of . . . Courts where Favoritism as well as Corruption prevails." Jefferson was crestfallen. The "Honour as well as . . . [the] Avarice," which he believed would preclude Americans from submitting to Barbary, European-style, had proved insufficient. Further predations were apparently needed to persuade his countrymen to act as a nation and defend themselves. "The states must see the rod," he ruminated. "Perhaps it must be felt by some of them." In the interim, Jefferson could only watch disgustedly as the bribe was proffered to Algiers.[10]

To conduct this delicate transaction, Congress chose John Lamb, a Connecticut businessman with no diplomatic experience, but who had once worked in the Mediterranean, trading mules. "His manners and appearance are not promising," Jefferson worried, but then consoled himself with the hope that Lamb, after all, was a "sensible man" with "some talents which may be proper in a matter of bargain." Lamb's incompetence was swiftly revealed, however, the moment he arrived in Algiers, in February 1786. Misled by the French consul Jean-Baptiste de Kercy, who supported the United States while secretly denouncing it to Hassan Dey, Lamb failed to secure the release of a single American hostage. Instead, he received a list of additional ransom demands, which included a portrait of General Washington, whom the dey professed to admire. The *Dauphin*'s imprisoned captain, Richard O'Brien, a witness to this debacle, wished, "I hope never to see Captain Lamb in Barbary again except to buy horses and mules."[11]

America's first diplomatic initiative in the Middle East had ended in failure, but the fiasco in Algiers did not impede the United States from pursuing treaties with the other Barbary States. In fact, while Lamb was debasing himself before the dey, another American was attempting to negotiate with Tripoli, the principal city of modern-day Libya. The opportunity arose when the personal representative of the pasha of Tripoli, a nobleman named 'Abd al-Rahman al-Ajar, offered to host John Adams, America's minister to Great Britain, in his London chambers. Adams hesitated to accept the invitation, fearful that the discussion would revolve solely around tribute. The news of the mounting threats to America's Mediterranean trade, however, convinced him of the need to make peace with at least one North African state.

To Adams's censorious eye, 'Abd al-Rahman at first appeared alien and ogreish, an "ominous" figure suggestive of "pestilence and war." That initial aversion passed, however, as the envoy welcomed his guest with a pipe and a demitasse of strongly brewed coffee. In a hodgepodge of Italian, Spanish, and French, he questioned Adams about this new country, America, and the minister happily replied with detailed descriptions of his nation's government and people, climate and soil. 'Abd al-Rahman pronounced this "very great," but then, without pause and to Adams's astonishment, he characterized the United States as Tripoli's enemy. The Barbary States were "sovereigns in the Mediterranean," the Tripolitan explained, and "no nation could navigate that sea without a treaty of peace with them." That peace, moreover, came at a price: 30,000 guineas, plus a 3,000-guinea gratuity for himself. A similar sum would be necessary for conciliating Tunis, 'Abd al-Rahman estimated, and twice that sum for Morocco and Algiers. The total came to nearly one million dollars, about a tenth of America's annual budget.[12]

"It would scarcely be reconcilable to the Dignity of Congress to read . . . of the Ceremonies which attended the Conference," a dumbfounded Adams reported. "It would be more proper to write them for the . . . New York Theatre." Notorious for his vanity, the minister was outraged by the impertinence that 'Abd al-Rahman, the agent of a powerful but primitive kingdom, displayed toward the enlightened United States. He bemoaned the fact that "Christendom has made cowards of all their sailors before the standard of

Mahomet" and grieved over the prospect of paying off "unfeeling tyrants" who cared no more for their subjects' lives "than . . . so many caterpillars upon an apple tree." Adams shared Jefferson's belief that America's honor would be best served by resisting the pirates, but he continued to doubt the economic practicality of war. Factoring in the loss to U.S. shipping, rising insurance rates, and the vastness of America's debt, Adams concluded that it was safer to offer "one Gift of two hundred Thousand Pounds" than to risk "a Million [in trade] annually." Adams was defiant in vowing, "We ought not to fight them [the Barbary States] at all unless we determine to fight them forever," but battling the pirates, he still feared, was "too rugged for our people to bear."[13]

Jefferson, the populist, professed to have a greater feel for the American "temper" than the rather aloof Adams and remained certain that the American people would fight against North Africa if given the means and the option. Nevertheless, as a statesman, Jefferson did not dismiss the possibility of a diplomatic solution to America's piracy problems, should the opportunity arise. Thus, in March 1786, Jefferson joined Adams in London for one last attempt to prevent "a universal and horrible War" and reach an accord with Tripoli.

Before 'Abd al-Rahman, the Americans reaffirmed the affection with which the United States viewed all the nations of the world, including Tripoli. The American people were eager to avert bloodshed, they said, and to this end, and under reasonable terms, were willing to offer a treaty of lasting friendship with Tripoli. 'Abd al-Rahman appeared to listen intently to these representations, but when it came his turn to speak, he merely reiterated his original million-dollar demand. He then voiced a credo that would someday sound familiar to Americans, but left these founding fathers aghast:

It was . . . written in the Koran, that all Nations who should not have acknowledged their [the Muslims'] authority were sinners, that it was their right and duty to make war upon whoever they could find and to make Slaves of all they could take as prisoners, and that every Mussulman who should be slain in battle was sure to go to Paradise.

Adams had heard enough. The North Africans were guided solely by greed, he determined, and negotiating with them only "irritate[d] the Appetite of those Barbarians" and brought shame on the United States. Dubious of America's willingness to fight, though, Adams still believed bribery to be the country's only option. Jefferson similarly concluded that "an angel sent on this business . . . could have done nothing" to pacify the Tripolitans and he opposed further efforts to induce them monetarily. But Jefferson also persisted in asserting that Americans would take up arms to preserve their honor and well-being, and that peace with Barbary was attainable only "through the medium of war."[14]

Congress, still reeling from the aftereffects of the Revolution, wanted to avoid war and, in June 1786, instructed Jefferson, together with Adams and Franklin, to negotiate a peace agreement with Morocco. The ruler of that empire, Sidi Muhammad bin 'Abdallah, claimed to have been the first monarch to have recognized American independence and the first Muslim leader to seek a formal treaty with the young Republic. Congress dallied, however, and managed to offend the emperor. In retaliation, the Moroccans began seizing American ships, starting with the *Betsey* in October 1784. This indeed gained the Americans' attention, and now, "Armed only with Innocence and the Olive Branch," Jefferson, Adams, and Franklin set off to appease the emperor's wrath. In exchange for a "gift" of $20,000, the negotiators secured the *Betsey*'s release as well as a Treaty of Peace, Friendship and Ship-Signals. Thus began the longest-standing contract in American diplomatic history and the first one to bear an Arabic inscription and the Islamic date ("The Ramadan Year of the Hejira 1200"). The American consulate in Tangier, established under the treaty, would become America's oldest legation building and its only national landmark abroad.[15]

Though he was one of its negotiators, Jefferson feared that the treaty with Morocco would remain meaningless as long as America lacked the "public treasury and public force" necessary to ensure compliance. He consequently recommended suspending all further negotiations with North Africa until the United States undertook "measures . . . which may correct the idea . . . of impotency in the federal government." In the interim, the other Barbary States were quick to emulate Morocco's method for extracting American conces-sions. No sooner was the *Betsey* released than it was once again impounded, this time by Tunis, and its name officially changed to the *Mashuda*.

These ignominies weighed not only on Jefferson but also on George Washington, the most revered American of the time. Having struggled to surmount his country's powerlessness in 1776, Washington now felt "the highest disgrace" in seeing Westerners "become tributary to such banditti who might for half the sum that is paid them be exter-minated from the Earth." Like Jefferson, he believed that the Ameri-can people preferred confrontation with Barbary to blackmail, but they still lacked the warships to fight. "Would to Heaven we had a navy to reform those enemies to mankind, or crush them into non-existence," he confided to his former comrade-in-arms Lafayette.

Yet the reality remained that the United States had no navy, nor even a constitutional instrument for constructing one. "Without a national system of government, we shall soon become prey to the nations of the earth," the Massachusetts *Sentinel* editor Benjamin Russell wrote to John Adams. "Our sufferings are beyond . . . your conception," wrote Captain O'Brien, marking the two years that he and twenty-one crew members of the *Dauphin* and the *Maria* had languished in Algerian jails. A sense of national exasperation, of humiliation, spread. David Humphreys, a wartime aide to General Washington as well as a seasoned diplomat and poet, captured that vexation in verse:

> *See what dark prospect interrupts our joy!*
> *What arm presumptuous dares our trade annoy?*
> *Great God! The rovers who infest thy waves*
> *Have seiz'd our ships, and made our freemen slaves.*[16]

Under the specter of imprisoned sailors in North Africa and imperiled American ships, delegates from twelve of the thirteen states gathered in Philadelphia in May 1787. Their purpose was to consider replacing the Articles of Confederation with a more central-ized national charter—to rectify the very weakness that had humbled the United States before Barbary. As honorary chairman of this Constitutional Convention, Washington urged representatives to refrain from all "talk of chastising the Algerines" until "the wisdom and force of the Union can be more concentrated and better applied." This request from the venerated hero of the Revolution could not be lightly ignored, and the participants in the convention avoided all mention of Barbary. But as citizens of a trading nation, they could not entirely evade the question of creating the navy necessary to protect that trade. James Madison, the diminutive Virginia aristocrat widely regarded as the assembly's most dynamic participant, spoke for many of those present by reiterating his fear of a strong, standing navy, yet he nevertheless recognized America's paramount need for naval power. "Weakness will invite insults," he reasoned. "The best way to avoid danger is to be in [a] capacity to withstand it."[17]

Though downplayed during the Constitutional Convention, the connection between the Middle East and the American federation figured prominently in the impassioned state-level debates on ratifying the proposed Constitution. The Reverend Thomas Thacher reminded the Massachusetts convention that the enslavement of "our sailors . . . in Algiers is enough to convince the most skeptical among us, of the want of general government." Nathaniel Sargeant said it was "preposterous" to think that the United States could continue under the ineffectual Articles of Confederation and still defend itself from "piracies and felonies on ye high seas." Support for the Constitution as a framework for protecting American trade emanated from across the country, not only from maritime New England. Hugh Williamson of North Carolina, a distinguished physician and astronomer, wondered, "What is there to prevent an Algerine Pirate from landing on your coast, and carrying your citizens into slavery?" The Kentucky attorney George Nicholas asked, "May not the Algerines seize our vessels? Cannot they . . . pillage our ships and destroy our commerce, without subjecting themselves to any inconvenience?" The only answer, both Williamson and Nicholas averred, was union.[18]

Such forceful reasoning could not, however, allay the concerns of those who still feared the expansion of central power, and many of the debates became protracted and bitter. In a determined defense of the Constitution, Madison joined New Yorkers John Jay and Alexander Hamilton to produce a series of essays that were later anthologized as *The Federalist Papers*. These, too, stressed the necessary linkage between trading vessels and warships. "If we mean to be a commercial people . . . we must endeavor as soon as possible to have a navy," Hamilton, the mercantile-minded realist, maintained (*The Federalist* No. 24), and warned (No. 11) that without a "federal navy . . . of respectable weight . . . the genius of American Merchants and Navigators would be stifled and lost." Specifically referring to the North African threat, Madison affirmed (No. 41) that union, alone, could preserve the nation's "maritime strength" from "the rapacious demands of pirates and barbarians." Jay's private letters reveal an even more pugnacious approach. Arguing "the more we are ill-treated abroad the more we shall unite and consolidate at home," the secretary actually welcomed pirate attacks that would compel the states to rally against "the . . . dangers from . . . Algerian Corsairs and the Pirates of Tunis and Tripoli."[19]

A more imaginative, if less remembered, attempt to marshal the Middle East in defense of the Constitution was mounted by Peter Markoe. Affectionately monikered "Peter the Poet," the St. Croix–born and Oxford-educated Markoe had gained a reputation as one of Philadelphia's leading bards and publicists. At the outset of the ratification debate, in 1787, he published *The Algerine Spy in Pennsylvania*, a satirical piece of Federalist propaganda. Presenting himself as Mehmet, an Algerian agent sent to scout out America's defenses, Markoe praised political and economic freedoms guaranteed by the United States, but then mocked its lack of national cohesion. "Totally ruined by disunion and faction," the states "may be plundered without the least risqué, and their young men and maidens triumphantly carried into captivity." To hasten America's despoiling, Markoe had Mehmet recommend seizing all of Rhode Island, the only state that boycotted the convention, and transforming it into a base for Algerian operations.

Publications like *The Federalist Papers* and *The Algerine Spy* helped tip the balance in the Federalists' favor. The Constitution officially adopted on March 4, 1789, empowered Congress to declare war and "to provide and maintain a navy." A threat from the Middle East had played a concrete role in creating a truly *United* States, a consolidated nation capable of defending not only its borders at home but its vital economic interests overseas. "In an indirect sense, the brutal Dey of Algiers was a Founding Father of the Constitution," the historian of American diplomacy Thomas Bailey wrote. Whether Americans would actually use their newly forged federal powers to fight, however, was still questionable.[20] A vocal portion of the public continued to object to the notion of a large standing navy and recoiled from engaging in foreign conflicts. Many were reluctant to take up arms under almost any circumstances, preferring the "Innocence and the Olive branch" approach to Barbary to an "erect and independent attitude."

Impotence and Indignation

Pacing the floor of his small Broadway office in New York, Thomas Jefferson continued to wrestle with America's reluctance to wield power. After departing Paris at the end of 1789, he accepted an appointment as secretary of state, a post that accorded him an annual salary of $3,500, five assistants, and the primary responsibility for resolving the Barbary crisis. The promotion brought little change in Jefferson's opinion of the pirates—"sea dogs," he called them, and a "pettifogging nest of robbers." Jefferson was typical of the Americans who later viewed the region as the repository of despotism and backwardness, a kind of inverse mirror of their own democracy and enlightenment. Certainly, to his mind, a band of Muslim holy warriors bent on enslaving innocent American sailors was far more deserving of whiffs of grapeshot than bags of hard-earned gold. But with much of American opinion still opposed to using force, Jefferson had no alternative other than to continue negotiating with North Africa for the hostages' eventual release.

Through the good offices of Mathurin monks, members of a French order devoted to redeeming Christian slaves, Jefferson offered Algiers a substantially reduced ransom plus sundry *douceurs*, or "softeners." The dey, however, rejected these gestures, and when revolutionary authorities in France suppressed the Mathurins, Jefferson lost his go-between. Months passed in which he received agonized letters from the imprisoned Americans, many of whom were mortally ill with the plague. Suffering "perpetual anxiety for our captives," the secretary felt that American policy was at an impasse, possessing the constitutional means to fight Barbary but still unwilling to employ them, "suspended between indignation and impotence."

Finally, in December 1790, a dismayed Jefferson recommended that America go to war. "The liberation of our citizens has an intimate connexion with the liberation of our commerce in the Mediterranean," he explained to Congress. "The distresses of both proceed from the same cause, and the measures which shall be adopted for the relief of one, may . . . involve the relief of the other." Jefferson had championed Congress's right to a say in determining foreign policy, likening the executive's exclusive prerogatives in that field to those of an "Algerine" pasha, but he now regretted that stance. The Senate again rejected Jefferson's call for war and instead earmarked the unprecedented sum of $140,000 for the purposes of ransoms and tribute. The task of proffering the bribe fell to the secretary of state.[21]

Begrudingly, Jefferson complied, but selected as his courier the man he believed would never buy peace from Barbary. The first American officer to raise the Revolution's flag, John Paul Jones had earned a reputation as a skilled, if mercurial, captain. Jefferson, in recognition of his valiant service to the United States during the War of Independence, had helped secure Jones a commission in the Russian navy. Jones went on to score major victories against the Ottoman Turks and to develop a deep aversion to Middle Eastern rulers. Only by making war against the pirates could Americans become "a great People who deserve to be Free," Jones maintained. Jefferson's plan was to send Jones to Algiers with $25,000, a paltry sum that the dey was almost certain to reject. Congress, spurned, would then appropriate sufficient funds to create a full-time Mediterranean squadron. "John Paul Jones with half a dozen frigates would totally destroy their [the pirates'] commerce," the secretary reckoned, "cutting them to pieces by piecemeal." Jefferson dispatched his instructions to the Paris hotel where Jones was billeted, but they arrived too late. The forty-five-year-old captain had contracted a mysterious illness and died.[22]

Jefferson's next choice as courier, Thomas Barclay, a veteran of the negotiations with Morocco, made it as far as Lisbon before he, too, succumbed to sickness. A third envoy, David Humphreys, was sent, the same warrior-poet who had mourned "The rovers who infest thy waves . . . and made our freemen slaves." Humphreys reached Gibraltar, only to learn that Algiers had waylaid eleven more American ships, shackling an additional 119 sailors. There seemed little sense in entreating for the freedom of the *Dauphin* and *Maria* crews while Algiers was bushwhacking others, so Humphreys headed home.

A full fifteen years after declaring its independence, the United States still faced a devastating threat from the Barbary pirates. Some American merchants were reduced to counterfeiting the "passes" that Barbary issued to tribute-paying countries, which immunized their ships from attack. Others were forced to hire Dutch or Spanish gunboats at exorbitant rates to escort them across the Mediterranean. So acute was the danger that Treasury Secretary Alexander Hamilton wondered "whether on acc[oun]t of our situation with the Algerines it may not be advisable to procure a foreign vessel" to transport John Jay to Britain.[23]

Popular opinion on the Barbary issue was changing, however. Americans were growing sick of the threat of hijackings, of skyrocketing insurance rates for their shipping, and, above all, of the debasement of their pride. George Washington, now in his role as president, swore to use everything in his power for "the relief of these unfortunate captives" in Algiers. He was also concerned about the latest war in Europe—revolutionary France versus Britain and other conservative states—and the presence of foreign gunboats close to America's shores. "If we desire to avoid insult, we must be able to repel it," Washington told Congress in December 1793. Agreeing with the president, Congress finally opened a debate on creating a navy.[24]

Representatives who still thought that warships were too costly to build and, once constructed, were too threatening to peace and liberty opposed the motion. "Bribery alone can purchase security from the Algerines," argued Abraham Baldwin of Georgia, while the Virginian John Nicholas conceded "we are no match for the Algerines at sea." Citing the need to hire "a Secretary of [the] Navy, and a swarm of other people in office," New Jersey's Abraham Clark warned that "the Combined [European] powers would find [an American fleet] a much better pretense for war." To minimize America's risks and expenses, Clark proposed that Portugal be hired to fight the pirates.

Such "pusillanimous measures," however, were repugnant to John Smith of Maryland and inconsistent with "the maxims of the Republics of all former ages." Another Marylander, William Vans Murray, recalled that the corsairs had "been at war with the United States ever since the end of the Revolutionary war" and had left Americans no choice but to fight. Fisher Ames from Massachusetts, a champion of unrestricted trade, waxed especially ominous: "Our commerce is on the point of being annihilated, and, unless an armament is fitted out, we may very soon expect the Algerines on the coast of America."

In addition to financial and strategic considerations, the debate over the navy also took on a constitutional dimension, pitting the proponents of a strong central government against its many detractors. In a startling reversal of policy, Jefferson, allowing his fear of federal power to override his long-held desire to confront Barbary militarily, opposed the shipbuilding measure. His colleague and admirer James Madison even questioned whether the country possessed sufficient timber for the purpose. On the other hand, the Federalist leader John Adams, who had always doubted the American people's willingness to fight the pirates, paradoxically supported the plan. The deciding factor, ultimately, was neither economic nor political but rather psychological. The majority of the members of Congress, irrespective of their feelings toward federalism, could no longer bear the disgrace of kowtowing to Barbary. The legislation passed narrowly, by a vote of fifty to thirty-nine, and only on the condition that the construction of warships cease the moment peace was attained with Algiers.

On March 27, 1794, Washington signed into law a bill authorizing an outlay of $688,888.82 for the building of six frigates "adequate for the protection of the commerce of the United States against Algerian corsairs." With a maximum armament of forty-four guns—less than half those mounted on Europe's ships of the line—the vessels would nevertheless be lithe and formidable, ideal for battling pirates. The U.S. Navy thus was born, a contentious but honorable birth, intended not to rule the waves but to free them.[25]

The Navy nevertheless proved exceedingly slow to emerge. The frigate-building project became bogged down in contract disputes between the states and quickly exceeded its budget. American leaders who hollered, "Millions for defense but not one cent for tribute," in response to French demands for protection money, still seemed willing to consider some form of payoffs to North Africa. Letters from the captives meanwhile reached the United States and began to appear in the press. Samuel Calder, master of the schooner *Jay*, wrote of being brought to Algiers in chains, naked and starved. "Death would be a great relief and more welcome than a continuance of our present situation," he cried. Another captain, William Penrose, asked, "What in the name of GOD can our countrymen be about?" He warned that his crew's imminent death would forever remain "a stigma on the American character."

A guilt-ridden government was once again forced to scrounge around for redemption money—the Dutch first promised a loan, then reneged on it—and watch as churches and so-called benevolence drives rallied to raise the sums. Finally, in the summer of 1795, David Humphreys was ordered to try once more to "soothe the Dey into a peace, a ransom," and negotiate a peace with Algiers.

Sensual looking, with an elegant nose, finely arched brows, and lips playfully pursed, Humphreys seemed well-suited to the sumptuousness of Portugal's court, where he served as America's minister. But diplomacy in the West bore scant resemblance to its practice in the Middle East, Humphreys soon discovered. Hassan Dey was coarse, rude, and temperamental. "If I were to make peace with everybody, what should I do with my corsairs?" he humored the American. "Surely they would take off my head." Fears of mortality did not, however, deter Hassan from demanding a monumental ransom of two million dollars for the hostages. He also insisted on receiving two frigates from the United States, each with thirty-six guns. Further negotiations seemed futile.[26]

In spite of his delicate appearance, Humphreys was a spirited bargainer. He managed to reduce Hassan's demands and, on September

5, 1795, to obtain his signature on a Treaty of Amity and Friendship. The agreement was far from an American victory, however. Under its terms, the United States was still required to provide Algiers with a frigate, plus an assortment of *douceurs*—"25 chests of tea of 4 different qualities . . . 6 Quintal of loaf sugar refined. . . . Some elegant penknives. Some small guilt thimbles, scissor cases . . . a few shawls, with roses curiously wrought in them"—worth more than $650,000.

Still, Hassan refused to release the captives until he had received his payment up front. To procure the cash, the U.S. government turned to Joel Barlow, a friend of Humphreys's and a fellow poet who had been living in Paris. Utilizing his European contacts, Barlow scoured the Continent for specie, but failed to find the quantity needed to satisfy the dey. "You are a liar and your government is a liar," Hassan berated the broad-nosed, wide-browed Barlow when he returned empty-handed to Algiers. "I will put you in chains . . . and declare war." Only at the last minute did Barlow manage to find a Jewish businessman in Algiers willing to lend America the cash and a ship to evacuate the hostages.

"Our people have conducted themselves in general with a degree of patience and decorum which would become a better condition than that of slaves," Barlow attested in February 1797, after delivering the surviving eighty-eight Americans to Philadelphia. Much of the city descended on the docks to greet the liberated sailors, showering them with flowers and feting them with cakes and assorted spirits. "No nation of Christendom had ever done the like for their subjects in our situation," a grateful John Foss exclaimed. "The United States have sent an example of humanity to all the governments of the world." The dey, too, was delighted, and volunteered to help mediate similar treaties between the United States and both Tunis and Tripoli.

The two regencies were in fact open to agreement and quick to follow Algiers's example of first attacking the Americans and then negotiating with them from an advantage. Tripoli's Murad Ra'is— formerly Peter Leslie, a Scottish renegade—lost no time in pillaging three American ships, while Tunisian corsairs sacked the *Eliza*, a Boston schooner. Frigate-less, the United States could not respond forcibly to this aggression; it could only send Barlow back to North Africa for another round of talks. He eventually hammered out treaties with both Tunis and Tripoli, at a total cost of $160,000.

The government was now diverting as much as 20 percent of its yearly revenues to the Barbary states, paid out in gold or precious stones or, more perversely, in cannon, powder, and gunboats—the very wherewithal of piracy. So vast were the payments that the Europeans began complaining that the United States was overindulging the corsairs and driving up the cost of ransoms. "To what height is this Barbary system to be carried?" Barlow, disgusted, queried Jefferson. "And where is it to end?" The diplomat predicted that it was only a matter of time before the regencies again raised their tribute demands and renewed their war against America. But rather than heed Barlow's warnings, Congress declared that peace with North Africa had been achieved and reduced the budget for building warships.[27]

Outside of the legislature, however, many Americans had grown dismayed with their country's policy of admonishing the pirates verbally while simultaneously coddling them with bribes. The mounting criticism was especially reflected in the arts. In 1797, Royall Tyler, a respected New England jurist with a penchant for novel writing, published *The Algerine Captive*, the fictitious diary of a ship surgeon named Updike Underhill. Captured and enslaved by the corsairs, Underhill endures "hunger, sickness, fatigue, insult, stripes, wounds and every other cruel injury." Yet none of these inhibits him from excoriating persons who make "degrading treaties with piratical powers" and who furnish them with the weapons for extracting even more humiliating concessions. Tyler concluded his tale with an exhortation worthy of *The Federalist Papers*, reminding Americans of "the necessity of uniting our federal strength to enforce a due respect among other nations" and that "our first object is union among ourselves."

Other writers joined Tyler in failing to understand why America, now constitutionally fortified and supposedly building a navy, was still bowing to North African dictates. "What, give it up tamely, and yield ourselves slaves, to a pack of rapscallions, vile infidel knaves?" protested Susanna Rowson, the nation's most prominent female playwright and author of *Slaves in Algiers; or, The Struggle for Freedom*. A similar question was posed by an anonymous poet, a veteran of the Battle of Bunker Hill and of captivity in Algiers, who also supplied an answer:

> *Does Columbia still disdain to own*
> *A well try'd patriot and a free-born son? . . .*
> *Then steer the hostile prow to Barb'ry's shores,*
> *Release thy sons, and humble Africa's powers.*[28]

Tyler, Rowson, and the nameless composer would all be disappointed. President John Adams, still doubtful of the American people's readiness to resist Barbary, continued to pay tribute and even appointed permanent representatives to each of the regencies. As if to emphasize the subordinate position of the United States, the liberated captive Richard O'Brien became the consul in Algiers and James Cathcart was sent to Tripoli. The position in Tunis, by contrast, went not to a former prisoner but to a government employee who had never before visited the Middle East or expressed any opinion about the pirates. William Eaton, a bluff and audacious young man, was nevertheless destined to become Barbary's most passionate foe.

The consuls assumed their posts in March 1799, shortly after America finally launched the first three of the six frigates commissioned by Congress. Floating a total complement of 124 guns and strengthened with detachments from the newly created Marine Corps, the *United States, Constitution,* and *Constellation* represented a small but robust force. The young navy proceeded to acquit itself worthily in an undeclared "quasi-war" with France in the Caribbean, where Napoleon's gunboats tried to block America's neutral trade with Britain. With the confidence gained from victories near its coast, America was poised to tackle even more complex and distant challenges abroad.

In spite of this assuredness, though, the nation was still uncertain whether or not to use its newly acquired power against North Africa. "These barbarians say that they have often heard of American frigates, but they have never seen any," Cathcart submitted in one of his first dispatches from Tripoli. "The conclusion they draw is that either we have none or would sacrifice considerable sums sooner than send them into the Mediterranean." Would the people of the United States continue to pay tribute, to emulate Europe, and to endure shame, or would they become, as David Humphreys hoped, "the Authors of the System for exterminating the pirates"?[29]

America's involvement in the Middle East had thus far centered on questions of power, both economic and military. But not all Americans were drawn to the Middle East for commercial or strategic reasons. Others were lured by romantic visions of the region, by their lust for adventure and their longing for new frontiers. The first of these Americans was John Ledyard, the world traveler and inveterate adventurer introduced in the prologue. For five months in 1788, Ledyard reported vividly of his experiences in Egypt, the heartland of the Arabic-speaking world. His descriptions would instill stark and astonishing images of the Middle East in the minds of many Americans, among them Ledyard's close friend—and soon to be president—Thomas Jefferson. Previously, he, like the vast majority of his countrymen, regarded the region as a bastion of infidel-hating pirates as well as a realm of exotic wonders. The Middle East, for Jefferson and his contemporaries, was not merely the precinct of power but, more alluringly, a theater of myth.

2

THE HOSTILE AND
ETHEREAL ORIENT

THE TERM "MIDDLE EAST" WAS COINED BY AN AMERICAN admiral in 1902. Before that time, Americans (and Europeans) spoke of the area as simply "the East" or, more commonly, "the Orient." The term vaguely referred to the landmass that stretched between Morocco and Egypt and curved scimitar-like through Arabia and the Levant before tapering, finally, in Turkey. But the designation was never entirely geographical—Casablanca, in fact, lies far to the west of Madrid, Marseille, and Rome. The Orient, rather, described a region unified by a distinct civilization, typified by unique modes of government, social structure, architecture, and dress. Its inhabitants, known to Westerners by an assortment of interchangeable names—Arabs, Levantines, Algerines, Moors, and Turks—were presumed to be hostile to foreigners and spoke languages grating to the American ear. More than by its political, artistic, or linguistic qualities, though, the Orient was distinguished by its religion, Islam. The followers of this faith, generally called Musselmen, were perceived by eighteenth-century Americans as the ultimate Other, a colorfully garbed but amorphous mass, the descendants of once venerable but long decayed civilizations, primitive, sordid, and cruel.

An Object That Promiseth and Deceiveth

Inimical images of the East passed to the New World in the minds of the first Europeans to probe it. "As . . . enemies of the sect of Mahomet," Christopher Columbus set out discover a new route to the Holy Land in 1492—he even took along an Arabic interpreter for the purpose—and so that "all the gain of this my Enterprise should be spent in the conquest of Jerusalem." Little more than a century later, George Sandys, soon to become treasurer of the Virginia colony, traveled to the Middle East and found a region rife with bloodthirstiness. "I think there is not in the world an object that promiseth so much . . . [yet] so deceiveth the expectation." The shield of Virginia governor John Smith bore the likeness of the Turkish heads he severed while serving as a mercenary against the Turks. Along with incipient notions of equality, the idea of Western superiority over the Orient landed with the Pilgrims at Plymouth. A rock near the colony reportedly bore the inscription: "The Eastern nations sink, their glory ends, And empire rises where the sun descends."

Though early America prided itself on religious tolerance, that forbearance rarely extended to Islam, which was scarcely considered a religion at all. Prominent colonial theologians such as Cotton Mather and Jonathan Edwards regularly denounced Islam as a false and morally degenerate faith. Muhammad, according to the Harvard president Samuel Langdon, was a counterfeit prophet and, worse, "an emissary of Satan." The jaundiced impression of Islam was reinforced by tendentious translations of the Quran. The "newly Englished" *Alcoran* of Alexander Ross, published in 1649, set out to expose the "contradictions, blasphemies, obscene speeches and ridiculous fables" in the book, so that the Christian "so viewing thine enemies in their full body . . . maist the better . . . overcome them." Similarly, the 1734 version by the lawyer George Sales, a copy of which was found in Thomas Jefferson's library, aimed at enabling Protestants to "attack the Koran with success" and hoped that "for them . . . Providence has reserved the glory of its overthrow." The purpose of the most popular colonial-era book on Muhammad, written by Humphrey Prideaux in 1697, was unambiguously announced by its title, *The True Nature of the Imposture Fully Displayed.*[1]

The farrago of fact and misinformation about the Middle East to which colonial Americans were exposed is reflected in the first short story written in the New World, a farce titled "Father Bombo's Pilgrimage to Mecca." Authored in 1770 by Philip Freneau and Hugh Henry Brackenridge—classmates of James Madison at Princeton and his fellow Jeffersonian Whigs—the story describes how the Prophet Muhammad appears before a plagiarizing student named Bombo and orders him "to change thy religion and profess Mahometanism and become a zealous musselman." Donning "Turkish habit," Bombo dutifully embarks on a six-week trip to the Meccan mosque that contains the Prophet's body. There the pilgrim washes his hands and feet and removes the rest of his garments. "I prostrated myself on the bare pavement, naked, with my face towards the East, begging the prophet to pardon my crimes." The text shows that Brackenridge and Freneau clearly knew something about Islamic rituals, but they also misconceived of Muhammad as a Jesus-like figure who, though interred in a sacred sepulcher, occasionally materializes to penitents and dispenses personal salvation. Muhammad indeed responds to Bombo's prayers and forgives his sins so that he can finally return to New Jersey.

Negative depictions of the Middle East also reached America through the memoirs of European diplomats and travelers, over a hundred of which had been published by the late eighteenth century. Though most of these books were in French, a few, including James Bruce's *Travels to Discover the Source of the Nile*, were available to English readers. These depicted the Middle East as an alien realm, at once romantic and threatening. The women of the region were often portrayed as lustful and the men as free-ranging and noble. The sixteenth-century geographer Leo Africanus, a Muslim convert to Catholicism, described the area's inhabitants as "savage" plunderers who "pluck out the eyes and cut off the hands and feet" of their prisoners. The Ottomans, according to Oxford's Richard Knolles in his *General History of the Turks* (1603), were "the present terror of the world." The French voyagers Savory and Volney conveyed more equitable impressions of the Orient, as did the classical writers Herodotus, Thucydides, and Homer. Nevertheless, apart from the snippets gleaned from returning merchants or from Arabic-speaking slaves, Americans of Ledyard's time had scant access to information about the Middle East, and the little they possessed was exceedingly unreliable and biased.[2]

This near-total absence of any real knowledge about the Middle East left a vacuum that was easily occupied by rumors about the region, regarding not only its alleged enmity toward anything Western but also its immeasurable marvels. The image of the area as an ambit of visual and sensual delights derived from many sources, the richest of which were available on the colonial American bookshelf. The Bible, a text that almost all early Americans knew intimately and regarded as immutable truth, was the principal source of Middle Eastern fantasies. The Old and New Testaments presented a panorama of lofty towers and temples, of hanging gardens and shimmering oases and, most majestically, the desert. The passages describing such spectacles, when recited in drab Pennsylvania meetinghouses or in wind-pierced frontier cabins, could induce Middle Eastern reveries even in the most puritanical parishioners. Many dreamed of witnessing those wonders firsthand.

After the Bible, one of the most widely read books among early Americans was *A Thousand and One Arabian Nights*. It too served as a fertile source of Middle Eastern illusions, although illusions of a most unscriptural kind. An anthology of medieval Persian romances, *A Thousand and One Arabian Nights* first appeared in English in 1708 and instantly achieved popularity throughout the British Empire, especially in the American colonies. The reasons were not difficult to gauge. The escapades of Ali Baba, Sindbad, and Aladdin, and the pathos of Scheherezade storytelling for her life, transported Americans from their arduous lives to a tantalizing world of hidden treasures and minaret-orbiting rugs, of veiled but available odalisques. One might only imagine the sensory swoon produced in the prim New England cleric or stately southern prig by this excerpt from the book's introduction:

A secret gate of the Sultan's palace opened all of a sudden, and there came out of it twenty women, in the midst of whom marched the Sultaness. . . . [They] threw off their veils and long robes, that they might be more at freedom, before ten black servants . . . and each of them took his mistress. The Sultaness, was not long without her gallant, she clapped her hands . . . and immediately a black came down . . . and ran to her in all haste. This amorous company continued together till midnight and, having bathed altogether in a great pond . . . they dressed themselves, and reentered the palace.[3]

Biblical marvels and carnal allure together endowed the Middle East with a dreamlike aura. But would the image of an ethereal Orient suffice to attract Westerners to visit the region and to risk encountering its less splendorous qualities? The answer, for Americans more than for Europeans, was straightforward: the Middle East represented an opportunity for movement. As citizens of a nation already famous for its individualism and energy, a people so restless that, as one foreigner remarked, even their chairs had rockers, Americans craved movement. Pioneers by the thousands pressed inland, in search of untrammeled space. For some, though, not even the vastness of the North American continent could satisfy their wanderlust. They looked not only to the wilderness west of the Ohio River and beyond the Mississippi, but also in the opposite direction, eastward. For them, the Orient meant more than a mere phantasmagoria; it was an uncharted horizon, ripe for penetration and discovery. For Americans like John Ledyard, romantic and peripatetic, the Middle East was the ultimate frontier.[4]

A Connecticut Yankee in Egypt

Ledyard crossed into that frontier in the first week of July 1788, when his ship docked in Alexandria, Egypt. A congested, dusty warren into which six thousand residents were packed, stagnant and chaotic at once, the city bore no vestige of its ancient grandeur and no resemblance to the Middle Eastern myths Ledyard had imbibed. "Alexandria at large presents a sight more wretched than I have witnessed," he began in a harrowed letter to Jefferson. The local afflictions were almost too numerous to list: "Poverty, rapine, murder, tumult, blind bigotry, cruel persecution, pestilence!"

The dissolution Ledyard encountered was symptomatic of the

Ottoman Empire, to which Egypt, at the end of the eighteenth century, still belonged. Often called Turkey or the Sublime Porte (a reference to the door of the grand vizier's palace) by Westerners, the empire had arisen in the fourteenth century and steadily expanded to dominate the Middle East and huge swaths of Central Asia and Eastern Europe. The fierce Ottoman army launched repeated forays against Christian Europe, culminating in the 1683 siege of Vienna. That offensive proved to be a high-water mark, however, and thereafter the empire's fortunes declined. By the 1780s, the Ottomans seemed less like frightful specters to the West than incorrigible has-beens. The Viennese who once quaked at the thought of the "Moorish hordes" and the "terrible Turk" at their gates now regaled in "Turkish" fashions and thrilled to *The Abduction from the Seraglio*, a Mozart opera about a Spanish woman's rescue from an Ottoman harem, a comedy.

In few areas was the empire's downslide more pronounced than in its Arabic-speaking provinces. Once the seat of rich and enlightened kingdoms, global leaders in science and mathematics, these lands were, by the end of the eighteenth century, reduced to semifeudal backwaters. Life for the vast bulk of their inhabitants had changed little since the Middle Ages. There were no printing presses, no clocks, no modern academic institutions. Roads were scarce and, in the absence of a strong central authority, travelers were exceedingly vulnerable to attack. Few Europeans dared to penetrate this inhospitable region, confining their presence to port cities, where they cowered under consular protection. The local population had no such recourse. As Ottoman hegemony weakened, the peasants were exposed to the whims of provincial satraps and the scourge of brigand bands.

Conditions were especially dim in Egypt. Some three to four million natives lived in subsistent conditions and were annually ravaged by famine and disease. Rather than relieve this misery, the country's Ottoman governors engaged in a relentless power struggle with the local Mamluk dynasty, devastating the countryside and trampling over its hapless peasantry. In 1788, with Mozart about to compose another opera set in an imaginary Middle East, *The Magic Flute*, and shortly after the United States placed a pyramid on the reverse side of its Great Seal, the genuine Egypt, civilization's cradle, had fallen to an unprecedented nadir.[5]

This was the abysmal Egypt that Ledyard encountered in Alexandria. Yet he refused to believe that the city's decay was endemic to the entire country and, in search of the mythic Middle East, he departed for Cairo. The journey required five days' sailing on the Nile, an experience he had cheerfully anticipated, but that, too, disappointed him. "*This* is the mighty, the sovereign of rivers, the vast Nile, that has been metamorphosed into one of the wonders of the world?" The river, he reckoned, was little bigger than the Connecticut.

In Cairo, Ledyard presented his royal letter of introduction to a Signore Rosetti, the Venetian consul who represented British interests in the city. Ledyard learned that, much as Westerners referred to all Middle Eastern peoples as Orientals, Middle Eastern Muslims regarded Europeans and Americans alike as "Franks," a pejorative term left over from the time of the Crusades. For his own safety, the consul warned, Ledyard should keep a low profile and travel in native dress. The suggestion that a Christian should have to dissemble his identity just to please Muslims was, to Ledyard's mind, "very, very humiliating, ignominious, and distressing." He complained to Jefferson of "the shame to the sons of Europe, that they should suffer such arrogance at the hands of a banditti of ignorant fanatics," and yet Ledyard ultimately accepted the consul's advice. Trading in his breeches and three-cornered hat for pantaloons and a turban, he succeeded in spending three productive months, unmolested, probing the Nile.

Throughout these excursions, Ledyard proved himself a careful observer of Egypt's landscape. He noted the height of pyramids, the extent of urban sprawl, and speculated on the length of caravans. He bemoaned the common people's squalor, ranking it "infinitely below any Savages" he had ever seen. Ledyard's curiosity also lured him onto the field of battle, where the Mamluk and Ottoman armies were indecisively locked. Flustered by the stalemate, the Mamluk commander finally asked Ledyard to lead his troops. "This was about as far as a Connecticut Yankee could get from home," the American noted, "being offered a post in Egypt's civil war."

The extent of Egypt's disintegration deeply saddened Ledyard. He blamed Russia for Egypt's predicament, for weakening Turkey with war—a residue, perhaps, of his lingering bitterness toward Catherine. Yet he also faulted the "Mahometans" for being "a superstitious, warlike set of vagabonds," and Islam, which "does more mischief than all other things." On the other hand, he admired the Muslims' ability to combine piety and commerce as well as their "invincible attachment to liberty." The image of the camel-borne nomad who roams the desert unencumbered by governments or borders—an image akin to that the colonial frontiersman and, later, the Western cowboy—would become a recurrent theme in American writing on the Middle East, and a persistent influence on U.S. policy toward the region.

Apart from the myth of the liberty-loving nomad, however, Ledyard found little romance in the Middle East, certainly none of the strand spun by *A Thousand and One Arabian Nights*. "Nothing merits more the whole force of burlesque, than both the poetic and prosaic legends of this country," he complained to Jefferson. He contrasted the lustrous trees with the "dust, hot and fainting winds, bugs, mosquitoes, spiders, flies, leprosy, fevers, and almost universal blindness" seething in their branches. Like Jefferson, Ledyard viewed Middle Eastern society as a mirror image of America's, raising a left hand of darkness and hate to the right hand of American enlightenment. "Sweet are the songs of Egypt," he concluded, "on paper."

Meanwhile, Ledyard prepared for his passage upriver into Africa. He consulted with the Mamluk commander Ismail Bey, who warned him about brigands capable of morphing into wild animals and advised him to travel lightly, without valuables. He then secured a place on the next caravan to Sennar, over a thousand miles to the south. In a last letter, dated November 15, 1788, Ledyard advised Jefferson never to come to Egypt and to take all those wondrous depictions of the East—by Savary, Thucydides, and Homer—and "burn them." In a scarcely disguised understatement, he confessed, "I have passed my time disagreeably here." Then, with his trademark drama, Ledyard said good-bye to his most devoted and illustrious American friend: "I go alone. . . . Do not forget me. I shall not forget you. Indeed, it would be a consolation to think of you in my last moments. Be happy."[6]

The farewell was indeed to be final. Perturbed by a delay in his departure, Ledyard launched into a nervous fit that brought on what contemporary accounts called "a bilious complaint." As a remedy, he swallowed quantities of vitriolic acid and resorted to the "strongest tartar emetic." The patient consequently began vomiting blood and was then subjected to the "skill of the most approved physicians in Cairo." Twenty-four hours later, the man who had recently assured his mother that he was in "full and perfect health" and had "trampled the world under his feet, laughed at fear and derided danger," died.

John Ledyard was buried in the sand dunes lining the Nile, in a modestly marked grave, the location of which is unknown today. He left behind an unpublished manuscript, "A Eulogy to Women," which lauded the opposite sex as "kind, civil, obliging, humane, tender beings," but few other personal effects.[7] The precedent he set, however, was enormous. For the first time a citizen of the United States had traveled to and meticulously reported on the Middle East, an area then known to his countrymen almost exclusively from the Bible and myths.

The impact of that precedent was already evident in 1792, when Henry Beaufoy recounted Ledyard's exploits in *Ladies' Magazine*, a leading Philadelphia monthly. The article inaugurated a series of mawkish stories on Middle Eastern themes, *Arabian Nights*–like vignettes about Eastern women who, "although generally tender and timid, become bold and ungovernable when the passion of love takes possession of them." But there were also informative studies on the customs of the Egyptians, the Circassians, and the Druze, and descriptions of Middle Eastern cities that confirmed John Ledyard's impressions. "He who is new to all these objects is dazzled with their variety," an anonymous traveler wrote. "Every idea he has formed to himself vanishes, and he remains absorbed in surprise and astonishment."

As the century waned and a new one opened, other Americans followed Ledyard's example and embarked for the Middle East. One such voyager was the Charlestonian Joel Roberts Poinsett, a future war secretary and discoverer of the flower that still bears his name. As a guest of a Persian khan in 1806, Poinsett was entertained with "handsome" dancing girls in "long red pantaloons . . . their heads covered with a veil," and shown a pool of petroleum, a "Land of Eternal Fire," which he speculated might someday be used for fuel. Twelve years later, George Barrell of Boston, "having perused Eastern Tales," became "beguiled" by "the idea of . . . listening to the Moorish flute and the enchanting voice of some fair Circassian." He subsequently journeyed to Anatolia, but discovered that the flute sounded like a "badly played bagpipe" and that fair Circassians could be found only in the slave market. Still, Barrell urged all Americans to cast aside their "unhappy prejudices" and retrace his path to the Orient.

Such accounts, even when demystifying, sustained American fantasies of the Middle East, luring growing numbers of men and women into Syria, Palestine, and Mesopotamia. Those who remained at home, meanwhile, would continue dreaming of the region. Some thirty travel books on Egypt were published in the United States in the first quarter of the nineteenth century alone. No fewer than four American cities were named for Cairo, and three for Baghdad and Medina. There were also two Meccas, an Aleppo, and an Algiers. Illuminated by Ledyard's travels, the Middle East remained a source of intense interest for many Americans, adventurers as well as decision makers, including Thomas Jefferson.

Jefferson had all along assumed that Ledyard would return from Egypt and proceed with his plan for traversing America by foot in search of the Northwest Passage. That expectation was dashed in March 1789, when Jefferson read of his good friend's demise in one of the Paris newspapers. He anxiously wrote to Tom Paine, who had since relocated to London, asking him to confirm the reports with the African Society. "Ledyard was a great favourite with the Society," Paine consoled him. "They . . . lament him with affectionate sorrow." Sir Joseph Banks, one of Ledyard's principal patrons from London, extolled the late explorer's gifts both as an author and as an enlightened thinker. "That man," Banks said, "was all Mind."[8]

Jefferson would eventually realize his dream of mapping a course across North America, with the help of the explorers Lewis and Clark. For now, though, he was less concerned with exploring his country's interior than with forging its policy overseas. Among the most pressing and complex issues facing the future president would be America's relations with the Middle East. Here, certainly, Ledyard's observations proved valuable. They had enabled Jefferson to view the region through American eyes—incisive, proud, and discriminating—and further disabused him of any lingering romantic notions. As president, Jefferson would deal with the Middle East in a fashion distilled of illusions and focused solely on might.

A CRUCIBLE OF AMERICAN IDENTITY

THE SON OF AN UPSTANDING PRINCETON DOCTOR, A deckhand at fifteen and a captain before he turned twenty, beloved husband and father of four, respected by both his officers and his crew, William Bainbridge might well have been bound for greatness had it not been for his pervasive bad luck. Encountering two enemy frigates during the quasi-war with France, for example, he was forced to surrender command of the schooner *Retaliation*, without ever firing a shot.

Ill fortune again rained on Bainbridge in September 1800, when he received orders to sail the frigate *George Washington* to the Middle East. For over three years, the United States had been paying a major share of its national budget in the form of tribute to the Barbary States. North African ports were frequently hosts to American ships unloading cargoes of lumbers, spices, naval stores, and guns intended to appease and enrich the local rulers. The hold of the *George Washington* contained some $500,000 worth of tribute goods, all of it destined for Algiers.

For Bainbridge, the ignominy of delivering this bribe was compounded by the fact that the *George Washington* was the first U.S. Navy ship ever to enter the Mediterranean. Still, as a representative of his country's flag, Bainbridge expected to be shown respect. Instead, he received disparagement. "You pay me tribute, by which you become my slaves," Hassan Dey berated him. Though largely autonomous from the Ottoman Empire, Algiers still paid tribute to the sultan and Hassan now ordered Bainbridge to transport this booty to Istanbul. When the captain refused, the dey reminded him that the *George Washington* was moored directly beneath city's cannons and within range of the *Crescent*, the thirty-two-gun frigate that President Adams had given to Algiers. "To save the peace . . . to prevent captivity and detention to the ship, officers, and crew . . . and pillage and slavery to the citizens of the United States," Bainbridge complied.

The *George Washington* was summarily crammed with 150 sheep, twenty-five cows, five horses, and four each of antelopes, tigers, and lions, along with assorted ostriches and parrots. To this menagerie was added a million dollars in gold, jewels, and goods, the Algerian ambassador and his family, and about one hundred African slaves. A proud man, though not yet thirty, stout and full-faced and crowned with a stylish pompadour, Bainbridge railed against this imposition. More demeaning for him than the stench and discomfort was the sight of the American flag being struck and replaced by the pennant of Algiers. "[Such] mortifying degradations . . . make me ponder on the words, *independent United States*," he grumbled, and vowed never again to bring tribute to Algiers "unless authorized to deliver it from the mouth of our cannon."

The three-week passage to Istanbul was "as unpleasant as could well be imagined," wrote Bainbridge. His crew found sophomoric relief by tacking hard during the Muslims' prayers, laughing as the prostrate worshippers slid across the deck and struggled to keep oriented toward Mecca. The laughter ceased, however, as the ship exited the Aegean and entered the heavily fortified Dardanelles Strait. Lacking a *firman* (imperial decree) to pass the batteries, Bainbridge cleverly ordered the firing of an eight-gun salute, waited for the fort to return the gesture, and then, in the smoke and confusion, made full sail across the Sea of Marmara. Ahead of him lay Istanbul, the imperial capital, or Constantinople, as Westerners still insisted on calling it. Bainbridge thus became the first American serviceman to behold the epicenter of Ottoman power.[1]

The view, by all accounts, was spectacular, a glittering montage of minarets, bastions, and domes. Beneath that majesty, though, lay an infrastructure corroded by decades of corruption and misrule. An effort to stem the empire's decline had recently been launched by the young sultan Selim III, who initiated far-reaching reforms and attempted to modernize his army. He required his officers to learn French and consulted with European experts, among them an innovating artillery officer named Napoleon Bonaparte. Napoleon repaid Selim's attentions by invading Egypt in July 1798 and advancing up the Syrian coast in the largest European penetration of the region since the Crusades. With Russians, Austrians, and the British encroaching on the empire from all sides, and European merchants exploiting the extraterritorial privileges—"capitulations"—granted to them by the Porte, Istanbul was not especially welcoming of Westerners.

Bainbridge, though, was a citizen of the one Western country the Ottomans respected—an island kingdom, they thought, which had successfully freed itself from European rule and had never coveted their lands. They had seen the Stars and Stripes hoisted only once, from the mast of a visiting French schooner on Bastille Day, 1793, but that single glimpse made a durable impression. Now, sighting that same flag as the George Washington made its way past Seraglio Point, the sultan purportedly likened its stars to the "heavenly bodies" on Turkey's own emblem and deduced that the two nations were celestially linked.[2]

Bainbridge's reception in Istanbul was accordingly warm, even fraternal. Admitted to the court of the capudan pasha, the chief of the Ottoman navy and the sultan's brother-in-law, the captain regaled his listeners with descriptions of his native land. Duly impressed, the capudan wrote to William Loughton Smith, America's first minister designate to the Porte, describing his pleasure in hosting "Capitaines Vilon Bien Bridg et George Valziton," and of his hope for similar visits in the future. He lavished gifts on Bainbridge and, at the captain's request, revoked the death sentence on the Dardanelles commander who had allowed the Americans to pass. The

George Washington was royally saluted as it exited the straits and set a course for home.

The hospitality shown to him in Istanbul could not, however, mitigate the insult that Bainbridge had sustained in Algiers. His rage continued unabated even after he returned to the United States and received a medal for heroism. If only Americans knew the "weakness" and "effeminacy" of the pirates, they would surely opt for war, Bainbridge fumed. "I am sure they would not long be tributary to so pitiful a race of Infidels."[3]

Triumphs and Tribulation

The umbrage was no longer Bainbridge's alone. The dey's effrontery had, according to Secretary of State James Madison, "deeply affected the sensibility" of the people of the United States, as well as of their new president, Thomas Jefferson.

In the fifteen years Jefferson had been dealing with the issue, his attitude toward the Barbary States had remained essentially unchanged. "There is no end to the demand of these powers," he insisted. "Nor any security in their promises." He continued to believe that force, rather than bribery, was a "more economical & more honorable" response to the pirates and declared himself "an enemy to all these douceurs, tributes and humiliations." He swore, as president, never again to submit to blackmail. Rather, he determined "to dispatch American frigates to the shores of North Africa" and "send the powder and ball wanting for Algiers."

Yet, ever the man of contradictions, Jefferson came into office extolling America's isolation from international affairs and reiterating his opposition to military entanglements. He proceeded to decommission a number of the Navy's ships and to reduce its contingent of officers. Remarkably, Jefferson maintained the hope of building an international coalition against Barbary, of working "in rotation" with the European powers to rid the Mediterranean of corsairs.

The Europeans, however, had never abandoned their initial aversion to Jefferson's proposed alliance. Meanwhile, North African "insolences," as the president called them, multiplied. Tripoli looted two American brigs, the *Catherine* and the *Franklin*, and demanded an additional $100,000 in tribute. Tunis also clamored for more—forty cannons and a stand of 10,000 muskets, plus a frigate of thirty-six guns. James Cathcart, America's consul in Tripoli, summarized the situation by asserting that "to buy peace with Tripoli is to bid for war with Tunis." The choice before the United States was now simple: either give up on the Mediterranean entirely or unilaterally prepare for battle.[4]

Jefferson opted for battle, but in doing so he came up against a daunting legal obstacle. The U.S. Constitution, created, in part, in response to the Barbary threat, reserved the right to declare war not for the president but for Congress. Uncertain whether Congress would make such a decree, Jefferson determined to sidestep the legislature and order a policing operation that fell just short of all-out war. The Navy was consequently instructed to enforce the existing treaties with North Africa, but also to "chastise" any aggression by the pirates "by sinking, burning or destroying their ships."

By circumventing Congress and personally authorizing military action in the Middle East, Jefferson set a precedent for future American presidents. In his case, however, the maneuver proved superfluous. While Jefferson was determining to act, tensions with Tripoli erupted. "A delay [in payments] on your part cannot but be prejudicial to your interests," Yusuf Qaramanli, the pasha, warned the American consul, Cathcart. On May 14, 1801, Qaramanli's troops marched to the American consulate and, in the traditional Tripolitan manner of announcing hostilities, cut down its flagpole. For the first time since gaining its independence, the United States was the target of a formally declared war.[5]

The country did not wait for further aggression from Tripoli, but quickly dispatched a squadron to the Middle East. The frigates *Essex, President,* and *Philadelphia,* together with the twelve-gun sloop *Enterprise,* reached Gibraltar, where they kept the *Mashuda*—formerly, the ill-fated *Betsey*—bottled up in port. They then crossed the Mediterranean to blockade Tripoli harbor and lob a few shells into the city to "amuse" Qaramanli. In the course of these operations, the *Enterprise* chanced upon the *Tripoli,* an enemy ship bearing fourteen guns. Employing a ruse then considered acceptable in naval warfare, the *Enterprise* ran up a British flag and drew within point-blank range. Then, hoisting suddenly the Stars and Stripes, American gunners raked the *Tripoli*'s deck with canister, slicing its sails and rigging. A boarding party under Lieutenant David Porter cast the pirates' guns and cargo into the sea and stripped their commander, Reis Muhammad Sous, of his sword. The *Tripoli* was allowed to limp home, where Sous was publicly flogged and pelted with tripe. Of his eighty-man crew, thirty had been wounded and thirty killed, but not a single American was hurt.[6]

America's first military engagement in the Middle East was an unqualified triumph, but its success proved maddeningly brief. Tripoli's captains, in their fleet and shallow-drafted vessels, handily ran the blockade. Even the *Mashuda* managed to slip its cordon. The squadron's commodore, Richard Dale, a seasoned fighter who had been captured twice and wounded three times in the War of Independence and had sailed under John Paul Jones, was flummoxed. Damning the "whole tribe, Algereans, Tunisians and Tripolians," Dale could see no means of protecting American commerce without maintaining a permanent Mediterranean force of four frigates, at least. The United States would otherwise have no alternative but to resort, once again, to bribery.

"Shall we buy peace?" the temperamental Jefferson, his reddish complexion darkening, harangued his cabinet. Victory, he realized, could not be achieved without a much larger fleet, but that would require a declaration of war—the very congressional act the president had originally intended to skirt. Surprisingly, though, Congress now proved amenable. "I am fully persuaded that our fellow-citizens who are engaged in commerce have an equal right to protection with the planter who remains at home upon his farm," the representative from Virginia, John Stratton, explained. On February 6, 1802, Congress passed an Act for Protection of Commerce and Seamen of the United States against the Tripolitan Corsairs, a de facto declaration of war.[7]

The squadron, expanded to five frigates and a schooner and bolstered by a contingent of Marines, was permitted to use its "best exertions to keep the enemy's vessels in port" and to "subdue, seize, [and] make prize of" any attempting to escape. Nevertheless, much like the first expedition against Tripoli, this mission, too, was doomed.

A portent of that failure occurred on the night of May 25, when eleven wheat-laden feluccas foundered on Tripoli's coast. A landing party under Lieutenant Porter managed to set fire to half of the boats and scatter their undisciplined crews. "Twas good sport I must confess," Midshipman Henry Wadsworth, uncle of the poet Longfellow, recalled. But the Tripolitans managed to regroup and lay down a withering fire that left Porter wounded in both thighs and fifteen sailors dead. America had suffered its first military casualties in the Middle East, but with little gain to show for them. Tripoli's boats continued to evade the frigates or, when sighted, to scurry landward for the safety of the city's guns. The Americans' frustration was aggravated by their commander, Richard Morris, who spent much of his time dining with British officers in Gibraltar, in the company of his wife and son. Rather than rally his forces for a concerted offensive, Morris stepped onto Tripoli's shore waving a white flag and a $5,000 "inducement" for the pasha.

Described by Cathcart as a "venal wretch destitute of every honorable sentiment," Yusuf Qaramanli was a cold-blooded ruler who had seized power by murdering one brother and exiling another. He would not be inexpensively bought. Nor was he easily intimidated. "I do not fear war, it is my trade," he informed Morris. The pasha had already concluded that Americans were no different from Europeans, that they "will talk a great deal and do nothing, and at last come cap in hand and sue for peace upon my own terms." He accordingly sought $200,000 in gifts from the United States, plus a $20,000 annuity. Dumbfounded by these demands, and fearing that Qaramanli might arrest and hold him for ransom as well, Morris fled back to his ship. The Navy subsequently court-martialed him for "inactive and desultory conduct" and stripped him of his commission.[8]

Jefferson had sworn to "rest the safety of our commerce on . . . our own strength and bravery in every sea," but pledges of that sort, by 1803, rang hollow. Emboldened by Tripoli's defiance of the United States, Tunis and Algiers also upped their tribute demands, and Morocco abruptly declared war. "Our security against the Barbary Powers must depend on force and not upon treaties, upon ships of war instead of presents and subsidies," Rufus King, America's minister to Britain, counseled his government. Jefferson certainly agreed, but debt-ridden by his purchase of Louisiana from France, he was hard-pressed to maintain even two frigates in the Mediterranean, much less mount a full-scale attack.

The president did have one notable advantage: a new commodore. Edward Preble, a forty-two-year-old naval martinet from Maine, was obsessed with discipline and hygiene. Numerous ailments contracted in a British prison ship during the Revolutionary War had done little to diminish Preble's predatory appearance, his fiery red hair and talonlike nose, or his desire to meet the pirates in battle. "The Moors are a designing, artful, treacherous set of villains," he growled and swore "to beat . . . his savage highness," the pasha, "into a disposition more favorable to our views."[9]

Sailing under Preble was William Bainbridge, the luckless captain of the *George Washington*, who had since recovered from his humiliation in Algiers to command one of America's premier frigates, the thirty-six-gun *Philadelphia*. Shortly after entering the Mediterranean in August 1803, Bainbridge engaged the *Mirkoba*, a Moroccan man-of-war that, on inspection, proved to be the captured American brig *Celia*, with its crew in chains belowdecks. "I sincerely hope that this capture may be productive of good effects to the U.S.," the captain reported, and stressed the "lenity" and "humanity" shown to the Moroccan prisoners "to impress on their mind a favorable opinion of the American Character."

Preble, meanwhile, anchored in Tangier and demanded to speak with the emperor. "Are you afraid of being arrested?" Sulaiman asked as Preble approached him without bowing or removing his sword. "No," the American answered. "[And] if you presume to do that, my squadron . . . will lay your batteries, your castles and your city in ruins." Morocco at once agreed to renew the 1786 treaty, unconditionally.

Preble's expedition began auspiciously but, like previous operations, it, too, ended in defeat. On the afternoon of October 31, while chasing a Tripolitan polacca close to shore, the *Philadelphia* struck a reef and foundered. Frantic efforts to dislodge the ship—cutting the foremast, heaving equipment overboard—or even scuttle it proved futile. With his guns pinned at useless angles and nine enemy gun-boats closing in, Bainbridge resigned himself to surrender. He and 307 crewmen were stripped of their uniforms and left shivering outside the former U.S. consulate, while the victors, wielding cables, pried the *Philadelphia* loose and tugged it triumphantly into port. The ship, Qaramanli boasted, would be enlisted in Tripoli's navy and renamed *The Gift of Allah*.

"It is with deep regret that I inform you of the loss of the United States frigate *Philadelphia*," Bainbridge wrote the secretary of the navy, thus announcing America's worst military disaster since the Revolution. He revisited the indignity of his first Middle Eastern voyage, recalling how "to strike [colors] to any foe was mortifying, but to yield to an uncivilized enemy . . . was humiliating." To Preble, though, he adopted a more aggressive air. In a note penned in vanishing lime juice, Bainbridge implored his commander to deny Tripoli its prize and to destroy the *Philadelphia* at once.[10]

Preble scarcely needed persuading. "Would to God that the officers and crew . . . had one and all determined to prefer death to slavery." He prepared an audacious plan in which the Americans would sail a recently seized Tripolitan ketch into the harbor, quietly board the *Philadelphia*, and torch it. To command the operation, Preble turned to the son of a U.S. naval hero, a young lieutenant lionized by one fellow officer as "chivalrous in temper, courteous in his deportment, and adding grace of manner to an attractive person." His name was Stephen Decatur.

With his slim, delicate nose and sensuous mouth, his doelike, long-lashed eyes, Decatur looked more like a poet than a swashbuckler. Yet, ever since childhood, when he purportedly swung from jib booms and defended his mother against ruffians, he had cultivated a reputation for physical daring. In a duel on Malta earlier that year, he killed an English officer and had to flee the island. Now, at twenty-five, Decatur was serving on the USS *Essex*, where he received Preble's orders to lead the mission. "We are now about to embark on an expedition which may terminate in our sudden deaths, our perpetual slavery, or our immortal glory," he said while asking for volunteers. The entire crew stepped forward.

At nine-thirty on the night of February 16, 1804, under a young moon, Decatur set out. With him on the ketch, now rechristened the *Intrepid*, were sixty-seven volunteers dressed as Maltese sailors. Ahead of them lay the double-shotted guns of the *Philadelphia* and all of Tripoli's batteries, a total of more than 150 muzzles.

With the help of an Arabic-speaking helmsman, the *Intrepid* managed to penetrate the harbor and make fast to the *Philadelphia*'s hull. Decatur then whispered the command to board. The volunteers swiftly overran the ship, killing twenty of its defenders and setting it alight. "Americans!" Tripoli's sentries cried—too late—for the fire had already ignited the *Philadelphia*'s cannons, blasting the city. Twenty minutes later, Decatur and his men stared, mesmerized, as fire consumed the frigate. "The flames . . . ascending her rigging and masts, formed columns of fire," one crew member recounted. "Whilst the discharge of her guns gave an idea of some directing spirit within her."[11]

The operation was hailed throughout Europe. Britain's Lord Nelson called it "the most bold and daring act of the age," and Pope Pius VII claimed that the U.S. Navy had "done more for the cause of Christianity than the most powerful nations of Christendom have done for ages." But for all of Decatur's fearlessness, Preble was still left with the burden of redeeming Bainbridge and his crew. The man who had once pledged to "spend [his] life in the Mediterranean" rather than pay "a cent for tribute or peace" now offered the pasha a staggering $100,000 in ransoms. Qaramanli only scoffed at the proposal, though, and demanded more than $1.5 million for his captives.

Dishonored, enraged, Preble resumed his offensive, bombarding and raiding Tripoli's port. In one poignant action, Decatur and fifteen men armed with "bayonet, spear, saber and tomahawk" charged through the "promiscuous hissings of round and grape" onto the enemy's boats. Though speared in the arm, he succeeded in shooting a pirate captain and in dodging another corsair who tried to decapitate him. His brother, though, also an officer with the fleet, was less fortunate and died from a gunshot wound to the head. By day's end, the Americans could claim forty-seven Tripolitans dead and fifty-six taken prisoner. "Some of the Turks died like men, but much the greater number like women," Decatur vaunted, but Preble quashed his brio. Learning that Decatur had captured "only" three gunboats, the commodore upbraided him, "Three, sir! Where are the rest of them?"

Preble had good reason to be piqued, for after six months and thousands of cannon balls, Tripoli lay largely unscathed. "Such attempts served rather to encourage than intimidate the Tripolitans," observed Dr. Jonathan Cowdery, the captive surgeon of the *Philadelphia*. The American prisoners, meanwhile, were reduced to a daily allowance of "eight oz. of bread and a little bad oil" and were repeatedly beaten and dragged into the desert to work. Hopes for alleviating their plight further diminished on August 7, when Preble was relieved of his command. "I cannot but regret that our naval establishment is so limited as to deprive me of the means and glory of completely subduing the haughty tyrant of Tripoli," he griped. But before departing, Preble determined to make a last, desperate grab for victory.[12]

The *Intrepid* was now primed with 15,000 pounds of gunpowder and packed with grapeshot and shells. A childhood friend of Decatur's, Captain Richard Somers, along with two lieutenants, Wadsworth and Joseph Israel, and ten sailors, volunteered to guide the ship into the harbor. Lighting a fuse, they would then descend into a rowboat and escape before the ship exploded, destroying the pasha's fleet.

The squadron watched as the *Intrepid* disappeared into the moonless, misty night of September 3 and was watching still, two hours later, when a detonation "loud and terrible" split the horizon. One witness, Midshipman Robert T. Spence, described seeing shells blazing in the air "like so many planets" and "a vast stream of fire . . . ascending to heaven." Short of its target and for causes unknown, the *Intrepid* had exploded, killing all hands. The next morning, Bainbridge, limping from a wound received from one of the navy's barrages, was taken down to the beach to view the scorched and mangled bodies. He begged permission to bury them, but the bey refused, insisting that the remains be left for the dogs.

"You have done well not to purchase peace with the enemy," Sir Alexander Ball, Malta's British governor, wrote to Preble, but the commodore would not be consoled. He was still beset by the triumph that eluded him and by thoughts of those who remained captive in Tripoli. To the American public, though, Preble was a hero. The celebrations that greeted his return to Washington, D.C., in January 1805 nearly upstaged those of Jefferson's second inauguration, which were held that same day. Decatur was also feted, decorated with a golden sword and promoted to captain, the Navy's youngest.[13]

Accolades alone, however, could not disguise the fact that America had gone to war in the Middle East but had so far failed to win. Nor did the United States have an excuse for failing, now that the Navy possessed enough warships to defeat all of the corsair fleets combined. "[P]eace with Tripoli was for a long time in our power and almost on our own terms," Madison averred, but other prominent cabinet members remained hesitant about applying that might. The Swiss-born treasury secretary, Albert Gallatin, reasoned that by bribing the pirates the United States would merely "share the dishonor . . . with so many nations as powerful and interested as ourselves," and save the $900,000 price of maintaining a Mediterranean squadron. Public opinion also remained divided about resorting to force, unsure of the relative costs of waging war and purchasing peace.

The dearth of support for military action, both within his government and among Americans at large, weighed on Thomas Jefferson. Entering his second term, the president listed the crisis in the Middle East as the nation's highest foreign relations priority. The loss of the *Philadelphia*, he wrote, "was the most serious one which has happened to the present administration," a "national stain" that threatened to expose America's weakness to the world. Particularly distressful to Jefferson were the efforts of American diplomats in Europe who had taken it upon themselves to request French, Russian, and even Ottoman assistance in redeeming the captives. By "begging alms in every country," these representatives threatened to deprive the United States of its "just desires of revenge," Jefferson worried, and to leave its "honor prostrated." In order to preclude that disaster, the president would have to permit American warships to "beat . . . [the Algerians'] town about their ears," but he still lacked a popular mandate for doing so.[14]

For one American, however, the absence of public enthusiasm for the use of force was irrelevant. As consul to Tunis, William Eaton had learned that paying tribute to pirates merely earned disdain for America and intensified their appetite for more. Experience had taught him that in the Middle East power alone was respected and that, in order to gain peace, the United States had no alternative but to wield it.

A Modern Africanus

Though his portrait depicts finely sculpted, almost idealized features, Eaton was described by one contemporary as "a great bulldog of a man—in appearance and personality." That pugnacity was manifest at age sixteen, when Eaton fled his father's Connecticut farm to fight in the Continental Army. He later attended Dartmouth, studied Latin and Greek, and memorized the campaigns of Caesar and Alexander the Great. The student also gained proficiency as a knife thrower, accurate at eighty feet, and dreamed of someday returning to battle. "No man will hereafter love you as I do," he confessed to a certain widow he was courting, "but I prefer the field of Mars to the bower of Venus." Eaton subsequently reenlisted in the army and served as a captain under General "Mad Anthony" Wayne, fighting Native Americans in Ohio.

Though he considered himself "a man not overly meek, scrupulously pious . . . [or] implicitly credulous," Eaton was an egoist who had trouble taking orders. Discharged from the corps, he found employment as a clerk in the Vermont legislature, where he might have languished if not for a family connection with Timothy Pickering, John Adams's secretary of state. In 1799, Pickering selected Eaton to serve as America's first-ever consul to Tunis, an assignment seemingly more suited to his character.[15]

Like John Ledyard before him, Eaton was at first flushed with romantic notions of the Middle East. He swore to uphold his belief in a tolerant "Universal God" and vanquish "the idea that Mahometans and Christians are *natural enemies*." His instructions were to help turn Tunisians away from piracy to more peaceful vocations, such as agriculture. Yet the gifts he bore with him to North Africa, including two American-made warships, conveyed the oppo-

site message—namely, that piracy paid. The bey of Tunis accepted
the bribes, then promptly threatened to renew his war with America.
Eaton had to entice him with bolts of precious cloth, gold watches,
and gem-studded canes, at a cost of $6,000. In return, the bey pre-
sented him with a humiliating bill for $800, to pay for the gunpow-
der used in saluting the new consul's arrival.

"A year endured is longer than an eternity *enjoyed*," Eaton was
caviling by 1800. "Is this not enough to constitute hell?" That short
period sufficed to eradicate the consul's original fantasies and to
leave him thoroughly disgusted. His grievances against Tunis seemed
almost too numerous to be cataloged—"foetid vapor of stagnant
lakes, exhalations of putrid carcases . . . mad rays of a ve[r]tical sun
. . . hotter than tobacco & rum . . . brutal turks, swindling jews, per-
fidious Italians . . . lazy cammels, churlish mules and savage arabs."
Though he made an impressive effort to learn about the local culture, mastering four dialects and traveling widely throughout the
region, Eaton could find nothing redeeming about the Middle East—
a "land of rapine and sodomy," he concluded, whose people knew
"no restraints of honor nor honesty."

More stinging than the physical discomforts, though, was the
shame Eaton experienced in watching America transfer its honestly
earned wealth to the despots of North Africa. "Genius of my country! How art thou prostrate!" he groaned after learning of Captain
Bainbridge's humiliation by Algiers. His indignity was again aroused
by Tripoli's declaration of war against the United States in May 1801
and by the Navy's repeated failure to protect American trade. Were
there no Americans "whose nerves convulse, blood vessels bust, and
heart indignant swells" at indignities inflicted on them by corsairs,
he asked. "Are we then reduced to . . . bartering our national glory
for the forbearance of a Barbary pirate?"

Eaton proposed an audacious answer to his own questions. One
thousand U.S. Marines would invade Tunis and overthrow the bey,
striking fear into other Barbary rulers. Secretary of State Madison
rejected the plan, however, and instead authorized Eaton to conciliate the bey with an inducement of $20,000. "[The] Government may
as well send *quaker meeting houses* to float about this sea as
frigates," the consul groused, and suggested that the symbol of the

United States be changed, from an eagle wielding arrows to one clutching "a *fiddle* bow or a *cigar*." Eaton could not comprehend how the president and the Congress failed to realize that paying tribute and refraining from the use of force merely emboldened the pirates and further endangered American ships. "There is but one language which can be held to these people," Eaton wrote, "and this is *terror*."[16]

Eaton had nearly despaired of America's fecklessness when, in September 1801, he met Hamid Qaramanli, the exiled brother of Tripoli's sovereign. Impressed by his nobleness and courage, Eaton now suggested that the United States help Hamid reclaim his rightful throne and retain him as a trustworthy ally. Only by changing Tripoli's regime could Americans "redeem their national honor with *steel* and not with *gold*," Eaton explained, but the principled, if often reticent, Madison once again balked at the idea. Though the consul was free to apply his "zeal and . . . calculations" on Hamid's behalf, Madison replied, the United States would not interfere in another nation's domestic conflicts.

Eaton was livid. The government seemed bent on "buy[ing] oil of rose to perfume that pirate's [Qaramanli's] beard" rather than "gun batteries to chastise his temerity." He warned that in ten years the pirates would be raiding towns on America's coast, raping their women, and abducting young boys. Officials in Washington might as well start dressing as slaves, Eaton jeered.

Later generations of Americans would remember Eaton as a hero, a trailblazer, and a maverick, preferring to forget that he was also a misanthrope, a curmudgeon ruthlessly critical of his fellow consuls, and a bigot. He defamed Treasury Secretary Gallatin as "a cowardly Jew" and Jefferson as a "whipt Spaniel" cowering before the lash of Barbary.[17] The malevolent Eaton was also conniving in his financial deals—a penchant that increasingly displeased his superiors as well as his Tunisian hosts. These schemes finally provided the bey with a pretext for banishing the consul, and in April 1803 Eaton returned to the United States.

Eaton did not give up on his plan for replacing Yusuf Qaramanli with Hamid and as soon as he reached Washington, began lobbying for congressional support. He assured legislators that the people of Tripoli, "those harmless sun-brown children of credulity," would rally to the pretender's cause. Meanwhile, word arrived of the *Philadelphia*'s seizure by Tripoli and the capture of its entire crew. News of the disaster pitched Eaton into anguish. If America's position in the Middle East was humiliating before, it now seemed thoroughly hopeless.

Eaton's campaigning finally paid off in May 1804, when he was appointed U.S. agent to the Barbary States. At the first opportunity he sailed for Egypt, where the fugitive Hamid had last sought refuge from his brother. "God ordained that you should see trouble," Eaton wrote, comforting him. "We believe he hath ordained also that your troubles shall now have an end."[18]

Eaton's troubles, however, had scarcely commenced. Traveling up the Nile in the company of Lieutenant Presley Neville O'Bannon and his small detachment of Marines, Eaton braved rapids, Bedouin raids, and shakedowns from corrupt Ottoman officials. He located Hamid, forlorn and beleaguered, at a place called Arab Tower, about 150 miles from Cairo. There, on March 8, 1805, Eaton assembled his army.

The force was motley in the extreme, composed of nine Americans, ninety Tripolitans, sixty-three mercenaries from Europe, and 250 Bedouin. Armaments were scarce. "I shall be compelled to draw on the enthusiasm of Arabian resentment . . . as a substitute for field artillery, muskets, cartridges, [and] flints." Gathering his troops, Eaton explained that all men were considered equal in the United States, irrespective of creed, and valued solely for their honesty. He also doled out large quantities of gold—"Cash," he grunted, "is the only deity of Arabs"—and pledged to do his utmost to establish Hamid in power. Hamid, in turn, promised to maintain peaceful relations with the United States once he became pasha and to release all of the American prisoners in Tripoli. Eaton then promoted himself to general, donned a spanking white uniform of his own design, and set out to accomplish what no commander since antiquity had even contemplated: marching five hundred miles across the sun-hammered Western Desert.

The trek, he wrote, "o'er burning sands, and rocky mountains . . . through an inhospitable waste of world," indeed proved agonizing. After twelve days, the men were reduced to eating half-rations of rice, uncooked for lack of water. But the cruel terrain and dwindling provisions were the least of Eaton's obstacles. More menacing were the fights that broke out between Muslim and Christian contingents in his army, and also the Bedouin who, in their daily demands for higher wages, threatened to desert or revolt. "They have no sense of patriotism, truth nor honor," Eaton complained. "And no attachment where they have no prospect of gain." Hamid, too, proved to be a nuisance, incessantly whining about his fears of Yusuf and about his lack of faith in America. Tensions climaxed when Hamid joined the Bedouin in storming the supply train, only to be repulsed by a firing line formed by Eaton and the Marines.

Surmounting these crises, Eaton and his force staggered, utterly parched, to the Bay of Bomba, about thirty miles west of Tobruk, where an American warship was supposed to be waiting with supplies. The bay, however, was empty. Days passed, and death seemed certain for all four hundred men when a sail miraculously appeared on the horizon. The USS *Argus* had arrived, loaded with victuals and water. Refreshed, Eaton's army continued its westward march to Darna (or Derne), the region's second-largest port and an ideal launching site for a final thrust at Tripoli. On April 25, Eaton galloped up to Darna's gate and demanded the city's surrender. "Let no difference of religion induce us to shed the blood of harmless men," he called out to the governor, assuring him that his sole objective was to enthrone a rightful sovereign. The governor's response was laconic: "My head or yours."

Eaton could no longer tarry; a large contingent of Qaramanli's men, he discovered, was rushing to Darna from Tripoli. While the *Argus*, along with the *Hornet* and the *Nautilus*, hove within range and began bombarding Darna's defenses, Eaton drew his sword and signaled for a frontal assault. Two Marines were killed and Eaton was shot through the wrist, yet the attackers managed to breach the walls and storm the city. The fighting was hand-to-hand, but after four hours the Stars and Stripes fluttered over Darna. The battle was far from concluded, though. Three thousand of Yusuf's troops appeared and immediately counterattacked. The charge was broken at the cost of sixty of Eaton's men. Still, the self-proclaimed general remained confident of his soldiers' ability to weather the siege and to continue the march to Tripoli. Then, in late May, the USS *Constellation* appeared offshore with a most astonishing message from the commodore, Samuel Barron. The U.S. government was withdrawing its support for the campaign to install Hamid, having concluded a favorable agreement with Yusuf.[19]

Though this was never revealed to Eaton, Jefferson had all along doubted the feasibility of changing Tripoli's leadership by force. Searching for a diplomatic option, the president turned to Tobias Lear, a forty-two-year-old former aide to George Washington, who was then serving as consul to Santo Domingo. Long-faced, businesslike, and grim, Lear was not the type to spur a mercenary army across the desert to attack an enemy fort, preferring negotiations instead. He dismissed Eaton as an egotistical romantic and ridiculed Hamid as a moral weakling incapable of signing any treaty, much less of keeping one. Rather, Lear would deal only with Yusuf, offering to exchange one hundred Tripolitan prisoners of war for the *Philadephia* captives and to pay Tripoli a "balance" of $60,000.[20]

Yusuf, now threatened by a major enemy force in Darna, eagerly received the deal. He even agreed to let Hamid return to Tripoli, if Eaton would withdraw with his men. With the decision finalized, on June 4, 1805, the USS *Constitution* sailed into Tripoli harbor. It cruised alongside the charred wreck of the *Philadelphia* and was welcomed by a twenty-one-gun salute. Assembled on the dock were Bainbridge and 296 of his men (six had died, five had converted to Islam), freed after nineteen months of grueling captivity.

News of the arrangement spread throughout North Africa. Algiers dropped its demands for additional tribute and Tunis reaffirmed the Treaty of Amity and Friendship. A goodwill delegation of Tunisian envoys also traveled to Washington, where they ran up bills for wine and the services of one "Georgia, a Greek," and enjoyed themselves so much that three of them refused to go home. Back in Tripoli, meanwhile, American carpenters fashioned a nautical spar into a new flagpole for the U.S. consulate. Delighted with the fruits of his diplomacy, Lear expected that America's peace with Barbary would be "so unusually honorable" that all of Europe would admire it.[20]

Eaton, in contrast to Lear, was crestfallen. He had traversed one of the world's harshest deserts, fought pitched battles against superior forces, and spent ninety days in the same uniform, only to be told to retreat. Better that the *Constitution* were "covered with blood and death," he swore, "than to see a few contemptible turks triumph over a crew of pale Americans." He warned Commodore Barron that Jefferson's decision had irreparably impaired America's deterrence power and that the pirates would now strike again and more viciously. But the commodore had his orders to abandon Darna. Sneaking under darkness to the beach, Eaton and his Christian troops were evacuated by American ships. The Bedouin, Eaton recalled, "some uttering shrieks, some execrations," destroyed what remained of the camp.[21]

Eaton would never forgive what he regarded as Lear's treachery and Jefferson's double cross. "Honor recoils and humanity bleeds," he complained to his friends in Congress, and accused the administration of abetting "patricide, fratricide, treason, perfidy . . . and systematic piracy." In spite of his petulance, many representatives considered him a hero, a modern incarnation of Leo Africanus, the sixteenth-century geographer of the Middle East. "You have acquired immortal honor and established the fame of your country in the East," Commodore Preble lauded him. Yet even Eaton's firmest supporters were uncomfortable with the notion of overthrowing a legitimate monarch and jeopardizing what promised to be a lucrative peace.[22]

A similar sense of realism, it seemed, had also motivated Jefferson. He had achieved his long-sought goal of creating a military force capable of imposing America's will on Barbary, but at the same time, he learned that the use of power in the Middle East could be fraught with moral compromises. Qaramanli had indeed been vanquished, but in the end he was also paid. The United States had humbled a Middle Eastern ruler, gaining immensely in terms of its pride and freedom of trade, but it had yet to eradicate the practice of tribute.

The qualified nature of America's victory was evident in Jefferson's annual address to Congress in December 1805. Never at a loss for paradox, the president who had once dismissed dozens of naval officers and opposed the construction of frigates now proposed an unprecedented expansion of the nation's maritime defenses. Seaports would be fortified and waterways regularly patrolled, he announced.

A campaign would be mounted to recruit new captains and to begin building massive, seventy-four-gun vessels, America's first ships of the line.

Jefferson unveiled this plan and then revealed how "an operation by . . . a small band of our countrymen . . . gallantly conducted by our late consul Eaton" had created the "impression" necessary for reaching an agreement with Tripoli. As a result, America's prisoners had been liberated and its merchants freed from peril. Though the United States still needed to maintain vigilance in the Mediterranean, Jefferson concluded, the rulers of Barbary "seem generally disposed at present to respect our peace and friendship."[23]

Jefferson's words no doubt aroused a thunderous ovation. Nevertheless, many congressmen might have been discomfited by the president's use of qualifiers like "seem" and "at present." Some, too, may have noted the absence of any guarantee for permanent peace with North Africa, or for an end to payments of tribute. A few may even have predicted that America's Navy, expanded and reinforced, would someday have to fight Barbary again.

Powder and Balls

On June 22, 1807, the thirty-six-gun frigate *Chesapeake* departed Norfolk, Virginia, en route to join America's squadron in the Mediterranean. Once outside territorial waters, the ship encountered the *Leopard*, a British double-decker with fifty guns. Britain, short on sailors for its war with Napoleon, had demanded the right to search American ships for so-called British deserters and to impress them into the Royal Navy. The *Leopard* closed in, but the American commander, James Barron—the younger brother of Samuel Barron—held fast. The battle proved embarrassingly one-sided. Short of fuses to ignite their cannons, the Americans managed to fire only one broadside to the *Leopard*'s seven, before surrendering.

Occurring so briefly after the North African successes, the *Chesapeake*'s defeat dealt a stinging blow to the Navy's and the nation's pride. Barron was convicted of negligence by a court-martial board that included David Porter and Stephen Decatur. More ignominious still, the Navy was forced to reduce the size of the Mediterranean Squadron in order to reinforce America's shores. In spite of his recent boasts of triumphs over Barbary, Jefferson now quietly recommended making additional payments to Algiers "to secure peace there while it is uncertain elsewhere."

Algiers, not surprisingly, was eager to exploit America's disadvantage. In February 1809, its corsairs sacked the Philadelphia brig *Sally*, enslaving fifteen of its crew. "They fired several shots at us, and then boarding us sword in hand, commenced an outrageous attack," Seaman Thomas Nicholson of New Jersey remembered. "They unmercifully beat and maimed us and . . . confined us 48 hours, without food." Once again, the Americans were pelted with refuse and paraded through the streets, prior to being sold at auction. Those who tried to escape received the customary punishment, as Nicholson harrowingly described:

After they had stripped the sufferer naked, they inserted the iron pointed stake into the lower termination of the vertebrae, and thence forced it up near his back bone, until it appeared between the shoulders, avoiding the vital parts. The stake was then raised in the air and the poor sufferer exposed to the view of the other slaves, writhing in . . . insupportable agony.

America's ability to respond to these outrages was definitively undermined in June 1812 by the eruption of war with Britain. Three months later, Algerian pirates snatched the *Edwin*, a Salem-based brig, and its eleven-man crew. "My policy and my views are to increase, not to diminish the number of my American slaves," the dey, Hadj 'Ali Pasha, explained. "And not for a million dollars would I release them." Algerian recidivism was soon replicated in Tripoli and Tunis, both of which resumed their attacks on American merchantmen and declared their allegiance to the British crown.

Though armed with some fifty warships, the United States now faced a Royal Navy of eight hundred vessels, a quarter of them ships of the line, and could not spare a single frigate for the Mediterranean. "Should our differences with Great Britain be so accommodated as to admit of sending a naval force into this sea . . . *Algiers will be humbled to the dust,*" Tobias Lear predicted.[24] But Britain would not accommodate the United States by ending the war and President James Madison saw little alternative, once again, to bribing the pirates.

The concept of paying tribute was now exceedingly unpopular among Americans, however, and to execute that unsavory task the administration selected an extraordinary man, Mordecai Manuel Noah. At age twenty-seven he had already excelled as a journalist, a playwright, and a politician, and had established friendships with public figures such as Stephen Decatur and Joel Barlow. Descended from Portuguese Jews, Noah also distinguished himself as a defender of Jewish rights and identity. As such, he seemed uniquely qualified to intercede in the Barbary affair. Jews, even those from European backgrounds, were widely regarded as natural intermediaries between the Christian West and the Islamic Middle East. Indeed, another American Jew, Colonel David Franks, had served as George Washington's personal representative in the treaty negotiations with Morocco in 1786. Madison acted on that precedent by naming Noah as the U.S. consul to Tunis and by authorizing him to spend $3,000 for the redemption of each captive. This money, the consul was to explain, had been donated by the prisoners' families and was in no way connected to the federal government.

Noah embarked for the Middle East—appropriately, aboard the *Joel Barlow*—in May 1813 and immediately made contact with the Algerian dey. He secured pardons for six Americans, but at the exorbitant cost of $25,910. Appalled by this expense, and afraid that the public would learn of it, Madison sought some excuse to recall the consul to Washington. "It might be well to rest the reason pretty much on the ascertained prejudice of the Turks against his Religion," the president ventured, "and it having become public that he was a Jew." Though no one in Tunis had ever expressed any such sentiment, Noah was forced to come home.[25]

Madison had helped establish a tradition of appointing American Jews to Middle Eastern diplomatic posts, but his initial liberalism was sullied by the persistent practice of paying ransoms. Similar lapses were liable to occur as long as America remained powerless to resist the pirates' demands and to respond to their depredations forcefully. The United States was unable to muster that might, however, while hostilities with Great Britain continued.

The War of 1812 threatened not only America's security—the British burned the nation's capital—but also its hard-won unity, as New Englanders opposed to the war contemplated secession. Nevertheless, through the resilience of ground commanders such as Andrew Jackson, a leader later to play a pivotal role in America's relations with the Middle East, disaster was averted. The Navy, especially, excelled. Applying the experience they had acquired fighting Barbary, American crews braved Britain's naval juggernaut, sinking and capturing several enemy ships. The score with Algiers remained unsettled, though, until the war's end with the Treaty of Ghent, signed on Christmas Eve, 1814. Public opinion in America clamored for retribution against the pirates and it fell to the president to decide when and how to exact it.

James Madison did not make decisions easily. At sixty-four, he was a wizened and frail man, cerebral and shy, and often at odds with his cabinet. Now, caught between popular pressure for revenge against Barbary and his reluctance to wage another war so soon after peace had been restored, the president waffled. Nearly three months passed before he went to Congress and asked for—and promptly received—a formal declaration of war. The commander of the expedition, Stephen Decatur, received instructions to threaten to inflict "serious disasters" on the rulers of North Africa and achieve nothing less than "a just and lasting peace."

Decatur departed New York on May 15, leading a powerful squadron of ten ships, including the forty-four-gun frigate *Guerriere*, recently captured from the British. One month later, near the coast of Spain, the *Guerriere* engaged Algiers's forty-six-gun flagship, killing its captain, Reis Hammida, and thirty of his crew. Decatur's force next chased aground another hostile brig, the *Estedio*. A total of five hundred prisoners had been taken, at a cost of seven Americans who were killed by a misfiring cannon.

On the morning of June 28, Omar Pasha, Algiers's new dey, awoke to the sight of ten American warships debouched in his harbor. Panic-stricken, he appealed to the British, recalling how they had assured him "that the Americans would be swept from the seas in six months" and pointing out that now "they make war upon us with some of your own vessels!" But the tables had effectively turned. Britain was no longer at war with the United States, and Algiers, alone, could not defend itself against the American fleet. The dey had no choice but to receive Decatur, together with the new U.S. consul designate, William Shaler. Cuban born and Princeton educated, Shaler was a shrewd and hard-nosed negotiator whose opinion of the North Africans closely echoed Eaton's. "Islamism, which requires little instruction, . . . seems peculiarly adapted to the conceptions of barbarous people," he wrote, amazed that so "worthless a power should have been so long permitted to vex the commercial world and extort ransom."

Shaler and Decatur presented the dey with what they styled "liberal and enlightened" terms, "dictated at the mouths of our cannon." Not only would Algiers cease receiving tribute from the United States; it would pay a $10,000 indemnity and unconditionally release its American captives. "If you insist in receiving powder as tribute," Decatur warned the Algerian ruler, "you must expect to receive balls with it." Omar made an unctuous appeal to Madison, addressing him as "the Emperor of America . . . our noble friend . . . the pillar of all Christian sovereigns, the most glorious among princes . . . the happy, the great, the amiable," but his effusiveness was wasted. "It is a . . . settled policy of America, that as peace is better than war, war is better than tribute," the president replied. "The United States, while they wish for war with no nation, will buy peace with none." Madison's adamancy was further demonstrated that July when the ship of the line *Independence* positioned itself off Algiers. Commanded by William Bainbridge, it would remain in the North African area as the mainstay of the Mediterranean Squadron, America's first permanent overseas force.[26]

By that time, Decatur had advanced to Tunis and Tripoli, demanding compensation for seized ships and the release of any remaining hostages. The fleet returned to the United States with the flags of twenty-nine enemy vessels—the banners were stitched into a mat and presented to First Lady Dolly Madison—and with seven Tripolitan prisoners who were exhibited as "real bona fide imported Turks" in several New York theaters. So concluded more than three decades of struggle between United States and North Africa. The pirates of Barbary who had captured a total of thirty-five American vessels and seven hundred sailors, and who had threatened America's survival and tarnished its pride, were crushed.

Yet the question could still be asked: was that struggle justified? In purely financial terms, the answer was an unequivocal no. The price for battling Tripoli alone between 1802 and 1805 came to three million dollars, a sum far greater than the tribute America paid to all four Barbary States in those same years. John Adams was correct in his estimate that fighting the pirates would prove costlier than bribing them. Strategically, however, America's gain vastly exceeded its outlay. By realizing Jefferson's ideal of an "erect and independent attitude" in the Middle East, the United States shielded itself from blackmail and garnered respect internationally. "The name of an American is now the proudest in the world," trumpeted the widely read *Niles' Weekly Register*. "We are greatly mistaken if this war with Algiers does not give it additional influence in the councils of Europe." The boast was far from empty. A year after the American expedition, a combined Anglo-Dutch fleet followed Decatur's example by pummeling Algiers into submission. As one British contemporary huffed, "It was not to be endured that England should tolerate what America had resented and punished."

The Barbary Wars altered European perceptions of the United States, but, more decidedly, the victory also transformed Americans' image of themselves. The war infused them with reinvigorated emotions of national pride and a galvanized sense of identity. Patriotic symbols such as flags, bald eagles, and effigies of Uncle Sam proliferated. The *Niles' Weekly Register* extolled the "energy which liberty gives to its champions, [and] that renders its cause invincible when opposed to tyranny." The audiences that once cringed at Susanna Rowson's jeremiad on American impotence, *Slaves in Algiers*, now thrilled to *The Siege of Tripoli*, James Ellison's paean to American valor. They delighted to the words of the poet Joseph Hanson, who exulted in *The Musselmen Humbled*:

The poor Bashaw [Pasha] must shortly be disturbed,
By an unwelcome visit from his enemy. . . .
Within a hundred fathoms of his castle they approach;
And in the nautick way most handsomely salute it;
Powder and ball, without reluctance is bestow'd
For they well know the great Bashaw deserves it.[27]

The Barbary Wars ended in triumph for the United States, but not for some of its principal American participants. Stephen Decatur returned to yet another hero's welcome and to notoriety for coining the phrase "my country right or wrong." Five years later, however, the commodore was killed in a duel with James Barron, the former captain of the *Chesapeake* who never forgave Decatur for court-martialing him. Though Decatur's remains were later interred at the U.S. Naval Academy at Annapolis, they were originally entombed in Philadelphia alongside those of the negotiator Joel Barlow. Appointed America's representative to France in 1811, Barlow accompanied Napoleon on his calamitous invasion of Russia and died of exposure in Poland. William Bainbridge met a more prosaic end, dying of natural causes after commanding the navy yards of Boston and Philadelphia. He never surmounted his sense of ill for-tune in the Mediterranean, carping, "I have been deprived of the opportunity of either fighting or negotiating" with Barbary. Publicly hounded for his role in the Tripoli treaty, even years after the event, Tobias Lear took his own life in Washington, in October 1816.

Eaton, too, never recovered from his North African trauma. Though the experience enabled him to appreciate the United States, where "the lamp of God is permitted to illuminate the mind," he remained an embittered man. Vengefully, in 1806, he joined Aaron Burr's treasonous plot to conquer the Louisiana Territory, but later turned state witness against Burr. Overlooking this disrepute, the Massachusetts legislature, "desirous to perpetuate a remembrance of heroic enterprise," granted Eaton ten thousand acres of farm-land. There he remained, idle and hermitlike, salving his biliousness with drink. "I am closely besieged," he confided to an old army friend in 1810. "The Field Martial of Death has driven in my out posts [and] is drawing lines . . . about my citadel." He died the following year.

From his hilltop estate at Monticello, the aging Thomas Jefferson followed the news of Decatur's victories in North Africa and the fall of the Barbary corsairs. Restoring ties with his old friend and nemesis John Adams, Jefferson wrote of his pride in the U.S. Navy, which he called America's "wooden walls," and its commitment "to keep the Barbary States in order." In spite of bitter opposition to its construction and setbacks in its early engagements in the Middle East, the Navy had emerged as a world-class fighting force. The Mediterranean Squadron was, in fact, on permanent patrol at the time of Jefferson's and Adams's almost simultaneous deaths, on July 4, 1826, their nation's fiftieth birthday.

The legacy of America's Barbary Wars would live on in America—in Preble County, Ohio, in Eaton, New York, and in Tripoli, Iowa, as well as in the twenty municipalities named for Stephen Decatur. U.S. Marines still hymn "to the shores of Tripoli" (though, in fact, they reached only Darna) and brandish a scimitar-shaped sword reminiscent of that presented by Hamid to Lieutenant O'Bannon. The nation's oldest war monument, situated at Annapolis and commissioned by an act of Congress, commemorates the victory over North Africa. Another memento is the bell of the USS *Philadelphia*, retrieved from the sea and returned to the United States in 1871. The most prominent symbol of the war, however, is perhaps the least acknowledged. First composed for Bainbridge and Decatur in 1805 and set to an old English drinking tune, the anthem for which Americans rise at ballgames and other public occasions originally described "turbaned heads bowed" to the "brow of the brave" and "the star-spangled flag of our nation." Only after the Battle of Fort McHenry in the War of 1812 were the lyrics revised by their author, Francis Scott Key.[28]

A HALF century after its founding, the United States was still on its own, but fully capable of defending its trade. Freed from piracy, American commerce thrived. Mediterranean ports registered a four-fold increase in visiting American ships in the 1820s. The United States now supplied the region with some twelve million gallons of rum annually and purchased most of Turkey's opium crop. "What a reproof to the Christians of America," mourned one Yankee missionary after landing in Anatolia. "Anticipated by her merchants, finding a market for their poisons!" Most Americans evinced no such qualms, however, but rather reveled in their newfound strength. Addressing Congress on December 2, 1823, President Monroe prohibited further European intervention anywhere in the New World. The audacity of that doctrine would surely have sounded blusterous in earlier years, before the Barbary Wars and the flexing of America's muscle in the Middle East.[29]

These remarkable accomplishments in the field of foreign affairs could not, however, conceal the contradictions that continued to trouble the United States at home. Though the country's population more than quintupled in its first fifty years of independence, reaching eleven million, nearly a fifth of that number remained slaves. If the Barbary Wars enabled Americans to rally in the face of foreign and internal challenges, then the issue of African American slavery increasingly and irreparably divided them. Yet even this most divisive conflict would be influenced by the Barbary saga and by the experience of American captives in North Africa.

Few events in the post-independence period had a more transformative impact on America than its war in the Middle East. A dire threat from the region prompted former colonies to coalesce and pool their resources, to create naval strength and project it far from America's shores. By choosing to fight rather than cosset the pirates and by departing from the European norm, the country had asserted its national character. Its citizens would never again have to endure the "mortifying degradations" suffered by William Bainbridge back in 1800, nor would they, like Bainbridge, hesitate to ponder the words "independent United States." Through the crucible of this thirty-year conflict, Americans had defined themselves.

Exhibiting their newly gained élan, Americans ventured throughout the Middle East, beyond North Africa to Arabia, Anatolia, and the Fertile Crescent. For growing numbers of them, the objective was no longer the pursuit of profit or security, or even the validation of myths. Their purpose, rather, was to bring salvation and enlightenment to the region, to remake it in America's image. Eschewing romance, disavowing "powder and balls," these young men and women would instill their ideals solely through Bibles and textbooks, in schoolrooms and clinics, by faith.

4

ILLUMINATING AND EMANCIPATING THE WORLD

PEOPLE CRAMMED INTO THE PEWS AND PEERED THROUGH the mullioned windows of Boston's Old South Church. They had long anticipated this day, October 31, 1819, convinced that it inaugurated a new era, a new world, perhaps. Their murmurs, converging into a drone, might have presaged the arrival of some august theologian. Yet, when the doors opened, neither a reverend nor even a deacon strode down the aisle, but two unassuming preachers, both aged twenty-five. The crowd fell silent as one of them, short, broad-nosed, and bespectacled, stepped up to the pulpit. His name was Levi Parsons, and the topic of his sermon was not the Gospel, not the Resurrection, but the Jews.

"They who taught us the way to salvation were Jews," Parsons began. They had faithfully preserved the Bible, had worked, suffered, and died defending "our" religion, he attested. "Our God was their God. Our heaven is their heaven." Most crucially, Parsons recalled, they had provided humanity with its Savior. "Yes, brethren, he who now intercedes for you before the throne of God . . . is a Jew!" To show their gratitude for the Jews' munificence, he concluded, Christians must strive to restore that people to sovereignty in its ancestral and biblical home.

Parsons explained how the Jews had been living for eighteen centuries in political limbo, homeless, and shorn of independence. The
time had now arrived, however, to redress that inequity. "Admit," he
said, "there still exists in the breast of every Jew an unconquerable
desire to inhabit the land which was given to the Fathers; a desire,
which even a conversion to Christianity does not eradicate." That
land was Palestine, once splendorous but now not an independent
state nor even a distinct province, but a sparsely inhabited Turkish
backwater waiting for its rightful owners to regain it. And reclaim it
they would, Parsons ventured. Were the Ottoman occupation of
Palestine to vanish, "nothing but a miracle would prevent their [the
Jews'] immediate return."

Parsons was not advocating conquest, of course—even after its
victory in the Barbary Wars, America was in no position to fight the
Ottomans—but rather a program of peaceful persuasion. Christian
missionaries would journey to the Middle East, to the "consecrated
walls" of Jerusalem, and there perform deeds of such spectacular
righteousness that the Jews would be enticed to return home and
"receive Him"—that is, Jesus. The emergence of a Messianic Jewish
polity in Palestine would fulfill the conditions necessary for the Second Coming, Parsons affirmed. Consequently, not only the Jews but
Muslims and even the misguided Eastern Christians would bask in
the sacred light. The millennial age of peace and spiritual solidarity
would commence and the Ottoman Empire—indeed all empires—
would bow before the sovereignty of Christ. "Every eye is fixed on
Jerusalem."

The congregation received these tidings openly, raptly, and waited
with mounting frisson as the next man rose to preach. This was Pliny
Fisk, taller and more presentable than Parsons and less loquacious.
He, too, spoke of the need to work wonders in the Holy Land, to
help bring about redemption, whatever the hazards involved. "And
now, behold, I go bound in the spirit unto Jerusalem," he proclaimed, and the parishioners burst into tears.

Viewed from a twenty-first-century perspective, Fisk, Parsons, and
the people who lauded them might seem radical in their beliefs and
peripheral to American society. The contention that they alone could
save the Jews, Muslims, and other Middle Eastern peoples would

surely sound naïve, if not arrogant, to many Americans today. After all, why should the descendants of ancient civilizations and the inheritors of some of history's most venerated traditions embrace the faith of these alien upstarts, emissaries of a Protestant sect less than three hundred years old and a country scarcely more than fifty?

These Americans, however, were anything but marginal. The doctrines of the Methodists, Presbyterians, and Congregationalists commanded massive followings in the United States, transcending all barriers of class, education, and gender. Among the missionaries and their supporters were farmers and merchants, doctors, and artisans, the minimally educated and graduates of the country's finest colleges, women and men. Deeply imbued with American ideals of individualism, civic virtue, and patriotism, they viewed themselves as the direct inheritors of the Revolutionary tradition. In that same Old South Church forty-five years earlier, the Sons of Liberty had gathered before marching out in Native American garb to dump British tea into Boston harbor.

Enthusiasm for the crusade proposed by Fisk and Parsons gripped not only long-settled Americans but also more recent immigrants. Nor was the excitement confined to Boston or even to the so-called Bible belt of New England. Embarking on a countrywide tour to solicit donations for their journey, the young preachers would be welcomed by congregations throughout the South and in frontier chapels west of the Alleghenies. "The spirit of missions is beginning to command the influence and wealth of the American churches," Parsons rejoiced.

Common to all of these communities was the conviction that America had a divinely assigned role to act as a "light unto nations," and to strive for global peace. "They went determined to lift mankind to a higher and better plane of living," the historian Oliver Elsbree wrote of Fisk, Parsons, and the thousands of young women and men destined to follow them. "They sought to take the best America then had to offer to the heathen world." The missionaries had the unique quality of being both guileless and patronizing, haughty and unaffected, yet thoroughly well-intentioned at the same time. Their arrogance was essentially benign.

The parishioners left Old South Church, to the peals of a bell forged by Paul Revere, with their thoughts far from New England. They were thinking of a distant corner of the Ottoman Empire and of the monumental events soon to unfold there. Levi Parsons and Pliny Fisk, meanwhile, traveled to Washington, D.C., where Secretary of State John Quincy Adams supplied them with letters vouching for their probity. Thus equipped, the young preachers were ready to become the first American missionaries to the Middle East, those lands where, they believed, "great transactions" had shaped the destiny "of all ages and all nations for time and eternity."[1]

John Ledyard had journeyed to Egypt in search of adventure, and men like William Eaton and Stephen Decatur had defended their country from North African corsairs. For Fisk and Parsons, though, the sole purpose for voyaging to the Middle East was to disseminate their faith. How, then, did they and vast numbers of their countrymen come to believe that, by exporting evangelical Protestantism to the predominantly Muslim Middle East, the entire world could be saved? Why were they so confident that young citizens of a new United States could convert the ancient and venerable peoples of the region and so redeem humanity?

"As Like as Like Can Be"

The answers to those questions could be found two hundred years earlier, embedded in the founding ideas of America.

"Come let us declare in Zion the word of God," proclaimed William Bradford, the future governor of the Plymouth Colony, as he stepped off the *Mayflower* in 1620. Bradford was quoting Jeremiah, but "Zion," for him, was not the old Promised Land of Canaan but its new incarnation, America. Its inhabitants were not the ancient Israelites but the 101 passengers who had arrived with Bradford, his fellow Puritans.

Bradford's remarks reflected not only the discovery of a New World but also the rediscovery of the Old Testament. Starting with the Reformation, the people of England gained access to the books that the Catholic Church had long deemphasized—the Pentateuch, Judges, Prophets, and Kings. The effects of this encounter were metamorphic. England swiftly appropriated the biblical narrative, from the story of Abraham to the Book of Daniel, as its national epic, wedding what the poet Matthew Arnold called "the genius and history of us English to the genius and history of Hebrew people." Biblical phrases enriched the English language and scriptural concepts of social freedom and justice helped strengthen parliamentary government. Numbers of Englishmen, clergy and laymen alike, became proficient in Hebrew and christened their children with Old Testament names like Jesse and Sarah, Samuel and Rebecca.

The urge to embrace the Old Testament past was particularly fierce among the Puritans, the most unbending of England's reformists. In their search for a pristine religion unsullied by hierarchies and politics, and for parallels to their own persecution, the Puritans remembered the Jews and their ancient faith. They believed that God had spoken directly to the chosen people, kept His covenant with them, and delivered them from bondage. The Puritans concluded that they were the heirs to that contract, a New Israel embarked on a second Exodus from slavery to freedom, destined for a Promised Land. Impelled by that sense of chosenness, the Pilgrims journeyed from England to Holland and from there to Plymouth Rock, their stepping-stone to salvation.

Having stamped their own identity onto that of the Jews, the Puritans superimposed the map of the old Canaan over the new one they now settled. "In no country are the Scriptures better known or more highly prized," observed Edward Robinson, a nineteenth-century descendant of those Puritans and the father of biblical archaeology. "The names of Sinai, Jerusalem, Bethlehem, the Promised Land, become associated with [an American's] earliest recollections and holiest feelings." More familiar with the geography of the Holy Land than with their new and strange environs, Americans would give scriptural names such as Salem, Shiloh, and Zion to over a thousand towns and cities in North America. The study of Hebrew was mandatory at many New World colleges such as Princeton, where James Madison majored in the language, and at Yale, Dartmouth, and Columbia, which placed Hebrew logos on their emblems. Even Native Americans, whose lineage many colonists traced to the Lost Ten Tribes, were imprinted onto the biblical palimpsest. "Jerusalem was, New England is," the Reverend Samuel Wakeman told a Hartford congregation in 1685. "They were, you are . . . God's covenant people." Peter Fogler, Benjamin Franklin's grandfather, couched the thought more colloquially: "[In] New England they are like the Jews, as like as like can be."[2]

By the mid-eighteenth century, colonial America's certainty in its own divine election helped ignite the Great Awakening of revivalist faith. New churches were established—Baptist, Methodist, and Presbyterian—and new colleges such as Princeton and Dartmouth founded to assist in spreading their doctrines. Old Calvinist notions of predestination were cast off and replaced by a more indigenously American confidence in the individual's ability to save him or herself through vigorous devotional action. Yet Christians were to seek not only their own redemption but also that of others, by guiding them to spiritual rebirth. Assured of their ability to fulfill this task, a great many Americans looked forward to a new millennium, a golden age in which "every nation shall be a free people," as the theologian Jonathan Edwards predicted, and "the whole earth may be as one community, one body in Christ." That event would be heralded by Protestant America, envisaged by its founders, quoting Matthew (5:14–16), as "the light of the world," the incomparable "city on the hill."

The colonists' image of themselves as the New Israel attained special poignancy during the War of Independence. Casting King George III in the role of pharaoh and the Atlantic acting as the Red Sea, patriot writers likened George Washington to Moses, and John Adams to Joshua leading their people to freedom. For Alexander Hamilton, an Episcopalian who had learned to read Hebrew in his youth, the destiny of America was not unlike that of the Jews, a people whose history was "entirely out of the ordinary course of human affairs" and "the effect of some great providential plan." The Yale president Ezra Stiles noted that the number of Israelites present at Mount Sinai—three million—was precisely the population of the United States at the time of independence. Harvard's Samuel Langdon suggested that "instead of the twelve tribes of Israel, we may substitute the thirteen states of the American union." The image of those tribes crossing the wilderness to Canaan adorned the Seal of the United States proposed by Franklin and Jefferson.[3]

The passion of religion in America, though, did not prevent the young Republic from separating its churches from the state. In the 1796 treaty with Tripoli, for example, the United States declared that it was "not founded in any sense on the Christian religion" and had "never entered into any war . . . against any Mahometan nation . . . arising from religious opinions"—an assertion unanimously endorsed by the Senate. Faith, nevertheless, continued to pervade every aspect of American life, including government. Congressmen, cabinet members, and even presidents would often advocate for missionary activity both within North America and abroad.

Enlivened by frontier freedoms and unfettered by a national church, Protestantism in America continued to spawn original denominations, new venues for its spiritual creativity and might. By the end of the eighteenth century, the torrents of religious energy converged in a Second Awakening which emphasized the return to fundamentals and the belief in imminent redemption. "We have now entered upon that period which is immediately preparatory to the Millennium," one Connecticut minister announced in 1815, describing a period in which all wars would cease, every community would have its church, and every family have its daily consecration. Particular emphasis was placed on evangelizing the Jews, on uniting the Old Israel with the New. Proselytizing organizations, such as the Female Society for Promoting Christianity among the Jews, flourished and expectations of mass conversions soared. A popular prophecy held that "the tabernacle of God is [soon] to be pitched among men," and in towns and villages across New England and New York young people were prepared to devote their lives to transforming that vision into reality.

The Second Awakening called on Americans to revel not only in their spirituality but also in their national pride. "The Christian . . . ought to cultivate patriotism to a high degree," advised Pliny Fisk. "What could be more suitable, than the glowing fire and burning zeal of political enthusiasm *consecrated* to Christ?" This symbiosis of love of country and devotion to God struck Alexis de Tocqueville as one of America's most extraordinary qualities. Writing in 1835, the Frenchman concluded that Christianity exerted "a greater influence over the souls of men . . . in America" than anywhere else in the world and that only in the United States was religion linked to "democratic instincts" and the "spirit of individual independence."

Infused with this blend of piety and patriotism, numerous Americans were prepared to save the world spiritually, by teaching the Gospel, as well as politically, by promulgating freedom. The urge to pursue that mission would remain a constant in the country's foreign relations, providing a hefty counterweight to its flight from foreign entanglements and a rallying point for its disputatious leaders. For all their disagreements on spiritual matters, the founding fathers were virtually unanimous in their commitment to America's secular, civic faith. To Jefferson, a deist, the United States was "an object so valuable to mankind," one that would bring together "all nations for a free intercommunication of happiness." For Adams, the Unitarian, America was "a great . . . design of Providence for the illumination of the ignorant, and emancipation of . . . the earth."[4]

America's commitment to its vision of global betterment, secular and religious, crystallized in 1808, at Williams College in Massachusetts. Caught in a sudden summer electrical storm, five students tested their confidence in God by selecting the most vulnerable shelter imaginable, a haystack. "Though you and I are very little beings," the students' leader, Samuel J. Mills, told them: "We must not rest satisfied till we have made our influence extend to the remotest corner of this ruined world." All five survived the experience, drenched but ablaze with the desire to preach the Gospel abroad. Word of the Haystack Incident, as it was later hallowed, spread to other colleges—Harvard, Brown, Union—and especially to Middlebury and the Andover Theological Seminary, where both Levi Parsons and Pliny Fisk would study. Soon the students were petitioning their home churches to sponsor missionary efforts overseas, pressuring their elders to act.

The elders responded swiftly enough. In 1810 they established the American Board of Commissioners for Foreign Missions. Composed of clergymen from various denominations, together with industrialists, physicians, businessmen, and lawyers, the board sought to foster missionary centers or "stations" throughout the non-Protestant world. "Only the extension of Christian love could bring nearer to humankind the millennium that would wipe out poverty, injustice and oppression," opined one of the board's founders, the Reverend Samuel Hopkins.

Such evils were to be eliminated, initially, in the American Southwest, and later in Africa, India, and China. But of all the fields for evangelical action none aroused the board's excitement more than the Middle East. Here was a region that had yet to be claimed by any European power, but which lay at civilization's crossroads—a region blessed, moreover, with the holiest land of all. Listening to the bells of Middlebury College signaling the end of the War of 1812, Levi Parsons claimed to hear "the groans of the eastern world, which are wafted to heaven for deliverance." "Zion," he rejoiced, "will prosper!"[5]

If "Zion," for the Pilgrim leader William Bradford, referred to the new Promised Land of America, then for Levi Parsons two centuries later it meant the old and original Land of Israel, which was now called Palestine. While conversions might be made elsewhere in the world, only in Palestine, the missionaries believed, would they have an immediate and millennial impact. Only there would the Protestant's longing to reunite with their spiritual forebears, the Jews, converge with their yearning for the Messiah's reappearance.

The fascination that many American Protestants displayed toward the Jews did not stem from any extensive contact with them—some four thousand Jews lived in the United States at that time, roughly .04 percent of the total population—nor did it derive from a desire to befriend them personally. Indeed, some early evangelical writing contained comments that would certainly sound anti-Semitic today, including their insistence that all Jews ultimately be baptized. Yet whatever feelings they bore them as fellow citizens were distinct from the affection with which the evangelists held the Jews as their cousins in faith and as the agents of future redemption. By expediting the fulfillment of God's promises to repatriate the Jews to their homeland, Christians could re-create the conditions of Jewish sovereignty that existed in Jesus' time and so set the stage for his reappearance. This was the concept of "restorationism," and its impact was immense. Christian theology had once portrayed the Jews' loss of sovereignty as punishment for their rejection of Christ's first coming, but the evangelists now saw the revival of Jewish statehood as a pre-requisite for His second visitation on earth.

Restorationism was neither new nor unique to American Protestantism. Evocations of the idea can be found in Sir Henry Finch's 1621 treatise, *The World's Great Restauration, or, The Calling of the Jews,* as well as in the poems of John Milton and the philosophy of John Locke. En route to the New World, the Puritans took the concept with them to Holland, where they petitioned the Dutch government to "transport Izraell's sons and daughters . . . to the Land promised their forefathers . . . for an everlasting Inheritance." Colonial American theologians such as John Cotton, the leading minister of Massachusetts Bay, and Increase Mather, Harvard's first president, called for the destruction of the Ottoman Empire to make way for the Jews' return. By the Second Awakening, the dream of reinstating Jewish rule in the Holy Land was fast becoming doctrine. Ezra Stiles of Yale forecast that "the return of the twelve tribes to the Holy Land" would spark an outburst of spiritual energy sufficient "to convert a world." Another New Haven cleric, David Austin, took this prediction literally and spent his life's savings building docks, inns, and warehouses in preparation for the Jews' departure. "When that empire falls . . . the Jews will begin to be restored [to Palestine] . . . and Christ will take to himself his power and reign," proclaimed Asa McFarland, a Massachusetts Presbyterian, in 1808, at the time of the Haystack Incident.[6]

Restorationist fervor, it must be noted, arose without any thought for the physical existence, much less the political or religious desires, of the thousands of Arabs then living in Palestine. Rather than focus on faceless populations, Americans preferred to concentrate on the momentous Middle Eastern events—Napoleon's penetration of Egypt and the defeat of the Barbary pirates—which seemed to portend Palestine's liberation. Once the "weak and imbecile" Ottomans were ousted, an 1816 issue of the *Niles' Weekly Register* speculated, the Jews would swiftly make the deserts "blossom like a rose," and Jerusalem would again "rival the cities of the world for beauty, splendor and wealth." The Continental Congress president Elias Boudinot, a founder of the American Bible Society, predicted that "the mighty power of God" would soon summon the Jews from exile and repatriate them "to their beloved . . . land of Palestine." More ardently still, John Adams envisioned "a hundred thousand Israelites . . . [as] well disciplined as the French army" marching into Palestine and conquering it. "I really wish the Jews again in Judea an independent nation," the ex-president wrote Mordecai Noah, America's former consul in Tunis, in 1819. That same year, Pliny Fisk and Levi Parsons boarded the brig *Sally Ann* and finally embarked for the East.[7]

The Day of Small Things

They followed the path long used by American merchants in the Mediterranean, a six-week voyage from New England to Smyrna (modern-day Izmir) on Turkey's Aegean coast. One can scarcely imagine the sense of shock and alienation experienced by the two young preachers as they entered this ancient Middle Eastern city, the presumed birthplace of Homer. In contrast to the uncluttered and well-ordered Boston they left behind, Smyrna, "the Pearl of the Levant," was a bedlam of meandering alleyways, strange smells, and discordant music. "There seems to be hardly similarity enough between this country and the U.S. to entitle them to be considered as belonging to the same world," one contemporary American visitor observed. Nevertheless, Smyrna's Greek Christians, who made up nearly half of the city's population, greeted the Americans cordially. They spent the next two months acclimating themselves and studying the local dialect and customs. "Do nothing rashly, nothing inconsiderately or inadvertently, or needlessly expose yourselves to resentments," Samuel Worcester, secretary of the American Board, had commanded them. Complying with these orders, Fisk and Parsons spent $48 on "Oriental dress" and $6.50 for Arabic lessons.

Beginning in March 1820, the pair set out on a 300-mile trek through Asia Minor, visiting each of the seven cities toured by Saint Paul and reconnoitering the region for "missionizing." Though few Jews were settled there, the area was densely populated with Eastern Christians, Greek Orthodox, and Armenians, whom Protestants regarded as spiritually misguided and especially ripe for rebirth. There were also Muslims, followers—so the Americans thought—of a spurious, even sinister, faith, and desperately in need of salvation. "WHAT GOOD CAN BE DONE?" Worcester wrote in capitals to Fisk and Parsons. "BY WHAT MEANS?" The questions pertained not only to Jews but also to Muslims and Christians, and not only in Palestine but "in Egypt, in Syria, in Persia" as well.

Yet Palestine, "the scene of great transactions," remained their primary objective and the preferred site of their first permanent station. Parsons elected to go first. "The permission to *anticipate* the spiritual welfare of Zion is an unspeakable privilege," he wrote. "With the spirit of Moses I can lead the armies of Israel to the spiritual Canaan." He would not travel lightly, but laden with five thousand religious tracts, including Bibles in nine languages. From his English missionary friends, Parsons received Polonius-like advice: "Go in the character of literary gentlemen . . . exercise in the morning, eat sparingly of fruit at first, dress warm, wear a turban." They also recommended that he travel only during the Easter and Passover pilgrimages, when foreigners were less conspicuous in Palestine.[8]

Though not a distinct country at that time or even a designated province, Palestine was an object of special Ottoman attention, if for no other reason than its status as the interface of major religions. The authorities showed particular sensitivity to Jerusalem, where the recognized religious communities, or *millets*, enjoyed far-reaching autonomy, and foreigners were forbidden to reside. Neither the governor nor community heads were apt to look amiably on an outsider from a breakaway Christian sect seeking to upset the age-old equilibrium. Remembering his goal—in Worcester's words, "the recovery of the world to God, to virtue, to happiness"—Parsons nevertheless strode out of Smyrna in December 1820 and three months later, frozen and footsore, entered the sacred city.

Parsons claimed to be the first American missionary ever to access those "consecrated walls." In contrast to the rest of the country, which Western travelers often found backward—even relative to other areas of the Middle East—underpopulated, and impoverished, Parsons was dazzled by Jerusalem. Climbing the Mount of Olives, he gazed down at the Old City to the west, and the Dead Sea to the southeast, and decided that "no place in the world commands a finer prospect or is associated with events more sacred and sublime." He received a surprisingly congenial welcome from the established churches, especially the "Latins," but was unsuccessful in evangelizing any of the city's estimated ten thousand Jews. More distressing, Parsons learned that Islamic law forbade the building of new churches and prescribed beheading as the punishment for proselytizing Muslims. The only promising candidates for conversion, then, were the Greeks and Armenians, the "Christians in name," as the missionaries called them, the adherents of a "long corrupted Christianity." These native communities, Parsons hoped, would provide Protestants with a natural link to Jews and Muslims and inspire them by their dedication to Christ. "This is indeed the center of the world," he reported to Fisk after spending some eighty days in Jerusalem. "The station must not be relinquished. The door is already opened."

Parsons reunited with his partner in the spring of 1821, but the situation in Smyrna had meanwhile deteriorated. Greece, an Ottoman possession since the fifteenth century, rose in revolt, and the rebellion quickly inflamed the Greek communities of Anatolia. Giving vent to ancient hatreds, Turkish soldiers swept through the area, burning and massacring indiscriminately. The two missionaries were forced to take shelter in the visiting USS *United States*—the first of many instances in which the agents of American power in the Middle East would help rescue the representatives of American faith. Though now secure, Parsons was sick with dysentery. Yet he remained optimistic, confident that "the present commotions will . . . secure all kingdoms to Christ." Until that time, however, the Americans resolved to leave Anatolia and retreat to the relative safety of Alexandria.

Parsons barely survived the passage and had to be carried, shivering, from the boat. Throughout the winter months of 1822, Fisk stayed by his companion's bedside, ministering to him and praying for his recovery. His efforts proved futile. Parsons had often written of his longing for martyrdom and in February his wish was honored.

News of his passing stunned the American Board. One young preacher, himself an aspiring missionary, penned an epitaphic verse:

Thy spirit, Parsons, lur'd by seraph's song,
Spreads its untiring wing and upward flies. . . .
Who now like him shall toil for Judah's race?
And who like him destroy Mohammed's sway.[9]

The missionary movement would not be disheartened, though, and neither would Pliny Fisk. He sailed to Malta to receive the shipment of a printing press from the board and to rendezvous with Parson's replacement. This was the Reverend Jonas King, a professor of Oriental languages at Amherst College, burly and garrulous, who had volunteered three years of service to the missions. The two, in turn, met up with the Englishman Joseph Wolff, a rabbi's son who had first converted to Catholicism before becoming an Anglican and marrying the daughter of an Oxford earl. "Suffer not your minds to be discouraged," read the party's new instructions, which urged the missionaries to persevere in "the diffusion of light and life in the regions of darkness and moral death." Fisk, King, and Wolff then departed for Egypt, intending to press on to Palestine.

Following the Nile upriver to Thebes, the missionaries distributed 900 Bibles and 3,700 religious tracts, and "disputed" with any religious figures they found, rabbis, sheikhs, and priests. They met the exiled Lebanese potentate, Bashir II, a convert from Islam to Maronite Christianity, who was elated to hear that his guests were Americans. "He gave us a salutation," Fisk recorded, "and an expressive look, which flattered our national pride." No less impressed by the missionaries' background was a Druze prince who invited them to visit his castle in Lebanon. Accepting the offer, the Americans hired a guide and thirteen camels to take them across the Sinai Desert, singing and discoursing as they went, and up the Mediterranean coast into Palestine, where their reception was decidedly cooler. Jonas recalled how "the Arabs poured down on us like a torrent . . . with drawn swords, guns, and heavy clubs . . . setting up a terrible yell, like the war-whoop of the savages of North America." Fisk was injured, though only superficially, in the head. The troupe survived, but instead of turning inland on the dangerous road to Jerusalem, they kept to the coast and eventually reached Beirut.[10]

The city, with its population of eight thousand and its white-washed houses and churches clinging to the hills over the bay, was more orderly than Jerusalem and Smyrna, and safer. Though adjacent to the Holy Land, it had little of Palestine's political instability and was situated on the sea, facilitating escape. British diplomats, moreover, were well established in Beirut and eager to extend their protection to people who shared their religion and culture but none of their imperialist goals. Most enticing for the missionaries was the presence throughout Syria's Mount Lebanon district of large numbers of Eastern Christians and Druze and even a small Jewish community, a reservoir of potential converts.

While King returned to the United States and Wolff continued on his wanderings, Fisk settled in Beirut. He had already traversed much of the region, attained fluency in Arabic and Greek, and supplied the *Missionary Herald* back home with detailed accounts of his travels. Now, at last, he resolved to answer to Samuel Worcester's questions "What good can be done?" and "By what means?" If a missionary could not convert the people of the Middle East, he could at least educate their children. By teaching them to read and write according to American methods, Fisk believed, he could open young people's minds to the possibility of salvation through Christ. Fisk's school, the first of many American institutions destined to alter the Middle East, opened its doors in 1823.

That year also saw the arrival of fresh reinforcements from America—Isaac Bird, a recent Yale graduate, and William Goodell from Dartmouth. The two brought their wives as well, reflecting the board's awareness of the potential role for women in the missionary enterprise. Bird and Goodell aided Fisk in running the school and joined him in preaching forays into many Middle Eastern cities, from Damascus to Antioch and Aleppo.

The sheer vitality and optimism evinced by the missionaries was reason for celebration in Boston. The American Board boasted of success in proclaiming the Gospel to "Druses, Maronites, Syrians and Greeks," and in establishing stations in "that most interesting portion of the world," Palestine. "The standard of truth and right-eousness has been erected," the commissioners bragged, "never to be permanently removed." Sereno Dwight, a noted biographer and chaplain of the U.S. Senate, envisaged the day when "missionaries loaded with books will feel their way into the farthest retreats of Mohammedan darkness" and when "the tidings of salvation will be proclaimed," in "Egypt, Arabia, and Persia."

Such self-congratulations were, in truth, unwarranted. Despite their unflagging efforts, the missionaries had succeeded in converting only a small number of Eastern Christians, most of whom were des-titute and had no choice but to accept employment or charity from the church. In Lebanon, opposition to the Americans' activities mounted from the Maronites, a Catholic sect traditionally associated with France and which ran its own lycée-style schools. "It is by no means expedient to teach women to read the word of God," one Maronite prelate asserted. "They are quite bad enough now, with what little they know—teach them to read and write, there would be no living with them!" The archbishop threatened to excommunicate any Maronite who attended Protestant services and to destroy all of the missionary publications, Bibles included.

The obstacles were equally immense in other parts of the Middle East. "The missionaries speak with no confidence of the conversion of a single native," admitted the recent Yale graduate Elnathan Grid-ley after arriving in Smyrna in 1825. "Scarcely ten [even] pretend to listen to the preached gospel." Eli Smith, a talented linguist who would soon spark a revival of Arabic letters and who toured the region for the American Board, painted a more dismal picture. Lamenting this "land of darkness, and of the shadow of death . . . [of] ignorance, indifference and wickedness," Smith recounted an incident in Egypt involving a Muslim man and his wife, who had recently converted to Christianity:

She was brought before the magistrate and condemned to be drowned in the Nile. . . . She continued to cry "I die a Christian"; but this only enraged her executors and hastened her death. In the mean time a fire was built on the shore to burn her husband, but . . . he saved himself by embracing the Mohamedan faith. This he could do having never been a Moslem, but for his wife no such resort was left.

A similar fate almost befell Pliny Fisk in Jerusalem. Arrested for distributing religious tracts in 1825, put in chains and tormented, he was released only after a personal appeal from the British consul. Given such adversity, Fisk wondered, would Christ himself have prevailed?[11]

Fisk by this time was exhausted, ill stricken, and demoralized. The pupils at his school, most of them Jews, had sold their New Testament texts for paper and one of his few converts, Assad al-Shidyak, was arrested for apostasy and left to die in jail. Harassed by both Muslims and Maronites, Fisk also felt hounded by the board, which he accused of editing his reports to downplay the friendliness of Greek bishops and the difficulties he encountered trying to convert the Jews. Due for home leave in October 1825, he made one last trip to Nazareth, but en route was waylaid and beaten by Arab brigands. Fisk was borne back to Beirut, treated with leeches and mustard poultices, and died an agonizing death.[12]

"One might rewrite the . . . [Book of] Hebrews with [the] well-known names . . . of Christian workers in Bible lands," an anonymous clergyman posited. "Foremost among these should come the names of Pliny Fisk [and] Levi Parsons." In spite of recalcitrant students and the opposition of Maronite prelates, the school that Fisk established not only survived but even grew. By the late 1820s, nine schoolhouses were operating in Lebanon, with an enrollment of six hundred pupils, over a sixth of whom were girls. The Beirut station assured the board that "our prospects of usefulness never wore a brighter aspect" and that "a wide and effectual door does indeed seem to be opening to us." Bolstered by this confidence, the board sent additional missionaries to Mount Lebanon and, from there, throughout the region. Samuel Worcester had once warned Fisk and Parsons "not [to] despise the day of small things."[13] Though seemingly small, their accomplishments had opened venues for the introduction of American faith—religious and civic—to the Middle East.

———

THE FOLLOWING decades would constitute a pivotal period for both America and the Middle East. Destabilized by the irreversible weakening of the Ottoman Empire, by the attempts of local leaders to seize independence and of the great powers to carve out areas of exclusive European control, the Middle East would be plagued by almost ceaseless upheaval and bloodshed. American settlers, meanwhile, would press westward to California and Oregon, and to Florida and Texas in the south. The Union's incorporation of newly delineated territories, some slave-owning and others free, revived the question of whether these areas could remain within a common polity, whether these United States could stay, indefinitely, one.

Out of American expansion and Middle Eastern unrest would emerge a new and deeply interconnected relationship. Aided by innovative technologies, borne by revolutionary forms of transport, Americans in unprecedented numbers would travel to the Middle East and penetrate some of its most inaccessible quarters. The peoples of the region would generally welcome these visitors and engage them on a multitude of levels—commercial, educational, and strategic.

In the centrifuge of this dynamic relationship, the once distinct themes of power, faith, and fantasy in America's interaction with the Middle East would inexorably meld. Instead of single-minded adventurers like John Ledyard, wielders of power like William Eaton, and preachers like Pliny Fisk, would come crossbreeds of trader-evangelists, missionary-sailors, and statesmen-explorers. American policymakers would for the first time be forced to choose between the furtherance of the country's commercial and strategic interests in the Middle East and the pursuit of their ethical and spiritual ideals.

Part Two

The Middle East and Antebellum America

5

Confluence and Conflict

IN JUNE 1821, UNDER THE PUNISHING SUDANESE SUN, an Egyptian officer paused to drink from the Nile. He had been traveling for nine months, hazarding boat-smashing rapids, hostile tribesmen, and heat. On barges laden with cannons, ammunition, and supplies, he and his troops haltingly advanced. Their mission was to subdue brigands disrupting Egyptian trade in the African interior and to broaden the influence of Egypt's ruler, Muhammad Ali. The officer, who called himself Muhammad Effendi, was described by acquaintances as a "pale, delicate-looking man"—an uncommon complexion in the Middle East—but with "the grave and calm look of the Turks." Kneeling, he cupped his hands beneath the water and raised them to his encrusted lips, but before sipping he uttered a benediction, or so he later wrote: "To the prosperity of the great and liberal republic of the United States."

Muhammad Effendi had been born thirty-four years earlier, at the time of the Constitutional Convention, in Cambridge, Massachusetts, and received the Christian name of George Bethune English. A member of the Harvard class of 1807, he first studied law but then switched to divinity and Hebrew. Like Levi Parsons, Pliny Fisk, and many seminarians who studied the Pentateuch at the time, English developed a deep reverence for the Jews and a desire to rectify "the infernal wickedness and diabolical inhumanity" done to them by Christians. He went well beyond seeking penitence, however; his encounter with the Old Testament led him to doubt the historical and theological veracity of the Gospel. It also prompted him to read a 1688 Italian translation of the Quran. He concluded that "Mahometans, who are the most numerous sect of religionists now in the world," possessed a superior claim to the biblical prophecies and had better fulfilled the Mosaic prohibitions against idolatry—"the worship of angels, and dead men, universal throughout three quarters of Christendom." Not surprisingly, these heresies sparked counterattacks from the Harvard Transcendentalist William Ellery Channing and from Edward Everett, the later senator and secretary of state. English, however, would not be dissuaded and he left Cambridge seeking new sources of excitement and substance in the world.

He went "out West," which at that time meant Ohio, and tried his hand at journalism before settling on the banks of the Wabash River as a member of the puritanical Harmonie sect. Tiring of utopianism, though, English journeyed in 1817 to Washington, where he called on an old family friend, John Quincy Adams, the new secretary of state. Adams obtained a posting for English in the Mediterranean Squadron and a commission as a first lieutenant in the Marines. But service aboard ship also bored him—the Barbary Wars were over— and after arriving in Egypt, English resigned from the corps.

The Middle East seemed to offer the young contrarian all that was lacking in his life—exoticism, adventure, and the religion that had previously inspired him in school. Rather than return to mundane Massachusetts, George English remained in Egypt, converted to Islam, and adopted the name Muhammad.[1]

From Harvard to Sennar

Open-minded to the point of heresy, English was hardly typical of the Americans of his day. Yet, in his attachment to the Middle East, he exhibited the same characteristics found in figures as diverse as John Ledyard, Levi Parsons, and William Eaton. Inspired by the

Bible, charmed by Oriental myths, and impressed by the caparisons of power, English represented a fusion of the motifs in his country's Middle Eastern involvement, an increasingly common amalgam.

By 1820, English was fluent in both Arabic and Turkish and ready to place his talents at the service of the Egyptian state. Through the good offices of the British consul, he was able to obtain an interview with Isma'il Pasha, a son of Muhammad Ali. English's varied experiences impressed Isma'il, but none more so than his brief stint in the military. Egypt was just then working to modernize its army and, to that end, eager to recruit European advisers. Though he had served in the U.S. Navy and had never risen above the rank of lieutenant, English emerged from the meeting with Isma'il with the title of *topji bashi*, or general, in command of Egypt's artillery.

If expanding Egypt's offensive capabilities was Isma'il's objective, English, with his penchant for romance, seemed unlikely to achieve it. Rather than modernize his regiment, the American tried to revive one of Egypt's oldest weapons, a chariot with blade-studded wheels for cutting down infantry. The experiment failed thoroughly and, before he could mount another, English was ordered into action against Sudanese rebels. While Isma'il and his vanguard proceeded overland, English and the bulk of the force were to follow on water, up the Nile. Starting in September 1821, English and his six thousand troops—Turks, Bedouin, North Africans—boarded barges at the Wadi Halfa cataract and set off for regions unfamiliar to most Egyptians and utterly unknown to Westerners.

The journey, through one hundred miles of roiling whirlpools and falls, proved to be harrowing. "The side of the boat approached to within a yard of the white foam," English remembered. "Our *rais* [helmsman] tore his turban from his head, and lifted his clasped hands to heaven, exclaiming, 'We are lost!' The rest of the boatmen were screaming to God for aid." The explorer survived the ordeal only to contract a severe case of "opthalmia," which blinded him for days. Still, English managed to recover and to come through with all but one barge, disembarking at Bahar al-Abiad, the headwaters of the White Nile.

Like William Eaton fifteen years before him, English had led a major expedition across a desolate stretch of the Middle East, and, like John Ledyard, he left vivid descriptions of everything he saw, from ramshackle villages to the bleak, unforgiving terrain. He noted the plight of slaves, the arrogance of bandits, and the patent discomfort of twenty-year-old tribesmen who had recently undergone circumcision. Especially fascinating for him were the ruins "now prostrate and confounded with the dust of their worshippers" that lined the riverbank and that he often explored at night, sneaking off from his convoy. "A voyage up the Nile may be considered as presenting an epitome of the moral history of man," English attested. "We meet at almost every stage with the monuments of his superstition and his tyranny."

From Bahar al-Abiad, English led his troops through a countryside freshly ravaged by Isma'il's cavalry, past incinerated hamlets and untilled fields strewn with corpses. He abhorred the behavior of Egyptian soldiers—"The luckless fornicators," English dubbed them—who looted and pillaged. Horrified, he watched as forty of them "engaged in driving, with repeated strokes of heavy mallets, sharp pointed pieces of timber, six or eight inches square, up the posteriors of some insurgents." More detestable scenes awaited English in Sennar, the same city that Ledyard had fruitlessly tried to reach over thirty years earlier. In place of the bustling and colorful caravanserais he had imagined, English found a cluster of four hundred filthy grass huts inhabited by "detestable" people who ate cats and rodents, and women who were, he claimed, "universally, the ugliest I ever beheld."

English, himself half-starved and ragged, was scarcely in better shape. The expedition, though, was judged successful and Egypt extended its suzerainty over the Sudan. Recuperating back in Alexandria, English became acquainted with the missionary Joseph Wolff, the converted British Jew, who tried to persuade him to return to Christianity. English also met Pliny Fisk, grieving over the recent death of Levi Parsons. The missionary joined in the effort to save the wayward general, only to find himself stymied. "Obstinate hostility to the truth is the prevailing temper of your soul," Fisk berated English. "I consider your case as one of the most deplorable and dangerous that I have ever known."

Though uninterested in resuming his former faith, English did yearn for his original home. At the end of 1822, he left Egypt and boarded a ship back to the United States. He published a memoir of the Sudan expedition that earned him—and the Middle East—much attention. "A few American steam boats . . . would soon make the Nile as navigable as our Hudson, Patomac or Mississippi," the aged John Adams observed after reading the book.[2] The former president's son, John Quincy, was also impressed and happily received English at the State Department. The secretary invited his old friend to reenter government service. His task was to apply his uncommon skills in securing the first-ever treaty between America and the Ottoman Empire.

Bribery and Brass

Relations between the world's oldest existing empire and its newest republic had, since the late eighteenth century, languished in ambiguity. Regarding the Porte as vital to American commerce and as "the Theater of Politicks in Europe," President Adams in 1798 named the South Carolina congressman William Loughton Smith as the country's first minister to the Ottoman Empire. Smith declined the offer, however, and the post remained unmanned. Jefferson, too, thought it "expedient" to put the United States "on the footing with the Porte" at least on a par with Prussia, but never followed up on the plan. The country would defeat the Barbary pirates, quadruple its trade with the Middle East, and furnish it with hundreds of missionaries—all without official relations with the region's preeminent power.

The absence of a treaty between Washington and the Porte owed much to anti-Islamic sentiment in America, but it also reflected anti-American policies in Europe. Fearing a challenge to their economic primacy in the Middle East, Britain and France worked to obstruct any negotiations between the sultan and the president. "There is no benefit for the Porte to make a trade treaty with the [American] republic because such a treaty would irritate Great Britain," concluded an official Ottoman report, prepared for Sultan Mahmud II, in December 1820. The author also noted that the Americans had demonstrated warlike behavior during the recent conflict with the Ottoman regencies of Algiers, Tunis, and Tripoli. American merchants operating in the Middle East were consequently subjected to exorbitant tariffs and exposed to arbitrary arrest by Ottoman agents and police. "Our countrymen, not having an ambassador at the Porte, remain at the mercy of the natives," recalled Boston's George Barrell after visiting Istanbul in 1818. There was, however, one American who sought to protect his countrymen's interests, a former Philadelphian named David Offley.

Although no portrait of Offley has survived, one might imagine him wearing the simple black waistcoat favored by his Quaker tradition and an expression that was at once stern and enterprising. Another hybrid type, Offley had been drawn to the Middle East not only by his religious convictions but also by his love of profit. After establishing a trading house in Smyrna in 1811, however, he soon found his business crippled by massive custom duties. Disgusted with paying what he termed "Imaginary Protection against Imaginary dangers," Offley drank dozens of cups of coffee and smoked innumerable waterpipes with Ottoman officials until he finally reached the court of the capudan pasha, the commander of the imperial navy. There, in 1815, Offley paid two thousand dollars in "bachsheesh" to obtain the same extraterritorial rights for Americans as those enjoyed by Europeans. Much of the process had to be repeated the following year, however, after the capudan's execution for treason, but by then Offley had learned what he considered to be the rules of Middle Eastern diplomacy, a combination of "bribery and brass."

Offley prospered, eventually handling two-thirds of all American ships calling at Smyrna, storing their cargoes and servicing their hulls. He even jailed their disorderly sailors for a fee of sixty dollars per year. Yet he could not issue passports or even protect American property. Offley's efforts to establish real diplomatic relations between the countries of his birth and that of his chosen residence continued to founder on European opposition.[3]

Hopes for a breakthrough seemed feeble until 1819, when the idea of achieving a U.S.-Ottoman agreement fixed in the dexterous mind of John Quincy Adams. Called by the historian John Gaddis "the most influential American grand strategist of the nineteenth century," Adams seemed to radiate intelligence from his expansive, high forehead to his determined mouth and inquisitively arched eyebrows. As a younger man, he had represented his nation in some of Europe's most illustrious courts and could now, as the fifty-two-year-old secretary of state, understand the value of formalizing America's relations with Istanbul. Such a treaty would safeguard the Middle Eastern trade that Adams, as a New Englander, appreciated and provide added security for the missionaries with whom the secretary, as a faithful Christian, sympathized.

Adams proceeded quietly, selecting as his agent in the matter a trusted but cunning New York lawyer named Luther Bradish. Like Offley, Bradish was both successful commercially and fervid in his beliefs, a future president of the American Bible Society. Disguised as an innocent sightseer, he boarded the USS *Spark* and planned to sail to Istanbul. At the Dardanelles, however, the ship was barred from entering the Sea of Marmara. Bradish had to disembark at Smyrna and to make his way overland to the Ottoman capital.

Portly and stiff-lipped, Bradish was ill-suited for the unrefined diplomacy of the Middle East. He was scandalized by the need to keep bribing Halet Effendi, the Ottoman foreign minister, while avoiding European interference. Yet the Ottomans appeared interested in concluding a deal, especially if it included gifts of American armaments and warships. "Though once only a minor republic," a memorandum presented to the sultan averred, "America is today almost as powerful as Britain. Their cannon foundries, ammunition stores, gunpowder factories and arsenals are in very good condition." On the basis of these demands, Bradish estimated that the treaty would cost nearly $50,000, including $7,000 "to preserve him [Halet] in his present opinion," and, if concluded, was likely to place violent strains on America's relations with Britain.[4] Adams may have found this price prohibitive—the record is silent—but, in any case, the entire question of U.S.-Ottoman agreement was soon rendered moot. First Halet was assassinated, and then, starting in 1821, the Ottomans were preoccupied with a rebellion in Greece.

NINETEENTH-CENTURY WESTERNERS regarded Greece as a southern European country situated on the Near Eastern cusp. Politically, though, as an integral part of the Ottoman Empire, Greece exerted an influence on events throughout the Middle East, as the war for independence soon demonstrated. Fighting between ethnic Greeks and Turks broke out in Smyrna as well, and nearly took the lives of Levi Parsons and Pliny Fisk. For the United States, the crisis became a source of constant dilemmas, pitching its relationship with the region into quandaries unequaled since the Barbary Wars. While the struggle against North Africa compelled Americans to choose between bribing the pirates and fighting them, the Greek war posed an even more fundamental question. Should the United States give precedence to its economic interests in the Middle East or should it forget financial considerations and uphold its democratic ideals?

America's reaction to the Greek revolt was in large measure an outgrowth of Philhellenism, or "love of all things Grecian," a political and intellectual movement dedicated to ancient Greek civilization. Like Lord Byron and other cultured Europeans of that time, educated Americans were thoroughly versed in the classics. They named their children after the heroes of Greek history and mythology, and their towns after the Hellenic cities of Athens, Sparta, and Troy. Grecian motifs were discernible in virtually every aspect of American life, from art and architecture to literature and government. In a letter to his elderly friend John Adams, Thomas Jefferson expressed his longing to "see the language of Homer and Demosthenes flow with purity, from the lips of a free and ingenious people." Many Americans shared that dream, viewing Greece, along with biblical Israel, as their cultural birthplace and Greece's quest for freedom as identical to America's own recent struggle against misrule.

The Greek revolt appealed not only to Americans' romantic side but also to their religious convictions. Large segments of the American population viewed the conflict as a showdown between Islam and Christianity, and the Greeks as latter-day crusaders. Even a nominally secular publication like the *North American Review* could claim, "Wherever the arms of the Sultan prevail, the village churches are leveled to dust or polluted with the abominations of mohametanism." A group of New York women pressed the point by erecting a monumental cross, inscribed with the words "Sacred to the cause of the Greeks," on Brooklyn Heights, where it was easily glimpsed from Manhattan. In his reply to Jefferson, John Adams confessed, "My old imagination is kindling into a kind of missionary enthusiasm for the cause of the Greeks."

The intensity of American Philhellenism and opposition to Islam was undoubtedly known to the provisional Greek government when it asked the "fellow-citizens of Penn, of Washington, and Franklin" to help "purge Greece from the barbarians, who for four hundred years have polluted its soil." The response could scarcely have been more exuberant. "Such an appeal . . . must bring home to the . . . American the great and glorious part which this country is to act in the political regeneration of the world," declared Harvard's Edward Everett. William Henry Harrison, the frontier general and future president, called for a nationwide mobilization for Greece. "Humanity, policy, religion—all demand it," he decreed. "The star-spangled banner must wave in the Aegean."

Thousands of Americans subsequently responded to that challenge. Societies dedicated to Greece's freedom were formed at Yale and Columbia, and fundraising parties or "Greek balls" were thrown in Albany, Richmond, and Savannah. State legislatures passed resolutions recognizing Greece's right to liberty, and citizens' committees arose to find homes for Greek orphans and collect donations for the rebels' relief. "A meeting was held here for the benefit of the Greeks," the Connecticut pastor Thomas Robbins informed his diary. "There was a full [house] and a collection of $60." In all, Americans raised some $100,000—about $2 million today—and helped finance the building of the sixty-four-gun frigate *Hudson*, Greece's flagship.

Mere philanthropy did not suffice for some Americans, who were willing to give of their livelihoods to Greece and even, possibly, their lives. Samuel Gridley Howe, abolitionist, physician, and pioneer in educating the handicapped as well as the husband of the "Battle Hymn of the Republic" author, Julia Ward Howe, volunteered his medical services to Greece. The memoirs of Howe's experiences, vivid with descriptions of Greek men massacred "like wild beasts, in the streets," of priests executed, and women and young boys carted off "to serve the brutal lusts of the rich," inspired others to follow in his path. Among them was the New Yorker George Jarvis, who served as a lieutenant general in the Greek army, and James Williams, an African American from Baltimore who had fought alongside Stephen Decatur in Algiers and who now battled the Turkish navy for Greece.[5]

Popular support for the Greek insurrection meant that Congress could no longer ignore the issue. The Kentucky congressman Henry Clay insisted that the United States consider recognizing the independent Greek state. "I have in mind the modern not the ancient, the alive and not the dead Greece . . . a Greece fighting for its existence and for the common privilege of human existence," declaimed Massachusetts' representative, Daniel Webster, who urged not only diplomatic assistance but also military aid to the nobly struggling Greeks. Yet not all Americans endorsed these recommendations. Many of Webster's own New England constituents, recalling their difficulties during the Barbary Wars, opposed any policy that might provoke the Porte into interfering with the lucrative Mediterranean trade or with missionary work in the Ottoman Empire.

How could the interests of merchants and missionaries in the Middle East be reconciled with the Philhellenism displayed by much of the American public? This was the predicament that now confronted John Quincy Adams. While he recognized the immense material and spiritual benefit of maintaining cordial relations with the Porte, the secretary believed that Islam was a "fanatic and fraudulent" religion, one that was founded on "the natural hatred of Mussulmen towards the infidel" and the "subjugation of others by the sword." He aspired to be the architect of the first U.S.-Ottoman treaty, but he simultaneously agreed with those Americans who viewed the Greek war as the latest phase in the millennial struggle between Christendom and the "[Muslim] doctrine of violence and lust."

Adams had yet another doctrine to consider when formulating his policy toward Greece. He worried that by intervening on the European continent in favor of Greece America might undermine its opposition to further European conquests in the Western Hemisphere, as stated in the Monroe Doctrine. So pressing were his concerns that when President James Monroe announced his intention to pledge American military assistance for the rebellion, Adams worked hard to dissuade him. The Europeans would certainly exploit such a statement to renew their colonizing efforts in South America, Adams argued, and to dominate the Caribbean trade. His arguments finally swayed the president. Even though the United States "cherished sentiments . . . in favor of the liberty and happiness" of Greece, Monroe told Congress, it would not intercede in an internal European affair.⁶

America's decision to withhold aid from the Greeks significantly augmented its image in Istanbul. At the same time, the Europeans' support for the rebels caused their influence to ebb in the Porte. The time was ideal for Adams to renew his search for a U.S.-Ottoman treaty and to call, once again, on the talents of George Bethune English.

An American Mussulman in the Capital of Islam

"You will inform me, by private letter, of your progress and success," Adams instructed English, after hiring him as America's secret envoy to the Ottomans. "[You] will communicate, as often as you shall have convenience and safe opportunities, any information, commercial or political, which may come to your knowledge, and which may be interesting to the United States." English's first assignment was to gain access to the new capudan, Husrev Mehmet Pasha, if not with the sultan himself.

Traveling, he wrote, as an "American Mussulman who has come from a far distant country to visit the Capital of Islam," English entered Istanbul on November 5, 1823, donned local dress, and rented rooms in the city's oldest quarter. Cautiously, he began building connections—first with the sultan's librarian and then with more senior factotums. Each connection brought him closer to his target, but at the price of becoming one himself. "My situation is full of danger and disquietude," he confided to Adams. "I frequently hear myself being denounced as a Greek spy in disguise, and my own servant when I go out of doors will not follow me in order . . . not to partake of a shot meant of me."

On January 4, English at last gained admittance to Husrev, a man preoccupied with the military situation in Greece and "much engaged in taking measures to preserve his head and his place." Husrev was also concerned about European demands for pieces of his empire and about designs on Middle Eastern markets. English therefore assured him that the United States had no desire for Ottoman lands, but only for open and mutually beneficial trade. America, moreover, was a country that respected all religions, Islam included, where "a mussulman citizen . . . would have precisely the same privileges as a Christian." Impressed by this presentation, the capudan agreed to discuss formulating a treaty, but do so only clandestinely, aboard ship, to avoid European intrigues. Maintaining the meeting's secrecy, English understood, also guaranteed that the capudan received all of the bribe money and would not have to share it with others. "I have thus far got on pretty well," the envoy guaranteed Adams.

Yet Adams was not reassured. English's penchant for cloak-and-dagger tactics and his liberal use of bribes discomfited the straitlaced secretary and led him to distrust the agent's ability as a negotiator of international treaties. Accordingly, he demoted English to the role of interpreter for John Rogers, commander of the Mediterranean Squadron. Adams instructed Rogers to follow through on the meeting with the capudan, to obtain terms with the Ottomans similar to those enjoyed by Britain and France, and to take care that none of his actions were construed as for or against the Greeks. The commodore could also promise Husrev that "his good offices will be duly estimated in the transaction."[7]

Rogers, a decorated veteran of the Barbary Wars, was a by-the-book officer appointed to rid the fleet of drunkenness and duels, not to conduct sensitive talks with Ottoman leaders. His lack of diplomatic finesse, compounded by Husrev's preoccupation with Greece, delayed further discussions on a treaty. Not until July 5, 1826—two and a half years after English arrived in Istanbul—did the commodore and the capudan finally meet, rendezvousing between the islands of Tenedos and Lesbos. Dressed in white Moorish costume, sailors from the USS *North Carolina* and the *Constitution* boarded the Ottoman flagship and regaled its crew with choruses of "Hail Columbia." Gifts were exchanged—silks and a waterpipe for Rogers, and for Husrev, jewel-encrusted rings, pistols, and a snuffbox. With English interpreting, the two men agreed that Rogers would proceed to Smyrna and await word of the treaty's approval. The capudan then cast off, saluting with his guns and flying the sultan's personal pennant, which was an honor never before bestowed on Westerners.

Rogers indeed proceeded to Smyrna, where, as Offley's guest, he attended soirees and entertained minor officials. He waited for more than a year but still received no reply from the Porte. Adams had meanwhile advanced to the presidency and was better placed to press for a treaty. But if "Old Eloquence," as he was known, had been an imposing statesman, his performance as head of state proved far less sterling. Instead of placating the Turks, his administration issued repeated declarations in support of Greek independence, giving rise to rumors that the United States was secretly arming the rebels. "See how these Franks never keep their promises," the Sultan complained. "It is wiser to respect the position of Great Britain and to delay the Americans with politics." Adams further alienated the Turks by proclaiming his sympathy for the "suffering Greeks" in "that most unequal of conflicts" and by wishing them "the triumph of humanity and freedom."

Adams managed to antagonize not only the Ottomans but also George English, who criticized his rashness and blamed him for undermining any remaining hopes for a treaty. It was the wrong moment to assail a president frustrated by years of failure to procure even a limited agreement with Istanbul. His opinion of English was hardly improved by David Offley, who traduced him as an unstable turncoat secretly in league with the sultan. The imprecations stuck. Accusing him of "misconduct . . . most mortifying" and of "eccentricities approaching to insanity," Adams resolved to sever all ties with his personal emissary and longtime friend. "I can now no longer sustain him," he wrote. English sailed back to America and tried, unsuccessfully, to plead his case at the White House. Unemployed, the former divinity student, ex-Marine lieutenant, and Muslim general died on September 20, 1828, not in Islam's capital but in that of his native United States.[8]

Annus Mirabilis: 1830

English's death coincided with a seemingly unstoppable downswing in the Middle East's political situation and a further reduction in the chances for a Turkish-American treaty. Exploiting the Ottomans' imbroglio in Greece, provincial rulers throughout the empire began to assert their autonomy. The great powers, meanwhile, feared that Greece's secession from Ottoman rule would inaugurate the Ottoman's total disintegration and trigger a European war over its pieces. They sought, therefore, to maintain the status quo in Greece. But the Porte, resenting what it regarded as alien interference in its internal affairs, sent a combined Ottoman and Egyptian fleet to southern Greece. French, British, and Russian gunboats intercepted the flotilla and on October 20, 1827, near Navarino Bay (present-day Pylos), sank three-quarters of the sultan's ships.

The Turkish defeat at Navarino emboldened the Greeks in their quest for independence and inaugurated the very scramble for Ottoman lands that the powers had hoped to avoid. Thus, in 1829, the Russians conquered a huge swath of the Bulgarian frontier and a year later France landed 24,000 troops at Algiers, initiating a 130-year occupation of the country. The so-called Eastern Question—what to do with the disintegrating Ottoman Empire?—destined to plague Europe throughout much of the next century, precipitating one war (in the Crimea) and contributing to the outbreak of another (World War I), commenced.

So, too, did the notion of an Arabic-speaking Middle East free of Ottoman rule. Muhammad Ali, a former Albanian mercenary who had been sent to Egypt earlier in the century to help liberate the country from Napoleon, was furious over the loss of his warships and the Ottomans' refusal to pay him for his services in fighting the Greeks. Independent in all but name from Istanbul and generously backed by the French, Muhammad Ali prepared to march his army into Anatolia and to establish his own empire.[9]

The amputation of entire Ottoman provinces by the European powers and their local allies hardly seemed conducive to an agreement between Ottoman leaders and those of another Western nation, the United States. Americans, moreover, had cheered the European triumph at Navarino; a Wisconsin town was even named for the battle. The Ottomans, though, in urgent need of a diplomatic counterweight to Europe and a source for replenishing its warships, were willing to ignore these slights. "However you may act towards us, the Americans will be our good friends," the Ottoman foreign minister reportedly told a British merchant. "And an American ship . . . is worth two of yours of the same size." While European consuls fled Istanbul in fear of reprisals, Americans were welcomed in the capital and told of the sultan's renewed interest in a treaty. Anti-Turkish sentiment in the United States, however, continued to inhibit a positive response to that offer until 1830, by which time a new tenant occupied the White House.

A penniless orphan and child soldier who forged himself into an outstanding lawyer, senator, and hero of the War of 1812, Andrew Jackson could scarcely have differed more from his privileged predecessor. He also had none of Adams's commitment to diplomatic protocol and conducted his foreign affairs less with "Old Eloquence" than with "Old Hickory." Jackson wanted trade with the Ottoman Empire and was unwilling to let any obstacle hinder him, not even popular sympathy for Greece. As one of the first foreign policy decisions of his administration, Jackson declared his determination to "leave no proper means unemployed to acquire for our flag the same privileges [in Ottoman lands] that are enjoyed by the principal powers of Europe," and to seek a formal treaty with the Porte.

Jackson's choice as negotiator was, fittingly, David Offley, who was accompanied by U.S. Navy Commodore James Biddle and the New York merchant Charles Rhind. The three began discreet discussions in Istanbul in February 1830 only to encounter the usual British obstructions. The Americans persisted, nevertheless, and on May 7 signed America's first-ever Treaty of Navigation and Commerce with the Ottoman Empire. This granted extraterritorial rights ("capitulations") to the United States and permission to trade in the Black Sea. Presenting the treaty to Congress, Jackson praised "the most friendly feelings . . . entertained by the Sultan" and the "enlightened disposition . . . evinced by him to foster the intercourse between the two countries." America, for its part, pledged to furnish the Ottoman navy with a variety of gunboats, including "two-deckers, frigates, corvettes, and brigs," all at discount prices.[10]

The year 1830 should then be remembered as the turning point in antebellum America's relations with the Middle East. It was the year in which the United States attained a legal and commercial status in Ottoman lands equal to that of Europe, the year in which the president established the precedent of selling American weaponry to the region. A navy yard, described as "entirely under American control and American regulations," was soon operating in Istanbul, churning out eleven ships of the line and twelve frigates, as well as the world's largest battleship, the 934-ton *Mahmud*. American officers were permitted to serve as advisers aboard these ships, while Turkish cadets seeking "improvement in seamanship and naval tactics" received instruction on American vessels. In addition to reoutfitting the Ottoman navy, the United States also armed its ground force with Harpers Ferry rifles, Colt revolvers, and American-style cannons.

Arms sales, though, accounted for only a segment of the boom in American commerce with the Middle East that began in 1830. Protected by the new treaty, merchants traversed the empire bearing the latest products of American industry, from false teeth to a machine capable—so its inventors swore—"of projecting balls without gunpowder." American-made "chairs and tables, books and book-cases, Yankee clocks and glass windows" were just some of the products that, according to a missionary stationed in Anatolia, the United States exchanged for consignments of dates, figs, and carpets. American textiles were especially valued throughout the area. One American visitor to Damascus reported seeing bolts of American cotton being borne on caravans bound for Asia Minor and another noticed bales in Anatolia bearing the stamp "Tremont Mill, Lowell, Mass." A common word for cloth in the Persian Gulf area was *merkani* and in Turkey, *americano*.[11]

HAVING ESTABLISHED themselves throughout the Ottoman realm, American businessmen began to venture beyond its boundaries. In Yemen, at the tip of the Arabian Peninsula, they purchased half of the annual coffee crop, and in Muscat (modern-day Oman) they bought gum Arabic, rhinoceros horn, and ivory. In 1832, a New Hampshire entrepreneur named Edmund Roberts, sailing aboard the USS *Peacock* with a trove of quality arms, maps, and mint-condition American coins, set out for Mocha and Muscat. He gained entrance to the fortress of Sultan Sayyid Sa'id, who was recovering from wounds suffered during a recent war with the Wahhabis. "The lumps of dirt and the spots on the wall were the blood and brains of many a victim," Roberts wrote. Sa'id signed a trade agreement with the United States, the first between his country and the West, and donated a pair of lions to the Washington Zoo. He also sent his personal emissary, Na'aman, to New York, where curious crowds followed his tours of monuments, clubs, and the newly built Long Island Railroad. Visiting Sa'id's fortress in 1833, a British diplomat found that its walls were no longer bloodstained but, more disturbingly, bright with paintings of American victories in the War of 1812.[12]

The expansion of America's trade through an increasingly unquiet Middle East meant a broadened role for the U.S. Navy. Citing the "salutary effect" that the Mediterranean Squadron continued to make on North Africa, Jackson believed that American consuls in the region "cannot be too sparing of their allusions to it." To emphasize the point, the USS *Concord* was dispatched in 1832 to Alexandria, where its commander, Matthew C. Perry, destined to open Japan to the West, became the first American commodore to visit Egypt. The following year, the USS *Delaware*, captained by the Barbary War veteran Daniel Patterson, paid calls to Cairo, Jaffa, and Beirut. Writing from Lebanon, an American missionary described how at least forty thousand people, "Christians, Moslems and Druzes . . . peasants, priests, sheikhs and emirs," toured the ship and were hosted by its spotlessly uniformed crew. One Arab nobleman, impressed by the spectacle, repudiated his previous image of Americans as a "savage and uncivilized people" and instead pronounced them "superior in every respect to other nations . . . in politeness and kindness towards us strangers." America, in the eyes of many Middle Eastern observers, would soon challenge the naval supremacy that the British had long enjoyed in the area. Ibrahim Pasha,

Muhammad Ali's son, went so far as to declare that Britain had only the second-best fleet in the Mediterranean, "after the American."[13]

Increased commercial and naval activity in turn necessitated a bolstered American diplomatic presence in the Middle East, but in responding to this need, the United States remained dolefully sluggish. There were few American consulates in the area, most of them manned by ill-paid and unqualified foreigners, some of whom could not even speak English. American-born consuls often proved even more incompetent. In Tangier, Consul James Leib, a notorious drunk, would nightly wrap himself in Old Glory and beckon to imaginary U.S. warships offshore, while his counterpart in Tunis, the failed actor John Howard Payne, succeeded only in composing the famous ditty "Home Sweet Home." "Our whole consular system is radically wrong, disreputable, and injurious to our character," carped one New Yorker after visiting the region in the 1830s. "The . . . American flag is waving over the houses of Greeks, Italians, Jews, and Arabs, and all the mongrel population." No flag flew over the Dardanelles, however, because the consul there was too poor to buy one.[14]

Such sparse and flawed representation was clearly inadequate for a country with broadening interests in the Middle East. The Jackson administration acted promptly to rectify the problem. In 1831 it appointed as America's first chargé d'affaires in Istanbul a most extraordinary—and ornery—man.

The Devil and David Porter

Known as Sindbad to his friends, David Porter arrived at his post after a storied, if occasionally notorious, career. The son of a Revolutionary naval captain, Porter had led the boarding party that captured the *Tripoli* in 1801, was wounded in a daring coastal raid, and was captured with the crew of the *Philadelphia*. Later, in the War of 1812, he became the first American captain to seize a British warship and the first to sail around Cape Horn. But Porter also had an impulsive side. He had killed a man in a bar brawl, served as a witness for Stephen Decatur's fatal duel, and attacked a Puerto Rican fortress that had failed to return his salute. An impenitent curmudgeon, he left his wife in Chester, Pennsylvania, to live on the Marmara Coast with his sister, and bombarded the State Department daily with rambling, misnumbered dispatches. Short, dark, and weather-beaten, with imperious, penetrating eyes, Porter was inhospitable to visitors and intolerant of the Middle East. "Salaams are an infernal nuisance," he snapped after one unctuous audience with Sultan Mahmud II. "Why the devil can't the man be satisfied with a decent salute?"

Similar to Andrew Jackson in temperament, Porter also shared his president's determination to enhance America's relationship with the Ottomans. He derived particular satisfaction from introducing his hosts to the wonders of American industry. "There is no part of the world so famous for men of ingenuity and useful mechanical Talents, as the United States of America," he reckoned. As proof of this genius, Porter proposed presenting the sultan with a swan-shaped steamboat, "the head and neck fixed to the bow, the wings to the guards of the wheel, and the tail to the stern," but the State Department rejected the idea in favor of the usual gem-studded snuffboxes. But Porter did arrive with made-in-Boston rocking horses for the children of the sultan's harem and U.S. Army caps for his troops. The first memento was delightfully received; the second, somewhat less so.[15]

Ensconced in a handsome villa overlooking the Bosphorus, Porter proceeded to overhaul America's diplomatic representation in the Middle East. Wherever possible, U.S. citizens were now appointed to the consular posts, and their performance was regularly monitored. The former captain also helped supervise the naval yard, supplying it with the finest New England carpenters and shipments of live oak, and assuring that its products surpassed the exacting standards of America's Navy. Duly impressed, Mahmud II elevated Porter from chargé to ambassador—America's first in the Middle East. "[I]t does not appear that any of the Diplomatists here have any idea that there is any thing like American influence," he wrote, adding modestly, "Had I the talent of a Metternich or a Talleyrand . . . I would not stand higher in the [Turks'] estimation."[16]

Porter was perfectly willing to wield that prestige, even in criticizing Ottoman policies. When a number of Syrian Jews were arrested and tortured on spurious murder charges—the so-called Damascus Blood Libel of 1840—Porter officially denounced the "barbarous" and "atrocious cruelties." He reminded the Porte that the United States made "no distinction between the Mohammedan, the Jews and the Christian," and wished to "protect that persecuted race among whose kindred are found some of the most worthy and patriotic of our citizens." Porter established a tradition that would continue well into the twentieth century, of extending America's protection to Middle Eastern Jews. This time the intervention succeeded. Buckling to protests from Britain and France as well, the Ottomans worked to suppress the libel and to secure the prisoners' release.[17]

Porter's most vexing difficulties, however, involved not Middle Eastern Jews but rather his Christian countrymen. By trying to convert Arab Christians to Protestantism, American missionaries in Syria and Mount Lebanon had provoked the ire of local churchmen, in particular the Maronite patriarch. In 1841, he petitioned the Porte to banish the evangelicals from the empire and, to issue the expulsion order, the Porte turned to the American ambassador.

Though hardly a religious man, Porter nevertheless professed a begrudging admiration for the missionaries and their pioneering work in education. "A reading nation," he believed, "cannot be long in understanding what are its true interests . . . [and] will not be long in acting." But upholding the U.S.-Ottoman treaty, not promoting American ideas, was Porter's primary responsibility. His efforts, however, were increasingly frustrated by the missionaires and their contempt for Ottoman authority. "Avoid doing anything . . . likely to offend . . . the musselman," he scolded them, emphasizing that the treaty did not protect Americans who "excite[d] the . . . inhabitants to change their rites and religion." If the missionaries persisted in proselytizing Ottoman subjects, Porter warned, they did so "at their own risk, and on their own responsibility."

In reproving the missionaries and showing sensitivity to the Ottomans' concerns, Porter was merely carrying out the Jacksonian instructions that had enabled the United States to establish itself as a friendly and economically significant power in the Middle East. Unfortunately for the ambassador, though, a new administration was now in office, with an imperious secretary of state. Daniel Webster, the veteran Philhellenist and unwavering critic of Turkey, had little patience for what he regarded as Ottoman intolerance. Though pilloried by a later writer as a godless man who had sold his soul to politics, Webster was, in reality, an upstanding Congregationalist and an honorary member of the American Board of Commissioners for Foreign Missions. In the board's opinion it was Porter, not Webster, who trucked with the devil by refusing to protect the missionaries. These Americans, the commissioners pledged, had always lived peacefully as "Frank residents of Beyrout" without converting the Maronites or violating Ottoman law. Webster was convinced and in a stinging dispatch dated February 2, 1842, he upbraided Porter for his inaction and ordered him to "omit no occasion . . . to extend all proper succor" to the missionaries.[18]

The reprimand left Porter deeply embittered, but not for long; the sixty-three-year-old salt died in 1842. His legacy, however, would live on in the many family members—Porters, Heaps, Farraguts, and Browns—destined to play prominent roles in the Middle East, and in the paradigms he established for America's relations with the region. In addition to selling arms and introducing American technology to Middle Eastern rulers, Porter solidified America's image as a regional power on a par with Europe, but one which, unlike the Europeans, had no territorial ambitions in the area. Thanks largely to David Porter, American diplomacy in the Middle East had advanced immeasurably since the days when clandestine agents like George English were compelled to sneak incognito through Istanbul's streets and conduct their negotiations in secret. And yet, while successful in establishing friendships with the Ottomans, Porter ultimately failed to maintain amity with his countrymen who were most active in the area. More than the statesmen, servicemen, and merchants from the United States, missionaries would exert a far-reaching influence on the relations between the Middle East and antebellum America.

MANIFEST
MIDDLE EASTERN
DESTINY

THE BRAZENNESS DISPLAYED BY AMERICAN MISSIONARIES in challenging Porter was evidence of the emerging alliance between church leaders and decision makers in the United States. The missionary movement had grown significantly since the early 1820s, when its first emissaries to the Middle East, Levi Parsons and Pliny Fisk, failed to attract converts and died forsaken deaths. Even the modest accomplishments of Fisk's successors—Isaac Bird, William Goodell, and Eli Smith—in establishing schoolhouses in Syria could not account for the missionaries' ability, a mere ten years later, to impact American policy toward the Middle East. The process through which small groups of women and men who journeyed thousands of miles into inhospitable territories managed to transform their country's relationship with an entire region and profoundly alter the region itself, is a remarkable story. It is a saga steeped in hardship and blood.

Stations of the Cross and the Sun

Through their schools, the missionaries had gained a foothold in Syria by 1827, but the ultimate goal of evangelizing Palestine remained elusive. That year, however, the American Board and the Boston Female Society for Promoting Christianity among the Jews decided to launch another mission to Jerusalem and, to spearhead it, chose a thirty-year-old pastor from the Berkshires named Josiah Brewer. "Marked," according to one of his professors, "with mildness, modesty, good sense and unaffected piety," Brewer was charged with succeeding where Parson and Fisk had failed by establishing a permanent station in the Holy City and initiating the ingathering of the Jews. "Our *Pilgrim mothers* [would] have exulted . . . had they foreseen that . . . their daughters should be sending back the gospel to Jerusalem!" Brewer declaimed as he departed Massachusetts, confident of his ability to supplant "the blood-red flag of the crescent with . . . the white banner . . . of peace," on Jerusalem's walls.

Peace, however, was the last thing Brewer discovered in Palestine. He landed in the country just after the disastrous Ottoman defeat at Navarino in 1827, portending the empire's dissolution. The vast majority of Palestinian Muslims at the time still viewed themselves as devoted Ottoman subjects and still considered all Westerners, whether Americans or Europeans, as "Franks" who threatened the Islamic state. Brewer's attempts to remind the natives that the U.S. Navy was not even present at Navarino and that America in fact respected Ottoman sovereignty proved ineffectual. Even less convincing were the protestations of goodwill toward Islamic culture that he uttered while distributing New Testaments. Evicted from two Galilean villages, lice-ridden and enervated by disease, Brewer finally curtailed his mission. He hobbled back to Boston in disgrace.[1]

The American Board nevertheless remained hopeful that some kind of station could eventually be erected in Jerusalem. Board elders pointed to improved conditions in the Holy Land since 1831, the year that Muhammad Ali, furious over the Ottomans' refusal to compensate him for his losses at Navarino, sent Egyptian troops to occupy Syria and Palestine. The modernizing Egyptians granted unprecedented privileges to the non-Muslim *millets* of the area. Eager to take advantage of this enhanced situation, the board authorized the launching of a new Palestine mission. Chosen to lead it were William and Eliza Thomson, a young couple who had met in Princeton, New Jersey, where he was studying Bible and she was teaching school. The two married in 1833 and promptly volunteered as evangelists.

Not all of Palestine's inhabitants welcomed Muhammad Ali's reforms, however. The Muslim majority deeply resented the equal rights that Egypt had granted to the local Christians and Jews and the openness it showed to foreigners. Anger at the occupiers escalated and then, following attempts to tax Muslim peasants and draft them into the Egyptian army, exploded in a violent revolt. The bloodshed peaked in Palestine in 1834, just as the Thomsons reached Jerusalem.

Eliza was then nine months pregnant and unable to flee the city. William Thomson felt he had no choice but to leave her behind and try to secure help in Jaffa. "I have not heard one syllable from Mrs. T. since I left," he fretted, haunted by rumors of atrocities. Eliza, in fact, had bolted herself indoors, panicked by the "roar of cannon, falling walls, the shrieks of the neighbors, the terror of servants and constant expectation of massacre." In spite of this trauma, she managed to give birth to a boy, Thomas. The father returned on July 22, following a column of Egyptian reinforcements, only to find Jerusalem in ruins and his wife desperately ill. She died two weeks later.

"The wreck of a country, and the dregs of a people," Thomson wrote despondently of Palestine. "The Jordan would scarcely be dignified with the name of river in America." His caviling could not, however, deter other missionaries from trying to work in Jerusalem. George Whiting and Betsey Tilden arrived shortly after Eliza Thomson's death, but neither could endure the privations. The numinous Palestine of the Bible was revealed to be "a land of devils," in the opinion of the veteran missionary Isaac Bird, "no longer the blessed but accursed." By the end of 1834, the American Board was finally compelled to admit that "not a single soul" in the Holy Land had been "brought to a sense of sin, and converted to God," and resolved to abandon all futher expeditions to Palestine. Henceforth, the missionaries' attention would be directed elsewhere in the Middle East, especially around the area of Mount Lebanon.[2]

The Bird and Goodell families continued to expand their schools and build new ones in and around Beirut, but conditions in the city began to deteriorate following the Egyptian invasion of 1831. Fighting erupted between pro-Egyptian Maronites and the Druze who remained loyal to the Porte, producing crossfires so intense that the Americans feared to step outdoors or even sit by open windows. The Maronites also exploited the chaos to press their anathemas against Protestantism and their opposition to evangelical schools. "The Turks . . . exhibit more excellent traits of character than the Christians," protested William Goodell. "The idea of not acting dishonorably seems very rarely indeed to visit the bosom of a Christian." Isolated and physically threatened, the missionaries concluded that they could no longer hold out in Lebanon. Beginning with the Bird family, evacuated by an Austrian schooner, the entire community fled.

The situation in Syria and Palestine had become insufferable for Americans, but even in Smyrna, a largely Christian city and the missionary's gateway to the Middle East, the atmosphere had grown adverse. The first attempt to establish a station in Smyrna, by the amateur mountaineer Elnathan Gridley in 1826, failed after the young preacher went climbing, caught pneumonia, and died. Gridley's replacement was Daniel Temple, painted by one biographer as "gloomy, austere, [and] sanctimonious," a diehard who had worked his way up from rural poverty to scholarships at Dartmouth and Andover. But nothing in New England had prepared Temple for the Middle East, where consumption quickly killed his wife and two of their four children. The devastated missionary returned to America, together with his surviving sons. "The thought of their being educated in this deeply depraved and ungodly part of the world is truly distressing," he wrote.

Temple nevertheless managed to overcome his revulsion to the Middle East and in 1833 he once again sailed for Smyrna, this time with a new wife and a printing press. His Bibles and textbooks were soon being studied in a school for Christian girls established by Joshua Brewer—the same Joshua Brewer who had retreated from Palestine five years earlier—now sponsored by the Ladies Missionary Society of New Haven. "If then the sword should not open a door . . . to the Christian preacher in Mahometan lands, may we not hope that the gradual progress of civilization will?" Brewer asked. The answer seemed clearer by 1838, by which time over two hundred girls had enrolled in the school.[3]

The missionaries' success in Smyrna remained exceptional, however, and the lack of even basic security precluded evangelizing efforts elsewhere in Ottoman lands. The American Board accordingly set its sights on a region beyond the empire's borders, on the Lake Urmia district of northwest Persia and on the community of Nestorian (Assyrian) Christians rumored to be living there. The task of accessing this nebulous realm fell to Harrison Gray Otis Dwight, a recent Andover graduate, and to the seasoned Lebanon missionary Eli Smith. The men rendezvoused in Smyrna in May 1830, disguised themselves in turbans and robes, and set out to become "the first Americans who have trod the soil of Armenia."

Before them, however, lay a trail as travail ridden as any across the American frontier. Heading eastward to Erzurum, the pair trudged for three weeks through a waterless countryside without encountering a single village. The slight and scholarly Smith complained of having to sleep in stables with "every species of dirt, vermin and litter," and of waking up rheumy eyed and feverish. Stricken with cholera outside of Tiflis, he was soon unable to walk and had to be strapped to a donkey cart by Dwight. In March, however, the Americans at last attained their goal and staggered into Urmia.

The city, compared with the turbulent Beirut and Jerusalem, at first seemed Edenic. Under the relatively open-minded Qajar dynasty, Persia was then experiencing an interlude of internal stability and freedom from the great-power encroachments of Russia and Britain. In Urmia, the missionaries found that the government did not interfere with their preaching and that the Nestorians' Bible-based theology was not unlike their own. "I felt a stronger desire to settle among them at once . . . than among any people I have ever seen," Smith blithely reported.

Settling in, the Americans erected a schoolhouse where forty students were soon receiving instruction in math, English composition, and Psalms. New missionaries arrived to reinforce the station—Justin and Charlotte Perkins in 1832 and, three years later, Asahel and Judith Grant. A native of Utica, New York, the twenty-eight-year-old Asahel was reputedly a swarthy man of medium height and unusual energy, "his eye bright, his aspect friendly, with a dash of enterprise and enthusiasm." He was also a country physician who inaugurated what would become an exalted missionary tradition, providing free medical care to Middle Eastern populations. In his first year in Urmia, Grant treated ten thousand patients. He fulsomely recalled, "The sick, the lame, and the blind gathered round by the scores and hundreds, and my fame soon spread abroad through the surrounding country."

Grant's endurance enabled him not only to care for the sick but also to explore the wastelands as far south as Kurdish Mesopotamia, braving bandits and punishing terrain, in search of more Nestorians. Back in the United States in October 1840, the doctor assured the board's commissioners that the Urmia station was thriving and that a new mission should be undertaken in the region of what is today called Iraq. The commissioners agreed and presently dispatched Colby C. Mitchell and Abel Hindsdale, together with their wives, to Mosul.⁴

American evangelists had registered their first unqualified Middle Eastern triumph, but then multiple disasters struck. Blinded and deranged by a sandstorm, the Mitchells succumbed to typhoid fever, and though the Hindsdales managed to reach Mosul, they arrived too debilitated to work. Disease also claimed the lives of Elizabeth Dwight, her son John, and all five of the Perkinses' children. Charlotte Perkins, suffering from epilepsy, returned to the United States. Sarah Smith, Eli's wife, drowned in a shipwreck near Cyprus, and his second wife, Mary Ward Chapin, died of dysentery.

"Enfeebled health and shortened life are among the sacrifices necessary to the work of the missions," Eli Smith confessed, referring not only to Urmia but to the entire Middle East. Women, often weakend by childbirth, were especially vulnerable "I sometimes fear that this sickness is a judgment upon me for improving so little my great blessings," wrote Mary Van Lennep, who in 1843 left Hartford, Connecticut, for the barrens of Anatolia. "I try to pray that . . . I may be willing to suffer." Missionaries were subject to physical attack by brigands and vigilantes and accorded only negligible protection by the Ottomans. "A man's hat is always more safe in America than a man's head is in Turkey," William Goodell quipped. Disease, however, remained the most efficient killer, responsible for a death rate among American missionaries in the Middle East that exceeded that of settlers on the western frontier. A third of all missionaries who left the United States for the Middle East between 1821 and 1846 died while on duty, most of them shortly after arriving. "The hour is near when you expect to leave the shores of your native land with the probability that you will never see them again," departing young seminarians were told. Mary Van Lennep was dead within a year.

What had begun as a glimmering vision of stations in the Middle Eastern sun had produced little but suffering and death—stations, rather, of the cross. Not even Asahel Grant was spared. In a short span of time, the doctor lost his wife and two of their three children. He nevertheless managed to retain his faith and to erect the mission near Mosul, but this, too, came to ruin. Late in the spring of 1843, Kurds and Turks attacked the Nestorians there, killing eight hundred and banishing thousands more. Grant rejected charges that the missionaries had provoked the massacre by encouraging the community to seek independence from Muslim rule. "Let us have the great consolation that we have been instrumental, in some measure, of awakening an interest and a spirit of prayer," Grant declared, struggling to comfort the Nestorians and also, perhaps, himself.

How, in the face of all these ordeals and defeats, did the missionaries come to enjoy such influence in the United States and, to a remarkable extent, determine the country's policies overseas? What factors enabled these Americans to recover from their agonizing setbacks, to replenish their ranks, and to rebuild all that had been devastated? "You Americans think that you can do everything . . . that money can buy or that strength can accomplish. But you cannot conquer Almighty God," an Arab guide taunted one newly arrived missionary.[5] The preacher certainly agreed that God could not be vanquished, but determination and wealth might still, he believed, achieve miracles, especially in the Middle East.

Resurrection

The turnaround for the missionaries began in 1840 when the European powers, fearing for the integrity of the Ottoman Empire, forced the Egyptian troops out of Syria and Palestine. Relative stability was restored to the area, but without reducing the rights that the minorities had achieved under Muhammad Ali. On the contrary, in gratitude to the Europeans for retrieving his lands, Sultan Abdul Mejid pledged to respect the "liberty, property, and honor of every individual subject, without reference to his religious creed." Foreign nationals were now permitted to reside permanently in Jerusalem and the empire's Protestants were finally recognized as a legitimate *millet*. For the missionaries, these events were nothing less than the handiwork of God. Exclaimed one of them, "Whereas, but a few years ago, there still existed . . . an obstinate bigotry and unrelenting spirit of persecution . . . there is now perfect toleration!"

The easing of restrictions had an immediate impact on missionary activities in Syria and Mount Lebanon. The Birds and the Goodells were able to reestablish themselves in Beirut and to welcome a new generation of evangelists, led by William Eddy and Henry Jessup. Returning to Lebanon from Urmia, Eli Smith began an Arabic translation of the Bible and developed the first Arabic-language movable type, "American Arabic." Within a decade, Smith's presses were producing some fifty thousand volumes per year in fourteen local languages, including translations of the *Dairyman's Daughter*, *Pilgrim's Progress*, and the region's first elementary school primers. Smith's only setback resulted from his attempt to adapt native music to the Protestant liturgy. "Not only do we find the singing of the Arabs no music to us, but our musicians have found it . . . impossible to . . . imitate their tunes," he conceded.[6]

THE MISSIONARIES' newfound success was an outgrowth of enhanced circumstances in the Middle East, but also of the radical transformations that were remaking America. The 1840s saw the rise of the Manifest Destiny ideology, a grander and more militant version of the old Puritan claim to a God-given right to the new Promised Land, which Americans now espoused to justify their conquest of the entire North American continent. Under the Manifest Destiny banner, the nation's population of 17 million inexorably fanned out across the existing twenty-six states and into the vast territories west of the Mississippi and north of the Rio Grande, uprooting Native American communities and ousting the Mexicans on route. But the concept also had a worldwide, educational dimension. According to the New York journalist John O'Sullivan, who coined the term, Manifest Destiny also ordained America "to establish on earth the moral dignity and salvation of man," to disseminate its principles, both religious and secular, abroad.

The global and edifying aspect of Manifest Destiny accorded well with the missionaries' sense of purpose and reenergized the movement precisely at its dimmest juncture. "The destiny of America is inevitably bound up with the destiny of the world," declared Dwight Marsh, the head of the Mosul mission. "America is only safe in the salvation of mankind." The evangelists were inspired by the dynamism animating their country and by the spirit of scientific inquiry it evinced. This was the America of breakthrough technological innovations, of Charles Goodyear's vulcanized rubber and the dependable brass movement clock of Chauncey Jerome. Among the newfangled products that American missionaries introduced to the Middle East were the camera, the sewing machine, and a revolutionary communications device invented by the son of an American Board member, Samuel Morse. "I do love to give a shock to these [native] people," confessed William Goodell. "It seems to move them a step forward toward the millennium."

Far more than its technical aspects, though, the image of military strength projected by the United States throughout the Manifest Destiny period electrified the missionaries. Middle Eastern peoples, averred the otherwise bookish Eli Smith, "ought to know that we are a powerful nation. And there is no other way to teach them this but to make them feel it." Much like the preachers on the American frontier who, when threatened with Indian attack, summoned the U.S. Cavalry, Smith and his fellow evangelists called on the federal government, its diplomats, and even its warships to protect them from irate Muslim rulers. Replacing David Porter as America's ambassador in Istanbul, Dabney Carr came into office in 1842 declaring his intention to protect the missionaries "to the full extent of [his] power," if necessary "by calling the whole of the American squadron in the Mediterranean to Beyrout." Carr, a grandnephew of

Thomas Jefferson, proved true to his proclamation. A year later, the USS *Independence* conducted a high-profile tour of Egyptian and Syrian ports. Its orders were to "inquire into the safety and prosperity of the Missions . . . and to extend to them such assistance as they may require."

The confluence of divinely ordained missions and state-sanctioned might was emblematic of the Manifest Destiny era both in North America and in the Middle East. Still, in contrast to the missions that often formed the nuclei of future forts, towns, and cities in the American West, the stations established by American evangelists in the Middle East never served to stake out territorial claims. Nor were they identified with big business interests, in the manner of the American missionaries in Hawaii. The absence of imperialist and economic agenda distinguished the Middle East missionaries not only from their counterparts in the United States, but also from the European preachers who often doubled as government agents. "I am persuaded that their [the Americans'] sole motivation was religious," concluded a French consul in Beirut after a scrupulous investigation. "I simply do not perceive any ulterior political motive."

American missionaries in the Middle East viewed Manifest Destiny not as a blueprint for conquering territory but rather as a warrant for capturing souls and minds. They continued to disparage Islam as a fraudulent, retrograde faith and dismissed all forms of Eastern Christianity as decadent and outmoded. Their approach to the peoples and cultures of the region remained rife with arrogance and yet their hubris was tempered with beneficence. Confronting a crowd of indignant Lebanese, William Goodell could with all sincerity declare, "We have come to raise your . . . population from that state of ignorance degradation and death which you are fallen, to do all the good in our power."

Millions of Americans now supported that salvational effort. From the modest grassroots campaign that began after the Barbary Wars, the missionary movement had blossomed in the four decades leading up to the Civil War into a national passion. Support for the missions flowed not merely from congregations across the country, but also from the mainstream press, from Congress, and even from the White House. Inspired by the Manifest Destiny vision, farmers and factory workers, the graduates of single-room schoolhouses and alumni of the nation's leading universities, northerners and southerners alike, reported for evangelizing duty overseas. There was never a shortage of volunteers. Perhaps the keenest gauge of Manifest Destiny's influence on the missionary enterprise was the annual budget of the America Board, which had soared from a mere $10,000 in the days of Fisk and Parsons to $250,000 by midcentury.[7]

The impact of improved conditions for missionaries working in the Middle East, together with the revitalization of the evangelists' zeal, was illustrated by the case of Cyrus Hamlin. Born in Maine in 1811, Hamlin had been orphaned at an early age and forced to work as a farmhand. But he also studied compulsively and ultimately won a scholarship to Bowdoin College, where he became the favorite student of Henry Wadsworth Longfellow and graduated at the top of his class. Startlingly handsome, if outlandishly whiskered, Hamlin was the embodiment of the Manifest Destiny age, described as "indomitably self-willed," "querulous," and "despotic." Forgoing the pulpit, he prepared for a career in the missions, but resolved to combine evangelizing with the genius of the industrial age. Manufacturing, for Hamlin, was more than just a process of production; it was also a means for purifying souls. Landing in Istanbul in 1840, he set out to instruct local youth in the rudiments of mathematics and grammar and induct them into the sacraments of work.

His arrival coincided with the new openness in the sultan's attitude toward the West. As a result, Hamlin obtained permission to construct his school in Bebek, a mere five miles from Istanbul. By 1842, some forty pupils were enrolled at the institution, spending half of each day in the classroom and the other half fashioning Franklin stoves and Boston-style rattraps and operating a flour mill. The only resistance to this innovative curriculum came from the Armenian patriarch, whose flock supplied most of the students, and from Muslim villagers who pelted the school with stones, making it, Hamlin carped, "rather leaky." Still, he managed to repair any damages and conciliate the patriarch. A contented Hamlin informed the board that "a decided impression" had been made on Ottoman education and "a general spirit of inquiry" aroused. "The old unchangeable East had begun to move," he asserted, but without realizing how profound that shift would prove. Hamlin had no inkling that his modest school would someday evolve into Turkey's first modern university.[8]

FROM A SITUATION of near-annihilation in the 1830s, American missionaries had recovered fully and, by the end of the antebellum period, were thriving. Hundreds of Muslims, Christians, and Jews were studying in missionary institutions throughout the Ottoman Empire, reading textbooks produced by American religious presses and absorbing American ideas. "This country is among the greatest civilized countries [in the world]," explained the pioneering Egyptian educator Sheikh Rifa'a Rafi' al-Tahtawi. "Its inhabitants . . . freed themselves from the grasp of the English and became free and independent on their own . . . [W]orship in all faiths and religious communities is permitted." Responding to a request from Sultan Abdul Mejid, missionaries also established an America-style school for Ottoman military cadets. With the language skills they learned, the young officers could read the latest U.S. Army manuals, as well as the more provocative works of Jefferson, Hamilton, and Paine.

Along with proselytizing and educating Middle Easterners, the missionaries also enlightened their countrymen back home. Through their innumerable letters, articles, and reports, the evangelists furnished Americans with images of Middle Eastern life that were far more detailed—and less varnished—than any culled from the Bible or *A Thousand and One Arabian Nights*. Missionary correspondence also served as a primary source for Edward Salisbury of Yale, who in 1841 became the nation's first professor of Arabic, and for the American Oriental Society, founded the following year and dedicated to the study of ancient and contemporary Middle Eastern cultures. Salisbury, in turn, joined the missionaries in promoting progressive education in Syria and in other Ottoman lands. "The countries of the West, including our own, have been largely indebted to the East for their various cultures," the scholar attested, "the time has come when this debt should be repaid."

In spite of their striking accomplishments, the missionaries continued to face numerous hazards in the Middle East and to grapple with daily frustrations. "There are no rail roads here and ideas as well as burdens move by camel trains," the Beirut-based William Eddy complained. Some of the most formidable opposition to the missionaries emanated not from the Middle East, however, but from their own American Board. Many board elders felt that the focus on schoolbooks and medicine had obscured the missions' original purpose of salvation. "Could Christianity be presented to men in its simplicity, without the technics of the schools, it might obtain a more ready and general reception," Dr. John Thornton Kirkland, a former Harvard president, concluded after visiting Syria in 1842. The missionaries replied that the services they provided helped gain the natives' trust, while generating a physical and intellectual atmosphere conducive to future conversion. Kirkland's wife, Elizabeth, whom we will presently meet as a pioneering traveler to the Middle East, disagreed with both her husband and the board and took the missionaries' side. "These worthy people have turned their attention to the establishment of schools as preparatory to the introduction to Christianity," she asserted. "Generally speaking the American missionaries are held in most respect."[9]

The question would be settled neither by the American Board nor by the missionaries but rather by the peoples of the Middle East, through their mounting demands for modern education and health care. If unresponsive to the missionaries' religious message, they would remain appreciative of their philanthropy and generally accepting of their presence. Taking advantage of that openness, increasing numbers of Americans would follow their spiritual impulses to the region. Among them were two hybrid types, a missionary-scientist and a missionary-soldier, who journeyed to the Middle East, the land most venerated by Americans in search of sanctity and knowledge.

Adventures in Sacred Paradise

The rider stretched high on the hump of his camel and squinted into the dusty glare. Hardly the traditional adventurer—no broad-chested John Ledyard or redoubtable George English—Edward Robinson was, at age forty-six, wan, overweight, and nearsighted, a professor of Scripture at New York's Union Theological Seminary. Like so many desert images, though, that of Robinson as a weakling was mirage-like. In fact, he was capable of riding eight hours straight under blazing skies while navigating by his compass and Bible. He had spent the last month crossing the barren Sinai Mountains, uncomplainingly, marveling at their "strangeness and overpowering grandeur" and reminding himself that these were the same serrated peaks that Moses and the Israelites traversed. Finally, in March 1838, Robinson prepared to exit the desert and step into a "romantic and exciting" land. Peering through his grime-dimmed spectacles, he spied the lapis waters of the Gulf of Aqaba and, beyond, the Wilderness of Judea. "Although not given to the melting mood," he admitted, "I could not refrain from bursting into tears."

Robinson was part of a lengthening procession of Americans who, in the decades before the Civil War, streamed toward the Holy Land. To accommodate the traffic, the United States appointed consular agents to six major Palestinian cities, making it the most widely represented Western nation in the area. These legations were nevertheless overwhelmed by the onrush of missionaries, tourists, colonists, and researchers, all drawn by the news of enhanced toleration of foreigners in Palestine and by effusive descriptions of its wonders.

Many of those accounts were, to say the least, exaggerated. William Thomson, the missionary whose letters spoke so astringently of Palestine, and who later left the country for Beirut, went on to write *The Land and the Book*, a rhapsody of idyllic images. No longer desolate and harsh, the biblical landscape was, he claimed, a paradise of "lofty mountains, covered with snow," "wide plains carpeted with gay flowers," and "lakes, rivers, and streams baptized with beauty." The volume sold out thirty editions in the United States and helped perpetuate the dreamlike aura surrounding Palestine. That mystique would swiftly vanish, though, as arriving Americans often encountered a gloomier reality. "There is no other country in the world . . . of which so much has been written, and of which so little is really known," remarked the American consul in Jaffa, noting how "a feverish state of expectation" about Palestine frequently pitched his countrymen into a post-pilgrimage depression.[10]

Edward Robinson, however, was an exception. Though a fervent Congregationalist, he never let religious beliefs becloud his scientific judgment. As a child on a Connecticut farm, he dreamed of someday visiting Palestine's holy places and, as an adult, he determined to remove the "vast mass of tradition, foreign in its source and doubtful in its character," surrounding those sites. The Puritans had superimposed a map of ancient Israel over their new Promised Land, America, and now their descendant Robinson sought to repatriate that map and restore its historical veracity.

Together with the Arabic-speaking missionary Eli Smith, Robinson headed north, through the area known today as the West Bank. The countryside, marred by "stagnation and moral darkness," indeed depressed him, as did its inhabitants' "unreliable" nature. Yet these same squalid towns appeared familiar to Robinson, "as if the realization of a former dream." His sense of reverie intensified on April 4, 1838—Easter Day—when he and Smith, "like the Hebrews of old, at the time of Passover," at last entered Jerusalem. A party of eight missionaries and their families greeted them, the city's largest-ever gathering of Protestants.

Robinson did not dally, though, and the next dawn he was out, armed with a hundred-foot measuring tape, gauging Jerusalem's walls. Using the Bible and other classical accounts as his guide, he identified the Siloam Pool and, in spite of his myopia and bulk, succeeded in crawling 1,750 feet through a narrow rock-hewn tunnel to the Virgin's Fountain within the Old City. He also located the remains of a massive bridge that once led to Herod's Temple and that is today known as Robinson's Arch. Robinson then ventured out into the countryside in search of scriptural sites, convinced that their current Arabic names contained echoes of their Hebrew originals. Accordingly, in the Arab village of al-Samu'a, Robinson located the remains of biblical Eshtemoa. He found that al-Jish was the ancient Gush Halav, and that al-Jib had been Gibbon, where Joshua made the sun stand still. Robinson, "the greatest master of measuring tape in the world," as one of the missionaries dubbed him, had retrieved a legendary past and grounded it in present-day reality.

Edward Robinson would make a second expedition to Palestine, in 1852, publish two hefty volumes of his research, and become the first American awarded a gold medal by London's Royal Geographical Society. He founded an entirely new field, biblical archaeology, an "American science" that was accessible not only to scholars but to clergy and laymen as well. It also lured to Palestine other Americans who, like Robinson, alloyed their faith with an irrepressible urge to explore.[11]

William Francis Lynch was one such wanderer, a Navy commander and an "earnest Christian and lover of adventure" who had already probed South America and the Far East. He was the same age as Robinson, forty-six, but keen-eyed and trim, the vision of the stalwart Virginian. In May 1847, bored by the lack of action in the Mexican War, Lynch requested leave to visit Palestine. He proposed to be the first Westerner to navigate the entire length of the Jordan River, from the Sea of Galilee to the Dead Sea, to "promote the cause of science, and advance the character of the Naval service." Beyond its academic and motivational value, though, Lynch hoped that his expedition would strengthen America's ties to the Holy Land and, through them, hasten a worldwide redemption.

With his handpicked crew of five officers and nine seamen— "young, muscular, native-born Americans, of sober habits"—Lynch departed New York for Istanbul. He presented himself at the court of Abdul Mejid, caused a stir by refusing to remove his sword, but then regained the sultan's favor by presenting him with an album of American Indian prints, a gift from President James Polk. In return, Lynch received a *firman*, or imperial decree, granting him "protection against the Arabs." The commander did not rely on this, though, and on reaching Beirut, he acquired the services of Henry James Anderson, a missionary doctor. "In the event of gun-shot wounds," thought Lynch, "surgical aid would be indispensable." The Americans also hired several Bedouin guards and purchased an arsenal of carbines, Colt pistols, bayonets, Bowie knives, and a buckshot-spewing blunderbuss.

The weapons, along with scientific instruments and camping gear, were loaded onto pack animals. Two galvanized iron boats were lowered onto gun carriages and lashed to the backs of camels. Exiting the coastal city of Acre, the peculiar train trudged thirty miles through a countryside that the Americans found depressingly barren and uninhabited. They nevertheless kept their spirits up with choruses of "Hail Columbia," "Yankee Doodle," and "The Star-Spangled Banner," and with occasional infusions of grog. "We Yankee boys flinch not," wrote one of the sailors, Edward Montague. "We fear neither the wandering Arab nor the withering influence of disease . . . neither the heat of the sun nor the suffocating sirocco." The men were particularly enamored of their commander, "one of the best, most humane, thoughtful, and generous men in the world," according to Montague, a hero with "the resolute 'go-ahead' spirit of a real, true-born American."

Lynch, too, seemed uplifted by all he saw, from the Stars and Stripes streaming above his troop, to the view of the Sea of Galilee. The thought that he walked on the very same shores that Jesus had trod, and touched the waters on which he had walked, overwhelmed him. So, too, did the hospitality shown to him and his crew by the ancient Jewish community of Tiberias. A wealthy merchant named Chaim Weisman invited the Americans to lodge at his home and feted them lavishly. A week later, on April 10, 1848, Lynch and his men took leave of Weisman and launched their iron boats.

"It must have been a singular sight from the shore," Lynch recalled. "[T]he crews in man-of-war rig, with snow-white awnings spread, and their ensigns flying, the men keeping time with their oars, as we rowed along the green shores of the silent Sea of Galilee." Christened the *Fanny Mason* and the *Fanny Skinner* (after the daughters of the secretary of the navy and a senior commodore), the metallic craft were designed to withstand the Jordan's reported shoals and rapids. A wooden skiff was also acquired, fitted with the blunderbuss, and nicknamed *Uncle Sam*. The river indeed proved turbulent, and bands of armed natives gathered on the banks. The melodramatic Lynch recalled how he and his crew "were wanderers in an unknown and inhospitable wilderness," where the presence of "barbarous tribes of warlike Arabs . . . prompts one instinctively to feel for his carbine, or grasp . . . the handle of his sword."

Yet the scientist in Lynch also took pains to record the river's depths and temperatures and to describe its harsh environs. Like Robinson, he tried to locate the exact site of events mentioned in the Bible—where the Israelites crossed into Canaan or Jacob wrestled the angel—though with far less precision. All around him, Lynch imagined, lay a land "teeming with sacred associations" and "hallowed by the footsteps, fertilized by blood, and consecrated by the tomb, of the Saviour."

Six days passed before the sailors, fatigued but exhilarated, neared Jericho. Lynch believed that no Christian had visited the area since the Crusades and that a Bedouin attack was likely. In a maneuver he had learned from Indian fighters in the American West, he drew his men and boats into a defensive circle. The tactic proved unnecessary, though. The only intruders were several dozen Christian pilgrims, among them two Americans, who cast off their clothes and scampered into the Jordan.

Thereafter, the party completed the remaining twenty miles to its destination, the still and oleaginous Dead Sea. The men, wrote Montague, could "float with perfect ease upon it, and could pluck a chicken or read a newspaper at pleasure while so floating." Lynch was less amused, oppressed by the desolation of the surrounding desert and by the troubling lack of fresh water. "The curse of God is surely upon this unhallowed sea!" His only respite came at the luxuriant spring of Ein Gedi, which Lynch renamed "in honour of the greatest man the world has yet produced," George Washington.

Lynch spent the next three weeks conducting experiments on the Dead Sea waters, which he surmised might have medicinal qualities, and exploring the ruins of Qumran and Masada. He hiked to Kerak, in present-day Jordan, where members of the Christian community, descendants of once-proud crusaders, were sorely oppressed by the Muslim majority. Though frenetically busy, Lynch found time to relish the romantic desert nights, "the tents among the tamarisks, the Arab watch-fires, the dark mountains in the rear, the planets and the stars above them, and the boats drawn up on the shore." He also kept abreast of events at home, through mail forwarded by the American consul in Jerusalem. One such dispatch brought word that John Quincy Adams, the president who had tried to open the Middle East to Americans over twenty years earlier, had died. "The thought of death harmonized with the atmosphere and scenery," Lynch lamented. "We lowered the flag half-mast, and there was gloom throughout the camp."

On May 10, Lynch hoisted the same flag over a raft anchored in the Dead Sea and ordered the iron boats disassembled. He and his men then headed north toward Jerusalem, Nazareth, and Caesarea. His impressions of these and other celebrated sites were similar to those of many American pilgrims, a blend of aesthetic disgust and spiritual elation. The trek, meanwhile, proved debilitating, and by the time they reached Damascus, all of Lynch's men were delirious with fever. One officer, Lieutenant J. B. Dale, died at the Beirut home of Eli Smith and was buried by William Thomson.[12]

Lynch returned to New York and to an unexpectedly mixed reception. Critics who had assailed President Polk for sending the U.S. Army against Mexico now berated him for wasting $700 of the public's money on yet another superfluous expedition. Lynch's memoirs of the trip nevertheless sold briskly. It was a quirky volume, alternately descriptive and prescriptive, but consistently adamant in tone. The author was brutal in his portrayal of the Arab, alleging that "his ruling passion . . . is greediness of gold, which he will clutch from the unarmed stranger, or filch from an unsuspecting friend," yet he was equally zealous in touting Palestine's economic potential. Lynch proffered several ideas for developing the Holy Land, including a plan for resettling African Americans on plantations to be created in the Jordan Valley. The key to these programs' success, he ventured, was security. "Fifty well-armed, resolute Franks . . . could revolutionize the whole country," he wrote.

Lynch's book concluded with an impassioned appeal for restoring the Jews to Palestine. The Jewish people were "destined to be the first agent in the civilization of the Arab" and the means of rejuvenating the entire region. Dr. Anderson, the expedition surgeon, expanded on Lynch's proposal and, under the aegis of the American Geographical and Statistical Society, circulated a petition urging the

United States to promote Jewish colonization in Palestine. "Jewish influence brought to bear . . . in what is called Syrian Arabia," it stated, "would most effectually give a new impetus to the commerce of the East, as well as of the world."[13]

The Fullness of Time in Palestine

The proposition that the United States should actively assist the Jews in returning to Palestine was neither new nor, in the antebellum period, considered especially radical. The restorationist ideas once prevalent among the evangelical churches of colonial America had deeply penetrated the mainstream. While the more established Episcopalians and Unitarians continued to shun the notion, the masses of Methodists, Congregationalists, and Presbyterians embraced it. Many Americans believed that the Jews were already in the process of moving back to their homeland, an underpopulated area that, the missionaries assured them, could absorb millions—"A land without a people for a people without a land," in the slogan of Lord Shaftesbury, a contemporary British restorationist. "There appear to be unusual movements among the Jews, and a looking toward Palestine," Connecticut's Reverend Thomas Robbins informed his diary in June 1838. Sarah Haight, a Long Island woman who journeyed to the Middle East in the 1830s, was convinced of the imminence of the Jewish ingathering in Palestine. "God's own peculiar people shall again be brought . . . to rebuild and worship in their own temple," Haight predicted, foretelling what she called "the fullness of time of the Gentiles."

Restorationism found its broadest exposition in an 1844 treatise, *The Valley of Vision; the Dry Bones of Israel Revived*, by a New York University professor of Hebrew, the Reverend George Bush. The author of a biography of Muhammad that described him as a "pseudo-prophet" but also as a "man of superior cast of character," Bush called for "elevating" the Jews "to a rank of honorable repute among the nations of the earth" by re-creating their state in Palestine. Such restitution would benefit all of mankind, forming a "link of communication" between humanity and God. "It will blaze in notoriety," Bush foretold. "It will flash a splendid demonstration upon all kindreds and tongues of the truth." The book was not without its critics, however. The highbrow *Princeton Review* denounced the "belief in the literal Restoration of the Jews [that] has for years been gaining ground in Christendom." Yet a widening sector of the American public continued to believe with George Bush—a forebear of two later presidents of the same name—in the dream of Jewish statehood.

For Bush, as for most American restorationists, a Christian's role in reestablishing the Jewish polity was limited to prayer and, at most, providing the "carnal inducements" necessary to entice the Jews back to Palestine.[14] Some adherents to the doctrine, however, sought a more active role in that resettlement. They would personally travel to the Holy Land, take up residence, and prepare for the Jews' return.

An example of this activism was rendered by one of America's newest and most controversial sects, the Mormons. Joseph Smith, the movement's founder, was a committed restorationist, and in October 1841 he sent his personal Apostle, Orson Hyde, on a pilgrimage to Jerusalem. Climbing the Mount of Olives, Hyde erected an altar and beseeched God to "restore the kingdom unto Israel—raise up Jerusalem as its capital, and continue her people [as] a distinct nation and government." Mormons would later integrate that prayer into their liturgy and, on the site of Hyde's altar, build a branch of Brigham Young University.

An even more ardent activist than Hyde, Warder Cresson remained permanently in Palestine and devoted his life to repatriating the Jews. A father of six from Philadelphia who had once been a Mormon and, before that, a Quaker and a Shaker, Cresson took up restorationism at age forty-six, in 1844. That year, Cresson met Mordecai Noah, the onetime consul in Tunis who had since embarked on a campaign to revive Jewish sovereignty in Palestine. Having tried and failed to enlist other American Jews in the project, Noah began promoting it to Christians. "Where can we plead the independence for the children of Israel with greater confidence than in the cradle of American liberty?" he inquired. The question resonated with Cresson, who became convinced that God had created the United States specifically to succor the Jews and that the American eagle would, in fulfillment of Isaiah, "overshadow the land with its wings." Irrevocably, he proclaimed, "there is no salvation for the Gentiles, but by coming to Israel."

Cresson promptly wrote to Secretary of State John C. Calhoun and asked to be posted as America's consul in Jerusalem. The request coincided with the State Department's search for diplomats acceptable to the missionaries, and after receiving assurances of Cresson's "capacity & probity," Calhoun approved the appointment. Dark-bearded with penetrating eyes and flared nostrils—the portrait of a fiery prophet—Cresson set sail on June 22, 1844, bearing with him a U.S. flag and a white dove that he planned to release on arrival. "I left the wife of my youth and six lovely children . . . an excellent farm, everything comfortable around me," he remembered. "But the light . . . of God's precious promises, in reference to the return of the Jew . . . became so great . . . that I could no longer remain at home."

Arriving in Palestine, Cresson settled in Jerusalem, created a "consular seal," and extended America's protection over the city's Jews, many of whom were impoverished scholars dependent on charity from abroad. Calhoun, meanwhile, learning from sources in Philadelphia that Cresson was "very weak minded," and "what there is of [that mind] is quite out of order," rescinded the consul's appointment. Cresson merely ignored the instructions, however, and persisted in aiding the Jews. In a meeting with the visiting British satirist William Makepeace Thackeray, the author of *Vanity Fair*, he explained how his country, in concert with the European powers, would soon intervene to secure an independent state for the Jews. Cresson "has no knowledge of Syria but what he derives from prophecy," wrote Thackeray. "I doubt whether any government has received or appointed so queer an ambassador."[15]

Cresson continued to impress visitors with his visions of Jewish statehood and his bizarre, almost trancelike, behavior. But Cresson was not the only American restorationist to take up residence in Palestine at that time, nor was he necessarily the strangest. Equally unconventional, at least, was the novelist, singer, poet, and revivalist preacher Harriet Livermore.

The daughter of a New Hampshire congressman, Livermore had

grown from a rambunctious tomboy into a graceful and dark-eyed ingénue who, in the years after the War of 1812, jilted a long line of suitors. Rejected, in turn, by an army doctor, she gave up on romance altogether in search of a higher love. "Sick of the world, disappointed in all my hopes of sublunary bliss, I drew up a resolution in my mind to . . . become a religious person." Her quest took her first to Congregationalism and then to Presbyterianism and the Quakers, but wearying of them all, she eventually turned to Baptism and established her own sect, the Pilgrim Stranger. Livermore believed herself a theological prodigy, an apostle to the Indians, whom she believed were descended from the Lost Ten Tribes. These and other unorthodox notions featured in her novel, *Scriptural Evidence in Favor of Female Testimony in Meetings for the Worship of God*, which was financed by several influential Washingtonians, including Senator John Tyler and Dolly Madison. Her ministry reached its pinnacle in 1827, when Livermore addressed both houses of Congress. "She is the most eloquent preacher I have listened to," remarked John Quincy Adams, a connoisseur. "No language can do justice to the pathos of her singing."

The turning point in Livermore's life came ten years later, however, when reports of Jewish resettlement in Palestine lured her to the Middle East. Armed with a State Department letter attesting to her "high character, both moral and religious," she visited David Porter in Istanbul and then boarded a steamer for Beirut. South of the city, in the mountains of Sidon, she stopped in on Lady Hester Stanhope, a fifty-year-old British recluse who had once served as secretary to her uncle, Prime Minister William Pitt. Stanhope, too, had originally moved to the Middle East in the hope of encouraging Jewish resettlement in Palestine, but despairing of success, acquired a Crusader castle and refashioned herself as the Nun of Lebanon. As former belles and fellow restorationists, Livermore and Lady Hester should have bonded, but the two women in fact quarreled over which of them was the truly elect and which would accompany the Lord on His triumphal reentry to Jerusalem.

From Sidon, Livermore proceeded to the Holy City and rented a modest residence atop Mount Zion. From there, she planned to supervise the construction of an educational colony for returning

Jews. Like many restorationists, Livermore subscribed to the Jeffersonian notion that all states required an agrarian base and that Christians had a divinely enjoined duty to reacquaint the Jews with farming. Livermore sought to see the colony completed, and then retire to a life of prayer and contemplation, "to meet [her] lot, which . . . is martyrdom."

Funding the colony, however, proved more onerous than Livermore anticipated and her means were soon exhausted. Desiring only "to earn [her] bread, to pay [her] debts, and return to Mount Zion," she tried peddling printed copies of her sermons, but was finally reduced to begging in Jerusalem's streets. Yet even this effort foundered. Starving, Livermore withdrew from Palestine and returned, soul broken, to the United States. She died in 1868—a martyr, indeed, to some—in a Philadelphia poorhouse.[16]

The restorationist idea remained distinctly alive, however, as did the vision of transforming urban, mostly indigent Jews into Palestinian peasants. While Harriet Livermore was languishing in Jerusalem, another American preacher arrived in the city, robust and eager to begin the work of colony making. Tall and striking but described nonetheless as "criminally modest," James Turner Barclay was something of a Renaissance man—a physician, an inventor, and an architect. People marveled at his penmanship, which, according to one source, could render the Lord's Prayer in letters so minute "they could all be inscribed on a five cent piece." Barclay's premium achievement came in 1831, however, when he purchased Monticello, Jefferson's classical estate, which had long since fallen into disrepair. Barclay attempted to revive the plantation through silk production, failed utterly, and subsequently turned to religion. He became a Presbyterian and then joined the Cambellites, a millenarian movement committed to restoring Christ's rule on earth. To this end, in 1850, Barclay journeyed to Palestine.

Like Livermore, Barclay sought to establish a settlement for reeducating the Jews in agriculture but soon encountered a similar dearth of funds. Frustrated, he returned to architecture and obtained work renovating the Dome of the Rock. Barclay also authored a best-selling book, *The City of the Great King*, which, like William Thomson's before it, portrayed Jerusalem in dazzling terms and, like George Bush's, extolled the restorationist idea. "God hath not utterly cast away his people whom he formerly acknowledged; and neither should we," he asserted. Christians, rather, must embrace the Jews, saying, "We will go with you, for we have heard that the Lord is with you."[17]

Such exhortations helped divert attention from the restorationists' failure to establish permanent footholds in Palestine and assist in the Jewish return. Other evangelists sought to succeed where Livermore and Barclay had faltered and to carry on the work of colonizing the Holy Land. The most headstrong and colorful of these was Clorinda Minor. A lifelong Episcopalian and the wife of a well-to-do Philadelphia businessman, Minor in middle age became an Adventist and began preparing for the End of Days. "Many Christians profess great sympathy for the Jews, and are waiting . . . for 'the set time' to favor Zion," she observed. The "set time," Minor calculated, was imminent, and in 1851 she left her husband and set sail for Palestine: "The conviction of my soul increased every hour that God was calling me to go!"

Shortly after landing in Jaffa, Minor met John Meshullam, a British Jew who had converted to Christianity and who shared Minor's desire to introduce the Jews to the "active labors of love." Their efforts, though, like those before them, were hounded by a shortage of funds. Minor subsequently appealed to her friends in the United States, who responded by sending over seven volunteers and $256 worth of tents, tools, seeds, and medicines. A plot of cultivable land was purchased at Artas, near Bethlehem, and the Manual Labor School of Agriculture for Jews in the Holy Land was established. Additional support came from Baron Moses Montefiore, the Anglo-Jewish philanthropist, who welcomed any contribution to Jewish colonization in Palestine. In her prodigiously selling memoir, *Meshullam!; or, Tidings from Jerusalem*, Minor foresaw "that His time to favor Zion is come, and that He will now set his hand a second time to recover Israel." Her prophecy seemed destined for fulfillment.[18]

Within two years, however, the Artas group had disbanded. The rupture resulted, first, from the Jews' refusal to show even the faintest interest in farming, but more fatally, from the festering rifts between Meshullam and Minor. Still, "the Modern Tabitha," as Minor was sometimes called, remained optimistic. She moved from Artas to a small farm outside of Jaffa and gave it the name of Mount Hope. With an orange grove given to her by Montefiore, and with the help of two German missionaries, Johann and Frederick Grossteinbeck, she eked out a tenuous existence. "If any of our Hebrew friends in the United States will help, we will . . . return them an exact account of every expenditure," she appealed to the American Jewish paper *Occident*. "Let not the opportunity pass, and the sufferers perish." Few donations arrived, however. The farm failed, and Minor eventually went bankrupt. She died, aged forty-nine, in 1855.

Still, some evangelists persevered. Following Minor's death, Mount Hope was purchased by Warder Cresson, the idiosyncratic and self-appointed consul, who envisaged it as a "model American farm" for teaching Jews how to raise pineapples, bananas, and lemons. Nearby, Walter Dickson from Groton, Massachusetts, founded another colony for the Jews. Dickson hired the Grossteinbeck brothers who duly married his daughters, Almira and Mary. Repeatedly harassed by local Bedouin, the American Agricultural Mission, as Dickson styled it, sought help from the U.S. Navy, which supplied it with several Hall carbines and cartridges. The marauders were repulsed—temporarily—and the settlement managed to survive.[19]

OVER THE course of forty years, beginning with Levi Parsons and Pliny Fisk in 1819, Americans had persisted in their efforts to bring the tenets of their faith, both sacred and civic, to the Middle East, gaining purchase in some of its remotest provinces as well as in its Palestinian heartland. They were far from alone in this endeavor. Missionaries from France, Great Britain, Russia and Prussia also penetrated the region, building schools and clinics and even establishing colonies. "Europe is striving to outbid America for the privilege of teaching and preaching in this country," complained the evangelist William Eddy, from Lebanon. No nation, however, could rival the geographical scope, the professional breadth, and the investment of human and financial resources of America's Middle East missions.

The missionaries' dedication remained a reflection of the roles that early nineteenth-century Americans arrogated to themselves as the executors of Manifest Destiny, the bearers of industrial age fruits, and democratic benefactors of the world. The missionary fervor was also indicative of the still irrepressible American need for new frontiers, fresh experiences, and movement. Observing these urges in the 1830s, the French political thinker Alexis de Tocqueville remarked on the "unquiet passions" of Americans. An "all-pervading and . . . superabundant force" seemed to propel them, a "strange unrest" even "in the midst of abundance."[20] That restiveness was not particular to evangelists, however. An impressive number of Americans—housewives and professionals, artists and businessmen, and even an African American slave—ventured to the Middle East in the pre–Civil War period, drawn to the area by their religious convictions and, even more compellingly, by their dreams.

UNDER
AMERICAN EYES

"I AM ALMOST TEMPTED TO FANCY MYSELF IN THE PARA-
dise of Mahomet," sighed the poet, biographer, and master storyteller Washington Irving. The year was 1829 and Irving was already
America's most celebrated writer, the author of *The Legend of Sleepy
Hollow* and the creator of Rip Van Winkle and Ichabod Crane. But
he was also a lawyer, an officer during the War of 1812, a friend of
David Porter and Daniel Webster, and a diplomat who had been
recently posted to the U.S. embassy in Madrid. From there, Irving
was able to visit Granada, the once splendrous capital of medieval
Muslim kings, and the majestic Alhambra palace. The experience left
him intoxicated, disoriented, and feeling as though he were lost in a
kind of Oriental dream and "living in the *Arabian Nights*."

Irving had long been fascinated by the Middle East. The images of
bleak, desert castles and steamy harems appealed to his melancholic
and romantic sides, but for the curly-haired, boy-faced bachelor
from Tarrytown, New York, the region was also a venue for wit. In
1807, after viewing North African prisoners from the Barbary Wars,
Irving had invented the figure of Mustapha Rub-a-Dub Keli Khan,
the captain of an impounded Tripolitan ketch, who, from his captivity in New York, offered blistering observations on American soci-

ety. "I have been positively assured by a famous dervise (or doctor as he is here called) that at least one-fifth part of them have souls!" he enlightens Asem, the "principal slavedriver" of the Bashaw, on the subject of American women. "I have actually seen an exceedingly good-looking woman with soul enough to box her husband's ears . . . and my very whiskers trembled with indignation at the abject state of these wretched infidels." Serialized under the title *Salmagundi*, Mustapha's letters assailed not only impudent women but also corrupt attorneys, fulsome generals, "slangwhangging" politicians, and even President Jefferson, "a man of superlative ventosity, comparable to nothing but a huge bladder of wind."

The Middle East again served as humorous outlet in 1824, when Irving collaborated on *Abu Hassan*, a play derived from a tale in *A Thousand and One Arabian Nights*. "A mighty potentate like thee may have hundreds of mistresses," the protagonist tells his companion, the Caliph Harun al-Rashid. "[B]ut now I am fain to content myself with half a dozen! Oh Nature, Nature, how easily art thou satisfied!

But in 1829 Irving found nothing risible about Granada's ruins, only reverie and awe. Shortly after the visit, he began writing *The Conquest of Granada*, a history rife with "romantic adventures, picturesque forays through mountain regions; daring assaults of cliff-built castles . . . beyond the scope of mere invention." Next came *Alhambra*, which would rank among his most cherished works. An anthology of Arabian tales scintillating with sinister magicians, scimitar-slashing horsemen, and princesses perpetually in need of rescue, the book sought to blend "naked realities" with "illusions of the . . . imagination."[1]

Published in 1832, *Alhambra* served to perpetuate the myths that Americans continued to harbor about the Middle East. For some, though, merely reading about the region was insufficient and they determined to see this fabled land for themselves. Washington Irving also planned a Middle Eastern tour, sailing from southern Spain to Morocco, but diplomatic duties took him elsewhere. Others would not be so indefinitely diverted. Belying Henry David Thoreau's dictum "Eastward I go only by force, but Westward I go free," they set out to explore the "Orient."

Fun, Fight, or Frolic

Little stood in their way. Freed of North African pirates and patrolled by a permanent naval squadron, the Mediterranean no longer represented an obstacle to American travelers. On the contrary, the sea now served as a conduit for a steadily expanding flow of individuals eager to discover the Middle East. By the 1820s, the Smyrna merchant David Offley was already complaining about the impecunious American students who occasionally appeared at his doorstep, desperate for shelter and food. Other Americans in the region reported encountering countrymen who had been living in the area for some time. There was the New Yorker in Istanbul who had converted to Islam and become an imam and the New England hunter who cruised the Nile, shooting crocodiles and cats. The captain of an American merchantman calling at Mocha in 1819 told of meeting a Philadelphian who had been serving in the sultan's army for nearly twenty years, and Western visitors to Cairo in 1820s were sometimes guided by a backwoods Ohioan who went by the name of Nebby Daood—Arabic for David the Prophet.

While early nineteenth-century Americans embarked for the Middle East, priceless relics from the region found their way to the United States. The city of Boston received its first mummy in 1823, the gift of an American trader in Smyrna, and Baltimore obtained 689 Egyptian antiquities from Colonel Mendes I. Cohen, the scion of a prominent Jewish family, who had explored the Upper Nile. The Boston businessman John Lowell also managed to send artifacts home from Egypt in 1832, before perishing in a Persian Gulf shipwreck. Displays of ancient Middle Eastern art, amassed and donated by local merchants, also appeared in Salem, Massachusetts, and in Charleston, South Carolina. These collections helped stimulate interest in classical Egyptian forms, especially pyramids, sphinxes, and obelisks. Significantly, construction of the Washington Monument commenced in 1833, with marble contributed by the Ottoman Sultan.[2]

The growth of America's fascination with the distant Egyptian past was accompanied by a deepening curiosity about the contemporary Middle East. Not only wanderers and outcasts wanted to visit the region suddenly, not only pilgrims, scientists, and missionaries, but also professionals and venerable members of society. To them, the Middle East was no longer merely a battlefield, a Bible scene, or a marketplace; it was also an untrammeled region that any adventurous American, suitably equipped and bankrolled, just might pleasurably tour.

The numbers of American visitors to the Middle East climbed steadily throughout the 1830s. Under the terms of the U.S.-Ottoman treaty, they enjoyed the protection of U.S. consuls and were shielded from arbitrary arrest. Transportation to the region was facilitated as well, thanks to the advent of steam technology. Beginning in 1838, a spunky Bostonian could take a train to New York and board a steamship bound for Istanbul or Alexandria. With a carelessness that John Ledyard would have found unimaginable and with a speed that Pliny Fisk would have envied, Americans accessed the Middle East.

Yet the voyage still required immense physical stamina and the patience to endure multiple discomforts. The average passage took twenty-one days, with stops at London, Marseille, and Malta, and a standard fare of salted meat and hardtack. "There are no berths, no beds, no tables, no provisions, no dishes," William Henry Seward, a New York senator and future secretary of state, grumbled en route to Palestine in the late 1850s. "The cabin is filled with . . . ants, cockroaches, and all kind of vermin." Once ashore, visitors could be quarantined for as long as two weeks, often in conditions even more disagreeable than those at sea. In exchange for these inconveniences, passengers were required to pay about $190, the equivalent of a month's salary for a U.S. senator in 1840 or a year's wages for a manual laborer in the South.[3] Nevertheless, Mediterranean-bound vessels were almost always fully booked by vacationing Americans in search of exotic adventures.

One of these wayfarers was John Lloyd Stephens, a thirty-year-old New York Brahmin, Columbia graduate, and associate of Tammany Hall. After reading *A Thousand and One Arabian Nights*, he resolved to see for himself the "splendor and opulence [that] once made the Prophet smile" and, in December 1835, boarded a steamer for Egypt. Stephens was typical of the sixty Americans who, on annual average, registered at the U.S. consulate in Alexandria in the three decades after 1830. Most of them lived in northern cities, but there were also some, such as the Mississippi-born bookseller James Cooley, who hailed from the South. American women also visited the Middle East in this period: two of them—Sarah Rogers Haight of Long Island and Elizabeth Cabot Kirkland, the forty-four-year-old daughter of a U.S. senator from Massachusetts—wrote grippingly of their experiences. The most exceptional of the travelers, however, was David F. Dorr, an African American slave from Louisiana who toured the Middle East with his master in 1854. Escaping later to Ohio, Dorr published an account of his travels, *A Colored Man round the World*, which he dedicated to his "Slave Mother" and to "the ruins of the ancestors of which he is the posterity."

Though their backgrounds were diverse, American travelers shared remarkably similar impressions of the Middle East. Accustomed to well-ordered and largely homogenous American cities, the tourists were disoriented—literally unable to find the East—by the labyrinthine layout of Middle Eastern streets and by their culturally diverse inhabitants. James Cooley's description of Cairo in 1842, for example, "narrow, gloomy . . . dusty, prison-like, and peculiar," was indistinguishable from Stephens's. While Stephens marveled at "the dashing Turk with his glittering saber, the wily Greek, the grave Armenian, and the despised Jews, with their long silk robes, their turbans," Cooley gaped at the "Arabs, Armenians, Copts, Egyptians, Greeks, Jews, Syrians, and Turks . . . in their native costumes . . . apparently happy in all their filth and tawdry rags." The same sense of anomie and shock struck Sarah Haight, on entering Istanbul in 1839. "I only saw a mass of irregular buildings, thrown together without any architectural rule, and in defiance of all good taste."

Alike in their initial perceptions of Middle Eastern cities, the Americans subjected Middle Eastern society to the same ruthless judgments. Most arrived in the region already biased against Islam and soon found their prejudices confirmed. Islam, for Stephens, was a "false religion" followed by "bigoted Musselmans" and "haughty and deluded fanatics" and, for Cooley, a creed of "ignorance and superstition" embraced by "lunatics, idiots, and imposters." Haight deplored the "Mohammedanism [that] . . . pulls down . . . every country in which it predominates," and even David Dorr, who at first praised Islam for its acceptance of black people, ended up fearing Muslims as bigots and "head-choppers of Christians."[4]

Cruelty, the Americans invariably assumed, was endemic to Islam and chronic throughout Middle Eastern cultures. In support of this charge, Stephens related his visit to a Cairo court where a seed-munching governor quietly ordered one of his subjects flogged. "When I heard the scourge whizzing through the air . . . and the first loud piercing shriek, I could stand it no longer," Stephens recounted, adding that the governor kept smiling throughout. Americans were especially distressed by what they considered the mistreatment of Middle Eastern women. Cooley claimed that Arab women were "kept like birds in a cage [and] fed like beasts in a den," and he recalled seeing one of them being bound and beaten by her husband while a crowd approvingly looked on. Yet not only women were treated brutally in the Middle East, the Americans discovered. Touring Morocco in 1842, Elizabeth Cabot Kirkland was stunned by the wholesale oppression of the Jews. "A rich Jew merchant is obliged to pull off his slippers before he passes the threshold of a Moor," she wrote, "and [the Muslims] drive them about the streets whenever they cross their path, much as you would a dog." Later, in Cairo, Kirkland encountered "a man lying stretched before us, the head severed from the body and placed between the legs." The victim, she learned, was guilty of engaging in politics.

Middle Eastern politics was another subject of fascination for Americans, and a focus of disgust. Convinced that America's democracy represented the highest form of human governance, the tourists regarded the region's autocratic rulers with a blend of abhorrence and contempt. Stephens denounced the Oriental system in which "life hangs by so brittle a thread that when you part from a man of power, in all probability you will never see him again," and Dorr pitied the sultan who "lives like a monarch, but will die like a fool." Dr. Valentine Mott, one of New York's most illustrious surgeons, was appalled by the coarseness of the Middle Eastern nobility he met in 1843. "His royal highness," wrote Mott of an Egyptian prince, a grandson of Muhammad Ali, "has evidently a greater quantum of adipose than cerebral matter." The editor and naval chaplain Walter

Colton, like Mott a liberal who looked for the positive in Middle Eastern life, nevertheless shuddered at the knowledge that the sultan could, with a wave of his hand, order a thousand decapitations. "Islamism," he concluded in 1836, was "the grave of inspired truth and liberty."

The Middle East suffered from many evils, these travelers agreed, all of which it could be rectified simply by abandoning Islam and embracing Western culture. "The same effort which lifts the Mussulman above the broken fetters of his despotism, will place him on the ruins of his religion," Colton ventured. "The scepter and the crescent, altar and throne, will sink together." Cooley also looked forward to a time when Muslims would adopt "a more enlightened and consistent faith" and so gain entrance to the family of "civilized nations." Haight went further by calling for an international "political crusade" to humble Islam and dismantle the Ottoman Empire. Presciently, she foresaw that Britain might someday take over Egypt and parts of Asia Minor and that France would occupy Syria and North Africa. But first Islam must "kick the beam," in Haight's quaint colloquialism, and disappear.

From a twenty-first-century perspective, the Americans who criticized the Middle East for its alleged corruption, cruelty, and bigotry were undoubtedly hypocrites. Their own nation enslaved nearly a sixth of its populace and, under the Manifest Destiny banner, forcibly uprooted numbers of native tribes. Hangings were still considered public entertainment in nineteenth-century America and political graft, epitomized by New York's Tammany Hall, flourished. Yet the memoirs of American travelers reveal little by way of introspection or a willingness to weigh their own country's foibles against those they attributed to the Middle East. Rather, their writings display an almost reverential love for anything remotely American. "There is a feeling of nationality among Americans abroad that I think belongs to no other people," averred Edward Joy Morris, a future congressman and ambassador to the Porte, who in 1841 planted the Stars and Stripes on the peak of an Egyptian pyramid. The artist William H. Bartlett, who came to Cairo in 1849 in search of "the city of Saladin and the Arabian Nights," ended up contrasting "Egypt, fallen and decrepit, bowed under oppression and . . . a false religion" with "America, daily rising in power, a land of light, freedom, enterprise, and Christianity!"

The United States, the paragon of liberty and virtue, had much to teach the Middle East, the tourists insisted. They looked forward to the day when missionaries, engineers, educators, and statesmen would, in the words of Sarah Haight, "penetrate the darkness that overshadows this heathen land" and remodel the region after America.[5] Oblivious to the lack of equality and justice that sullied their society back home, American travelers gazed into a Middle Eastern mirror, through its cracked and tarnished glass, and the image they saw was flawless.

AMERICANS VIEWED the Middle East through virtually identical eyes and they toured it according to almost uniform itineraries. After accessing the region either through Alexandria or Istanbul, they invariably journeyed to Cairo for a requisite junket to the pyramids and a cruise up the Nile. Because of the precariousness of the journey, they were obliged to hire armed guards and dragomen—sixteen men, in the case of Sarah Haight. Also for safety, Americans were advised to dress in native attire, which, in Stephens's case, consisted of "yellow slippers, blue sash, sword, and a pair of large Turkish pistols." When not fending off beggars and flies, the voyagers fixed their attention on the ruins lining the riverbank, a source of awestruck melancholy but also of cost-free souvenirs. Citing the needs of science, Mott chipped a piece from an ancient obelisk, and Stephens chiseled the relief of a hawk from a temple wall, saving, he said, "that precious fragment from the ruin to which it was doomed." The Americans also delighted in shooting wildlife—jackals, crocodiles, and birds. But the most titillating activity, at least for the men, was ogling Middle Eastern women.

In keeping with the nineteenth-century Western romantic perception of the Middle East as a fleshpot of bagnios, seraglios, and harems, antebellum American men roamed the region in a state of unflagging arousal. Accustomed to seeing women's faces but rarely their naked limbs, the travelers were obsessed with the sight of Middle Eastern women who, though usually veiled, often seemed indifferent to body covering. Dorr told of locking eyes with one masked maiden ("I would have given five pounds to lift her veil") and trying to buy another for twenty-five dollars. Chapters in his book detail the washing of harem girls by eunuchs, and the art of belly dancing. "Such a jingling and a screwing [and] . . . quivering of bodies is only to be imagined." Valentine Mott dwelt on the women's hennaed hands and long-lashed, kohl-blackened eyes, and Stephens fixated on the lips that, he imagined, nightly greeted the weary nomad. Few tourists were as libidinous as Nathaniel Parker Willis, however, an accomplished poet and publisher of Edgar Allan Poe. Traversing the Middle East in 1852, Willis tried "in vain to get a peep at the camel-driver's wife or daughter." He succeeded, finally, in catching a glimpse of a Jewish girl, "a graceful creature of fourteen, with a shape like a Grecian Cupidon," and an Arab slave whose "warm dark eye . . . lifted its heavy and sleepy lids, and looked out of the accidentally opened door." In both cases, Willis sighed, "In my life I have seen nothing so beautiful."[6]

From Egypt and the Nile, American tourists usually turned eastward, toward Lebanon and Syria. Because of the danger of rebellious tribes and highwaymen, here, too, they carried an array of weapons, including pistols, carbines, and sabers. "We kept our arms in readiness, never suffering the baggage to be out of our sight," wrote the poet Bayard Taylor, a translator of Goethe's *Faust*, while trudging toward Beirut in 1853. "I wore my Frank dress, a turban on my head, and over this a white cotton sheet which covered a considerable part of my face," recalled Elizabeth Cabot Lodge, while her husband, John Thornton Kirkland, the former president of Harvard, went about "armed with pistols." Hazards notwithstanding, the rustic, tawny villages and the medieval magic of Aleppo and Damascus enabled Americans to recover some of the romance they had lost in Cairo and Alexandria. Taylor, for one, pictured himself as a crusader marching into battle against Saladin. The very grass and trees, he mused, "heard the trumpets of the Middle Ages, and the clang . . . [of] European armor."

The climax of any Syrian tour was a pilgrimage to the castle of Lady Hester Stanhope, the same Nun of Lebanon who had hosted Harriet Livermore in 1837. The tradition of visiting Stanhope appears to have been established fifteen years earlier by a New Yorker named George B. Rapelje, a fifty-year-old "plain man, of steady habits" who spent several hours in the lady's company. Well entertained and victualed, Rapelje departed the castle with a sample of Damascene silk that Stanhope asked him to market in America. Unfortunately, by the time Stephens and Haight arrived, Stanhope was no longer receiving visitors. "Her friends have fallen away from her and her treasures have been exhausted by . . . wily Arabs, who . . . ridiculed her . . . religious creed," Haight explained. The American missionary William Thomson, one of the few people Stanhope still agreed to see, found her withered body in 1839 and gave it a pauper's burial.

Sailing the Nile, scaling pyramids, or eyeing Nubian beauties—none of these experiences compared with what was, for Americans, the zenith of any Middle Eastern trip: Palestine. The travelers' excitement mounted the closer they came to the Holy Land, measured by their ever frequent references to the Bible. For Cooley, the sight of Egyptian snake charmers evoked Ecclesiastes ("Surely the serpent will bite without enchantment"), and sharing a meal with peasants made him think of Matthew ("He that dippeth his hand with me in the dish"). "Can it be a . . . dream?" Stephens asked as he stood on the shores of the Red Sea, "the very spot where the chosen people of God . . . stopped to behold the divided waters," or atop Mount Sinai, "witness of that great interview between man and his Maker." Scripture and landscape melded the moment Americans entered the Holy Land. Here were cities they had heard and read about since childhood and from which many of their towns had taken their names. "All my historical recollections . . . came fresh to my memory," exclaimed Haight. "I saw in every face a patriarch, and in every . . . chieftain an apostle."

Yet the fantasy of Palestine, like that of Egypt or Lebanon before it, swiftly evaporated. Entering Nazareth and Tiberias, Jaffa and Bethlehem, the Americans were crestfallen to find not the idealized settings of the Bible but rather a backwater of thistles, ruins, and dust. "How deplorable is [the Holy Land's] condition now!" the same Sarah Haight bewailed. She was especially shocked by the sparseness of the population and its extreme poverty, even by Middle Eastern standards. "The very face of the earth is reduced to a . . . howling wilderness." Jericho, Dorr determined, "is not worth mentioning," a boring wasteland "covered with broken bricks and stones." Most disappointing were Bethlehem and Jerusalem, their holy sites dominated, Stephens roared, by minarets and decorated with "parti-colored marble and . . . gaudy ornaments." Dorr spent over two weeks in Jerusalem and departed "wishing never to return again."

Without exception, Americans returned from their Middle Eastern journeys bereft of any sense of reverie or illusion. Dorr, who once envisaged the Middle East as his ancestral homeland, in the end found nothing kindred about the region, only an abundance of dogs, snake charmers, and camel drivers contemptuous of anything Western. "Nothing denotes that the country or man is marching forward," a disappointed Valentine Mott complained. "There is no appearance of intellectual or moral elevation." Most disenchanted of all was John Lloyd Stephens. A month after setting out to find "gorgeous pictures of Oriental scenes," the once boyish-looking and clear-eyed Stephens had been transformed into an embittered, fault-finding grump. Misogyny, gluttony, indolence, bad manners, and an utter lack of hygiene were just some of the native characteristics of the Middle East he now found insufferable. "I never saw among the wanderers of the desert any traits . . . which did not make me . . . value more the privileges of civilization."[7]

In spite of the dim and often hideous pictures they painted, the books written by these American travelers proved exceptionally popular. John Lloyd Stephens, later to gain fame exploring Mayan temples in the Yucatán, published his *Incidents of Travel in Egypt, Arabia Petraea, and the Holy Land* in 1837 and sold an impressive 21,000 copies in two years. Critics also praised Colton's *A Visit to Constantinople and Athens* as "replete with information . . . on Oriental life and manners," and called Cooley's *American in Egypt, with Rambles through Arabia Petra and the Holy Land* "a novelty quite unique in its plan, and containing a great deal of . . . amusement." Haight's "precious volumes" were so "vivid and lifelike" that one reviewer imagined himself traveling to "those intensely-interesting regions" together with "the gifted-lady author." Following the success of his book, Bayard Taylor went on a lucrative tour in which, dressed as an Arab, he lectured American audiences on Islam. David Dorr also gained a modicum of fame, the *Cleveland Plain Dealer* judging his work "graphic and racy [and] an exceedingly interesting work."

Rather than tarnishing American illusions about the Middle East, the travelers' testimonies only burnished them. The more sordid the portrayal of the region, it seemed, the more alluring its appeal to Americans. Writers in the United States continued to dwell on Middle Eastern themes. Edgar Allan Poe, who had lauded Stephens's book for its "freedom . . . frankness, and . . . utter absence of pretension," had himself written a poem, *Al-Aaraaf*, inspired by *A Thousand and One Arabian Nights*, and went on to author *Tales of the Grotesque and the Arabesque*. Washington Irving, too, returned to Islamic subjects. In 1850, he published a two-volume study, *Mahomet and His Successors*, which, though not uncritical of the Prophet, nevertheless extolled "his enthusiastic and visionary spirit" and the "striking and sublime" quality of his "luminous path."

These works, both literary and anecdotal, further thickened the procession of Americans steaming toward the Middle East. By midcentury, the United States was second only to Britain in the number of its citizens visiting Egypt each year, and in Syria it was unsurpassed. "I have taken a thousand American gentlemen through Syria," boasted Yusef, an Arab dragoman who escorted the famed Kentuckian writer, artist, and frontiersman J. Ross Browne in 1853. "Yes, sir. . . . I like the Americans! . . . Up to everything—fun, fight, or frolic."[8]

YUSEF'S DESCRIPTION would not, however, apply to the most troubled, pacifistic, and depressive American traveler, who was also the most ingenious. The self-educated son of a bankrupt New York merchant, he had worked as a cabin boy and a whaler, had served in the U.S. Navy and lived among South Sea cannibals before settling on a western Massachusetts farm. In December 1856, with little more than a toothbrush and a single change of clothing, Herman Melville sailed for the Middle East.

Call Me Ishmael

Ill, despondent because his recent book *Moby Dick* had sold a mere three thousand copies, the thirty-seven-year-old Melville was desperate to recapture his readers' ardor. Images of the Middle East, many of them conjured from *A Thousand and One Arabian Nights*, had long captivated him, and both Stephen Decatur and David Porter had figured in his fiction. The huge and haunting "Arabian traveler" who moves the protagonist of Melville's *Redburn* to decamp for "remote and barbarous countries" was probably modeled on John Lloyd Stephens, and John Ledyard, "the great New England traveler," was mentioned in *Moby Dick*. Now Melville, who had exhorted his readers, "Call me Ishmael"—according to the Bible, the father of all Arabs—resolved to see "stony Arabia" for himself. His objective was to find inspiration for a Middle Eastern version of *Typee*, his most popular adventure story. "I am full (just now) of this glorious *Eastern* jaunt," he excitedly told his journal. "Think of it!— Jerusalem & the Pyramids."

Like Sarah Haight twenty years earlier, Melville entered the Middle East via Istanbul and was instantly overwhelmed. "Imagine an immense accumulation of the rags of all nations, & all colors rained down on a dense mob, all struggling for huge bales & bundles of rags, gesturing with all gestures & wrangling in all tongues." Like Stephens and Cooley, he shuddered at the nameless, meandering streets with their "horrible grimy tragic air" and "rotten & wicked looking houses," visualizing "a suicide hung from every rafter within." He, too, was astonished by the ethnic diversity and sexual intensity of the city, imagining that "out of every other window look faces (Jew, Greek, Armenian)," and "out of old shanties peep lovely girls like lillies & roses growing in cracked flower-pots." Along with the many American visitors before him, Melville was dumbfounded by how millions of Middle Easterners could, "with one consent," reject the essence of Western civilization, "much of our morality & all of our religion."

Following the standard itinerary, Melville departed for Egypt. In Alexandria, he paused to view Pompey's pillar, which looked, he thought, "like a huge stick of candy after having been long sucked," then proceeded to Cairo, that "grand masquerade of mortality," and the pyramids. There, at the foot of those colossal monuments, Melville lapsed into an almost mystical trance:

> Vapors below summits. Kites sweeping & soaring around, hovering right over apex. At angles, like broken cliffs. . . . Arab guides in flowing white mantles. Conducted as by angels up to heaven . . . A feeling of awe & terror came over me. Dread of the Arabs. . . . The idea of Jehovah born here . . . something vast, indefinite, incomprehensible, and awful. These the steps Jacob lay at . . . Might have been created with the creation.

Such reveries were not infrequent for Melville, or unwelcome. He longed for transcendent experiences, moments of spiritual and metaphysical illumination that could lift him above this disingenuous life and afford him glimpses of truth. Having attained those heights in Egypt, he fully expected to match, if not surpass, them in Palestine, his next destination.[9]

"No country will more quickly dissipate romantic expectations than Palestine," Melville conceded shortly after arriving in Jaffa. Joining a caravan of thirty Arab horsemen who delighted in discharging their revolvers into every puddle and cactus, tormented by insects and the piercing sunlight, he ascended into the Judean hills. "Is the desolation of the land the result of the fatal embrace of the Deity?" he asked himself, then answered, "Hapless are the favorites of heaven." Rather than uplifting him, the scenery pitched Melville into an ominous, hallucinatory gloom: "Whitish mildew pervading whole tracts of landscape—bleached—leprosy—encrustation of curses—old cheese—bones of rocks,—crunched, knawed, & mumbled—. . . You see the anatomy—compares with ordinary regions as skeleton with living & rosy man."

Darkening as he rode, Melville's depression overshadowed his initial sight of Jerusalem, which, he wrote, "looks at you like a cold grey eye in a cold old man." Nothing enchanted him, not the Mosque of Omar nor the Holy Sepulcher, which smelled to him "like a dead house." He sneered at the tour guides who pointed out the steps where Christ spoke and, in the same breath, the restaurant that served the best coffee. A descendant of Puritans who considered Americans to be "a peculiar, chosen people—the Israel of our time," Melville felt little affinity for the Jews he encountered. He described them as lingering "in the emptiness of the lifeless antiquity of Jerusalem," like "flies that have taken up their abode in a skull."

The very concept of restorationism was odious to Melville: "that preposterous Jew mania," he called it. He refused to believe that Palestine, a desert country, could ever sustain a state and that the Jews might be remade into farmers. Nor did he have much confidence in the ability of missionaries to transform Eastern Orthodox Arabs, much less the Muslims, into American-style Protestants. "Might as well attempt to convert bricks into bride-cake as the Orientals into Christians," he laughed.

Melville's attitudes toward Jews and missionaries did not endear him to the first American he met in Palestine, Warder Cresson. The former consul turned farm owner had also embarked on a physical and spiritual journey. By creating a Jewish state in Palestine, he came to believe, the United States could still save itself from dissolution over the issue of slavery. "God hath chosen Zion . . . as the center of the whole world . . . and there cannot be unity and harmony . . . without this concentration," he wrote. At the same time Cresson's "researches" into the New Testament and his extensive contacts with Jews had led him to question his own beliefs and to identify with those of the people he had come to baptize. Abandoning what he called "the sawdust of Christianity" for "the genuine article of good old cheese itself," Cresson became a Jew, underwent circumcision, and adopted a Hebrew name, Michael Boaz Israel.

Cresson's "model American farm," meanwhile, was failing, and in an effort to secure donations, he returned to his native Philadelphia. His wife greeted him not with affection but with a civil suit aimed at procuring his remaining American assets and adducing his conversion as proof of mental incompetence. The trial was a public event, with more than one hundred witnesses, among them Mordecai Noah, called to testify. The defendant won, "settling forever," Philadelphia's *Public Ledger* declaimed, "the principle that a man's 'religious opinions' never can be made the test of his sanity." Subsequently, Cresson—Israel—sailed back to Palestine, married a Jewish woman, and moved to Jerusalem. There, in January 1857, he met Herman Melville.

The encounter, for both men, perhaps, was uneventful. Melville wrote tersely of "Crisson," an "American turned Jew," who divorced his wife in Philadelphia and then married a Jerusalemite "Jewess." Beyond those words, however, his journal remained mute. Melville ultimately devoted only one word to describing the man who, Ahab-like, had forfeited everything in an obsessive pursuit. The single word was "Sad."[10]

Melville's interaction with restoration-minded Americans did not end with Cresson, though. He next visited the American Agricultural Mission, the colony maintained by Walter Dickson, the Grossteinbeck brothers, and several American families. Of these, the first to host Melville were the Saunderses, Charles and Martha, originally from Rhode Island. The pair, both in their mid-forties, had failed as gold prospectors in California before rediscovering their faith and sailing to Palestine. Mr. Saunders, portrayed by Melville as "a broken-down machinist . . . out at elbows," had been enervated by the Middle Eastern heat, "a man feeble by Nature, & feebler by sickness, but worthy." His daughter, too, looked ill, Melville thought, and homesick. Mrs. Saunders, by contrast, was studying Arabic with a neighboring sheikh and acting as a "doctress" to the poor, a plucky woman reading a "Book of Female Heroines," which Melville "took to be the exponent of her aspirations." Both of the settlers expressed bitterness toward the Jews who, they claimed, would "come, pretend to be touched & all that, get clothing & then—vanish." Charles Saunders had despaired of teaching even a single Jew to farm, much less of converting any, but Martha stayed sanguine. "She is waiting the Lord's time," Melville quoted her saying. "The Lord's work must be done."

From the Saunderses' house, Melville wandered over to that of Walter Dickson, a "thorough Yankee, about 60, with a long oriental beard, blue Yankee coat, & Shaker waistcoat." Also present was Dickson's starchy wife, Sarah. Melville inserted a transcript of his conversation with the couple, complete with biting asides, into his journal:

H.M. "Have you settled here permanently, Mr Dickson?"

Mr D. "Permanently settled on the soil of Zion, Sir." With a kind of dogged emphasis.

Mrs. D. (as if she dreaded her husband's getting on his hobby, & was pained by it)—"The walking is a little muddy, aint it?" . . .

H.M. to Mr D. "Have you any Jews working with you?"

Mr D. No. Can't afford to hire them. Do my own work, with my son. Besides, the Jews are lazy & dont like work.

H.M. "And do you not think that a hindrance to making farmers of them?"

Mr D. "That's it. The Gentile Christians must teach them better. The fact is the fullness of Time has come. The Gentile Christians must prepare the way."

The visit to Dickson's farm concluded the author's nineteen-day sojourn in Palestine, a profound but draining experience. The Middle East, that seductive region where Melville had hoped to rekindle his inspiration and revive his diminishing career, had proved an egregious disappointment. "The whole thing is half melancholy, half farcical," he groaned, "like all the rest of the world."

Twenty years would pass before the influence of Melville's Middle Eastern journey became manifest in *Clarel*, his vast epic poem. Spanning over eighteen thousand lines and couched in a dense tetrameter that readers and reviewers alike found impenetrable, the work tells the story of an American divinity student, Clarel, on the course of his pilgrimage to Palestine. In the Holy Land, where missionaries and merchants "in the name of Christ and Trade / Deflower the world's last sylvan glade," the youth meets a progression of devotionally charged and emotionally challenged characters. The most remarkable of these is Nathan, a "strange pervert" of Puritan stock who, like Warder Cresson, has changed his faith to Judaism. While Clarel strives to reclaim Nathan for Christianity, he also falls in love with the apostate's daughter, Ruth. The dichotomy between

Nathan and Clarel and the ambivalent treatment of the poem's many Jews—African and Indian Jews, Westernized Jews, wandering Jews—symbolized Melville's own spiritual wrestling. That conflict is left unresolved, however, by Nathan's murder at the hands of Arab bandits, followed by Ruth's heartbreaking demise.

Though clearly literary devices, the deaths of Nathan and Ruth were also grounded in Middle Eastern reality. A year after Melville's departure, on January 11, 1858, a party of five Arabs entered the Dickson farm, avowedly in search of a lost cow. The Americans came out to help in the search and were promptly set upon. Frederick Grossteinbeck ran back for his rifle but was shot in the groin. "Oh! Father forgive all my sins and help me to bear this dreadful pain," he cried to his wife, Mary, while bleeding to death on the floor. Mary was dragged, clinging to a broken bedstead, into the yard, where she was repeatedly and brutally raped. Sarah Dickson was also violated, and her husband was slashed and struck unconscious. Only their youngest daughter, Caroline, escaped unhurt, by playing dead in a corner. "We sat half an hour at least without stirring, in the dark," Mary remembered.[11]

The Dickson colony never recovered from the assault. The survivors fled to the United States, including Johann Grossteinbeck, who shortened and Americanized his name. His grandson, John, would go on to write novels, among them *East of Eden* and *The Grapes of Wrath*, of tragic, biblical proportions.

Ships of the Sea and the Desert

A flagrant attack against peaceful American families in the Middle East might have gone unanswered earlier in the century, but by the late 1850s Americans residing in the region could no longer be robbed with impunity. The status of Americans in the region had changed substantially since the days when George Bethune English had to change his name and religion in order to proclaim his patriotism on the Nile. The State Department rigorously protested the assault on the Dickson farm and demanded that its perpetrators be punished. But the Ottoman authorities dallied on the matter. Infuriated, Washington instructed its consul in Alexandria, Edwin de Leon, to proceed to Jaffa at once and lodge a protest with the governor.

De Leon was no ordinary consul. A former literary critic and correspondent from South Carolina, he had displayed both bonhomie and fierce indignation in his relations with Egyptian officials, and so gained their trust. De Leon was also a Jew, a member of a venerable Sephardic family who owed his post to the State Department's now established notion that Jews formed a natural link between Christian America and the Muslim Middle East. Deposited in Alexandria by the USS *St. Louis* in 1853, De Leon swiftly gained the confidence of Muhammad Ali's successors, Abbas Hilmi and Sa'id. Those connections proved useful when, following a series of pogroms against Russian Orthodox communities in the Crimea, De Leon secured shelter for the fleeing Christians in Egypt.

Charged with obtaining justice for the victims of the Dickson farm attack, De Leon determined to receive "prompt, stern and effectual" action from the Ottomans, "without which, American life and property will never . . . be safe in Syria, nor the American name respected." Arriving in Jaffa on March 5, 1858, he immediately demanded and received an audience with the governor, but refused to accept his gestures of hospitality.

"Are our countries at war that you treat us thus?" the slighted official asked.

De Leon answered brusquely, "We regard the murder of men and violation of women, when permitted and screened by Governors, as a declaration of war. You have commenced it, not we." If the governor refused to apprehend the assailants, the consul went on, the United States would send a warship to "throw shells many miles, and leave not one stone of Jaffa on another."

The governor at once relented and arrested several members of a powerful Bedouin tribe found in possession of Dickson's possessions. De Leon's demands had been met, but his problems suddenly multiplied. Hundreds of the prisoners' kinsmen, armed and demanding revenge, surrounded the city's walls. The consul was faced with the dilemma of either releasing the suspects or hunkering down for a siege. He chose neither.

Understanding "the Arab character well enough to know that any appearance of timidity on [his] part might imperil the success of my mission," De Leon assembled his vice consul, dragoman, and Janissaries—eight men, in all—and issued them horses and pistols. He then led his force out of the city and straight through the "wolfishly glaring" Bedouin. "The audacity of the act overawed them," he later boasted, adding that the Arabs from that day called him "majnun" (madman) which "carries with it in the East a kind of sanctity and immunity." The governor was less pleased, however, De Leon noted. A Muslim official had been compelled by a Jew "to punish 'true believers' . . . for the satisfaction of 'Christian dogs.' "

The suspects were subsequently tried and found guilty of murder, yet De Leon refused to consider the Dickson affair closed. "It is the nature of the Eastern Race, as of the tiger, after once lapping Christian blood to thirst for more," he posited. There would be further attacks against American citizens in the area, he believed, unless the United States acted demonstrably and with force. To safeguard the "unprotected heads of the Christians and Jews in Palestine," De Leon advised the government to send "an emblem of our power," a battleship, to the Middle East.[12]

The government heeded De Leon's advice and, in October 1859, the USS *Macedonian* appeared off the Syrian coast. The commander of the ship, Uriah Levy, was an exemplary figure, famous for declaring, "I would rather serve as a cabin boy in the American Navy than as a captain in any other service in the world," as well as for outlawing the Navy's long-honored practice of flogging. Prosperous in business as well, he had purchased Monticello from James Turner Barclay, the Jerusalem missionary, and restored its Jeffersonian charm. Most exceptionally, however, Levy had become the first American Jew to attain the rank of commodore.[13]

Thus it happened that two American Jews, De Leon and Levy, set out to protect American Christians in the Middle East—a paradoxical situation, no doubt, but one that reflected the self-assurance that the United States could now demonstrate in the region. More elementally, the episode indicated the extent to which the tools of diplomatic and military power could be wielded in the service of American religion in the Middle East, the ultimate amalgam.

STILL MISSING from that mixture, however, was the mythic component, but that, too, would soon to be supplied by another extraordinary American. Vermont-born and Dartmouth-educated, George Perkins Marsh had worked as a sheep breeder, miller, bridge builder, and quarryman before inheriting a fortune and devoting himself to art. He also found time, in 1840, to be elected to Congress, where he developed a close friendship with the aging congressman John Quincy Adams. Ten years later, Marsh left Washington to take over the American embassy in Istanbul. The Turks impressed him as "a rude people" and the Middle East as "a wretched place, full of villains of every description . . . rape, murder, robbery, and religious vendettas." He nevertheless became an effective ambassador, advancing the sale of American-made warships to the Porte and organizing the first Ottoman naval mission to the United States. In addition to exercising authority, though, Marsh, the son of a Methodist minister, also pursued his religious impulses and at the first opportunity visited Palestine.

The trip would prove transformative for Marsh, not least because of the illness that nearly took his life near Nazareth. While recuperating, he reflected on the pitiful state of the Holy Land, its hillsides long deforested and soil drained by centuries of unchecked cultivation, overgrazing, and neglect. America, too, would become desiccated, Marsh reckoned, if its citizens wantonly exploited their environment and their leaders remained indifferent. There, in Palestine, Marsh formulated the ideas later incorporated in his masterwork, *Man and Nature*, that called for government protection of wildlife and precious resources. The same urge to safeguard the United States from the ecological devastation of the Middle East led Marsh to pioneer the American conservationist movement and the creation of a national research institute on nature, the Smithsonian.

Conservationism was an outgrowth of Marsh's religious experience in the Middle East, but the region also stirred his rustic imagination. While riding to Jerusalem, he became fascinated by the animal that Melville once likened to "a clergyman in a stiff cravat" and "a cross between a[n] ostrich & a grasshopper"—the camel. Marsh had a different metaphor for camels, "ships of the desert," and he believed that, if imported to the United States, camels could thrive in the arid Southwest, delivering mail and maintaining supply routes between outposts. Most usefully, camel-borne cavalrymen could subdue "the Comanches . . . and other Rocky Mt. Bedouins" and "strike with a salutary terror the . . . savage tribes upon our border."[14] What began as a fantasy of camels would, Marsh believed, result in the projection of American power.

Marsh presented his vision of the camel corps at the Smithsonian in January 1855 and immediately made a convert of Secretary of War Jefferson Davis. "Napoleon, when in Egypt used . . . the same animal in subduing the Arabs, whose habits and country were very similar to those of the mounted Indians of our western plains," he reasoned. The result was the American Camel Company, created by Congress with a budget of $30,000. The sum was entrusted to three relatives of the late ambassador David Porter—Edward F. Beale, Gwinn Harris Heap, and Lieutenant David Dixon Porter—who in turn enlisted the help of Edwin De Leon in Egypt. In all, seventy-nine camels were purchased from various Middle Eastern ports and loaded onto the USS *Supply,* the same ship that delivered William Lynch to Palestine. "Americans will be able to manage camels not only as well, but better than Arabs," boasted the officer in charge of the consignment, Major Henry Wayne. "And they will do it with more humanity and with far greater intelligence." Wayne's bravado notwithstanding, five Arab "camel conductors" also boarded the ship, among them one Hadji Ali or, as the Americans nicknamed him, Hi Jolly.

Braving weeks of turbulent seas, on May 14, 1856, the camels reached their destination in Indianola, Texas. Their reception was no less stormy, as the sight of the bizarrely shaped beasts triggered a stampede of local mules, horses, and cattle. Camels, Americans learned, may conserve water, but they were also petulant, flatulent, halitosic, and liable to induce seasickness in their riders. The people of Galveston simply banned the animals from their city, with a fifty-dollar fine for violators. The caravan nevertheless completed its maiden trek, through alternating downpours and sandstorms, from San Antonio to Fort Defiance, Arizona. "What are these camels the representation of?" asked May Stacey, a trooper who accompanied the train. "The 'go-aheadness' of the American character," he answered himself, "which subdues even nature by its energy and perseverance."

Jeff Davis was exuberant. "These tests fully realize the anticipations entertained of their [the camels'] usefulness in the transportation of military supplies." The government decided to buy an additional one thousand camels, one of which was to have been presented to Congress by Lieutenant Porter. The plans, however, never materialized; travel by dromedary was soon outmoded by that of the iron horse. The surviving camels were either sold to mines and circuses or left to roam freely in the southwestern desert. The last of them, Topsy, died at the Los Angeles Zoo in 1934. Hi Jolly, who later became a prospector and a U.S. Calvary scout, would be honored by a pyramid-shaped memorial and an Arizona highway that still bears his name. America's brief romance with the camel would soon be forgotten, though, obscured by gathering storms in both the Middle East and the United States.[15]

IN 1860, long-smoldering ethnic tensions in Syria, perennially stoked by the Europeans, erupted in a nationwide conflagration. Druze warriors slaughtered some twelve thousand Maronite, Greek Orthodox, and Greek Catholic Christians. "The blood at length rose above the ankles, flowed above the gutters, gushed out of the water-spouts and gurgled through the streets," the American missionary Henry Jessup wrote of one massacre. "Not a body was buried." The unprecedented scale of the atrocities overwhelmed the evangelists, who were suddenly saddled with feeding an estimated fifteen thousand "terror-stricken, hungry and shelterless" refugees. Americans were once again caught in a Middle Eastern crossfire of which they had little understanding or warning. Fearing for their own lives, finally, the missionaries retreated to Beirut, where they, too, became objects of charity.

The enormity of civil strife in the Middle East, however shocking, was dwarfed by the massive rift cleaving America. The antebellum period in American history was hurtling toward a cataclysmic end. Also concluding was a crucial forty-year span in the country's relationship with the Middle East, an era characterized by fundamental and far-reaching change.

Building on their postcolonial legacy in the region—the Barbary Wars, the early searches for adventure, and the advent of missionary efforts—Americans had engaged the Middle East with a mixture of self-confidence, curiosity, and zeal. No longer supplicants, American diplomats approached Middle Eastern rulers from positions of strength and, increasingly, with friendship. At the same time, tourists and explorers traversed the region with alacrity and, through their writings, introduced thousands of their countrymen to a spectrum of Middle Eastern cultures. Popular fascination with the area was also fueled by American artists, who, eager for inspiration beyond that supplied by *A Thousand and One Arabian Nights*, drew freely from Middle Eastern motifs. American evangelists, meanwhile, recovered from tragic setbacks to lay the foundations of an educational network that would help instill local populations with republican and patriotic ideas.

Rather than merely attacking or reacting to the Middle East, Americans were for the first time interacting with it and on multiple levels—strategic, commercial, cultural, and scientific. And although their relations were not always mutually respectful or tension free, the people of the United States and those of the Middle East were participating in highly diverse and frequently fruitful contact. They had begun, however fitfully, to know one another.

While relations between the United States and the Middle East intensified, the major themes of American involvement in the region—power, fantasy, and faith—also intermingled, clashing at times, but ultimately, irrevocably, merging. At home, however, Americans were growing asunder. Jefferson Davis would soon be elected the president of a newly seceded Confederacy. William Francis Lynch, enlisting as a captain in the Confederate navy, would find himself at war with David Dixon Porter and Uriah Levy, both of whom remained loyal to the Union. Edwin de Leon would also serve the Southern states, while Johann Steinbeck took up arms for the North. David Dorr would be severely wounded, fighting for emancipation in Georgia.[16]

The constitutionally joined nation, produced, in part, by America's Middle East experience was tragically unraveling. The coming Civil War would alter the Republic in many and profound ways, yet it would also exert an enduring impact on peoples from Morocco to Syria to Anatolia. The region's first Western-style universities would be built and the latest technologies introduced to help modernize traditional societies. Strife in the United States would also play a crucial role in the construction of the Suez Canal, which would influence the region's politics for more than a century. While blue and gray battled over their country's future, American soldiers, churchmen, and travelers together transformed the Middle East.

Part Three

THE CIVIL WAR
AND
RECONSTRUCTION

The Middle East comes to the American Civil War: Union troops
dressed in the Algerian Zouave style marching in Washington, 1861.

FISSION

SLAVERY, THE ISSUE THAT INCREASINGLY DIVIDED THE American people in the period between the Revolution and the Civil War, bore no obvious connection to the Middle East. This was an American scourge and Americans, not Egyptians or Moroccans, had to confront and expunge it. And yet, from the earliest days of the Republic, the Middle East occupied a prominent and often pivotal place in the clash between slavery's opponents and protagonists. An illustration of that centrality appeared in a March 1790 edition of the *Federal Gazette*, in an article entitled "On the Slave-Trade." The piece was reputed to be the work of Sidi Mehemet Ibrahim, an Algerian prince who possessed a great number of slaves and wished to defend his right to retain them. That the prince's slaves were white Americans, rather than African blacks, was presented as merely incidental.

"If we cease our Cruises against the Christians . . . [and] forbear to make Slaves of their People, who . . . are to cultivate our Lands?" Sidi Mehemet asked. It was a rhetorical question, for the answer was obvious: in the absence of American captives, the Algerians themselves would have to toil. But the prince also expressed concern for the well-being of the slaves, worrying whether years of captivity had rendered them incapable of surviving independently. Once freed, he reasoned, the slaves were certain to become social burdens, subjected to inhumane working conditions, and the pitiless vagaries of nature. Rather than "sending them out of Light into Darkness," Sidi Mehemet wondered whether the American slaves would not be better off basking under the "Sun of Islamism" and enjoying Algeria's care. "Let us then hear no more of this detestable Proposition [of emancipation]," he concluded, "the Adoption of which would . . . create universal Discontent, and . . . general Confusion."

The article aroused considerable controversy throughout the young United States, not least because its author was, in reality, fictitious. Sidi Mehemet Ibrahim was the product of the aged but still agile mind of Benjamin Franklin. By citing the same arguments used to justify the enslavement of black people in the United States—their alleged inability to adapt to freedom or to survive without the munificence of whites—to defend the enslavement of Caucasians by Algiers, Franklin sought to expose the hypocrisy of American slave owners. His parody was timed to coincide with a vicious congressional debate over the legality of the slave trade, a contest that pitted state prerogatives against the inalienable rights of men—the Constitution against the Declaration of Independence. The gap between the anti- and pro-slavery representatives proved unbridgeable, however, and Congress resigned itself to the status quo. Franklin's last invention—he died three weeks later—failed to achieve its purpose. Throughout the next seventy years, slavery would increasingly polarize and ultimately fracture the American people.[1]

Peculiar But Kindred Institutions

Franklin was not the first American to draw a parallel between slavery in the United States and its practice in the Middle East. Years earlier, in 1776, the Reverend Samuel Hopkins decried the faithlessness of the slave-owning congregants in his own Newport, Rhode Island, church. "If many thousands of our children were slaves in *Algiers* or any part of the *Turkish* dominions . . . would any cost or labour be spared . . . in order to obtain their freedom?" he upbraided them. A future founder of the American Board of Foreign Missions, Hopkins wondered aloud why the same Americans who fretted over Christian prisoners in North Africa displayed total indifference to the plight of America's slaves. "The reason is obvious," he said. " 'Tis because they are *Negroes*."

Comparisons between the two brands of slavery, American and Middle Eastern, grew more commonplace after the United States gained its independence and Barbary began seizing Americans. Like the Reverend Hopkins before him, John Jay reproved his countrymen for showing sympathy for the sailors captured by Algiers but apathy toward their bond servants at home. "The American slaves at Algiers were WHITE people," he explained, "whereas the African slaves at New York were BLACK people." A correspondent for the *New Jersey Gazette*, calling himself Humanus, observed in September 1786, "Masters [of black slaves] doubtless shudder at the idea of slavery among the Algerines, and execrate them as barbarous tyrants, but are they less barbarous than the followers of Mahomet?" The following year, Martha Jefferson informed her slave-owning father, America's minister to Paris, of a Virginia sloop that had narrowly escaped seizure by Algerian corsairs, only to return to a country that permitted slavery. "Good God have we not enough?" she pined. "It grieves my heart . . . that these our fellow creatures should be treated so terribly . . . by many of our countrymen." Early opponents of slavery such as the Abolition Society of Pennsylvania urged the Constitutional Convention to regard the plight of Americans in Algiers as divine retribution for "the injustice and cruelty of which we are guilty toward the wretched Africans." Which was worse, an anonymous essayist asked his readers in 1789, the enslavement of Africans by Americans or the Americans' enslavement by Africans? The answer, he posited, was simple: "Six of one and half a dozen of the other."

The similarities between American and Middle Eastern slavery served as a popular theme for early American writers. Royall Tyler, the New England jurist whose 1797 novel *The Algerine Captive* had criticized American passiveness toward Barbary, also assailed America's hypocrisy regarding slavery. Before his seizure by pirates, Tyler's picaresque hero Updike Underhill serves as a surgeon aboard a slave transport—the cynically named *Sympathy*—where Africans were treated "like so many head of cattle or swine" and beaten, starved, and raped. "I thought of my native land and blushed." Later, after his own enslavement by pirates, Underhill vows that, if released, he will "fly to . . . the southern states . . . [and] on [his] knees conjure them to . . . cease to deprive their fellow creatures of [the] freedom which their . . . constitutions . . . have declared to be the unalienable birthright of man." The year 1797 also saw the publication of *The American in Algiers*, an anonymous poem by a "Patriot of Seventy-Six," who claimed to be writing from an Algerian jail. After describing the horrors of being dragged through the streets, insulted, and beaten and thrown at the feet of the dey, the poet likens his own ordeal to that of American blacks:

Does not that Sacred Instrument contain
The Laws of Nature, and the Rights of Man?
If so—from whence did you obtain
To bind our Africans in slav'ry's chain?
What then, are all men created free,
And Afric's sons continue slaves to be.[2]

Even more damning comparisons were made by those Americans who had personally experienced slavery in the Middle East. James Stevens, a seaman liberated from Algiers in 1796, denounced "the execrable practice [of slavery] in the United States" and asked "with what countenance then can we reproach a set of Barbarians, who have only retorted our own acts upon . . . our citizens?" Relentless in his condemnations of North Africa for its enslavement of Americans, William Eaton was no less restrained in denouncing the institution in his own country. "Barbary is hell," he proclaimed from Tunis in 1799, but "so, alas, is all America south of Pennsylvania; for oppression, and slavery, and misery are there!"

The most influential of these testimonies was that of James Riley, a thirty-eight-year-old sea captain from Connecticut, staunch Presbyterian and militia volunteer during the War of 1812. As skipper of the *Commerce* in 1815, Riley was shipwrecked off the coast of the Spanish Sahara, captured by Arabs, and driven across the desert. He ultimately reached the port city of Mogadore, where the British consul ransomed him, but not before the American had been severely flogged, parched, and reduced to a mere ninety pounds. Returning to Washington, D.C., Riley met President Monroe, who encouraged him to publish his story. Riley's *Sufferings in Africa* became a national sensation, selling nearly a million copies over the next forty years. Particularly appealing to readers was the final chapter in which the author, recalling with horror the black slaves he had seen on sale in New Orleans, urged Americans to cut down "the cursed tree of slavery" and to "shiver in pieces the rod of oppression." Among the book's most enthusiastic admirers was a young bibliophile who preferred reading to working on his father's Indiana farm. Later, as president, Abraham Lincoln would list *Sufferings in Africa*, along with the Bible and *Pilgrim's Progress*, as one of the books that had most shaped his life and thinking.

Lincoln was not alone in drawing abolitionist conclusions from the works of Americans who had witnessed Middle Eastern slavery firsthand. Some of the institution's most outspoken opponents, among them Horace Mann, Charles Wells Brown, and Theodore Parker, cited the barbarity of Middle Eastern slavery in their demands for freeing American blacks. Some even insisted that North Africa's slaves were treated more mercifully than those in the United States. In his 1847 polemic, *White Slavery in the Barbary States*, the Harvard Law professor (later Massachusetts senator) Charles Sumner compared "the Barbary States of America" unfavorably with those of North Africa and charged the South with demonstrating greater "insensibility to the claims of justice and humanity."[3]

The persistence and cruelty of Middle Eastern slavery proved particularly abhorrent to American missionaries serving in the region, most of whom were unswerving abolitionists. A boat crammed with black slaves sailing toward Cairo in 1823 seemed to Levi Parsons and Pliny Fisk "a sight which could not fail to excite the most painful emotions in our breasts." Twenty years later, from the crest of Mount Zion, Harriet Livermore prophesied "great national calamities" awaiting the United States as punishment for its permissiveness toward slavery.

Some of the most poignant comparisons, however, were made by

African Americans, who likened their plight in the United States not to that of Americans in Algiers but to that of the ancient Hebrews in Egypt. The Holy Land, accordingly, served as their symbol of freedom—an association illustrated by their churches, which were often named for Zion and other biblical sites, and celebrated in their music. "A keen observer might have detected in our repeated singing of 'O Canaan, sweet Canaan . . . ' something more than a hope of reaching heaven," the era's preeminent African American leader, Frederick Douglass, recalled. "We meant to reach the North, and the North was our Canaan."[4]

Curiously, those least disposed to link the two brands of slavery were the Americans who journeyed to the region. Beginning with John Ledyard in 1788, American travelers in the Middle East made a point of visiting local slave markets. They wrote with horror of the sights they witnessed, but never connected them to similar scenes in the United States. In Cairo, Dr. Valentine Mott was shocked to see a sale of white women, "the beau ideal of a race that is deemed the most perfect of human beings," and pronounced it a "heartrending spectacle," but never once mentioned the auction of black women in his native United States. Nathaniel Parker Willis pitied the eastern European slaves "chained together by the legs . . . dispirited and chilled" whom he passed in Istanbul, but made no mention of the human chains passing through America's Southern cities. Encountering a slave caravan in Jidda, in present-day Saudi Arabia, John Lloyd Stephens was "struck with the closeness of man's approach to the inferior grade of animal existence," yet failed to denounce the dehumanization of millions of his own countrymen.

Of the many American tourists who documented their journeys through Muslim lands, only two appear to have drawn explicit connections between Middle Eastern slavery and "the peculiar institution" back home. Both were originally from the South, yet their observations served to illustrate the divisions soon to rend the entire country. James Cooley contrasted the condition of slaves in the Middle East with that of blacks in his native state of Mississippi who, he claimed, were "well fed, happy, and civilized." A diametrical view was submitted by David Dorr, the self-described "Colored Man," who identified unreservedly with the bondsmen, black and white, he saw in the Middle East. Invoking the many years he spent as a slave and the millions in the United States who had yet to be liberated, Dorr dared to ask what so many of his countrymen had merely wondered, "Oh, when will we be the 'freest government in the world?' "⁵

North, South, and Middle East

Dorr's question was answered only after many blood-soaked battles, beginning on April 12, 1861, with the Confederate shelling of Fort Sumter. From that day until the South's surrender four years later, the American people were consumed by their internal cataclysm and had scant enthusiasm for Middle Eastern affairs. Apart from the Zouave uniforms—fezzes, pantaloons, sashes—adopted from French-Algerian troops and worn by several Northern units, Americans had almost no reminders of their antebellum involvement with the area. The paramount concern of both Union and Confederate leaders was to secure the support of the region's rulers for their cause or, failing that, to ensure their neutrality in America's conflict.

Secretary of State William Henry Seward worried that the governments of the Middle East, "accustomed as they are to wait upon power with respect, and visit weakness with disdain," would take advantage of the violently divided United States. Indeed, America's ambassador to the Porte in 1861, the Alabaman James Williams, tried to persuade the Porte to shun the Union and recognize the Confederacy. President Lincoln consequently replaced Williams with Edward Joy Morris, a Pennsylvanian, and assured the sultan of his desire to "continue to cultivate the friendly relations which have always so happily existed between the government of the United States and that of the Ottoman empire." But the Ottomans, who had long battled secessionist movements in Greece and the Balkans, needed little persuasion. In replying to Lincoln, Sultan 'Abdul 'Aziz reiterated his "friendly sympathies" for the North and his hope that its differences with the South "may be soon settled in such a manner as will preserve the Union intact." The sultan also took the extraordinary steps of renewing the 1830 treaty with the United States and forbidding Confederate privateers from operating in Ottoman waters.[6]

Generally stable, typified by mutual esteem, America's relations with the Middle East throughout the War between the States contrasted radically with the savagery that Americans displayed toward one another. And yet the perils of being perceived as weak in the region were illustrated by two relatively obscure, but nevertheless illuminating, episodes.

The first incident occurred in February 1862, with the journey of Henry Myers and Thomas T. Tunstall to Morocco. Myers, from Georgia, was paymaster of the Confederate cruiser *Sumter*, which managed to seize eighteen federal ships before putting into port in Gibraltar. Seeking supplies, Myers, together with Tunstall, an Alabaman who had served as a U.S. diplomat in Spain, boarded a French packet for Cadiz, but stopped en route for a sightseeing tour of Tangier. The allure of the Middle East proved costly for the pair, however, when their presence in the city became known to U.S. Consul James De Long.

A former judge from Ohio, De Long, fifty, was a fierce patriot with a penchant for impetuous action. Arriving at the dilapidated consulate building in November 1861, he immediately asked the State Department to send him a large American flag "with 34 stars," as well as gilt-framed portraits of Washington, Lincoln, and all the cabinet secretaries. Thus arrayed, De Long next demanded that the Moroccan government withhold recognition from the "so called Southern Confederacy" and forbid secessionist privateers from anchoring in Moroccan ports. Five days after receiving assurances to this effect, on February 20, De Long learned that "rebels" had landed in Tangier.

"American Citizens, may talk and plot treason and rebellion at home," the consul vowed, "but they shall not do so where I am, if I have the power to prevent it." Appealing to the "Moorish authorities," De Long had Myers and Tunstall arrested and clapped in irons in the consulate's uppermost floor. They repeatedly tried to escape, offering their watches to the Moroccan guards and attempting to saw off their chains with a knife hidden in Myers's pants leg, but in vain. De Long, meanwhile, requested assistance from the U.S. Navy in removing his prisoners from Tangier. "I want the presence of a

Federal man of war in this bay," he wrote, sensing that his action might prove controversial.

De Long was aware of an event that occurred four months earlier, when the Union warship *San Jacinto* impounded the *Trent*, a British merchant vessel, and captured two Confederate diplomats on board. Their arrest triggered an international crisis as London charged the United States with violating British neutrality. Fearing that Her Majesty's government might retaliate by recognizing the Confederacy, the Lincoln administration backed down. The prisoners were released and the captain of the *San Jacinto* was cashiered. De Long feared a similar fate, for he, too, had incarcerated Confederate officials on ostensibly neutral ground.

Indeed, France promptly denounced what it considered a flouting of its neutrality, arguing that Myers and Tunstall had sailed to Tangier under the protection of the French flag. The *Sumter*'s captain, Raphael Semmes, meanwhile accused "the unscrupulous Consul" of taking advantage of Morocco's "political ignorance," prompting the emperor, Muhammad IV, to close Tangier's harbor. In protest, De Long reminded the ruler of Morocco's Barbary past and asked him whether "70 years of uninterrupted friendship" between Americans and Moroccans would be ruined "for the sake of [Confederate] Pirates."

De Long's situation continued to deteriorate, however, and on February 27 became desperate as a crowd of three hundred foreigners, mostly Frenchmen, surrounded the consulate and demanded the prisoners' release. But the feisty Ohioan refused to give in. "I have heard of barbarian mobs in barbarian countries, but it is the first time that I have ever heard of nearly the entire Christian population in a semibarbarian country rising a mob to interfere with the acts of a Christian consul." Violence might have ensued but for the timely appearance of the USS *Ino*. With bayonets fixed, thirty U.S. Marines charged ashore—the first to land in North Africa since the Barbary Wars—and managed to press through the mob. De Long then issued an ultimatum: either Muhammad IV would reopen the port and permit the captives to be evacuated or the United States would close its consulate. Given the choice between placating the French and alienating the Americans, the emperor sided with Washington. Less than an hour later, guarded by a detachment of Moroccan troops and watched by "at least three thousand spectators," De Long and the Marines led Myers and Tunstall up the *Ino*'s gangplank.

A jubilant De Long informed his fellow consuls, "If temporary civil war is waging in my beloved country, we still have a Union and a Constitution, which we will in God's name preserve . . . through succeeding generations, and a flag . . . [that] shall not be insulted by a rabble European mob on the coast of Africa." His elation, however, was premature. Fearing a rupture of Union relations with France, Lincoln again relented and released both Tunstall and Myers from prison in Boston. And like the captain of the *San Jacinto* before him, De Long was replaced. The embittered former consul questioned whether Lincoln's leniency would backfire and cause Middle Eastern leaders to doubt America's strength.

De Long's dismissal did not, in fact, augur a decline in America's status in Morocco or elsewhere in the region. On the contrary, the Union's spirited opposition to Confederate privateers only enhanced Washington's standing throughout the Middle East. Proof of that elevation came in 1865, when the United States was invited to join nine European countries in establishing a lighthouse on Tangier. The convention, though minor by great-power standards, was a landmark for America—its first-ever multinational treaty.[7]

The Civil War did nevertheless place strains on America's relations with one Middle Eastern state, Egypt. The focus of the controversy lay far away from the region and even from the battlefields of Pennsylvania and Virginia. Rather, Egypt and the United States came to loggerheads—however improbably—in Mexico.

Ever since the issuance of the Monroe Doctrine in 1823, the United States had sought to prohibit further European interference in the Western Hemisphere. Forty years later, however, with its armies locked in internecine warfare, the nation was incapable of enforcing the policy. Taking advantage of that paralysis, Emperor Napoleon III of France conspired to create a New World empire, beginning in Mexico. In January 1863, he dispatched thirty thousand troops to Vera Cruz with orders to occupy Mexico City. With them marched a battalion of five hundred Egyptians whose services had been volunteered by the Egyptian ruler Sa'id Pasha, a fervent ally of France. The soldiers were mostly black Sudanese who, the French believed, were acclimated to Mexico's heat and resistant to yellow fever.

The Lincoln administration was outraged by Napoleon's aggression and keenly disappointed with Egypt. Relations between Washington and Cairo, if never especially close, had consistently been friendly. At the outset of the Civil War, the Egyptian government had acceded to the State Department's request to banish an American vice consul, Robert Wilkinson, who remained loyal to the South. The department, in turn, had lauded Egypt's "generous contribution" in aiding "the widows and orphans of the defenders of the Union," and the bravery of several young Egyptians who had volunteered to fight for the North. That goodwill was now jeopardized, however, by the presence of Egyptian forces so close to America's border, and in violation of its long-standing doctrine.[8]

The French went on to conquer much of Mexico and to install an Austrian archduke, Maximilian, as its monarch. The Egyptian contingent throughout served admirably, patrolling ports, and guarding railroad cars. About one hundred of them died, including their commander, Colonel Jabbar Allah Muhammad, ironically from yellow fever.

The United States remained powerless to intervene, at least until Appomattox in 1865 and the victory of Union arms. Only then could the State Department send its consul in Alexandria, Charles Hale, with an unequivocal message for Sa'id. "What the Pacha has done in Mexico at the request of another power, the United States might do in Egypt at the request of some friendly power," Hale warned him, and reminded him that the United States now had 100,000 black troops who, like Sudanese in Mexico, were well suited for Middle Eastern service. These soldiers could easily be landed in Egypt, Hale said, "if the vicious principle of interference which supports the empire in Mexico, to which the Pacha lends his soldiers, should at any time be retaliated by us."

Duly intimidated by this threat, Sa'id backed down and refrained from sending further reinforcements to Mexico. The French were eventually defeated by republican rebels who executed the hapless

Maximilian. The surviving Egyptians—the only Arabic-speaking Muslim soldiers ever to be deployed in the Americas—sailed home.[9]

THE CIVIL WAR had ended and the United States could once again interact with the Middle East as an undivided nation. The war had reminded Americans of the dangers of being perceived as weak by the region's rulers and of the need to project at least a semblance of power. Now, with its economy rapidly industrializing and a million men under arms, the United States could cast an unambiguous image of economic and military strength. The transformation was not lost on Middle Eastern governments, many of which were buying up Civil War surplus and looking to the United States as a potential counterpoise to European imperialism.

With their great-power status nearly established, Americans could resume their antebellum pilgrimages to the Holy Land and their pursuit of Middle Eastern myths. And Lincoln yearned to join them. Riding with the First Lady in a carriage on the evening of April 14, 1865, the president purportedly spoke of his dream of someday touring Jerusalem. Later, after they reached their destination, Ford's Theater and took their seats in the box, Lincoln again leaned toward his wife and whispered, "How I should like to visit Jerusalem!"

Shot during the course of the performance, Lincoln did not live to experience the Middle East, but one of the Southern sympathizers implicated in his assassination sought asylum there. A quondam Confederate courier and spy, Harrison Surrat Jr., was associated with Lincoln's murderer, John Wilkes Booth, and other members of his conspiracy. While federal troops quickly captured or killed the ringleaders, the twenty-one-year-old Surrat escaped—first to Canada, then to Britain and Italy, and finally to Egypt. Forewarned of Surrat's arrival in Alexandria, Charles Hale, the consul, watched disembarking passengers until he found one who "looked American" and had him arrested. On December 21, 1865, Surrat was led in chains aboard the USS *Swatara* and shipped back to Washington. Though the trial ended in deadlock—Surrat died, a free man, in 1916—the United States praised the "considerate and friendly disposition" of Egypt's government and presented it with a portrait of the late president.[10]

Though perhaps strange to twenty-first-century readers, the fact that this concluding chapter of the Civil War saga was set in the Middle East proved fitting. The cataclysm that first fractured and then welded the United States would also serve as the catalyst for economic upheaval in many parts of the region, for revolutionary advances in health and education, and unprecedented exposure to the West. Yet in few areas of the Middle East would the war's influence prove more irreversible and profound than in Egypt, a country largely unknown to antebellum Americans but which, in the age of Reconstruction, became a centerpiece of America's attention.

Rebs and Yanks on the Nile

The Civil War's long-term impact on Egypt could be compressed into one word: cotton. Long famous for its production of linen and other fine fabrics—the word "cotton" derives from the Arabic *qutn*—Egypt in 1820 imported a new Jumel strain of the plant. High-grade and long-staple, the new Egyptian cotton became a favorite among the textile manufacturers of Europe. Sales of the crop multiplied, enriching Muhammad Ali, who contrived to monopolize the market. "Practically every available acre in the Nile Valley was devoted to cotton," a Western visitor observed. "The fields were covered with white bulbs and every fellah dreamed in terms of cotton." William B. Hodgson, the first of a long roster of State Department Arabists, visited the country in 1834 and compared it "to a Southern plantation at home," luxuriantly fertile but worked by wretched peasants. Nevertheless, "this maladministration does not probably affect the quality of Egyptian produce," Hodgson assured his superiors, "which alone is of interest to the United States."

Egypt's cotton production expanded even further in 1837, with the import of the country's first cotton gin from the United States. The innovation so impressed Muhammad Ali that in 1846 he hired

Dr. James B. Davis, a South Carolina planter, to apply American methods of cotton growing. Davis arrived in Egypt, together with "four Negro field hands," eager to set to work, only to be frustrated by the infamous Egyptian bureaucracy. Davis returned to his Columbia home two years later, minus an eye lost in a work accident, and with nothing to show for his labors but nine Angora goats, gifts of Egypt's ruler.[1]

Still reliant on ancient methods of farming, Egypt could not compete with the massive and thus far cheaper yields of the Southern states, which continued to meet most European needs. The imbalance changed radically, however, with the outbreak of the Civil War. The Union blockade, a self-imposed Southern cotton embargo aimed at pressuring Britain and France to support the Confederacy, and the depredations of battle—all combined to deprive Europe's mills of their raw materials. The price of cotton quadrupled and so did the acreage Egyptians devoted to its cultivation. Federal leaders were delighted. "The . . . increase of cotton in Egypt is of . . . vast importance to our own country," Secretary of State Seward observed. "The insurrectionary cotton states will be blind to their welfare if they do not see how their prosperity and all their hopes are passing away, when they find Egypt . . . supplying the world with cotton." Washington went so far as to send an agent to Cairo to urge the Egyptians to grow even more of the downy crop. Thus, while countless bales rotted on Confederate docks, Egypt's exports skyrocketed from $7 million in 1861 to $77 million four years later, an elevenfold increase.

Much of this windfall accrued to one man, Muhammad Ali's grandson, Isma'il. Before ascending to power on the death of his uncle Sa'id, in 1863, the thirty-two-year-old Isma'il had made himself one of the largest private landowners in Egypt, applying the latest in agricultural technology. Shrewd, taciturn, and ambitious, the Saint Cyr–educated Isma'il resolved to use his—and Egypt's—expanding wealth to Europeanize the country. He adorned his cities with majestic palaces and thoroughfares, created a Western-style consultative assembly of delegates, and scored the desert with irrigation canals, train tracks, and telegraph lines. Lincoln-like, he abolished the corvée system under which nearly a fifth of the peasant population had been coerced into digging the Suez Canal, and helped ensure Egypt's unity by purchasing a hereditary title—khedive—from the Ottomans. None of these accomplishments were ends in themselves but rather the means to achieving Isma'il's ultimate goal of independence, not just autonomy, for Egypt. And for that he needed an army.

Accordingly, the khedive determined to acquire the most up-to-date weaponry and equipment for his troops, and a cadre of Western advisers to train them.[2] Egyptian rulers had traditionally employed French and British officers as military instructors, but Isma'il had begun to suspect the European powers of plotting to incorporate his country in their empires. The United States, by contrast, had recently acquired a reputation for military prowess equal to that of any state in Europe and yet it had never shown an interest in Egypt.

A Pleasant But Insouciant Past

In contrast to Syria and Palestine, both hubs of missionary activity, Egypt was never a focal point for Americans. Though the United States maintained consulates in Alexandria and Cairo, and American shipbuilders provided vessels for the Egyptian navy, trade between the two countries remained negligible. Missionary activity, too, was limited in the Land of the Nile, where, prior to 1861, not a single school or clinic had been built. The U.S. government, meanwhile, took little interest in Egyptian affairs, not even in the digging of the Suez Canal. When the canal founder Ferdinand de Lesseps invited the United States to take part in the project in 1857, predicting that the channel would "shorten by 2,000 leagues the maritime distance from Bombay to New Orleans, Boston, and New York," President Buchanan scarcely bothered to respond. Contacts between Cairo and Washington were limited to the occasional exchange of gifts, such as the miniature copy of the Sphinx that Buchanan "cheerfully received" and pronounced a "curious relic."

Though always cordial, U.S.-Egyptian relations were chilled by the presence of Egyptian troops in Mexico. But whatever annoyance Egypt caused Washington through its collaboration with France was more than outweighed by Egypt's contribution to the blockade of

Southern cotton. Charles Hale, the same consul who threatened Egypt with invasion, welcomed Egypt's enrichment through cotton sales. "Egypt's rulers have always been friendly to us," he wrote. "They have appreciated our position and respected our rights." A year after the landings at Vera Cruz, in December 1864, Lincoln informed Congress, "Our relations with Egypt . . . are entirely satisfactory."[3]

For Isma'il, though, merely "satisfactory" ties with the United States would not suffice. While closely monitoring the war, the khedive was amazed by the efficacy of American arms and the might of Northern industry. He noted the swiftness with which the United States had recovered from its rupture and reasserted its international standing. Americans were destined to play a prominent role in world affairs, Isma'il believed, and could assist Egypt in its quest for independence. American military advisers would not only modernize Egypt's army but also provide a human bridge between Egypt and this increasingly influential power. Fifty years earlier, Isma'il's great-uncle had hired the adventurer George Bethune English to update his artillery corps, but now the khedive sought to recruit many such officers from a land that was thousands of miles away and lacking any history of cooperation with Egypt. To assist him in this formidable task, Isma'il turned to a most unusual American.

He might have been plucked from an adventure novel—burly and bearded, dashing and extravagant. By the time he met Isma'il in 1868, Thaddeus Mott had already served as an officer in the Italian and the Mexican armies, mined for California gold and sailed the Far East, and commanded Union cavalry in Louisiana. He was also the son of Dr. Valentine Mott, the New York surgeon who had toured Egypt and the Middle East in the 1840s and who had since maintained a close rapport with Ottoman authorities. Following his father to Istanbul, Thaddeus married the daughter of a wealthy Ottoman landowner, learned to speak Turkish fluently, and established his place at court. There, during a royal reception, Mott met Isma'il and managed to impress him immensely. On the spot, the khedive offered him a generalship and a job enlisting former American officers in the Egyptian army.

Mott accepted the position and, returning to the United States, conveyed Isma'il's request to several former Confederate generals—Beauregard, Johnston, and Pickett—and to the Union brigadier Fitz-John Porter, a nephew of David Porter. None expressed the slightest interest in serving in Egypt or of helping to recruit qualified veterans who would. Porter did, however, introduce Mott to William Tecumseh Sherman, the bristly-bearded commander who was now the chief general of the U.S. Army. Though ruthless in putting down the Confederacy, Sherman was sympathetic to Egypt's efforts to secede from the Porte. He was also eager to find employment for the many demobilized but experienced officers who had served in the Civil War, both beside him and against him in battle.

One of those comrades, William Wing "Old Blizzards" Loring, would be chosen to lead the advisers. A one-armed survivor of battles against Comanches, Mexicans, and Mormons, a former lawyer and Florida politician renowned for his unshakable integrity, Loring was also a frontiersman who had once led a regiment 2,500 miles to Oregon without losing a single soldier. A plug of a man—short, stocky, and dark—he had stood up to a Yankee charge at Vicksburg, exhorting his troops to "give 'em blizzards, boys!" and later sustained a bullet wound in the chest. Loring was no stranger to the Middle East, having worked with the army's camel corps at Fort Defiance and then toured the Ottoman Empire shortly before the shelling of Fort Sumter. Now, bored by his employment as an investment consultant in New York, he leapt at Sherman's invitation.

So, too, did Charles Pomeroy Stone, a charismatic and brilliant West Point graduate and linguist whom history later scorned as a "soldier of misfortune" and "the American Dreyfus." Volunteering early for the Northern cause, Stone was placed in command of Washington's defenses, but was soon blamed for the Union defeat at nearby Ball's Bluff and imprisoned for six months without trial. Though physically and emotionally broken—his wife died during his confinement—he managed to return to active service only to be scapegoated for further Union setbacks. Stone finally secured work managing a Virginia mine, which was where Sherman found him, miserable and desperate for change, in 1869.

Loring would become the inspector general of the American advisory force and Stone its chief of staff. Joining them was an initial complement of eighteen officers, men like Colonel Samuel Lockett, poet, artist, and designer of the Confederate defenses at Vicksburg, and from the Army of Northern Virginia, Brigadier Raleigh E. Colston, and Captain William Briggs Hal, who once freed a slave ship near Africa but who then sailed valiantly for the South. Together with these ex-Confederates came a personal friend of President Lincoln, Major Chancellor Martin, and Colonel Vanderbilt Allen, a member of the parvenu Vanderbilt family, and Captain Eugene Fechet, from Michigan, a participant in every major battle from Shiloh to Atlanta.[4] Though visceral enemies only a few years before, these veterans boarded the same boats, suffered the same seasickness, and disembarked in Alexandria in August 1869, disoriented but reunited as Americans in the Middle East.

The Great Civilizers

The Americans' arrival coincided with an ominous time in Egypt. The economic boom ignited by the Civil War had suddenly, with the onrush of peace, been extinguished. The price of Egyptian cotton plummeted. The years of plenty had left Egypt a stunning architectural heritage exemplified by the Cairo opera house, where Verdi's *Aida* was first performed in 1871, and the nearby Ismailiya suburbs, with a sophisticated system of canals and bridges and a European-style spa at Helwan. Most spectacular of all was the hundred-mile Suez Canal, officially opened in 1869 with a three-day extravaganza of balls and banquets for Europe's royalty—one of the many effusive and incalculably expensive celebrations staged by the khedive. Yet, along with such splendors, Isma'il bequeathed his people a staggering $100 million debt. Now, with cotton no longer acceptable as collateral, the European powers were demanding an increasing say in Egypt's finances.[5]

None of this insolvency was evident to the Americans, though, as they transferred from Alexandria to Cairo and indulged in a two-day tour of the city. In addition to the pyramids, they visited the hall where, in 1804, Muhammad Ali supposedly entertained Commodore Barron and the men of the Mediterranean Squadron. The landmark made less of an impression on the latter-day officers, however, than did the teeming, fetid streets and the local bey who complained that too many Americans had arrived and that some would have to go home. James Morris Morgan, a twenty-four-year-old swashbuckler who had once delivered the Confederacy's seal to Britain and then served as Jefferson Davis's personal escort, responded by challenging the bey to a duel. "That was about as pretty a call of a bluff as it was ever my good fortune to witness," Stone approvingly recalled. The bey backed down and guided his guests to the Hotel Oriental, where an Italian tailor outfitted the officers entirely in black—"An exact reproduction of the coat of a Presbyterian parson," according to Morgan.

From the hotel, the officers were driven over the Nile, through palm-braced boulevards, and into another world—of colonnades, lush carpets, and chandeliers—at the Gezireh Palace. "The East with its luxury and its magnificence and the West with its civilization and taste had here met," gasped Lieutenant Colonel Charles Iverson Graves, a broad-shouldered Annapolis graduate who had taken the job in Egypt to feed his wife and five children on his failed Georgia farm. "[P]erfect harmony had combined to construct the most exquisite and perfect habitation since the Garden of Eden." Admitted, finally, to the inner court, struggling to imitate the chief of protocol's bows and supplications, the Americans at last beheld the khedive. The experience was anticlimactic. Diminutive and pudgy, Isma'il had the habit of closing one eyelid when he spoke—an affect that, together with his swarthiness, lent him a vaguely sinister air. His words, however, delivered in French and translated by Lieutenant Colonel Charles Chaillé-Long, moved the Americans deeply. Recalling their recent war service and the integrity of the United States, Isma'il praised the officers' "discretion, devotion, and zeal" in helping to establish Egypt's independence. "When this shall be accomplished, as it will be *Inshallah*!" he declared. "I will bestow upon you the highest honors."[6]

Such accolades would have to be earned, however, and the Americans set to work. Stone established his headquarters in the imposing citadel overlooking Cairo, in a wing once reserved for Muhammad

Ali's harem. There he created the first general staff in Egyptian military history, amassed a library of four thousand books and many more maps, and acquired a press for printing training manuals. Drawing on both American and British models, he drafted the Egyptian army's first code of conduct. Loring, meanwhile, performed a comprehensive survey of Egypt's defenses. The results were dismal. The army possessed few cannons, most of them obsolete, and almost no ammunition. The shore batteries were crumbling and all communications between them, by rail or wire, had collapsed. Most pathetic of all, however, was the army itself, described by Loring as "medieval"—forty-thousand ragged and disorganized peasants drilled by equally ill-trained officers, poorly executing tactics from the time of the Napoleonic Wars.

The task of rectifying this situation was gargantuan, and Stone and Loring divided it between them. The one-armed general assumed responsibility for defending the country's coast. With the help of the engineer and onetime Confederate gunboat commander Colonel Beverly Kennon, Loring designed a series of hidden forts along the strategic shoreline from Alexandria to Rosetta, covering it with large-caliber, precisely enfiladed guns. Stone took it on himself to revamp the army completely. Assisting him were Alexander Reynolds, a brigadier at the Battles of Chickamauga and Atlanta, and his son, Frank, who had graduated second in the West Point class in which George Armstrong Custer finished last—a Philadelphia family that had chosen to serve the South. Another rebel commander, Henry Sibley, the inventor of the single-pole conical tent and a former traveling companion of Ulysses S. Grant, took charge of Egypt's artillery. Stone and his staff sectioned the army into regiments and divisions, provided it with paymaster and quartermaster corps, and raised factories for the production of arms.

The Americans furnished Egypt with the foundations of a modern army and, through it the potential to one day preserve the country's independence. Yet, just as Isma'il realized that building parks and convening legislatures could not ensure Egypt's sovereignty, so, too, the Americans understood that uniforms and tactics alone did not make a united army. Needed were galvanizing ideas like the love of one's country and a commitment to civil society. Egyptian soldiers might experience difficulty in learning such alien notions, but without the ability to read a book or a newspaper—a skill lacking in 90 percent of the soldiery and a third of the officer corps—the task might prove impossible. To redress this deficiency, the advisers established an Arabic-language school at Abassiyah for some fifteen hundred commissioned and noncommissioned officers. Many of these Egyptians arrived with their sons, asking that they, too, be taught. Stone, upholding "the express right of a soldier to have his son educated," agreed. Nearly three thousand neatly attired Egyptian children were soon studying in grammar schools created by the former warriors of the Wilderness and Gettysburg. "The army here is the great civilizer," trumpeted Lockett. "And Generals Stone and Loring have been its teachers." Within three years, nearly three-quarters of the troops were literate.

The representatives of American power in the Middle East thus became conveyors of America's civil faith. Fantasy, too, seduced them. In their new dress blues, with golden epaulettes and belts, vermilion trousers and tarboosh—"I looked so much like a streak of lightning that one would have been justified in listening for thunder," Morgan swaggered—the officers were feted in a succession of galas, soirees, and operas. International parties in honor of Isma'il's children lasted as long as a week. For Colonel William McEntyre Dye, previously of West Point and the Twentieth Iowa Infantry, the "fantasia" of such spectacles was overwhelming. The "dazzling splendor" of ladies with their varicolored parasols and ambassadors in ribbon-festooned vests sipping sherbet under satin pavilions made him swoon. "The limits of the imagination were reached, everything dancing before the mind like a vision."[7]

The brilliance of that image soon dissipated, however. Much like earlier American visitors to the region, initially star-struck but eventually dismayed, the officers eventually wearied of Middle Eastern realities. Loring grew contemptuous of Islam, a religion, he charged, "born of the sword" and "opposed to enlightenment" that "crushes out all independence of thought and action." He complained that young Muslims were taught "the same barbarous lesson . . . that led their ancestors to rapine and plunder," and hoped that "some Arab Luther" would emerge to end the inculcation of hate. Lieutenant

Colonel Graves, by contrast, admired the Muslims' reverence for Jesus—"In this respect they are better than either the Jews or the Unitarians"—but came to deplore the Muslim subjugation of women. "All the efforts of His Highness can make to civilize his people will be useless until he abolishes all the Harems and eunuchs from the Land!" he predicted. William Dye, who once marveled at Oriental grandeur, soon despaired of modernizing the Egyptian who, in contrast to the American's "imaginative soul . . . winging . . . like a fairy scout into the future," was wedded solely to a cruel and obscurantist past. An officer who had fought against, but had come to admire, the Sioux, Dye found nothing laudable in the Egyptians' penchant for "lying, baksheesh, blackmail, bribery, forgery, theft and corruption . . . and murder!"

Such revulsion only reinforced the Americans' cultural insularity, their reluctance to learn Arabic or live in non-European neighborhoods. The lack of understanding was mutual. Reproached by James Morgan for praying each morning rather than cleaning his rifle, Ahmad 'Urabi, an officer destined to play a pivotal role in Egypt's history, responded by denouncing Morgan's "Christian prejudices." Morgan, in turn, aroused local indignity by openly flirting with the khedive's nineteen-year-old daughter, Fatma. When Cairo's chief of police ordered Morgan to fetch him a glass of water, the son-in-law of the last Confederate treasurer responded by hurling the water testily into the Egyptian's face.

None of these impediments, however, hindered the officers from carrying out their tasks. By 1873, Egypt had all the appurtenances of a late nineteenth-century Western-style army, including staff and naval colleges, commands for submarines and mines, and a system for conveying orders. "The army, both officers and men, are pretty well up to the standard of that of our country," Samuel Lockett pronounced.[8] So impressively had the officers acquitted themselves that Thaddeus Mott was sent once more to the United States to try to recruit others.

Unfortunately, this new military edifice rested on a rotting economic base, as Egypt's debts grew fathomless. Unable to count on either cotton or Suez Canal dues to relieve his bankruptcy, Isma'il grasped for his last possible source of income: conquest. Incalculable stores of gold, gum, and ivory lay south of the Sudan, in what is today Uganda, Ethiopia, and the Central African Republic. Many of these lands had been claimed by Muhammad Ali and remained under nominal Egyptian rule, but few had been charted, much less subdued. Establishing Egypt's control over these defiant regions, and evading French and British designs on them, was an assignment requiring exceptional courage, fortitude, and skill—in Isma'il's view, the Americans' qualities precisely.

Hearts of Darkness

Two expeditions were launched. The first, a scouting probe deep into the Sudan, followed much the same route taken by George English over fifty years earlier, along the Nile cataracts from Wadi Halfa. Leading the march was one of the most seasoned and respected of the American advisers, Raleigh Colston, a onetime professor of geology who had served prominently as a Confederate brigadier. Colston planned to travel four hundred miles upriver before turning southwest toward El-Obeid in the Sudanese heartland. There he would meet another party cutting inland from the Red Sea, this one led by a New York native with a handlebar mustache and the singular name of Erastus Sparrow Purdy.

The teams left Egypt in November 1874 and trudged for three months across the blistering provinces of Darfur and Kordofan, through impoverished villages populated, Colston wrote, with "strange and hideous specimens of humanity" and illegal markets for slaves. As many as eight of the Egyptian troopers died each day of exhaustion and disease, as did a far greater number of pack animals. Finally, Colston himself fell ill with an excruciating bladder ailment that paralyzed his lower body. He refused to be evacuated, though, and continued collecting geological and botanical specimens and filing reports. "Although I am prostrate as a result of a grave illness . . . which appears to be mortal," he informed Stone, "I nevertheless desire to do my duty until the last moment." Passing his command to a young New Englander, Major Henry G. Prout, Colson had himself lashed to his horse and driven in the direction of Cairo.

Purdy, meanwhile, succeeded in reaching Berenice, on the Gulf of Suez, before turning west toward Aswan, where, he speculated, a dam might someday be built. The opposite of the soft-spoken Colston, a voluble braggart, Purdy could nevertheless draw on his extensive experience surveying parts of Colorado and Baja California. He could also rely on his formidable assistant, Alexander McComb Mason, a Virginia aristocrat whose credits included mercenary work in Chile, Cuba, and the South China Sea, one of the few Americans to master Arabic. Purdy and Mason succeeded in rendezvousing with Prout and to survey hundred square miles of previously unmapped territory, measuring rainfall and tracing possible routes for railways. The area's economic potential was not deemed promising, however, because of the limitations of the local tribes. "In the philanthropist, and in the missionary, they may excite an intense interest," the expedition's final report surmised. "[B]ut as subjects of the Egyptian Government . . . they will never add . . . to the wealth, to the strength, or to the glory of the state!"[9]

The disappointing findings of the first mission only reinforced the importance of the second, far more ambitious incursion into Africa. As chief of this expedition, though, Isma'il chose an Englishman, Lieutenant Colonel Charles "Chinese" Gordon, as the governor of Egypt's so-called Equator Provinces. Engineer, evangelist, and suppressor of the Taiping revolt that gave him his moniker, Gordon was a ruddy and boyish-looking fifty-year-old, a complex man with a capacity for immense compassion and fearsome anger. Though ostensibly charged with stemming the slave trade and enforcing Cairo's monopoly on ivory, Gordon in fact aimed at establishing Egyptian control over the sources of the Nile before any claim could be staked there by Britain or France. To dispel any impression that he favored either of those powers, Gordon selected an international staff of officers and, as his second in command, chose the thirty-two-year-old Marylander Charles Chaillé-Long.

Gordon gave his assistant all of twenty-four hours to prepare and then, on February 21, 1874, departed on a journey that would take them—by train, steam, and almost three hundred miles of marching—to Berber, a trading town abutting the Nile. En route, relations between the two men soured. A frustrated poet and actor prone to embellish his war record, a dandy with a fondness for silken top hats and capes, Chaillé-Long struck many of his acquaintances as fraudulent, "a feeble fellow" who, in Gordon's view, dwelt "on what he *has* done, and . . . that does not help what has *to be* done now." Isma'il, however, did not share that opinion and considered the American a natural adventurer capable of penetrating the Ugandan wilderness and procuring a treaty with its king. Thus, while Gordon retired to Khartoum—he would die there a decade later, murdered by Muslim insurgents—Chaillé-Long set out on a two-month trek through "pitiless rain, mud, misery, malaria and the dread fevers of the jungle," to Rubaga, near today's Kampala, the capital of King Mutesa.

The American's reception was surprisingly warm. The turbaned, "copper-colored" Mutesa signaled with his scimitar for respect to be shown to his guest. "Prostrate upon their faces, their noses in the dust, lay ten thousand subjects," a flattered Chaillé-Long recalled. His gratitude instantly gave way to horror, though, when, in accordance with a macabre custom, a "number of warriors rushed in . . . [and] lassoed and choked to earth those within reach, and then beat out their brains with clubs."

Chaillé-Long nevertheless managed to contain his revulsion and to delight Mutesa with a demonstration of a mirror, a music box playing "Dixie," and an electric battery that literally shocked the king. Gifts were exchanged: from Egypt, precious silks and stones and a horse—the first ever seen in Uganda—and from Mutesa, an albino boy and eight young girls, including his own daughter. Then the treaty was signed. "The entire Nile basin passed under the protectorate of Egypt," Chaillé-Long congratulated himself, "and the chief object of my mission was accomplished."

His mission, in fact, was far from over. Eschewing the direct route home, Chaillé-Long detoured in an attempt to prove that the Nile flowed from Lake Victoria in southwestern Uganda to Lake Albert, along the border with what would become the Congolese Republic. The American and his escort of native canoes paddled for six grueling days through dense river overgrowth, only to emerge into open water and the sight of seven hundred hostile Bunyaro warriors. "Give it to them now, and let every shot tell," Chaillé-Long exhorted his men as he aimed his Number 8 rifle at the chest of the Bunyaro chieftain. With supporting fire from two fellow officers, he managed to repulse the natives, killing eighty-two, but not before a bullet grazed and burned his face. He further survived a visit with canni-balistic Niam-Niam villagers, a poison-arrow barrage from eight thousand Yanbari tribesmen, and a nocturnal attack by a leopard. Three months later a frayed and fever-stricken figure stumbled into Gordon's headquarters. "My hair hung in great damp locks around my shoulders," Chaillé-Long recounted. "My beard seemed to ren-der more cadaverous my emaciated face; while the painful wound upon my nose, and one eye closed and blackened, caused him [Gor-don] to doubt my identity." Back in Cairo, his American colleagues mistook him for a beggar.

Though British explorers scoffed at his discoveries, branding him an "American pirate and bush-whacker," Chaillé-Long had located Lake Kioga, had navigated one hundred miles of a previously unknown stretch of the Nile, and traced the river's route through Uganda. He had also extended Egypt's hegemony from the Sudanese deserts to the rainforests of central Africa, a vast and luxuriant empire. "This young officer . . . has done in a few days more for Egypt, than . . . an army accomplished in four years, with an expen-diture of two and a half million dollars," the khedive publicly praised him.[10] The Egyptian leader no longer had such sums of money, however, nor did he have much time. His European creditors were already repossessing much of his assets and pressuring him to declare bankruptcy. Urgently, he needed the means for exploiting the rich domains secured for him by Gordon and Chaillé-Long, an access to Africa far shorter and less tortuous than the 3,000-mile odyssey from Cairo.

Chaillé-Long, meanwhile, was determined to rest on his newly attained laurels and to recuperate from his travails in his home state of Maryland. He got no farther than Paris, however, where orders reached him to return to Egypt at once. In September 1875, he took command of thirteen hundred troops and sailed five hundred miles to the Gulf of Aden, to what is today the Somali coast. "I need not repeat to you that secrecy be maintained upon the destination of the mission," Isma'il cabled him. "I rely, Colonel, upon your zeal, upon your activity, and your intelligence." Without arousing British suspicions of his purpose, Chaillé-Long was to try to find a water route, by way of the Juba River, west into Uganda. Another expedition would land north of there in Abyssinia—today's Ethiopia—to vanquish the rebellious King John. If successful, these operations would effectively link East and Central Africa and secure them both for Egypt.

While Chaillé-Long conquered a fort belonging to Zanzibar's sultan and pressed on to the Juba, the Abyssinian campaign quickly floundered. The commander, a Danish colonel named Arrendrup, though warmly regarded by his peers, was totally devoid of battlefield experience. He nevertheless rejected the suggestion of Major James Dennison, his American adjutant, to consolidate his three battalions of troops and not enter a valley where an ambush might be set. Dennison, far younger than Arrendrup but a West Pointer and seasoned Civil War vet, proved to be prescient. In less than an hour, King John's troops decimated two thousand Egyptians, including the ill-fated Dane.[11]

To avenge the massacre, Isma'il dispatched a 12,000-man force armed with Remington breechloaders and polished Krupp artillery. Though ten years had passed since he had last led troops in the field, Loring was asked to serve as the chief of staff, and with him went other Americans—Lockett, Graves, and Dye, Army Surgeon James T. Johnson, and Captain David Essex Porter, another grandson of America's first ambassador to Istanbul. Yet, to quell public murmurings over the massacre of Egyptians under the foreigner Arrendrup, Isma'il thought it best to give overall command of the expedition to his waspish war minister, Ratib Pasha. Like Arrendrup, Ratib had never before led men in battle. He is a man, Dye observed, "as sensitive as his figure is delicate" and "as shriveled with lechery as a mummy is with age." The minister's main concern was not excelling in combat but rather assuring the comfort of Isma'il's effete and feckless son Hassan, who decided to accompany the troops.

Steaming to the Egyptian-owned port of Musawwa in February 1876, the force at once penetrated the Eritrean countryside, a region that reminded Dye of the Texas chaparral. The terrain proved deadly to the pack animals, however, hundreds of which succumbed to disease and thirst and the relentless beatings of their Egyptian drivers.

Over two hundred of the surviving mules were burdened with Hassan's sumptuous camp of tents, furniture, and wine, leaving only a few for carting vital supplies. Ratib, meanwhile, proved himself, in Loring's view, "morally and physically an arrant coward." He rejected alliances with friendly tribes and refused to send out scouts or pickets or even agree to a war plan. Rather, following Arrendrup's misguided footsteps, Ratib hunkered down with six thousand of his soldiers in the Gura valley, dominated by hills on all sides—"a splendid place for King John to creep down on us," Loring judged it, "as complete a *cul-de-sac* as any army ever got into."

Making the best of an eminently hazardous deployment, Loring asked Lockett to construct a blockhouse fort. "Loring has blockhouse on the brain," Dye complained, but the redoubt would soon save their lives. The work had scarcely been completed when the brawny and handsome King John, accompanied by two pet lions, reached Gura. Also with him was a popular army fifty thousand strong and the mutilated bodies of Arrendrup's soldiers, displayed as a warning to the Egyptians. Ratib, intimidated, rebuffed Loring's proposal for preemptive action and, citing his need to defend Hassan, retreated to the safety of the fort.

The attack, when it came on March 7, was devastating. The Egyptian line instantly broke and ran. Dye, badly wounded in the foot, watched helplessly as "surgeons and sheiks, infantry, cavalry and artillery, riderless horses and transport animals" stampeded past him. The soldiers crowded into a ravine where, in a manner reminiscent of the federal debacle at Petersburg, the Abyssinians methodically slaughtered them. "It is impossible to convey the sensation of horror . . . in witnessing this terrible sight," Loring, who was watching from the fort, recalled. "The Egyptians not only let themselves be killed by a handful of savages, but slowly . . . were marching into the enemy's clutches." Their only hope lay in the Egyptian field guns, which were under the command of one Osman Pasha and well within the enemy's range. Osman, though, afraid of drawing fire onto his own position, merely cringed behind the breastworks. The shiny Krupp howitzers stayed silent. Dye had no choice but to limp back to Loring and the other officers barricaded within the fort.

The defenders' situation was desperate. Loring, who claimed to have survived more battles than any other American—seventy-five by his reckoning—was terrified. He saw the valley suddenly come "alive with the moving mass" of glittering spears and shields, and heard "hideous . . . howls like the roar of wild beasts," as the Abyssinian warriors descended. They already had butchered the Egyptian wounded who had been left writhing on the field. Dye could hear their cries for mercy, none of which were heeded. "They escaped the bullet only to feel the scimitar, resisted the club only to be lanced . . . the frenzied barbarians reveled in blood." A massacre, similar to the one soon to befall American cavalrymen thousands of miles away, on the banks of Montana's Little Big Horn River, seemed imminent. Still, Ratib refused to order a counterattack, preferring instead to cower among sacks of cornmeal in the fort's pantry. The Americans were reduced to threatening to shoot their own troops if they did not stand and fight.

Thus prodded, the Egyptians managed to lay down effective fire from their Remingtons and to save the fort—and themselves—from annihilation. Loring recorded with horror, however, how the defenders then "rushed out of the fort and at once showed their prowess by killing the wounded of the brave Abyssinians, mutilating the dead, cutting off their hands and feet and scattering them about." In retaliation, King John executed another eight hundred of his Egyptian captives and tortured the remainder, including Dr. Johnson, whose leg had been shattered by a bullet.

The Americans braced themselves for another assault, most likely the last. Peering through one of the fort's gunports, Dye could see "one unsightly mass of crushed and disfigured forms . . . naked and bleeding bodies . . . dismembered trunks, cleaved and gasping heads and quivering flesh, all ghastly in human gore." The survivors might then have been overwhelmed handily by the tribesmen, but the shrewd King John concluded that he had less to gain from a massacre than from a negotiated cease-fire. Instead of delivering a coup de grâce to the Egyptians, he sent them an emissary of peace.

"No sooner had he entered the camp than a gay and festive scene began," Loring scornfully wrote. "Splendid repasts were spread at the prince's table, and all went as merrily as though nothing had happened." After an exchange of lavish gifts and embraces, Ratib agreed to withdraw. Hassan excused himself from the gathering, ostensibly to go out on a hunt, and hurried back to Musawwa, where his father's yacht waited to return him posthaste to Cairo. A ragged column of four thousand Egyptian troops, together with their battered American officers, followed several days later.

The ignominy of Loring and his men did not end in Abyssinia, however, but deepened with their return to Cairo. Ratib finagled to have himself declared a hero, while the artillery commander Osman, of whom Loring wrote "if he was in any other army in the world he would be tried by a drum-head court-martial and shot as a worthless coward," claimed to have personally killed a thousand Abyssinians. The only court-martials were of Americans—of Major Dennison, for his alleged culpability in the Arrendrup fiasco, and Dye, for slapping an Egyptian officer who refused to fight. Not even Chaillé-Long escaped censure. Criticized for his failure to find a route from Juba to Uganda—the river turned south, not west—he was also faulted for showing an "excess of zeal" in attacking the Zanzibar fort. Racked with malaria, the explorer returned home, as unheralded as the other American officers.[12]

The mistreatment of the khedive's American advisers was soon forgotten, though, in the crisis surrounding Egypt's foreign debt, now estimated at an astronomical $500 million. Isma'il was forced to sell Egypt's shares in the Suez Canal Company to Britain and to place the country's finances under broadening international control. In June 1878, Egypt's European overseers recommended far-reaching cutbacks in the budget. The schools for educating Egyptian soldiers and their sons were dismantled, and almost all of the American advisers were dismissed. "It was a crime against humanity which no words can properly stigmatize," Loring lamented.

So, after nearly a decade of service, they departed—Mott to Istanbul as an adviser to several sultans and Dye as the consultant to Korea's king. Chaillé-Long also entered the diplomatic service, after graduating from Columbia Law School. Lockett found employment as an engineer, designing Chile's rail system, and Prout as a railroad executive. Not all of the officers went on to successful careers, however; Sibley and Reynolds Sr., for example, drank themselves to death. Many of the Americans never recovered from the illnesses they contracted in Africa and several, including Colston and Purdy, died from them. All were owed money by the Egyptian government, in some cases for years, though eventually they received their back pay plus a pension of $6,000. The sum enabled Charles Iverson Graves to pay the mortgage on his farm in Georgia and even adorn it with a house. To the end of his life, he kept a pet donkey to remind him of his experiences in Egypt.

"Old Blizzards" Loring was perhaps the most fortunate of the advisers, returning to United States to write his memoirs and tour the western frontier. He died in New York in 1887, with Stone and Chaillé-Long by his bedside, and was buried in his native Florida, with ten thousand people attending. Alone among the officers, only Charles Stone remained in Egypt. Promoted to lieutenant general, he was still at his post in 1879 when Britain and France, fed up with Isma'il's refusal to relinquish total control over his economy, pressured the Ottomans to install a more amenable monarch in Egypt.

The Americans left, some with fond feelings, others with far less warmth. "Every man who has come out to Egypt has been deceived," Lockett, looking back, complained. "The whole confounded thing [was a] miserable humbug—all show, all bunk, all make-belief." Dye concluded that no one could accomplish anything in Egypt "unless he has unlimited power entrusted to him," adding, "No intelligent foreigner should ever serve under an Egyptian." Yet Stone begged to differ. "Egypt has been kind to us and generous to us all in our days of plenty," he affirmed. "And will again when plenty returns to her." Loring, too, recalled, "During the ten years of my residence in Egypt, in no single instance was I ever refused an interview [with Isma'il], nor was there ever lacking the most perfect courtesy and consideration."

A total of forty-eight Civil War officers, both blue and gray, worked, explored, and, occasionally, fought for Egypt. They built an army, erected schools, and blazed new trails into Africa. Dye, in his memoirs, lauded them: "They were men of established reputation . . . educators anxious to assist in the great work of civilizing . . . the classic land of the Nile, prompted by an earnest desire to acquire knowledge while imparting [it]."[13] And while some of their contributions proved transitory, the concepts of patriotism and citizenship introduced to Egypt by these Americans could not be reversed. Indeed, the army they helped create became the leading force for the liberation and modernization of Egypt and remained so for well over a century.

Yet the veterans were not alone in the effort to instill American-style ideas among the peoples of the Middle East. Elsewhere in the region, the missionaries were building similar schools and through them disseminating the same nationalist and civic notions. And no less than the officers who served in Egypt, American evangelists were also influenced by the Civil War, both by the horrors it engendered and by the hopes it improbably produced.

THE TRUMPET THAT
NEVER CALLS RETREAT

HAD IT NOT BEEN FOR SLAVERY AND FOR THE RACIAL prejudice that permeated even the ostensibly antislavery North, Edward Wilmot Blyden might never have visited the Middle East. Born in St. Thomas in the Danish West Indies in 1832, Blyden was slated to be a tailor like his father, but refused to abandon his dream of studying theology. He left home at age eighteen and moved to New Jersey, intending to enroll in Rutgers's Theological Seminary. Handsome, eloquent, and refined, he met all of the requirements of admission but one, his race. Edward Blyden was black. Rejected by Rutgers, he presumed that equality was unattainable anywhere in the United States and decided to emigrate to Liberia.

Founded in 1817 as a refuge for former slaves from the United States, Liberia emerged thirty years later as an independent state modeled on the American Republic, but which also imported some of America's prejudices, granting special privileges to the small immigrant community and denying them to millions of natives. Yet, once ordained by the Presbyterian Church, Blyden chose not to shun Liberia's indigenous tribes. He journeyed farther into West Africa, into Sierra Leone and the territories that today form Nigeria. There, for the first time, he encountered a different faith, Islam, about which Blyden was ignorant.

African Muslims, Blyden soon learned, were "self-reliant, productive, independent and dominant, supporting, without the countenance or patronage of the parent country." He credited Islam with saving native peoples from animism, with educating them and endowing them with pride. Most importantly for Blyden, Islamic civilization, conveyed to black Africans by "Arab missionaries" of similar color and cultural background, served as a bulwark against the slave hunters, most of whom, he alleged, were pagans.

Impressed by what he saw of Islam, Blyden desisted from further evangelical efforts and dedicated himself to building ties between Christians and Muslims in Africa. Once consolidated, he believed that the continent could serve as a nexus between the ancient societies of the Middle East and the Western civilization they spawned, a catalyst for "the spirit . . . to destroy race enmities . . . and to reconcile nation with nation." Visits to Egypt, Lebanon, and Syria, undertaken in the summer of 1866, only steeled Blyden's commitment to his dream.

That vision embraced not only Christians and Muslims but also Jews, whom Blyden regarded with "awe and reverence." He had acquired that respect growing up among the Jewish community of St. Thomas, and later in life Blyden believed that Jews were destined to ally with blacks in sowing brotherhood throughout the world. He further held that the reestablishment of Jewish statehood in Palestine would set an example for African liberation. "I would earnestly . . . entreat Israel to remember that land of their sojourn and early training," Blyden wrote, "[and] to assist Ethiopia to stretch forth her hands unto God."

William Blyden later served as Liberia's secretary of state and ambassador to Great Britain as well as an editor and a distinguished professor of classics. He aspired to become a liberator, in a league with Lincoln and the early abolitionists. "Not the author of the Fugitive Slave Bill will be immortal in the annals of the nation, but the writer of the Emancipation Proclamation," he decreed on one of several return visits to the United States. "Not the memory of Jeff Davis will send a thrill throughout humanity, but the recollection of the so-called insanity of John Brown."[1]

Subsequent generations would credit Blyden with inspiring Pan-Africanism and the Black Muslim movement. Few, though, would hold him up as a model for his evangelical contemporaries in the Middle East, all of whom were white and far less approving of Islam. Nevertheless, in his energy, determination, and dream of one day peacefully binding all Middle Eastern peoples in a network of shared ideals, Blyden indeed epitomized the movement. Like Blyden, the missionaries sought to unite Middle Eastern peoples by fostering common values and forging new identities. They, too, strove to transform the suffering wrought by racial hatred in the United States into a force for universal betterment. In their hearing, "the trumpet shall never call retreat," described in "The Battle Hymn of the Republic," heralded not only triumph over inequity in the United States but a new era of comity for the Middle East.

Grains of Mustard Seed

Traditionally, the missionary movement in the United States was closely identified with abolitionism, and tolerance of racial differences was among the values that evangelists took with them to the Middle East. If God, asserted Henry Jessup, "could place a Tammany ward politician side by side with a Negro Republican" at His own table, then missionary schools could accept all pupils, irrespective of race or ethnicity. In the missionary view, the Civil War came as a long overdue vindication of their tolerance as well as a necessary, divinely appointed step toward redemption. "This great struggle . . . is indeed His chosen method of removing from our land one of the foulest abominations that ever cursed the world," Justin Perkins, writing from Mosul, explained. "The war is needful to the liberties, and even the life of our nation." Of the 150 missionaries that Edward Joy Morris, America's ambassador to the Porte, estimated were serving in the Middle East at the outbreak of hostilities, not one sympathized with the Confederacy, not even those who hailed from the South.

While the war prompted most Americans to turn inward, focusing on the domestic crisis and all but ignoring international affairs, the fighting provided added impetus to the missionaries. "The providential history of this war will be marvelous," predicted the American Board secretary Rufus Anderson, and not without foundation. In spite of severe budgetary cutbacks and a shortage of army-aged volunteers, the Middle Eastern missions flourished. In Egypt, for example, a land formerly overlooked by evangelists, the Reverend John Hogg and his family sailed 1,160 miles up the Nile, visited sixty-three villages, and preached to an estimated seven thousand people. Reaching Assiyut, a Coptic city halfway between Cairo and Aswan, Hogg established a school for girls that later became one of Egypt's most prestigious educational institutions. Another school was opened in Jaffa by Mary Briscoe Baldwin, an austere and lantern-jawed Virginian, with funding provided by the Union admiral David "Damn the Torpedoes" Farragut, the adopted son of David Porter. The feminist pioneer Mary Mills Patrick established a women's college in Istanbul and the Eli and Sybil Joneses, a Quaker couple who had tended to Northern wounded during the war, inaugurated the American Friends School in Ramallah, in what is today the West Bank. By the end of the Civil War, Syria alone boasted thirty-three mission schools with a student population of one thousand, a fifth of them girls.[2]

Missionaries in the Middle East, reported Ambassador Morris, "enjoy[ed] a liberty of conscience that is not accorded to dissenters from the established faith in some of the most enlightened kingdoms of Europe." Exploiting that openness, American evangelists vastly expanded their activities in the region. Schools, clinics, and churches grew so numerous that by 1870 American Protestant denominations felt compelled to divide the Middle East into separate theaters of operation. The Congregationalists consequently assumed responsibility for missionary work in Turkey, while the Presbyterians claimed Syria, Egypt, and Iran. The smallest church, the Dutch Reformed, was left with the least populated and therefore least promising area, Arabia and the Persian Gulf.

The Middle East, as never before during the antebellum period, lay tantalizingly open to the missionaries, though large segments of the native population remained averse, and even hostile, to their presence. The Eastern churches persisted in rebuffing the Americans, disdaining them as arrogant upstarts. "We had the Gospel before America was born," the Coptic patriarch lectured the Reverend Hogg. "We don't need you to teach us." Evangelists had negligible success in their efforts to convert Jews and remained forbidden, at the pain of death, from proselytizing to Muslims. "Mohammedans, Muscovites and Monks furnish their full quota of opposition [to us]," a Presbyterian report of the 1870s complained, but the preachers had little hope of recourse, not even from their own government. Maintaining David Porter's original policy of avoiding unnecessary friction with the Porte, the State Department reminded missionaries that "no foreigner who objects to Ottoman law need live under it," and those that do "must also take the peril of their position" into account. The depth of those perils was once again illustrated in 1862, when two American missionaries, one in Adrianople (Edirne) and another in Alexandretta, were murdered.[3]

Native enmity indeed proved dispiriting for the missionaries, but not as demoralizing as their failure to produce converts. Four decades of punishing and often fatal labor by the Americans had saved no more than thirty souls in all of Syria and a comparable number in Anatolia. The average cost per apostate, the writer Baynard Taylor reckoned, was close to $16,000, "a sum which would have Christianized tenfold the number of English heathen." Another author, Henry Field, estimated that "Christian Missions make no more impression upon Islam than the winds of the desert upon the cliffs of Mount Sinai," and that "more converts are . . . made from the Gospel to the Koran in a day, than all our missionaries have made from the Koran to the Gospel in a century." Responding to these dreary statistics, the American Board reminded its evangelists of the difficulties they had already surmounted in the Middle East and of the vast rewards that the region would ultimately yield. In words seemingly culled from the Civil War experience, missionary leaders spoke of waging "offensive warfare" against the "citadels" of Islam and decadent Orthodoxy. "From the same battlefields a cry of help is raised again by those too few and too weak to sustain the . . . powers of darkness and sin."

Such saber rattling could not, however, hide the failure of American Protestants to remake the Middle East in their own devotional image or quell the debate over educating native peoples who had no intention of accepting Christ. Board members continued to insist that a missionary's job was achieving redemption and not running schools and hospitals, while the evangelists maintained that their "semi-secular" work was no less ethically imperative, a means of "letting in the light" to the Middle East.[4]

The controversy surrounding the missionary schools was especially intense in Istanbul, where Cyrus Hamlin, last seen teaching Armenian students to bake bread and make ovens as part of their moral education, sought to create the region's first modern university. Starting in 1860, Hamlin appealed to the Ottoman authorities for permission to open a new and significantly expanded school, but the sultan, under pressure from the Catholic and Orthodox churches, demurred. Fortunately, Admiral Farragut happened to be visiting Istanbul as the sultan's personal guest and managed to secure the necessary permits. Hamlin proceeded to purchase a plot for the campus in the Bebek hills, overlooking the Bosphorus, and acquired a small collection of books from Harvard. Only one obstacle remained, the largest: the American Board, which refused to bankroll any secular institution.

Hamlin consequently resigned from the board and in May 1861 returned to the United States intending to raise funds for the university himself. He hoped to draw on the connections of his cousin Hannibal Hamlin, Lincoln's first vice president, but was once again frustrated, this time by the outbreak of war. "No one was about to throw money into a risky foreign venture when the fate of the entire country was at stake," Hamlin admitted. He headed back to Istanbul, despondent, but while passing through Paris, he chanced to meet Robert Rhinelander Robert, an outstanding philanthropist from New York. Excited as much by Hamlin's vision as by the bustling missionary himself, Robert proffered an initial grant of $30,000—the first of many hundreds of thousands—to begin construction. Hamlin set to work, personally laying the foundations of the cupolaed hall that would later be named for him, the first structure in the Middle East to be built with American-made girders.

The doors of Robert College opened in 1863, the year of Gettysburg, Vicksburg, and Chickamauga, and admitted a mere four students. That number soon rose to over one hundred, however, as the school obtained the imperial imprimatur of Sultan Abd al-Aziz and a charter from the New York Board of Regents. Though primarily geared toward engineering and applied science—one of its professors introduced the telegraph to the Middle East—the college would serve as a conduit for the import of Western ideas and mold new generations of Turkish modernizers. Among its graduates would be five future prime ministers of Turkey, including the country's first woman prime minister. "The work has proved to have the divine leaven that diffuses itself," Hamlin, looking back on his achievement, reaffirmed. "It is the grain of mustard seed becoming a tree."[5]

Hamlin would not be the only missionary to witness a flowering of American-style education in the Middle East. A second and equally influential university would be built in Beirut, through the labors of Daniel Bliss.

"Their faces are so entirely devoid of expression," Bliss wrote of his first glimpse of Middle Eastern natives—Arabs, Armenians, and Jews—in 1855. "It is hard to realize that some of them have souls." Bliss had come to the region, together with his wife, Abby, to open a mission in the remote Arab villages of Mount Lebanon, a task that required extraordinary endurance. But physical strength was only one of the qualities that Bliss abundantly possessed. Like Hamlin, he had been orphaned at an early age and had worked on various farms and in factories in Vermont before earning a scholarship to Amherst. Now, at age thirty-seven, he trudged across the snow-encrusted peaks to reach his destination. Within five years, he had succeeded in learning Arabic and establishing separate primary schools for girls and boys.

Bliss had once again demonstrated the missionaries' determination to make an impact on the Middle East, irrespective of the dangers. But no amount of fortitude could protect them from the vicious fighting between Maronites and Druze that erupted in 1860. The violence compelled most of Syria's missionaries, Bliss among them, to seek shelter in Beirut. There, though destitute, Bliss made contact with veteran evangelicals like William Thomson, Henry Jessup, and

Harrison Dwight, and observed their schools firsthand. He saw how many of their students, immediately after graduating, left their country for America. For them, he noted, "the promised land is not now east and west of the Jordan, but east and west of the Mississippi." To reverse this trend, Bliss advocated a curriculum that would instill in pupils a love of their homeland and a commitment to civic duties. Native teachers should be trained as soon as possible, he urged, and their language of instruction should be Arabic.

On the first day of 1862, Bliss submitted to the American Board his proposal for furnishing the Arab world with its first modern college. The reception was characteristically tepid. Rufus Anderson regarded the project as yet another diversion from the missionary effort, but recognized its value in revitalizing the Syrian station, a "necessary choice of evils." Permission was ultimately granted, but Bliss had to raise much of the $100,000 endowment himself, soliciting contributions from a number of British and American donors, among them Mrs. Franklin H. Delano, an Astor family Brahmin and great-aunt of the thirty-second president. With the proceeds, Bliss purchased a plot of land overlooking St. George's Bay, "a home for jackals and a dumping place for the [city's] offal," and rented classrooms in existing buildings. Four years later, the missionaries in Beirut laid the cornerstone for the new Syrian Protestant College. Bliss, its first president, undoubtedly shocked many board members back home when he pledged that "a man white, black or yellow, Christian, Jew, Mohammedan or heathen, may enter and enjoy all the advantages of this institution . . . and go out believing in one God, or in many Gods, or in no God."[6]

Though he hastened to add, "It will be impossible for any one to continue with us long without knowing what we believe to be the truth and our reasons for that belief," Bliss had conceded what Hogg and Hamlin and most missionaries already knew but had never dared vocalize. Unable to import their spiritual beliefs into the Middle East, Americans would have to settle for instilling secular notions of patriotism, republicanism, and the preservation of individual liberties. These principles took root in the college's student body as it expanded from sixteen students to several thousand and, through them, percolated throughout the region. Among the early graduates were Ya'qub Sarruf and Faris Nimr, pioneers of modern journalism in Egypt, and Dr. Shibli Shumayyil, the Darwinian theorist and social commentator, and the lexicographers Nasif al-Yaziji and Butrus al-Bustani, who modernized written Arabic. Praising these accomplishments in a lecture to the college in July 1866, Edward Wilmot Blyden looked forward "to the day that students may be sent from Liberia to Syria to learn the Arabic language," and "the Syrian College [will] aid in evangelizing not only the West and South of Asia, but the North and West of Africa."

The college's most enduring contributions were not literary, however, but political. Its "great mission," according to Jessup, was to create a "new Phoenicia, a new Syria," based on brotherhood and loyalty to the motherland. This objective was predicated on the novel notion that the diverse peoples of Syria in fact constituted a distinct Arab nation. "No one can look upon these ungainly and heavy Turks, and feel that the susceptible and lively Arabs—the hardy mountaineer and the Bedaween rover—were made to be their subjects," maintained a contemporary missionary "Intelligence." The overwhelming majority of Syrians, though, defined themselves not in national terms but rather by religion, tribe, and district—usually in that order. They showed little promise of attaining internal cohesion, much less the unity necessary for independence.

The United States offered a model for achieving that solidarity. A country coalesced from many states and various ethnicities, America had successfully wrested its liberty from a world empire and had recently fought to preserve its union. "Oh that all the Christians in the Turkish Empire had the spirit that the Americans had in 1775!" Bliss yearned and his wish was presently granted. Growing numbers of Syrian Protestant College graduates embraced the American paradigm and declared themselves devotees of Arabism ('Aruba). Together with their Muslim neighbors, with whom they shared a common past and cultural heritage, these activists worked for the merger of all Arab lands into a single, sovereign state. The college, wrote the celebrated Arab historian George Antonius, had provided "the intellectual effervescence" for an "Arab revival," and one that would radically transform the region's politics. By failing to make Prostestants out of the local inhabitants, by fulfilling the dictates of

America's civic faith, the missionaries had helped fashion an entirely new identity in the Middle East. Fifty years after North African pirates prodded Americans into forging a federated and distinct United States, American educators were prompting diverse Middle Eastern peoples to unite into a unique Arab nation.[7]

OTHER MISSIONARIES, though, still refused to concede their original, evangelical goal. They continued to enjoy the support of a "very considerable and intelligent portion of the people of the United States," according to William Henry Seward, himself a spirited supporter of missions. The secretary of state, also known for his restorationist sympathies, went out of his way to extend American protection to the Jews of the Middle East. Following a series of pogroms against the Jewish community of Morocco in 1863, he instructed the consulate in Tangier to "exert all proper influence" to shield the "Israelites" from the "barbarous cruelties" of their government.

Like many Americans, Seward persisted in believing, in spite of the nation's calamity, in the imminence of Christ's return. For some American evangelicals, though, the carnage that had so recently ravaged America proved that faith alone no longer sufficed. Committed Christians, they held, must not only long for but also labor toward redemption. That conviction compelled one American, George Adams, to lead dozens of his followers to Palestine with the goal, once again, of colonizing the country and restoring its sovereignty to the Jews, of preparing the world for peace.[8]

On Eagle's Wings

Reports on his early life are sketchy. The best accounts place his birth in Oxford, New Jersey, in 1811 or 1813, a farmer's son apprenticed to be a tailor. By the time he turned thirty, though, George Adams, had abandoned his trade for the Shakespearean theater and wandered far from his home. Acquaintances described him as an intelligent-looking but contentious man, of medium build and dark eyes and hair, with "lips shut tight as a clamshell" and eyes so close-set "he could look down the neck of a Johnson's Liniment bottle without squinting." He also had a drinking problem and, after repeatedly showing up drunk for performances, was finally banned from the stage.

Adams would, at this juncture, seem an unlikely candidate to spearhead a revivalist movement in Palestine, a person with few or no religious beliefs. His journey to faith began in 1844, when Adams converted to Mormonism. He became friendly with Orson Hyde, the first Mormon envoy to Jerusalem, and dreamed of replicating Hyde's pilgrimage to the Holy Land. But before he could leave, Adams was excommunicated for lewdness and embezzlement. He next appeared in Springfield, Massachusetts, now a Campbellite minister, only to be defrocked once again for intemperance. Fleeing his reputation, Adams moved to Indian River, Maine. He married a local woman, strong-willed and stout, and established his own Church of the Messiah. From his pulpit and on the pages of his monthly, *The Sword of Truth and Harbinger of Peace*, Adams prophesied the Second Coming, an era of brotherhood and financial prosperity. The prerequisite for this golden age, he proclaimed, was the Jews' restoration to Palestine. "The reign of Christ on earth and the return of the Jews to Canaan are even now on the very eve of occurring."

Starting in 1862, while Union and Confederate forces gored one another on the fields of Shiloh and Antietam, George Adams remained in Maine, scouring the state for volunteers. "Palestine will soon shake herself from the dust of ages and arise in glory, as in the days of old!" he bellowed at revivalist rallies, his long hair flailing, a tenebrous glare in his eyes. Finally, he departed for the Holy Land, taking with him Indian River's postmaster, Abraham McKenzie, in order to assess its suitability for settlement. Their report was rife with praise. The soil of Palestine, Adams claimed, was excellent and its climate similar to California's. With the aid of American innovations—"Johnson's patent shifting mold-board" and "Smith's remarkable double-back-action drill"—the country could support thousands of colonists and myriads of tourists annually. Jews could be retaught how to farm.

Exploiting this felicitous news, Adams was able to recruit 156 Americans to his cause—artisans, fishermen, farmers, and traders, together with their wives and children. He changed his name to George Washington Joshua Adams, declaiming, "The great Restitution, as foretold by the Prophets and Apostles, has now commenced." Adams instructed his followers to pool their savings, a total of forty-two dollars, to pay for their passage to Palestine.[9]

Though clearly an outsider, Adams represented ideas that continued to engage key segments of American society, including some of its most preeminent figures. In a meeting with Abraham Lincoln in 1863, the leading Canadian churchman Henry Wentworth Monk protested the fact that Jews, unlike Negroes, had yet to be emancipated. "There can be no permanent peace in the world until the civilized nations . . . atone . . . for their two thousand years of persecution [of the Jews] by restoring them to their national home in Palestine," the reverend posited, and though never known for his piety, the president readily agreed. "Restoring the Jews to their national home in Palestine . . . is a noble dream and one shared by many Americans," he said, adding that once the war was won, Americans would again be able to "see visions and dream dreams" and lead the world in realizing them.

Lincoln's remarks indicated the extent to which the restorationist idea continued to captivate a broad cross section of Americans and the degree to which Palestine remained a national obsession. Tempered by the heat of battle, that fixation only hardened after the Civil War. Two years after Lincoln's assassination, Victor Beauboucher, the U.S. consul in Jerusalem, noted that five hundred Americans had entered Palestine during the preceding eighteen months and passage to the country was completely booked. A former Union soldier who had lost a leg at Cold Harbor, Beauboucher was impressed with the pilgrims' fervidness and their remarkable familiarity with the land. "This is the first country where I have felt at home, yet I have been in no country so unlike my own," confessed the Episcopal minister and Massachusetts congressman Henry White Warren after disembarking at Jaffa in 1868. "You come to the Holy Land with something of the feeling that you come to your home," wrote the celebrated Civil War correspondent John Russell Young. "Somehow you always belonged here." Americans' knowledge of Palestine, rooted in their daily Bible readings, could now be broadened by membership in the Palestine Exploration Society, dedicated to the study of Holy Land geography. They could also visit Palestine Park with its mock-up of the major sites—Nazareth, Bethlehem, Jerusalem—built on the bank of Chautauqua Lake. "We know far more about the land of the Jews," boasted *Harper's* magazine, "[more] than the degraded Arabs who hold it."[10]

A preoccupation with Palestine and the belief in its eventual restitution to the Jews were not, however, synonymous. Similar to Herman Melville's ridicule of Warder Cresson and the Dicksons was the dismissal by prominent theologians, particularly those from the more mainstream churches, of the restorationist idea. The Reverend Warren avowedly felt at home in Palestine, but the country's Jews gave him "the greatest temptation toward despising a brother a man ever encountered." Philip Schaff of the Union Theological Seminary could write rapturously of his first glimpse of Jerusalem in 1878, and then, a paragraph later, call for the destruction of the city's "squalid and forbidding" Jewish quarter. For Warren and Schaff, the pitiful state of the Jews was proof of the fulfillment of biblical prophecy and punishment for their rejection of Christ. The *Princeton Review* seemed to speak for them and other conservative ministers when, in 1866, it denounced restorationism as "radically false," contrary "to the whole drift of . . . New Testament teaching," and "injurious to the interests of true religion."

These detractors of restorationism, though often strident, rarely attained the force—or the popularity—of the notion's defenders. One such advocate, the Presbyterian Nathaniel Clark Burt of Ohio, returned from an 1867 trip to Palestine praying that the Jews "shall yet be brought home to that country once their own by divine promise and gift." The following year, Philadelphia's Reverend Henry Riley predicted that "His people" would soon "be gathered from their wide dispersion among the nations, and restored to the actual possession of Palestine." In books, especially, supporters of a Jewish-ruled Palestine enjoyed a patent edge over its opponents. In her best-selling memoir, *Hadji in Syria*, Sarah Barclay Johnson, the daughter of the missionary James Turner Barclay, expressed her hope of someday witnessing "the Hebrew race . . . returning to their ancient city, and . . . the land of their forefathers," and of Palestine's reverting to its "rightful owner." Even more widely read was William C. Prime's *Tent Life in the Holy Land*, a gushing journal of the author's experiences in Palestine. The editor of the *New York Journal of Commerce*, Prime rhapsodized that the country's past was "cast in holy radiance" and speculated how a future Jewish state would have to be initially provisioned with foodstuffs "imported by Jaffa and brought on camels from over the sea."

America's Palestine mania would deepen in the decades after the Civil War and, with it, the romance of Jewish restoration. "So much has been said for generations of the Jews regaining possession of Jerusalem, that it is agreeable to think that they are likely to do so at last," professed a *New York Times* editorial. "They certainly deserve Jerusalem." Few Americans would have embraced that sentiment more ardently than George Adams and his disciples who, in August 1866, boarded the steamer *Nellie Chapin* bound for Palestine. "The sons of Ephraim are now gathering home," Adams proclaimed.[11]

THE JOURNEY from Boston to Jaffa took forty-two days, roughly twice the usual duration. Still, the pilgrims refused to complain, one of them swearing that "he would rather sit himself on a plank and puke his way across the sea than miss the trip to Palestine." Yet far rougher ordeals awaited them after the *Nellie Chapin* landed. Following the violent demise of the Dickson colony and the friction it caused with the United States, the Ottoman government was loath to allow the establishment of new evangelical settlements. The Adams pilgrims were consequently forced to camp out on the beach, between the refuse heaps of local butchers and the graves of some two hundred recent cholera victims. "The exhalations through the porous sand from such a vast body of decomposition was very bad," a diarist among them recorded. "The shore was the world's privy."

In spite of their discomforts, the Americans' morale remained high. Sailors from the USS *Ticonderoga*, on shore leave in Jaffa in September 1866, found that the colonists were still optimistic about their chances for success. Adams excitedly described plans for constructing an American-style city, complete with "churches, hotels, [and] two colleges," and for rebuilding the temple, with a Rothschild family member serving as high priest. The first step toward realizing that vision seemed to materialize early in 1867 when U.S. Vice Consul Hermann Loewenthal, a German-Jewish convert to Christianity, secured the group ten acres of arable land just outside of the city. Though this was much less than the three million acres Adams promised them, the colonists set to work. Within days, seventeen prefab houses imported from Maine were reassembled and a meetinghouse raised. "We the colony now stand free from every government on earth," declared Adams, who now took to calling himself President Adams and who flew the American flag "every Lord's day."

The farmers' crops quickly fell prey to scavengers, however, and, with winter approaching, the community faced the specter of famine. Adams was frequently seen in drunken rampages, arguing fiercely with his wife, and denouncing Loewenthal as "a monster in human form" and a "wily Jew . . . [who] opposed all Christian progress." Less than six months after disembarking on holy soil, seventeen of the Americans were dead, the victims of exposure and dysentery. "Put your faith in God, and use a little wine or rum," Adams reassured the survivors, many of whom were already growing skeptical of his remedies.

Conflicting reports regarding the colonists' plight filtered back to the United States. In a letter to the *New York Times*, one settler denied allegations that the community was failing and insisted, "Mr. Adams has the good-will of the Latins, the Greeks, the Armenians, the Maronites, the Turks, the Arabs, the Jews, and the Mohamedans." Another told the *Bangor Times* that the Arabs were "our warmest friends," and that he thought "it a glorious thing to live in a country where once dwelt the prophets, patriarchs, and the Messiah himself." Other articles, however, dredged up Adams's repellent past and cast him as an "adventurer, a charlatan, and a scamp." Conflicting rumors described the settlers as either engaged in a miniature civil war or indulging in free love.

The settlement, meanwhile, became an attraction for American tourists. The Connecticut industrialist Charles Elliot portrayed the colonists as "unprotected as they would be on the Texas frontier," and the Reverend Henry Whitney Bellows, from New York's historic All Souls Church, declared Adams a "religious fanatic" with "a decided bee in his bonnet." And yet the sight of the prim, cottage-style houses, each with its well-tended garden, proved irresistible to the traveling correspondent John Swift. The colony, to his mind, was a "modern Mayflower," a community of "genuine Yankees" who, "with a new religion in one hand and American plows . . . in the other," were striving "to regenerate the land on American principles." He quoted Adams boasting of his plans to "civilize the benighted Arabs" by planting democracy among them and creating a Jewish state. Adams's wife, "the Presidentess," assured Swift that redemption was near now that the "American eagle of freedom" had "winged his glorious flight from the newest to the oldest land on earth."[12]

The question of whether Adams represented a point of pride for the United States or a potential embarrassment was placed, finally, before the State Department. Secretary of State Seward sent his friend the Reverend Walter Bidwell to investigate the colony. Bidwell reached Jaffa in March 1867 and, with the exception of a "pale faced and decidedly intellectual" woman who wanted to go home, found that the settlers were generally content and confident of a fruitful future. Indeed, compared with the hovels and trash heaps of Jaffa port, the colony seemed resplendent to Bidwell. A shockingly different impression, however, was submitted by J. Augustus Johnson, the American consul in Damascus. Married to the evangelical author Sarah Barclay, Johnson was partial to missionaries, but what he saw in Jaffa only sickened him. "American citizens," he warned Washington, would soon be "begging of Arabs . . . to avoid dying of starvation in the streets." Only by awakening to their senses and freeing themselves from Adams's spell could those Americans hope to survive, Johnson wrote.

The wake-up occurred in the summer, as the death toll among the settlers reached sixty. Desperate, twenty-two of them published "An Appeal! To Philanthropy and Common Humanity" in the American press, and beseeched the federal government to evacuate them. "How can we confide in the hand or heart of one who has staggered on his pulpit too drunk to read the word of God?" they asked the consul Beauboucher. In a letter to Maine's governor, Joshua Lawrence Chamberlain, they claimed that they were utterly destitute, bereft of food and medicine, their property stolen by "the vile imposter Adams." They reminded Chamberlain, a hero of Gettysburg, that many of them "had chased the bright folds of the Stars and Stripes over many a southern battlefield" and were deserving of their country's help.

Moved, finally, by these entreaties, the State Department allocated $3,000 to pay for the colonists' evacuation. The money sufficed for only sixteen of them, but others found passage on visiting American naval ships. Adams warned them that they would only "recede and become . . . paupers and beggars" in America, but then he, too, departed, presumably to raise money for the group in Britain. He would next resurface at a Baptist church in Philadelphia, in 1873, preaching the Gospel and denying any association between himself and the George Washington Joshua Adams of Jaffa.

By the summer's end, some fifty former settlers had returned shamefaced to Indian River. Abraham McKenzie brought with him a Bedouin tent and opened a business selling genuine "Palestine soil." But forty of them remained in Jaffa, only one of whom, Rolla Floyd, managed to find permanent employment guiding American tourists up to Jerusalem. Though the settlement continued to be known locally as *Almalikan*—the Americans' place—most of its buildings were purchased by German Adventists. Ownership of Adams's house passed to Platon Ustinov, a colorful Russian baron and antiquities collector, grandfather of the actor Peter. Thus, ingloriously, ended yet another attempt by American evangelicals to establish a colony dedicated to the Jews' return to Palestine. "The failure of the American settlement at Jaffa . . . is but a repetition of the fate of previous similar experiments," the local British consul, Noel Temple Moore, summed up. "There seems little hope of success attending these enterprises."[13]

The American eagle, which, in Mrs. Adams's imagery, was to have delivered the Jews to sovereignty in their ancient homeland, appeared to have folded its wings. Following the collapse of the earlier colonizing attempts of Harriet Livermore, Clorinda Minor, and the Dickson family, the disintegration of the Adams community discouraged many American evangelists from settling permanently in Palestine. Yet one family—the Spaffords, profiled in a later chapter—would still attempt to create an American colony in Jerusalem, while other missionaries would establish schools and clinics throughout the country. The surge of Americans to Palestine—indeed, to the entire Middle East—continued to swell, animated not only by piety but by an insatiable yearning for adventure.

11

AMERICAN
ONSLAUGHT

A TOUR OF THE MIDDLE EAST, ONCE REGARDED AS A reckless jaunt, had by the post–Civil War era become a thoroughly respectable excursion. The decades after 1860 witnessed a tenfold expansion in the volume of Americans sailing abroad—not only missionaries but, in vastly larger numbers, tourists as well. Nearly two thousand travel books were published in the United States in this period and luxury steamers were booked well in advance. Most of these travelers headed for Europe, but a significant share also explored the Middle East. A visitor to Syria, Dr. Jacob Freese, attested that "the number of American travelers [here] far exceeds . . . those of any other nation," a fact confirmed by the artist Frederick Church, a founder of the Hudson River School. Arriving in Damascus in 1868, Church discovered that Americans had snatched up every available hotel room. "The few Englishmen here stand with their hands in their pockets and exclaim 'most extraordinary—these Americans!' " In Egypt, too, the number of American tourists had risen from an antebellum rate of sixty per year to nearly five hundred. By the early 1870s, Bedouin guides at the pyramids were purported to be speaking American-accented English and nicknaming their donkeys Yankee Doodle.

Lured by a significant reduction in fares and the shaving of the sailing time from New York to Egypt to a "mere" seventeen days, Americans journeyed eastward. Still, the advent of this "nomadic era," as *Putnam's Magazine* called it, could not alone account for the unprecedented American exodus. Rather, Americans continued to be drawn by mythic images of the Middle East, by "the perfumes of Arabia, the colors of Paradise," in the words of the travel writer Charles Dudley Warner, "this full-blown fantasia." The old frontier restiveness also enticed Americans eastward, especially now that the western frontier was vanishing. Most pressing, however, was the urge, after four years of bloodshed and scarcity, to venture out into the world, to accentuate life and celebrate it. "Ah, you Americans!" Foreign Minister Nubar Pasha of Egypt told Henry M. Field, a Massachusetts correspondent, in 1878. "You are the true Bedouins!"

Americans could sate their wanderlust by roaming the Middle East, but not without risking their health, if not their lives. Tourists remained an appealing target for brigands; Americans were still encouraged to engage bodyguards and to pack personal sidearms and knives. Ignoring that warning, a certain New Yorker named Klein tried to ford the Jordan by himself, but was forced by armed Bedouin to pay an "escort fee" of $7,000, a vertible fortune in 1878. Travel in the region was especially perilous for women who, alone and unveiled, often felt sexually threatened by their surroundings. The nationally acclaimed actress Rose Eytinge, on tour throughout the Middle East in the late 1860s, bristled at the need to cover her head whenever she went outdoors or to arrange a male escort—practices that she found "most irksome for an American woman . . . used to coming and going as she pleases." More hazardous for American travelers than robbery or sexual harassment, however, was disease. Dysentery remained the leading killer, taking the lives of Martha and Helen Woolsey, the daughters of the president of Yale, while crossing Lebanon in 1870. The Middle Eastern climate was "unfavorable for the foreigner, and often fatal to the tourist," according to the Damascus consul J. Augustus Johnson, who testified that "the graves of modern travelers and explorers may be seen from Dan to Beer Sheva, and from Jerusalem to Damascus." The consul in Alexandria complained that most of his time was taken up repatriating the remains of Americans who perished while sightseeing in Egypt.[1]

Undaunted by these dangers, Americans persisted in traversing the Middle East with abandon and even alacrity. The "Yankees" whom the Londoner Eliza Bush saw in Egypt in the 1870s seemed to have "few ideas between them all, except those of getting over the ground as quickly as they could," while her countryman John MacGregor marveled how "these cousins of ours do their sightseeing so uncommon quick." Even the American officers serving in Egypt were astounded by the immense volume of American visitors in the country, on the one hand, and, on the other, by the shallowness of their tours. "They usually come in caravans," remarked one of them, "are packed into hotels like sardines and are led around the country like sheep."

About the only time, it seemed, that Americans dallied in the Middle East was to desecrate or pillage its monuments. On pyramids and temples, tombs and obelisks, Americans left their mark in the form of brilliantly rendered Stars and Stripes and hieroglyphs hastily chiseled off. They also specialized in graffiti; one inscription in particular, "Powell Tucker, New York, 1870," adorned dozens of ancient sites. And what they could not steal or vandalize, Americans were ravenous to buy. "They often think with their purses, admire with their cheque-books and appreciate with their yawns," a former Confederate officer observed. Another expatriate in Egypt, a New Jersey merchant calling himself "Antiquity" Smith, took advantage of this craze for relics and made his fortune selling artifacts—real and manufactured—to Americans.

The disrespect that Americans displayed for the classical past of the Middle East was only exceeded by their contempt for its contemporary society. Much like antebellum visitors to the region, American tourists of the post–Civil War period continued to revile what they regarded as the inherent depravity and cruelty of Middle Eastern life. The perceived mistreatment of women, judged by Charles Dudley Warner as "the conclusive verdict against the religion of the prophet [Muhammad]," was still especially repugnant. Even while rushing through the region, Americans remained immovable in their sense of cultural superiority to the native population and in their expectation of deference from it. Blocked by a Muslim guard from entering Jerusalem's Tomb of David, for example, the previously pacific Dr. Freeze raged at the "disgrace to the civilization of the age" shown by this "miserable fellaheen," and called on Christian America to redress it "either by diplomacy or the sword."

The "ugly Americans" had indeed made their appearance in the Middle East, yet not all visitors to the region from the United States were gauche, destructive, or dismissive of Middle Eastern cultures. "The people . . . are a perpetual study for the excellence and grace of their forms and motion," commented Ralph Waldo Emerson, in May 1872, while cruising up the Nile. "The lateen sail is the shadow of a pyramid; and the pyramid is the simplest copy of a mountain." Making the same journey some years later, Frederick Douglass imagined that the descendants of the pyramid builders could help "combat American prejudice against the darker colored races of mankind," how the fiercely independent Arabs, "half brothers to the Negro," would serve as a model for "raising colored people . . . in their own estimation."[2]

Such affirmative remarks about the Middle East are virtually absent from the pre–Civil War travel literature and they testify to the tolerance and broad-mindedness of these towering men of ideas. But they also intimate the deeper humility wrought by the national torment of war. That modesty, coupled with curiosity, energy, and a yearning for life, accompanied a great many Americans to the Middle East in the aftermath of Appomattox. Their ranks would include not only lawyers, writers, and the leisured rich but also, for the first time, workers, schoolteachers, and clerks—the democratization of American travel. Joining them, too, would be some of the country's most illustrious figures, the helmsmen and heroes of the Civil War.

A Gorgeous Gleaming Pageant

"To the oppressed masses," William Henry Seward once proclaimed, "the United States is the Palestine from which comes . . . political salvation." Now, at age seventy, the former secretary of state was setting out for the genuine Holy Land, making him the most prominent American ever to visit the Middle East. This would be his second trip to the region. The first, it may be recalled, took place before the Civil War, during which the then Senator Seward acquired three Arabian stallions from Baghdad, plus a box of "antiquities" and a Bedouin spear. Over the course of the next decade, Seward had achieved fame as a firebrand abolitionist, as the statesman who helped dissuade Britain and France from recognizing the Confederacy, and as the negotiator who parlayed the purchase of Alaska. He survived a serious carriage accident in 1865 only to be hideously injured in an assassination attempt—part of the Booth conspiracy—that left him bedridden for a year. His wife and daughter died during that period, but Seward rebounded and returned to office, serving until 1869. A feebler man might have retired at that juncture, but in spite of short stature and receding chin, Seward was anything but fragile. No sooner had he departed from government than he boarded a steamer for Egypt.

His reception in the land of the Nile was extravagant. A train of plumed cavalry accompanied him to the pyramids, and royal vessels conveyed him past the ruin-lined banks of the Nile and across the modern Suez Canal. Though flattered by this attention, Seward remained critical of many aspects of Egyptian society. The sight of multiple wives and Africans slaves reminded him, unfavorably, of Mormonism and the Confederacy. Still, he applauded the khedive's attempts at political and social reforms. Addressing groups of young officers, Seward stressed the need for universal education in Egypt and for the creation of a native cadre capable of assuming the government posts that were then held exclusively by foreigners. Only then could Egypt be freed from its "double thralldom"—"first, to the Ottoman Porte, and second . . . to the Christian nations of Europe."

Leaving Egypt, Seward sailed northeast until he spotted the American flag furling over the U.S. consulate in Jaffa. Muscle-bound Arab stevedores bore him from his dinghy to the shore, where an imperial proclamation welcomed him as the "former chief minister of the Government of the Republic of the United States of North America." In the company of Ottoman horsemen, Seward proceeded up to Jerusalem, where he toured the dim and dust-choked halls of the Holy Sepulcher, the Western Wall with its clusters of Jewish worshippers, and the gleaming Mount of Olives. He reveled in the sacred scenery. Most inspiring for Seward, however, was a Jerusalem synagogue that had been built with donations from American Jews. Attending Sabbath services, he watched, mesmerized, as "a remarkable rabbi, clad in a long, rich, flowing sacerdotal dress," intoned Hebrew prayers first "for the President of the United States" and "the deliverance of the Union from its rebellious assailants." Though he might have revealed that the prayer had at least been partially answered, the visitor sat quietly as the congregation chanted a final benediction, for "Mr. Seward's health, [and] . . . his safe return to his native land."

Seward indeed headed back to the United States, but not before making a memorable stopover in Istanbul. On July 4, 1870, he presided over the Independence Day celebrations at Robert College. Together with the college president, Cyrus Hamlin, 150 students were there to greet him—the boys in dress whites and straw hats, the girls in linen gowns and sashes—regaling him with "My Country 'Tis of Thee" and "The Battle Hymn of the Republic." In a banquet room bedecked with crossed American and Turkish flags, after a Yankee repast of turkey, baked beans, and doughnuts, Seward spoke. "It used to be thought that all great ideas must go from the East westward," he began, "but men have already begun to see good coming from the West to the East." He went on to explain that Robert College exemplified the generosity that Americans were capable of exhibiting, even in wartime, and urged them to remain altruistic now that their nation was reunited. "It is not enough that the corporate existence of our country is maintained, if its national spirit is not also preserved and developed."[3] After watching a baseball game, played against the backdrop of the Bosphorus, Seward left Istanbul for a six-month spree through Europe. He returned, finally, fulfilled by his extraordinary travels, to his home in Auburn, New York, where he died the following year.

Seward's voyage set a precedent for other Civil War–era personages eager to make semiofficial visits to the Middle East. The most acute and observant of these was George B. McClellan, the onetime commander of the Army of the Potomac and failed presidential hopeful. Arriving in Alexandria in late October 1874, McClellan embarked on a one-hundred-day cruise up the Nile, pausing to pick his way through timeless ruins and to sample Bedouin hospitality. None of these experiences thrilled McClellan more, though, than a chance encounter with two American officers, Raleigh Colston and Erasmus Sparrow Purdy, on their way to survey the wilderness of Darfur. McClellan sentimentally remarked that, though "one had fought in the war in the Federal army, the other in that of the Confederates," the two Americans now sat amicably, "side by side on the banks [of the Nile]."

An exacting man, slight and dapper—"Little Napoleon," critics called him—McClellan passed stern judgments on Middle Eastern society. Though the Egyptians, he maintained, were a "kindly, intelligent, and industrious race," Islam had transformed them into a nation of dissemblers and religious fanatics. Most Muslims, he ventured, had "little but life to lose in this world, and much to gain in the other by entering it from a conflict with the unbeliever." On the other hand, Westerners would never understand Middle Eastern peoples "so long as we . . . judge them by the rules we are accustomed to apply to ourselves . . . [rather than] weigh their actions by their own rules." McClellan nevertheless believed that change could be effected gradually in the region, through education and widening exposure to the West.[4]

The American public voraciously followed the accounts of Seward's and McClellan's visits to the Middle East. Neither excursion, however, matched the sensation generated by the voyage of one of the Civil War's most colorful, and controversial, commanders. In March 1872, seven years after he marched his victorious troops through Alexandria, Virginia, General Sherman landed in Alexandria, Egypt, proffering tokens of peace.

Sherman's first impressions of the Egyptians were enthusiastic. "Their Faith in Mohamet commands respect," he wrote his son, Tommy, a student at Georgetown. He recalled that "twenty years ago . . . a Jew or Christian dog was hunted and stoned . . . and the pious Mosselman thought they were doing an act that would entitle them to reward in the World to come." Now, however, the Egyptians welcomed the Westerners who, "skilled as Mechanics," bring "steam engines to help the poor laborers . . . railroads that skim over the dry

John Ledyard, "a new character to the world" and the first citizen of an independent United States to explore the Middle East.

America's second international treaty, signed by Thomas Jefferson and John Adams and bearing the imperial seal of Morocco with the Islamic date of "Ramadan, 1200."

Professor George Bush, Hebrew scholar and author of *Valley of Vision* (1844), which advocated renewed Jewish statehood in Palestine, and an ancestor of two later U.S. presidents of the same name.

"The rovers who infest thy waves have seiz'd our ships and made our freemen slaves"—the poet-diplomat David Humphreys, who negotiated the release of American hostages in the Middle East in 1795.

Painted by Herring, from the Original by Stuart, in Yale College: Engrd by G. Parker.

DAVID HUMPHREYS, LL.D.

Joel Barlow, America's special emissary to the Barbary pirates. The dey of Algiers warned him, "I will put you in chains and declare war."

JOEL BARLOW.

George Sandys, treasurer of the Virginia colony and veteran mercenary in the Middle East. "I think there is not an object that promiseth so much," he wrote of the region, "[yet] so deceiveth."

The explorer of Persia in 1806 who speculated that Middle Eastern oil might someday be used as fuel—and discoverer of the flower that bears his name— Joel Roberts Poinsett.

William Bainbridge, the ill-starred captain who was forced to transport Algerian tribute and who lost his warship to Tripoli's pirates.

EDWARD PREBLE. U.S.N.

Edward Preble

"The Moors are a trecherous set of villains"—Commodore Edward Preble, commander of America's Mediterranean Squadron, 1803.

"My country right or wrong"—Stephen Decatur, the Navy's youngest captain and hero of America's 1815 victory in the Middle East.

Decatur in battle, 1805, driving pirates off the captured *Philadelphia*.

Another Early Nineteenth Century Print Showing Decatur Leading His Men to Drive the Pirates Off the Captured "Philadelphia"

An early champion of Zionism, and the first of many American Jewish emissaries to the Middle East, Mordecai Manuel Noah.

David "Sindbad" Porter, painted after the Barbary Wars and before his appointment as America's first ambassador to the Ottomans. "Salaams are an infernal nuisance," he snapped after meeting the sultan. "Why the devil can't the man be satisfied with a decent salute?"

The Washington socialite and revivalist preacher Harriet Livermore, who attempted to establish an American colony in Palestine in 1837. John Quincy Adams called her "the most eloquent speaker [he had] ever listened to."

Cyrus Hamlin, the industrial-minded missionary from Maine who moved to the Middle East in 1842 and founded the region's first modern university.

Eli Smith, linguist and inventor of "American Arabic" type, who recommended frequent visits by U.S. warships to the Middle East. "They ought to know that we are a power," he said.

ELI SMITH.

Warder Cresson, the quirky Jerusalem consul who, in the 1850s, traded "the sawdust of Christianity" for the "good old cheese itself" and converted to Judaism.

James Turner Barclay, physician, scientist, architect, and missionary to Palestine in 1850. "We will go with you," he pledged to the Jews, "for we have heard that the Lord is with you."

George Perkins Marsh, father of American conservationism and founder of the U.S. Army Camel Corps, created in 1857 to strike "a salutary terror" into "the Comanches and other Rocky Mt. Bedouins."

Memorial in Quartzite, Arizona, to the U.S. Camel Corps and its famed Arab guide, Hi Jolly (Haji Ali).

"Earnest Christian and lover of the adventure," U.S. Navy Captain William Francis Lynch, who in 1847 became the first Westerner to navigate the Jordan River from the Sea of Galilee to the Dead Sea.

Ismail Pasha, the Egyptian khedive who hired Civil War veterans to modernize his army. "When this shall be accomplished," he told them, "as it will be *Inshallah*, I will bestow upon you the highest honors."

Thaddeus Mott, mercenary, gold miner, and American recruiter for a Middle Eastern army.

Veteran of seventy-five battles and inspector general of the Egyptian army from 1869 to 1875, William Wing "Old Blizzards" Loring.

Charles Pomeroy Stone, the "American Dreyfus" and Civil War "soldier of misfortune" who served as Egypt's chief of staff and as senior engineer in constructing the Statue of Liberty.

The swashbuckling James Morris Morgan, Jefferson Davis's former bodyguard and soldier of Egypt, circa 1870.

Charles Chaillé-Long, the effete but effective explorer of the Nile in 1874. "The entire Nile basin passed under the protectorate of Egypt," he proclaimed, "and the chief object of my mission was accomplished."

Soldier and explorer of the Sudan, Erastus Sparrow Purdy.

A native of Indian River, Maine, who joined the George Adams colony and moved to Jaffa in 1866, Rolla Floyd became the first American tour guide in Palestine, accompanying—among other dignitaries—Ulysses S. Grant.

MODERN ICONOCLASTS AT WORK ON THE MONUMENTS OF ANCIENT EGYPT

American tourists chipping souvenirs from an ancient Egypt temple, "saving precious fragments from the ruin to which they are doomed."

"America is the Palestine of political salvation," wrote Secretary of State and American Middle East traveler William Henry Seward.

"A glorious gleaming pageant." Ulysses and Julia Grant visit Egypt in 1878.

An African-American preacher of peace in the Middle East, Edward Wilmot Blyden.

Lew Wallace, Civil War hero, hunter of Jesse James, and author of *Ben-Hur,* America's ambassador to the Ottomans in 1881.

An advertisement for the memoirs of Mark Twain's Middle Eastern travels, which sold over half a million copies—"right along with the Bible," he quipped.

An American consul in Alexandria, Elbert Eli Farman, procurer of Cleopatra's Needle and staunch opponent of the British conquest of Egypt.

deserts and telegraphs that carry messages from Cairo to Suez in a minute." Modern science, the former warrior predicted, would break down all barriers between the Middle East and the West and eradicate all prejudices.

Sherman's initial displays of amity, however, soon gave way to impatience with the Middle East and the more mercurial sides of his character. Cairo, he complained, was "a hard-looking old-adobe town" crammed with "a conglomeration of men women and children of some twenty different breeds with camels, donkeys, horses, dogs and vermin." He claimed that "our Negroes when slaves had better houses" and that Egyptian women were "bought and sold—like animals." Especially infuriating for Sherman were the Egyptians who thought themselves superior to the Westerners and who paid less attention to him than to his military escort, Lieutenant Frederick Grant, the president's son. He swore to "undertake to move the pyramids" rather than show respect to "a race that . . . look . . . and talk and act just like our Indians."

Sherman's ire would be quelled, albeit temporarily, by a visit from Generals Loring and Stone and by the personal tour of the Suez Canal he received from Ferdinand de Lesseps. The khedive Isma'il made further amends by restaging the opera *Aida* for Sherman's benefit and presenting him with a diamond brooch, at a combined cost of $200,000. But the extravagance of Sherman's reception in Egypt was outdone by the lavishness showered on him in Istanbul. Treated as a visiting head of state by Sultan Abdul Aziz, Sherman reviewed parade after parade of royal guardsmen, all armed with Winchester rifles, and flotillas of American-made warships. He also rode in trolley cars that had been imported from the United States—a year before their debut in San Francisco—and made a perfunctory visit to Robert College.[5]

Like Seward's before it, Sherman's journey signified the continued blending of American fantasies about the Middle East with America's rising prestige as an economic and military power. Not only private citizens like Jacob Freese and Charles Dudley Warner were visiting the region but also high-ranking officials, former and incumbent. And no tour more spectacularly demonstrated that synthesis than that of the ex-chief of all Union forces and the past president of the United States, Ulysses S. Grant, the most famous American of his time.

Grant had come a long way since his days as a failed farmer, fire-wood salesman, and real estate broker, surviving bankruptcy, bouts of alcoholism, political scandals, and some of the grisliest combat in human memory. Now, at age fifty-five and a private citizen, Grant was still an international celebrity, the first American since George Washington to have held his nation's supreme military and civilian offices. To commemorate that triumph, as well as to escape lingering accusations of corruption during his presidency, Grant and his wife, Julia, embarked on a world tour. Starting in Europe in May 1877 and continuing eastward, the trip was billed as "the most remark-able journey in all recorded history . . . like a romance."

Romance, on January 5, 1878, became reality as the USS *Vandalia* delivered the Grants to Alexandria. Many hours passed before they could leave the ship, however, as a seemingly limitless procession of officials came on board to salute them. Wrote Julia, "One might eas-ily think we were bombarding Alexandria in place of making a plea-sure visit." The exuberant reception continued once the party went ashore, where the carriage route was lined with thousands of well-wishers waving torches and lanterns and hailing the "king of Amer-ica." An immense banner proclaimed "Welcome General Grant," with the *n* in "Grant" turned upside down.

If Seward and Sherman received exclusive treatment, the Grants' reception was, fittingly, presidential. The couple was given use of the fabulous Qasr al-Muzha—the Little Palace of Pleasures—and a full-time liveried staff. "We had only to clap our hands and lo! A servant dressed in white approached with noiseless steps," Julia recalled. The couple proceeded to visit the usual sights and provided Egyptians with some unprecedented ones, among them that of a former head of state and his wife bouncing toward the pyramids on donkeyback. They cruised up the Nile, shooting hyenas and crocodiles and croon-ing "Rally Round the Flag, Boys" and the "Star Spangled Banner."

Egypt, for the Grants, was a chiaroscuro of splendor and decay. Staring at the Sphinx, Grant remarked, "It looks as if it has kept on thinking through all eternity without talking too much," and concluded, "I have seen more to interest me in Egypt than in any of my travels." Julia, though, was less charmed. "One could not but reflect here on the emptiness, frailty and vanity of the works of man," she brooded. "Egypt, the birthplace, the cradle of civilization—Egypt, the builder of temples, tombs and the great pyramids—has nothing."

Ancient visages certainly excited Grant, but not as visibly as those from his own distant past. "Why there's Loring, whom I haven't seen for thirty years," he exclaimed, taking the remaining hand of the officer who had fought by his side in the Mexican War and against him in the war between North and South. "And there's Stone, who must have been dyeing his hair to make it so white." A less felicitous encounter, however, occurred between Grant and the daughter of General Robert E. Lee, Mary, who happened to be visiting Egypt as well. A spirited woman, she refused to dine with her father's former nemesis, snapping, "I wouldn't sit down at the same table with General Grant to save his life." Instead, she climbed to the top of the Great Pyramid and waved the Confederate flag.[6]

Following the traditional American path through the Middle East, from Egypt the Grants ascended to Palestine. Julia found Jaffa to be "a poor place and very dirty," but her husband continued to exude excitement. The Holy Land, he reckoned, could "feed all that portion of the Mediterranean," if only it were tilled by Americans. Guided by Rolla Floyd, the Adams colony veteran, the pair began the scenic climb to Jerusalem. Bedouin and villagers clothed in what looked to the visitors like biblical dress lined the road, cheering. "The General's head was bared nearly all of the time in acknowledgement of the salutes as we passed," Julia noted. The most remarkable sight, however, welcomed them outside the Old City walls: a double row of mounted soldiers and blaring military band, "a gorgeous gleaming pageant."[7]

Ulysses S. Grant departed Palestine for Istanbul, where, once again, he was regaled as royalty, feted nightly, taken for tours of the bazaar and reviews of Turkish troops armed with Civil War swords and carbines. His trip to the Middle East, like those of Seward and Sherman preceding it, established a paradigm for many such visits by American leaders over the next century and a half. The schedule would invariably be hectic and the need to maintain appearances unrelieved. For Grant, the only respite from the frenzied pace lay in reading a book he brought with him from home. Set largely in the Middle East, the volume was not, however, the Bible or a missionary's correspondence but rather the scathing travelogue by Samuel Langhorne Clemens, better known as Mark Twain.

Innocence Lost

Cairo, for Twain, was an Illinois city bordering the Mississippi River, the Grand Turk was a steamboat, and "Arab" was a derogatory name for dockworkers. A onetime Confederate militiaman, riverboat pilot, and prospector, he had spent much of his thirty-two years moving as far west of his native Missouri as possible, with scarcely a thought about turning back east, much less to the Middle East. Nor did he have any particular yearning to see the Holy Land. Though raised a strict Presbyterian and respectably versed in the Bible, he lacked "the necessary stock in trade—i.e., religion"—to become a preacher, and detested the missionaries who made people "permanently miserable by telling them . . . how blissful a place heaven is, and [how] nearly impossible it is to get there." Yet Twain also suffered from the frontiersman's restlessness, and, by the spring of 1867, in spite of his more than forty sea voyages and a recent junket to Hawaii, he was "tired of staying in one place." Just then, he learned of the first-ever luxury around-the-world cruise, with stopovers in Morocco, Egypt, and Palestine. The itinerary excited him, evoking images recalled from his favorite childhood book, *A Thousand and One Arabian Nights*. Elatedly he wrote his mother, "I . . . welcome the wind that wafts a weary soul to the sunny lands of the Mediterranean!"

By that time, the hawk-nosed, mustachioed Twain was fast gaining fame in San Francisco for his sardonic vignettes on American life and his lecturing as "the Wild Humorist of the Pacific Slope." The cruise, organized by "prominent Brooklynites" and billed as a "picnic on a gigantic scale" with public figures such as the Reverend Henry Ward Beecher and General Sherman participating, seemed the perfect grist for satire. Twain accordingly appealed to two papers, San Francisco's *Alta California* and the *New York Tribune*, offering to submit regular dispatches from the voyage in exchange for the $1,250 ticket. "Isn't it a most attractive scheme?" he reasoned. "Five months of utter freedom from care and anxiety of every kind, and in company with a set of people who will go only to enjoy themselves, and will never mention a word about business." The editors readily agreed and on June 8, toting "green spectacles, umbrellas, veils for Egypt . . . and substantial clothing for rough pilgrimizing in the Holy Land," Twain boarded the *Quaker City*, a sidewheel steamer equipped with every convenience, including cannon for saluting royalty.

Neither Beecher nor Sherman was among the passengers, however, and instead of celebrities, Twain found a number of innocuous Americans, most of them middle-aged midwesterners. More disappointingly, in place of license to "scamper about the decks by day, filling the ship with shouts and laughter," and at night to "dance, and promenade, and smoke, and sing, and make love," the passengers received Plymouth Hymnals and invitations to attend daily services in a cabin that Twain quietly dubbed "the Synagogue." The so-called Grand Holy Land Pleasure Excursion, the satirist complained, "was a funeral without a corpse," and recommended that its name be changed to "The Grand Holy Land Funeral Procession."[8]

Twain nevertheless managed to make friends with some of the passengers ("eight out of the sixty-five"), and especially with two women journalists, Mary Fairbanks and Emily Severance, who expunged his off-color correspondence and curbed his more raucous behavior. The ship, meanwhile, crossed the Atlantic to its first destination, Tangier, where Consul James De Long had arrested the Confederate emissaries Myers and Tunstall five years earlier. "Travel is fatal to prejudice, bigotry, and narrow-mindedness," Twain asserted, disingenuously, as he entered the exotic Moroccan port.

'Isn't it an oriental picture?" Twain began and went on to describe the "packed and jammed city . . . of snowy tombs" and the "swarms of humanity . . . foreign and curious to look upon." Like so many American writers before him, he castigated Middle Eastern regimes

for their presumed corruption, dismissing the emperor of Morocco
as a "soulless despot" who mistreated his subjects, even his wives.
"[He] thinks he has five hundred [wives] . . . a dozen or so, one way
or the other, don't matter." He resented the supposed refusal of Muslims to allow "Christian dogs" to enter their houses and mosques
and recoiled from the cruelty of cutting off the legs and hands of
criminals. "They slice around the bone a little, then break off the
limb. Sometimes the patient gets well; but, as a general thing, he
don't." Yet even a captious observer like Twain could not be immune
to the city's romantic lure. "Tangier is a foreign land if ever there was
one," he admitted, "and the true spirit of it can never be found in
any book save The Arabian Nights."

In his criticism as well as his revelry, Twain indeed resembled earlier American visitors to the Middle East, yet one characteristic distinguished his writing from that of all other tourists. Whereas his
predecessors looked at the region and saw in its brutality and backwardness an inverse image of their own tolerance and refinement,
the mirror, for Twain, showed Americans to be equally small-minded
and crude. Seven years earlier, before the Civil War, American readers might have objected to such an unflattering depiction. But the
violent deaths of 600,000 soldiers forced Americans to look at themselves, to question whether they indeed retained any claim to innocence or the right to call any other culture uncivilized. Twain advised
his countrymen to prefer a death sentence to residence in the Middle
East, yet he also consoled those Middle Eastern peoples overrun by
that "strange horde . . . that called themselves Americans and seemed
to imagine . . . that they had a right to be proud of it."[9]

Leaving Tangier, the *Quaker City* embarked on a meandering
course toward the eastern Mediterranean that brought it back to
Europe and the French port of Marseille. Twain took the railroad to
Paris and arrived in time to watch a parade staged by Napoleon III
in honor of the visiting Ottoman sultan. The event provided the
writer with a platform for previewing his impressions of the Turkish
empire, well before he even reached it. While heaping encomium on
the puny French autocrat who had so recently invaded Mexico—the
epitome of "modern civilization, progress, refinement"—Twain
unleashed an invective against Abdul Aziz:

. . . a short, stout, dark man, black-bearded, black-eyed, stupid, unprepossessing . . . the representative of a . . . government whose Three Graces are Tyranny, Rapacity, Blood. . . . Born to a throne; weak, stupid, ignorant, almost, as his meanest slave; chief of a vast royalty . . . who holds in his hands the power of life and death over millions—yet who sleeps, sleeps, eats, eats, idles with his eight hundred concubines . . . [and] who believes in gnomes and genii and the wild fables of The Arabian Nights, but has small regard for the mighty magicians of today and is nervous in the presence of their mysterious railroads and steamboats and telegraphs.

As a satirist and social commentator, Twain rarely had kind words for any ethnic or religious group, yet his disdain for Muslims was unrivaled. A "filthy, brutish, ignorant, unprogressive, superstitious people," he alleged, the followers of Allah were also deluded by the "wild fables of The Arabian Nights." Such imprecations reflected deep-rooted American prejudices against Islam, as well as Twain's tendency to impute to Muslims a belief in the Middle Eastern myths to which he, in fact, subscribed. The extent of those illusions would become unequivocally clear to Twain when the *Quaker City* anchored in Istanbul.

The sense of otherness again proved bewildering for Twain. The streets all seemed mazelike to him and the people, dressed "in all the outrageous, outlandish, idolatrous, extravagant, thunder-and-lightning costumes," appeared kaleidoscopic. He complained about the plethora of graveyards and mosques, the dearth of whiskey, and the omnipresence of freaks—"the three-legged woman and the man with the eye in his cheek . . . the dwarf with seven fingers on each hand, no upper lip, and his underjaw gone." No number of negative adjectives, it seemed, could express Twain's disgust. Especially revolting were the Turkish baths of which he had long dreamed, but which he now found "vast, naked, dreary," with "nothing of romance, nothing of oriental splendor." Still, while wandering through the outdoor market, ambling between hawkers and camels and waterpipe-smoking sheikhs, Twain could almost forget his disenchantment. "The picture lacks nothing," he relented. "It casts you back at once into your forgotten boyhood, and again you dream over the wonders of The Arabian Nights."

Twain's aversion toward all things Middle Eastern only thickened the more deeply he penetrated the region. The city of Damascus, which looked to him like "an island of pearls and opals gleaming out of a sea of emeralds" from the distance, up close became "the very sink of pollution and uncomeliness." The Syrian men he encountered were a "wretched nest of human vermin," a hodgepodge of "rags, dirt, sunken cheeks, pallor of sickness, sores, [and] projecting bones," and the women so ugly they "couldn't smile after ten o'clock Saturday night without breaking the Sabbath." He scoffed at the ignorance of his Bedouin guides and at their vexingly unpronounceable names. Despairing of Arabic, Twain simply referred to all natives collectively as "Ferguson" and to their villages as "Jonesborough." He admitted, unhappily, "To glance at the genuine son of the desert is to take the romance out of him forever."[10]

From Syria, Twain and his party followed the usual American route into Palestine, but there the confluence ended. Although few travelers had dared to describe the Holy Land in anything less than superlatives, Twain maligned Palestine as a "hopeless, dreary, heart-broken land," its villages "frescoed . . . with disks of camel dung" and its roads more rock strewn than the stony countryside. "If all the poetry . . . upon the . . . bland scenery of this region were collected in a book, it would make a most valuable volume to burn," he surmised. Like many Americans before him, raised on bigger-than-life Bible stories, Twain was disappointed by the minuscule size of Palestinian sites—the Jordan, which he estimated to be about half the width of most American streets, and the Sea of Galilee, which he deemed so tiny that he refused to pay the exorbitant boatfare across. "Is it any wonder that Christ walked?" Three Palestines, he reckoned, could fit comfortably into the state of Missouri, with possibly room for a fourth.

In Palestine, Twain's impudence rapidly descended into sacrilege and nowhere more blasphemously than in Jerusalem. Bereft of any holiness, the city was a "mournful and dreary and lifeless" place for Twain, "grimy and impoverished," and teeming with lepers, idiots, and the blind. He seemed to derive pleasure in deriding the pilgrims, the Presbyterians in particular, who vainly came searching for their dream of a Promised Land only to find this waste heap. He debated whether to lie to his readers and relate how he tore himself "reluctantly away from . . . Palestine," but then reconsidered and wrote, "One is *glad* to get away."

In the end, though, not even Mark Twain—caustic, iconoclastic, outrageous—could suppress his admiration for the men and women who "journeyed thousands and thousands of miles, in weariness and tribulation" in order to "sail upon the hallowed sea and kiss the holy soil that compassed about it." An avowed secularist who routinely scorned Scripture, Twain could not resist purchasing a leather-bound Bible in Istanbul and reading it throughout his trip, and buying a second for his mother in Jerusalem. Nor could he deny the sense of "vagueness and mystery and ghostliness" that occasionally seized him in Palestine: "I am sitting where a god has stood, and looking upon the brook and the mountains which that god looked upon, and am surrounded by dusky men and women whose ancestors saw him, and even talked with him, face-to-face."

Behind his glibness lurked Twain's longing for the unconquerable faith of his forebears, that purity which he and so many of his generation had lost. "I cannot comprehend this," he again confessed before departing the Holy Land. "The gods of my understanding have always been hidden in clouds."[11]

The *Quaker City* at last steamed out of Jaffa, but not before taking on board forty new passengers—children, old people, recently married couples—all of them Americans. These were the survivors of the Indian River colony, simple people who, Twain related, had been "shamefully humbugged by their prophet," George Adams. The sight of these dejected and half-starved naïfs symbolized for Twain the pitiful illusions with which Americans approached the Middle East and Palestine in particular. "Palestine is no more of this workaday world," he concluded; "it is dreamland."

Still, Twain made one last Middle Eastern stop, Egypt, which proved to be anticlimactic. With his vitriol toward Muslim civilization spent, much of Twain's denigration aimed at the American tourists who "infested" the hotels and the "American vandals" who chipped off pieces of Pompey's Pillar with sledgehammers. Departing

Alexandria, finally, the *Quaker City* turned toward home, its passengers outfitted in "Moorish haiks, Turkish fezzes, sashes from Persia." Other souvenirs included orange tree seedlings that one enterprising tourist managed to replant and cultivate in Florida and several mummies later put on display in P. T. Barnum's museum. Of all the Americans who disembarked in New York on November 19, 1868, however, none was more enriched by the Middle Eastern sojourn than Mark Twain. The book he wrote about that excursion soon made him America's most celebrated author.

Compiled from his dispatches, *The Innocents Abroad; or, The New Pilgrims' Progress* earned Twain more than $300,000, selling half a million copies—"right along with Bible," he quipped. The title was vintage Twain, glib and ironic, for the excursion was hardly a pilgrimage and its participants anything but innocent. Readers nevertheless embraced that paradox, this "gospel of sincerity," as one of Twain's early biographers labeled it, secure in their war-born worldliness. The Barbary Wars fifty years earlier had helped Americans define themselves and now, after a vastly bloodier conflict, an American in the Middle East had sharpened—and darkened—that definition.

The publication of *The Innocents Abroad* launched Twain's career as an immensely successful novelist, essayist, and social commentator. He also became the publisher and friend of Ulysses Grant, who had read the book throughout his Middle East travels. But Twain would never again write about the region. He began a farce about an American convert to Islam who establishes a harem on the Mississippi, and an *Arabian Nights* spoof in which Scheherazade saves herself by boring a king with her tales, but completed neither.[12] Having seen the reality, apparently, Twain could no longer romanticize about the Middle East, even humorously.

MARK TWAIN may have dispelled the fantasy of Americans *in* the Middle East, but he could not extinguish their fantasies *of* the Middle East. Full vent to these was given on September 26, 1872, at the inauguration of the Ancient Arabic Order of the Nobles of the Mystic Shrine, a fraternal offshoot of the Masons. Founded by Dr.

Walter Fleming, a former Civil War surgeon, and the actor Billy Florence, who had performed in Cairo and Algiers, the "Shriners" adopted the scimitar and crescent as their emblems and the fez as their headgear. Their first temple was called Mecca, and entering it, initiates greeted one another with the Arabic salutation "Es Selamu Aleikum"—peace be upon you. The organization, though initially focused on fun, eventually became philanthropic and, a century later, could boast of half a million members and twenty-two hospitals specializing in pediatrics and burn care.

For the broader American public, too, illusions of Middle East remained rife. Among the most popular attractions at the 1876 Centennial Exhibition in Philadelphia was the "Egypt-Soodan" pavilion. Under a banner proclaiming "the oldest people of the world sends its morning greetings to the youngest nation," visitors viewed a replica of Ramses' temple and two thousand samples of Egyptian cotton. Proceeding to the Turkish pavilion, they could sip bittersweet cups of coffee and purchase "genuine" Ottoman items such as carpets, swords, and, of course, fezzes. The most alluring display, however, was a domed Moroccan villa set with intricate, inlaid wood imported—so the sponsors claimed—"from Tangier, that somnolent country so ludicrously described by Mark Twain."[13]

Whether welcoming each other in Arabic, buying fezzes at a fair, or laughing at the satire in *The Innocents Abroad*, Americans were still enchanted by the Middle East, or rather by the mecca of myths that, in their imaginations at least, it remained.

12

RESURGENCE

AMERICANS COULD NOW AFFORD TO FANTASIZE. REUNITED after an excruciating fission, they stood on the brim of a second industrial revolution, much mightier than the first, a burst of production that would propel them to world leadership in the export of machinery, textiles, and oil. The country's population, enriched by waves of immigrants, would swell 40 percent in the decades following the Civil War and fan out across thirty-seven states. Though dispersed, the American people were linked by more than a quarter million miles of railway, telegraph lines, and, by 1880, some 133,000 telephones as well. In steel production, American mills were ambitiously closing the gap with Europe and allocating a growing share of their output to weaponry and armor-plated battleships. This great fusion of energy could hardly be contained by North America. Now, with its western frontier largely settled, the country cast its attention beyond its continental borders, toward Central America, the Pacific, and the Far East. If not yet an imperial power in France's and Britain's league, the United States nevertheless commanded a role in international affairs.

In the Middle East, that role had traditionally been one of liberator, a champion of minority rights and of the independence of

Ottoman provinces like Greece and Hungary. Having paid such an agonizing price for their own national integrity, the American people felt entitled—indeed, compelled—to secure those benefits for others. Their beneficence, moreover, would now be backed by military and economic muscle. In spite of the carpetbagging corruption associated with Reconstruction, not withstanding the persistent prejudice against African Americans in the North and racist legislation in the South, and the final suppression of Native American tribes in the West, Americans would bring freedom to the East.

Stars and Stripes in the Empire of the Half-Moon

Though the documentary record on the episode is vague, the first American attempt to assist the Arabs in achieving independence occurred in Syria in 1868. Charles Lamar, Andrew Romer, and a certain Colonel O'Reilly, all Civil War veterans, led eighty Arabs in a revolt against Ottoman rule. Armed with breechloading rifles and howitzers, the rebels clashed with a superior Ottoman force near the Syrian city of Hamma. The fighting was savage and, after the rebels' camels were killed, Romer and Lamar fell prisoner. The two were cast into tiny, dank cells situated next to privies and then sent in chains to Istanbul, where they languished behind bars for months. The Damascus consul J. Augustus Johnson worried that the incident would give Middle Eastern peoples the impression "that Americans sympathize with . . . efforts to overthrow despotic governments" and encourage them to revolt. In contrast to the European powers, Johnson stressed, America's mission in the area was "one of humanity and not policy."[1]

Johnson's admonition proved accurate: the image of Americans as freedom fighters indeed proliferated. By the late 1860s, nationalist forces battling against the Ottomans on the island of Crete were appealing to Congress for military and humanitarian assistance. The Baha'is of Baghdad sought America's help in rescuing their venerable leader, Baha'u'llah, from Turkish exile. Washington, meanwhile, continued to show solicitude for oppressed Jewish communities throughout the Middle East—in Palestine, Persia, and North Africa. President Rutherford B. Hayes told Congress in December 1880 that the United States had "lost no opportunity" to pressure the emperor of Morocco to respect the rights of his Jewish subjects. "It is to America, the great pioneer of liberty and equality, that this unfortunate people lift up their eye," the grateful Jews of Casablanca said in thanking the State Department. "The stars and stripes of America will shine brilliantly in the empire of the half-moon," the leaders of Jerusalem Jewry declared. "The United States will forever be blessed by the chosen people in the sacred spot of our common ancestors."[2]

American concern for the victims of Middle Eastern intolerance was especially keen in Bulgaria. Though never considered part of the Middle East, the country was still an Ottoman province when, in 1876, Turkish troops massacred some 15,000 Bulgarian Christians. To investigate the atrocity, the State Department sent an urbane diplomat, Eugene Schuyler, translator of Turgenev and recipient of Yale's first Ph.D., to Sofia and its environs. "In Paniguischte 3,000 people killed by . . . regular troops," read one of Schuyler's daily reports, dated August 14. "Almost all women ravished, also boys and old men." Similar dispatches were filed by Januarius Aloysius MacGahan, an American of quite a different stripe, a bearded, bear-like newspaperman from Pigeon Roost Ridge, Ohio. MacGahan's articles, reprinted in the *New York Times*, described "the remains of babes and little children slaughtered by the hundreds, of immense heaps of bodies of maidens—first violated and then murdered—of . . . churches packed full of corpses." The testimonies of Schuyler and MacGahan proved pivotal in turning international opinion against Turkey and emboldening the Russians to attack the Ottomans in 1878—a war during which MacGahan lost his life to typhus. Bulgaria subsequently attained its independence, adopting a constitution drafted by Schuyler and several graduates of Robert College, the American school on the Bosphorus.[3]

Not since the signing of the U.S.-Ottoman treaty fifty years earlier had the United States expressed such open displeasure with the Porte. The dissatisfaction, moreover, was mutual; Schuyler was declared persona non grata and banished from Ottoman lands. Such friction, however, never interfered with the daily conduct of diplomacy between the two nations or the pursuit of lucrative trade. On August 4, 1873, the Ottomans opened the first Middle Eastern embassy in Washington, while American warships visiting Istanbul were regularly received with cannonades and Turkish band renditions of "The Battle Hymn of the Republic." In 1877 alone, the United States imported some $167,000 worth of opium, spices, and various "bazaar items" from the Ottoman Empire and supplied it with over $4.5 million in oil and military goods. Cyrus Hamlin reveled in reporting that Turkey "now gets its . . . Martini-Henry rifles from Providence, Rhode Island, and its ammunition from New Haven, Connecticut!"

The United States was projecting its influence through other and more distant parts of the region as well. In December 1879, the USS *Ticonderoga* became the first American warship to pass through the Strait of Hormuz and enter the Persian Gulf. Penetrating what had previously been considered an exclusively British lake, the sloop steamed sixty miles up the Shatt al-Arab waterway to the ports of Basra and Bushire. For the *Ticonderoga* commander Robert Wilson Shufeldt, this display of American strength aimed not only to claim new markets but also to promulgate American ideas. "There is no place in the world where the physical manifestation of power is so necessary for the diffusion of the knowledge . . . of a civilized Nation," Shufeldt, who had previously captained the steamboat *Quaker City*, proclaimed.

America's ability to assert itself in the Middle East was illustrated by a diplomatic incident that took place in 1881 and which nearly ignited a crisis. The setting was the sultan's palace in Istanbul where Lew Wallace, a former Union general, had come to present his credentials as the new American ambassador. Ironically, Wallace had replaced the ex-Confederate commander James Longstreet, who had failed to make an impression on his Turkish hosts, and was determined to succeed in his post. But instead of gaining admittance to the palace, Wallace was kept waiting in the antechamber. Such discourtesy was standard practice, his dragoman explained, intended to teach Westerners their place.

A formidable presence, in spite of his bookish specs and whiskers, Wallace had fought in some of the bloodiest Civil War fighting, and, as New Mexico's governor, had once hunted Billy the Kid. In addition to physical bravery, Wallace evinced strong religious views, which, when combined with a fecund imagination, had recently inspired him to write the best-selling novel *Ben-Hur*. He was a man accustomed to dispensing—and receiving—respect, not to being denigrated. As if back in battle, Wallace brusquely pushed through palace guards, burst into the imperial chamber, and marched straight toward the sultan.

Unlike his reform-minded predecessors, Abdul Mejid and Abdul Aziz, the new sultan, Abdul Hamid II, was archly conservative and chronically suspicious of the West. He glowered at the brash intruder, ignoring the dragoman who kowtowed and begged forgiveness for his master's impudence. Wallace, meanwhile, remained at attention, with his hand rigidly proffered. Anxious moments passed before the sultan's scowl slowly curved into a smile. Then, stepping forward and declaring him *doghru adam dir*—a forthright man—Abdul Hamid shook the American's hand.[4]

Wallace would have other opportunities to protest Ottoman practices and to demonstrate American mettle in the Middle East. Throughout much of the remaining decades of the nineteenth century, however, the major challenge to American ascendancy in the region stemmed not from the Porte but rather from the European powers. Rankled by what they regarded as an alien encroachment into an exclusively European sphere, the powers would attempt to block Americans from expanding their influence virtually everywhere in the Ottoman Empire. A foretaste of that friction occurred in Egypt, where the Europeans opposed one American's attempt to acquire a Middle Eastern memento and to share it with his fellow citizens back home.

A Generous Mark of International Regard

This was no mundane American, but the railroad magnate William H. Vanderbilt, the embodiment of Mark Twain's "Gilded Age" of excess, wealth, and optimism. Impressed by the honors that Egypt had lavished on Grant and learning that Paris, London, and Rome had each obtained an ancient Egyptian obelisk, Vanderbilt asked the

State Department to help him procure a similar monument for his own native city of New York. The department agreed and instructed its consul in Alexandria, Elbert Eli Farman, to request an audience with Isma'il.

"The population of the United States is approaching fifty million, and the time is not distant when it will be double that number," Farman told the khedive, Isma'il. Many of these millions would eventually visit New York, the consul explained, and "should an obelisk be erected there . . . they would learn something of its ancient history, and [that] it was a gift of His Highness to the people of the United States." An Amherst-educated attorney from Warsaw, New York, Farman at forty-eight possessed the high forehead, sentient eyes, and copious beard of a philosopher. In the three years since his appointment, he had worked closely with American missionaries to help free African slaves from their Egyptian masters, to the annoyance of local authorities. Farman nevertheless succeeded in cultivating a warm and candid relationship with Isma'il and had no difficulty telling him outright of Vanderbilt's request. The United States had two obelisks in mind, the consul said, one at Luxor and the other at Karnak.

Indebted to the American officers and educators who had contributed to Egypt's defense and welfare, eager to diminish the status of his European creditors by raising that of the United States, Isma'il readily obliged. He mentioned an obelisk even more impressive than those at Karnak and Luxor—the 3,000-year-old granite monument that had once adorned the Temple of Caesar in Alexandria and that was popularly known as Cleopatra's Needle. The obelisk could be taken, free of charge, "another souvenir," he said, "of the friendship that has constantly existed between the Government of the United States and that of the Khedive."

News of Isma'il's offer captivated America. The needle, Farman stressed, was indeed of better quality and greater historical significance than the obelisks given to Britain and France, and its transfer to New York would "long remain one of the marked events of history." President Hayes triumphantly told Congress that the gift represented "a generous mark of international regard" for the entire nation.

In praising Egypt's generosity, though, the president failed to anticipate Europe's resentment of American inroads into the Middle East. First, the Italians claimed that they owned the property under the obelisk and objected to its removal. Britain and France next insisted that all Egyptian property, artifacts included, belonged to them as security against Isma'il's debt. "It is not for Europeans, whose capitals are enriched with the treasures of Ancient Egypt, to say that not a single monument should be taken to the United States," Farman protested. Public opinion in the United States was also incensed. The European powers, the *New York Herald* warned, would "point the finger of scorn at us and intimate that we could never rise to any real moral grandeur until we had our obelisk."

European interference in Egypt's internal affairs meanwhile escalated, along with demands for Isma'il's removal. The ruler finally received a letter addressed to the "ex-Khedive" informing him of his "abdication." The soft-spoken visionary who once aspired to transform Egypt into an independent, Western-style country, who built theaters and canals, and who brought American officers to help modernize his army was replaced by his more pliable son, Tawfiq. Also eliminated was America's chance to receive an obelisk. Vanderbilt, however, refused to truckle to European fiat. He sent a former naval officer, Henry Honeychurch Gorringe, to Alexandria with instructions to rebuff all attempts at interference and to retrieve the obelisk at once.

Like Vanderbilt, Gorringe, innovative and robust, personified the new American age. Earning an officer's commission under fire during the Civil War, he rose to the rank of lieutenant commander and, as captain of the USS *Gettysburg*, escorted Ulysses Grant on his Middle Eastern tour. Gorringe was also an enthusiastic member of the Masons and shared their attachment to ancient Middle Eastern monuments. Arriving in Egypt in October 1879, he spent the next nine months laboring to extract the obelisk and its fifty-ton pedestal. With the help of one hundred local workmen and a winch once used to build the Brooklyn Bridge, he dredged 1,730 cubic yards of earth from around the obelisk's base. Detached, the seventy-foot-long needle was then hauled overland to an Egyptian steamer and inserted into its specially perforated hull. The operation cost over $100,000, but Vanderbilt covered all expenses, and in July 1880 the obelisk was ready to sail.

"It would be absurd for the people of any great city to hope to be happy without an Egyptian Obelisk," the *New York Herald* now chimed. Ballasted by cannonballs and sliding on iron tracks, the cargo descended onto the docks of New York harbor at West Fifty-first Street. From there, a team of thirty-two horses dragged it across town to Fifth Avenue and up to Eighty-second Street, where the train entered the sylvan confines of Central Park. Restlessly waiting on Graywacke Knoll, behind the newly built Metropolitan Museum of Art, were twenty thousand exhilarated New Yorkers, among them Secretary of State William Maxwell Evarts.

A son of the secretary of the American Board, Evarts was a pious man and a zealous supporter of Middle Eastern missions. Rising to address the crowd, though, he adopted a tone that was less religious than philosophical. Looking out over the sea of derby hats, parasols, and bonnets, Evarts wondered aloud whether any country, even one prosperous enough to buy an obelisk, could resist the forces of decadence. "Can you expect to flourish forever?" he asked. "Can you expect wealth to accumulate and man not to decay?"

Evarts's gravitas was lost in the cheers of the crowd. His listeners were more captivated by the consequence of the moment than by the contemplation of history—more conscious of their country's achievements of the past twenty years than apprehensive about its future. Riven during the Civil War, the American people were once again united and rising to world prominence. In the Middle East, as elsewhere in the world, the United States would be acknowledged as a formidable economic and military force. European nations would no longer seek to deny Americans the right to pursue their interests in the region or to establish relations with native rulers. That ascendancy was now heralded by a ground-shaking thud as cranes lowered the 220-ton monolith into its original pedestal. America's obelisk was confidently erected, looming over the east.[5]

Part Four

THE AGE OF IMPERIALISM

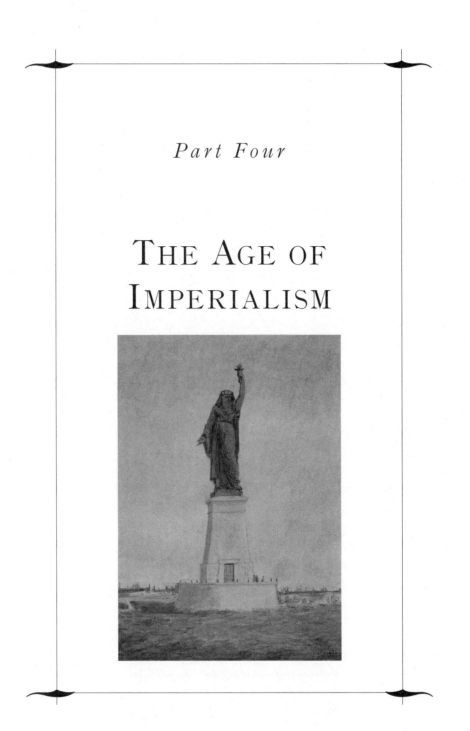

13

EMPIRES AT
DAWN

AWAKENING AT SUNRISE ON JULY II, 1882, THE INHABI-
tants of Alexandria, Egypt, could see an ominous line of silhouettes
stretched across the Mediterranean's horizon. Word of the mirage-
like sight filtered quickly through the city and soon throngs of curious citizens gathered on the docks. Peasants, clerks, and merchants
gazed wordlessly out at the specter hovering just beyond the harbor,
while platoons of anxious artillerymen scurried around their guns.
Many of them understood that the history of their nation, if not that
of the entire Middle East, was about to be altered. The political
upheavals that had long shaken Egypt, fracturing its pride and its
dreams of independence, were erupting.

The tremors had intensified over a three-year period, during
which the European powers declared Egypt insolvent, ousted Khedive Isma'il, and installed the more malleable Tawfiq. This flagrant
interference in Egyptian affairs sparked opposition from the swelling
ranks of Egyptian nationalists led by a charismatic colonel, Ahmad
'Urabi. Of peasant stock and a strict Islamic background, the
brawny, broad-nosed, and mustachioed 'Urabi was Egypt's highest-
ranking native officer. Vowing "Egypt for the Egyptians," he sought
to oust the Turkish elite that still controlled the army and free Egypt

of all its foreign debts. The khedive and his European creditors consequently conspired to have 'Urabi arrested. The colonel would not be silenced, however, and by 1882, he was threatening to unseat the khedive. Riots in support of 'Urabi broke out in Cairo and Alexandria and spread toward the Suez Canal. Fearing for the safety of its nationals in Egypt and, above all, for the security of its precious canal, Britain resolved to intervene.

The phantomlike forms aligned off Egypt's coast that July morning gradually came into focus: British battleships. At precisely 6:50 a.m., blinding flashes suddenly illuminated their decks. Seconds later, with deafening shrieks and numbing explosions, salvos of large-caliber shells smashed into the twisting alleys and elegant parks of Alexandria. The spectators on the docks instantly scattered and the city's famously bustling streets emptied. But the Egyptian army held its ground. Over one hundred guns, many positioned strategically in well-camouflaged bunkers built by the American Civil War veterans, raked the British fleet. Yet not even Alexandria with its redoubtable fortifications could withstand a concerted bombardment from the Royal Navy's ironclads. One by one, the shore batteries were silenced, and their shell-shocked defenders dispersed. By 5:30 that evening the battle was over. Hundreds of people—soldiers and civilians—had been killed and multiples of that number wounded. The British occupation of Egypt, destined to last some seventy-two years, had begun.

Ambivalent Legacy

Gruesome though it was, the invasion of Egypt was merely one milestone in an imperialist process that would bring about the conquest of a quarter of the world's landmass, seven million square miles of it by Britain and France alone. Europe's domination over vast tracts of land and numerous peoples presented the United States with fundamental dilemmas, particularly in the Middle East. If, during the Greek war of independence, Americans had to choose between pursuing their strategic interests with Turkey and preserving democratic principles, they now had to decide between their two strains of faith, sacred and civic. Should they side with Christian Europe against a despised and allegedly decadent Islam or with the victims of the same colonialism from which the United States had wrung its own liberation? Could the United States, a champion of freedom for Middle Eastern peoples, ingenuously condemn Europe at a time when Americans were settling their own continent and coveting territories in the Caribbean and the Pacific?

Americans began asking these wrenching questions as early as 1829, when the French invaded Algiers. David Porter, who was slated to man the U.S. consulate in the city, refused to serve under a French occupation and was instead made the minister in Istanbul. In Porter's place, the State Department sent Henry Lee, the grandson of the Revolutionary patriot Richard Henry Lee. The new consul professed nothing but esteem for "the Frenchman [who] fought by the side of Americans under the Standard of Washington" and hatred for the descendants of Algerian corsairs. "I do not know that I ever experienced a prouder glow of sympathy and triumph," Lee recalled, "than when I first beheld . . . the victorious Christian troops driving the Barbarian hordes before them."

Over the next fifty years, Europe's takeover of parts of the Middle East continued to arouse strong opinions among Americans. The memoirs of American visitors to the region were rife with expressions of support for dismantling the Ottoman Empire and dividing it between Britain and France. The yearning was particularly keen among American missionaries, many of whom enjoyed European consular protection and who regarded the imperialist powers as agents of divine will. "Only the hand that moves the world could accomplish all this," observed the veteran missionary Jonas King in 1865, referring to the buildup of British influence in Egypt and French encroachments on North Africa. But while Americans generally expressed support for Europe's penetration of the Middle East, some railed in protest. The Kansan Richard J. Hinton, commander of an African American infantry unit during the Civil War, declared that while "the United States must lead in the regeneration of Asia, we cannot follow in the footsteps of our European cousins, and become aggressors." The Reverend George Potts denounced Europe's "bloody conquests" in the East as a "great national sin, which calls for . . . a painful . . . retribution." Interviewed by the *New York Times* in November 1852, Potts, a Presbyterian, reminded Americans of their "duty as a just . . . and a God fearing nation to treat other nations as their neighbors, and not [to] emulate Europe's territorial lust."[1]

American ambivalence toward imperialism in the Middle East deepened in the closing quarter of the nineteenth century as the region pitched into protracted political turmoil. While the Europeans grappled with the Eastern Question—whether to preserve the "Sick Man of Europe," as they pejoratively called Turkey, or to safely dispose of its pieces—native nationalist movements from Cyprus to the Balkans sought freedom from Ottoman rule. In an attempt to stem or at least monitor the breakdown, the great powers met in Berlin in 1878. There, Britain received control over Cyprus, and Russia secured independence for the Ottoman provinces of Serbia and Bulgaria. The international situation appeared to stablize, but only briefly. Germany soon started supplying military advisers to Istanbul, while Italy laid claim to Libya. The Berlin agreements fell apart a mere three years later, in April 1881, when French troops crossed from Algeria into Tunisia, captured Tunis, and placed the entire country under a permanent trusteeship.

"It looks as though the French are coming here to stay," Dr. George Washington Fish, the American consul in Tunis, sighed. A sixty-five-year-old former Union Army surgeon, Fish had turned to diplomacy after his wife and two children died of typhus. Such hardships may have made him callused, but the sight of French troops decimating the peaceful Tunisians still appalled him. "In plain Anglo-Saxon language . . . the French are . . . using the [Tunisian] government for their own purposes," he protested. In contrast to Fish, though, the American press could barely contain its exuberance over the French offensive, with New York papers proclaiming, "Civilization gains whenever any misgoverned country passes under the control of a European race." *Harper's* magazine extolled the "brilliant and rapid campaign" that had "struck imaginations and revived memories of glorious periods of the past."[2]

If divided in their reactions to the French occupation of Algeria and Tunisia, Americans might have been more uniform in their judgment of Britain's invasion of Egypt. Unlike North Africa, Egypt had never waged war on the United States—relations between the two countries remained excellent—while Britain had twice fought the United States. On the other hand, the United States, with few educational and cultural institutions in the country and little interest in the Suez Canal, had always viewed Egypt as Britain's bailiwick. American administrations from Grant to Garfield accordingly rejected Egyptian appeals for assistance against British rapaciousness. "What folly it would be for our Government to meddle with the Egyptian Debt," declared Assistant Secretary of State William Hunter in 1879, adding that "there is not a man in America who is interested" in relieving Egypt's plight.

The bombardment of Alexandria again unleashed crosscurrents of sympathy and disgust in American attitudes toward imperialism. The Reverend Philip Schaff of New York hailed the British attack as a "triumph of the Cross over the Crescent," but the *Los Angeles Times* denounced it as "a shameful act of flagrant barbarity." Ulysses Grant predicted that Britain would emancipate Egypt as the Union had once freed Negro slaves, but Grant's wartime aide Major General Adam Badeau deplored the invasion as "a reproach to the English nation and an outrage on the civilization of the age." The depth of this confusion was best illustrated by the *New York Times*, which lauded the defeat of "fanatic . . . Arabs who might follow a new Caliph in a holy war," but also decried England's "everlasting shame," fighting, again, for "taxation without representation."[3]

Britain's incursion into Egypt once more compelled the United States to choose between its allegiance to Western civilization and America's legacy of anticolonialism. Were Americans, moreover, willing to stand by their anti-imperialist principles at the price of their own expanding global interests? Most Americans, viewing the events in Egypt from a distance of thousands of miles, could dwell on these ethical dilemmas. Others, though, witnesses to the British invasion, could not afford to deliberate. For them, ambivalence was an unaffordable luxury.

Reaping Egypt's Whirlwind

Charles Chaillé-Long, the dandyish American officer who sought fame exploring Central Africa, had just completed his legal studies and received a diplomatic posting to Alexandria when the crisis in Egypt flared. At the request of the State Department, he joined a squadron of four U.S. gunboats attached to Britain's Egypt-bound fleet. His task was to evacuate the small American community of Alexandria in the event of large-scale violence in the city. Though American warships were not involved in the attack, their very presence in Egyptian waters that July, genially exchanging salutes with British destroyers, indicated the degree to which Washington had resigned itself to Egypt's inevitable submission.

From the bridge of the USS *Galena*, Chaillé-Long observed the furious exchange of fire between British and Egyptian guns. The epic scene was soon eclipsed, however, by the specter of flames engulfing the city and driving thousands of its residents toward the sea. Taking advantage of the Egyptian army's defeat, rioters had rampaged through the most elegant Alexandrian neighborhoods, looting and torching houses and killing anyone they considered foreign—Frenchmen, Italians, Orthodox Christians, and Jews. British commanders, with orders only to bombard the city, not to occupy it, were powerless to stop these atrocities. But Chaillé-Long was incapable of merely watching. He mustered a force of 160 volunteers, sailors, and Marines armed with rifles and Gatling guns to try to secure the U.S. consulate and rescue as many of the survivors as possible.

The first forces ashore in the British incursion were, in fact, American. The scene that greeted them was grisly. "In the sea were a great number of ghastly bodies of men, women and children—swollen and inflated with gas," Chaillé-Long recounted. Most of the victims, he noted, were "Levantine Jews," slain as they ran from their burning houses, but among the estimated four hundred dead were also a number of Greek and Armenian Christians. "Men, women and children were seized, bound with ropes and dragged through the streets and after horrible torture and mutilation were killed, and the[ir] flesh . . . exposed for sale at mock auction."

The Americans lunged into the inferno. They managed to extinguish some of the more threatening fires, to cordon off the consulate building, and to convert it into a temporary clinic and shelter. They patrolled the city, restoring a degree of order until the vanguard of the British forces finally landed four days later. During that time, some three hundred refugees were shuttled back to the squadron. "I corralled them all in the poop, French, Italians, Greeks, Turks, Syrians," testified the captain of one of the U.S. ships, the *Quinnebaug*. "In the whole lot we had three Americans, two missionaries and a judge."

For this daring operation, the United States received the thanks of several European states. Great Britain, above all, paid tribute to the "sailors and marines who . . . contributed to the preservation of life and property in Alexandria . . . when [it] was in the hands of pillagers and incendiaries." But none of these governments supported Chaillé-Long's proposal for changing the name of the rebuilt consular district from Place des Consuls to Place des Etats Unis, or for erecting a plaque commemorating "the Americans . . . who saved many Christian lives and saved the city of Alexandria." Though he expressed a desire to stay on at the Alexandria consulate, the discoverer of Lake Kioga and the Ugandan source of the Nile was transferred to Korea. His request to remain in Egypt, explained one of the naval officers who befriended Chaillé-Long, must have been lost in the paperwork of America's mounting international interests. "We dominate one-half of the world, and, in spite of ourselves, we are involved in the colonial interests of the other half."[4]

Whatever his disappointments with the halfhearted reactions to his role in the British invasion, Chaillé-Long expressed no reservations about the attack itself. The khedive, he felt, was a corrupt and ineffectual ruler, and Egyptian nationalists were a bloodthirsty rabble of zealots. Not all the Americans residing in Egypt shared these judgments, however. Two men, in particular, both diplomats, adopted a radically divergent stance.

Elbert Eli Farman, the consul at Alexandria who had so adeptly procured Cleopatra's Needle for New York, was outraged at the injustices he saw committed against Egypt. Farman listed several perpetrators of these crimes, among them the "evil genius" Ferdinand de Lesseps and the "Shylock Jewish bankers" who lured the country into debt. His keenest resentment, however, was reserved for the "aggressive European Powers," which seemed determined to inflict "gross wrongs against small and weak countries." As early as 1879, Farman foretold that Britain and France would soon foment domestic unrest in Egypt, creating a pretext for invasion. Later he would claim that the 1882 riots were "instigated by an English subject."

If thoroughly disgusted with Great Britain, Farman expressed unqualified esteem for Ahmad 'Urabi. Farman was representative of the growing number of American diplomats who sympathized with native nationalism and abhorred European imperialism. He also subscribed to the romantic image of the liberty-loving Arab, a favorite among American travelers from John Ledyard to Mark Twain. 'Urabi, whose very name meant "desert-dweller" in Arabic, was a hero for Farman. "No patriot was ever more popular . . . [and] no patriot was ever less actuated by motives of personal ambition," the consul declared. "He was the idol of his people."

Farman was not alone in his adulation of 'Urabi. Another admirer was Simon Wolf, the U.S. consul in Cairo. The latest example of the now institutionalized tradition of assigning American Jews to diplomatic positions in the Middle East, the Bavarian-born Wolf was the biographer of Mordecai Noah and a Washington lawyer who had cultivated a close rapport with both Lincoln and Grant. Appointed at the White House the day before President James Garfield was shot—the assassin was another attorney, furious over his failure to receive a consular post—Wolf arrived in Egypt on September 9, 1881, the day that 'Urabi rebelled.[5]

New to the country and suffering from a stomach ailment that would plague him throughout his tenure, Wolf resolved to "act cautiously and feel [his] way slowly." The Europeans, he intuited, would seize upon the slightest provocation to occupy Egypt and, in the process, spark a massacre of its foreign population. "Here on this limited chessboard, the game of European diplomacy is more or less played," he informed the State Department, stressing that it was America's duty to protect its citizens in Egypt and strive to avert catastrophe. With these goals in mind, Wolf requested the presence of three American warships near the Egyptian coast and sought to make contact with 'Urabi.

The meeting took place on November 11, at the home of Lieutenant General Charles Stone, the lone remaining American adviser in Egypt. Wolf, solidly built with a shaved head, prominent nose, and handlebar mustache, may have noticed a certain resemblance between himself and 'Urabi, but the affinity was more than physical. Wolf shared 'Urabi's belief that the Egyptians were "the natives and owners of the soil" and deserved to be free from oppression. After assuring him that the United States was "in no way mixed up in European or Levant politics," and that he spoke as "a fellow-man, as an individual from . . . a free country . . . whose citizens had . . . themselves suffered tyranny and tasted the bitterness of an iron yoke," Wolf urged 'Urabi to show moderation and beware of "the Trojan Horse of French and English influence." The consul then delivered a speech which, even in a nineteenth-century context, surely sounded unique: "As an Israelite, a brother of the Arab branch of the human family, I fully appreciate all [the Egyptians] long for. I feel grateful to Mahammadens for their shelter and protection and [the] freedom my brethren had enjoyed for years in Moslem countries."

Impressed by this avowal, 'Urabi promised to exercise "management and wisdom" and the utmost restraint. Wolf was jubilant. "There is scarcely a native but knows . . . that the United States are their friend; that we are not here to plunder and oppress but to aid and encourage."[6] By late spring, however, the consul's autumnal optimism would seem baseless. Whatever self-control 'Urabi demonstrated proved insufficient to stave off the deterioration of Egypt's internal politics and to deny the British their justification for invading. In the ensuing melee, the American community in Cairo evacuated the city, with the exception of one family—General Stone's.

With his silvery Vandyke, gold-braided uniform, and sparkling medals, Charles Stone at fifty-eight presented the image of both the elder statesman and an éminence grise. Behind the formidable façade, however, lay a guileless and intensely loyal servant to the causes in which he believed. In Egypt, Stone had seen his American staff officers defamed and dismissed and his beloved Isma'il exiled.

He nevertheless remained faithful to Isma'il's successor, staying by his side when 'Urabi's rebels threatened to burn down the khedival palace and British warships neared the Egyptian coast.

General Stone had another, no less unshakable allegiance. Widowed during the Civil War, Stone had remarried a former Louisianan named Jeannie and raised a family of four children. The outbreak of crisis divided that family, standing Stone and his thirteen-year-old son, John, in Alexandria, cut off from Jeannie and the three teenaged daughters in Cairo. Suddenly, the general was faced with the choice of either deserting Tawfiq in order to reunite with his loved ones or staying with the khedive and leaving his womenfolk to fend for themselves. He elected to stay, hoping to dissuade the British from invading or, failing that, from opening fire before the city's eight thousand foreigners could be evacuated.

After seeing his son removed to the safety of the American warships, Stone spent the day of July 10 begging locally based British officials to intercede with their navy offshore. He found them "quietly eating their dinners in the city they were about to bombard, and jokingly discussing the probable effect of the heavy gun practice [on Alexandria]." Most British subjects had already left the city, Stone learned, and the bombardment was set to commence in twenty-four hours—too soon to withdraw all the foreigners from Cairo, 120 miles away. Stone now confronted an even more harrowing dilemma: whether to warn his wife of the impending battle and risk setting off a stampede of fleeing foreigners or to remain silent and pray for the best. "I felt that four ladies struggling in a railway station for [a] place, in the midst of a crowd of panic-stricken Europeans, would have but small chance [of survival]," he reasoned. Stone never sent the telegram.

Instead, he dashed heedlessly through the incoming barrage to visit barracks and hospitals, to tend to the wounded, and to urge the police to take action against the rioters. Everywhere chaos raged. "Crowds of women of all classes of society were rushing forth into the open country . . . the great number carrying each a small child and conducting other children; these, with old men who had hardly strength . . . to make their way." When not engaged in humanitarian work, Stone continued to serve the khedive, keeping abreast of the military situation through reports smuggled into the palace in pin boxes or rolled up in pistol cartridges. Throughout, he was haunted by the thought of his family and the unspeakable ordeals they might suffer.

He indeed had much to worry about. Rather than joining the exodus from Cairo, the Stones barricaded themselves indoors, together with armaments and three months' worth of provisions. Outside, in the street, Egyptian women ululated and pelted the house with rocks, while children cried "death to the Christians." Even long-employed servants cursed the Americans. Apart from the occasional staff officer who managed to break through to the home, the family had no contact with the outside world and no word from the general. Jeannie Stone, a feisty forty-three-year-old, would not be intimidated, though. "There never lived an Arab who could frighten me," she declared. Gathering her daughters in the kitchen, Mrs. Stone exhorted them to "be brave and face death like good soldiers" and to protect their virtue at all costs. "I expect you to save yourselves by putting a bullet through your heart," she said. "Don't leave it to me to do it."

After more than two weeks of confinement, Jeannie decided that the only way to save her children was to lead them out herself. The staff officers who heard this plan were thunderstruck, convinced that all four women would be murdered. Their warnings went unheeded. "For once in our lives we created a sensation," her youngest daughter, Fanny, recalled of the family's carriage ride straight through the center of Cairo. "Every man, woman and child seemed petrified with astonishment on seeing four Christian ladies driving boldly through the streets." On August 8, tired and dusty, but far from daunted by their experience, the Stones reached Port Sa'id, where their anxious father, waiting with outstretched arms on the bridge of the USS *Quinnebaug*, embraced them.[7]

That same month, a 20,000-man British expeditionary force under General Garnet Wolseley landed at Alexandria with orders to crush the 'Urabi revolt. The decisive battle took place on September 13, at Tel el Kebir, where the British decimated almost all of Egypt's army in roughly forty minutes. Captured, 'Urabi was at first sentenced to death for sedition, but later exiled to Ceylon. Wolseley received the thanks of Parliament and a peerage from the queen. Tawfiq honored him with the Order of the Osmanie, Egypt's highest distinction.

Elbert Farman, by contrast, was horrified. "Tel el-Kebir," he wrote, "was a slaughter, rather than a battle." He, too, was decorated by the khedive for meritorious service to Egypt, but could not stand to watch as Wolseley's troops invested Cairo. As soon as he completed his responsibilities helping to assess damages to the foreign community of Egypt, Farman returned to his law practice in Warsaw, New York, and became active in civic causes. Chaillé-Long also left Egypt an embittered man. 'Urabi, in his eyes, was "a very bad soldier and a very poor prophet," and the slogan "Egypt for the Egyptians" was little more than a "deception and a snare." Simon Wolf, too, departed Cairo and resumed his life as a Washington attorney and philanthropist, a friend to Presidents McKinley and Wilson. Disgusted by what he regarded as Britain's perfidy against 'Urabi, Wolf predicted that the Egyptian people would someday rise up and cast off their European yoke. "The cup is full to overflowing," he sermonized. "And he who sows the wind must reap the whirlwind."[8]

Among the last of the Americans to exit Egypt was the redoubtable General Stone. Though awarded the Star of Egypt medallion for his meritorious service during the revolt, he felt "that Egypt had become a British province and all hope had vanished as to the building up of an independent state." He continued to hold Britain responsible for provoking the massacre of Alexandria's foreigners, while disparaging 'Urabi's prowess as a leader. In December 1883, Stone took his family and what remained of his library and papers—most had been ransacked by the British—and returned to his home on Long Island. He resumed his previous career as a civil engineer and soon began work on his life's most monumental achievement, providing a timeless symbol for Americans and a beacon for the peoples of the Middle East.

Enlightening the World

The project was the brainchild of a man whom Stone had once met in Egypt, an Alsatian sculptor ten years his junior, Frédéric Auguste Bartholdi. The idea originated in Bartholdi's excursion to Luxor and his fascination with the area's ancient statues. "Granite beings of imperturbable majesty," the awestruck artist called them, remarking how their eyes appeared to be "fixed on the limitless future." At that moment, the handsome, dark-haired Bartholdi resolved to replicate that magnificence and so ensure his own immortality. Inspiration again graced Bartholdi at the lavish opening ceremony of the Suez Canal. He would carve the likeness of an Egyptian peasant woman holding aloft a torch of freedom. The monument, twice as high as the Sphinx, would guard the waterway's entrance and perhaps double as a lighthouse. Its name would be *Egypt (or Progress) Bringing Light to Asia.*

Bartholdi spent two years making sketches and terra-cotta models of his concept and persuading Khedive Isma'il to finance the construction. By 1871, however, Isma'il was bankrupt and incapable of servicing his debts, much less investing in statuary. Distraught, Bartholdi sought solace in a cruise to the United States. While sailing into New York harbor, he passed the egg-shaped Bedloe's Island and suddenly envisaged a new location for his icon—and a new meaning. Years of back-and-forth negotiations produced an arrangement in which the Americans would pay for the pedestal and France for the statue itself, to be constructed by Gustave Eiffel. There remained only to find a chief American engineer for the undertaking. Bartholdi remembered Stone.

The general, who had been imprisoned on Bedloe's Island early in the Civil War, knew the area well. He acquired the assistance of James Morgan and Samuel Lockett, both veterans of the Egyptian service, and began erecting the eighty-nine-foot-high pedestal and assembling the 350 pieces of Eiffel's copper colossus. Though originally scheduled to coincide with the centennial of America's independence, the dedication of the memorial did not occur until a decade later, in October 1886, a year before Stone's death.

The thousands of spectators who listened as President Grover Cleveland pledged "not [to] forget that liberty here made her home" gazed up at a creation that bore little resemblance to the one Bartholdi had visualized for Egypt. The Muslim peasant had been replaced by an idealized Western woman and the name of the piece changed from *Bringing Light to Asia* to *Liberty Enlightening the World*. Only the torch remained, unextinguished.

Over the next forty years, "Lady Liberty" would provide millions of immigrants with their first glimpse of America, kindling their hopes for better lives and beckoning them with the possibility of freedom. For Egyptians, though, as for the many Middle Eastern peoples destined to come under foreign rule during that period, there would be no such illustrious symbols. They, unlike these new Americans, would have few prospects for advancement and none whatsoever of independence. "When will you turn your face toward the East, O Liberty?" asked Ameen Rihani, an Arab American poet later to play a dynamic role in his country's relations with the Middle East. "Shall the future never see a statue of freedom near the Pyramids?"[9]

THE UNVEILING of the Liberty statue, with its message of universal emancipation, might have signaled an end to America's dilemma over imperialism. Yet that same event also inaugurated a rush for colonial acquisitions and the creation of an American empire extending to Cuba and Puerto Rico, Hawaii, and the Philippines. Departing from their long-established tradition of distinguishing themselves from Europe, particularly in the field of foreign policy, many Americans now subscribed to the popular European philosophy of social Darwinism, which asserted the superiority of the Caucasian race over all others. Under this theory's banner, the British assumed their "white man's burden" and the French their *mission civilisatrice* in Africa and Asia, while Americans asserted their Manifest Destiny to conquer not only their continent but also distant segments of the globe.

Notably excluded from that destiny was the Middle East. The United States had no need to conquer land in order to attain great-power status in the region, having bloodlessly achieved that rank through its educational and medical institutions. And even if they wanted to, Americans would have great difficulty acquiring territories in an area that was effectively dominated by Europeans. But while the United States lacked imperial ambitions in the Middle East, its experience there furnished an excellent model for expanding American hegemony overseas. As the historian James Field has posited, "The Muslim societies of North Africa and the Near East provided the school in which the American approach to the non-Western world was worked out." By encouraging missionary work, facilitating tourism, and stationing permanent squadrons to safeguard its trade, America laid the foundations of its Far Eastern and Caribbean empires.

Still, not all Americans supported their country's participation in the imperialist race. Prominent figures such as the industrialist Andrew Carnegie and the philosopher William James rejected the theory of social Darwinism and denounced the conquest of foreign peoples. Together they founded the Anti-Imperialist League and enlisted the support of colonialism's prickliest opponent, Mark Twain. Though he once considered himself a "red-hot imperialist" who "wanted the American eagle to go screaming into the Pacific," Twain had been disillusioned by the ruthless suppression of Filipino insurgents by U.S. troops in 1899. The United States, he felt, had lost track of its fundamental purpose in the world, to furnish, rather than to deny, freedom. "And so I am an anti-imperialist," Twain concluded. "I am opposed to having the eagle put its talons on any other land."[10]

Twain's views, however, appealed to relatively few Americans. A far larger portion of the public endorsed the imperialist enterprise and joined in the frenzy of "jingoism," a term meaning militancy in foreign affairs, coined during Britain's conflicts with the Ottomans. Americans on the whole still saw imperialism as a force leading to positive change in the Middle East and to improved opportunities for themselves. The Europeans would haul the region out of its obscurity and open it to more vigorous American pursuits—commercial, cultural, and, above all, religious.

In no sector of American society was support for imperialism more exuberant than among those who would today be called faith guided. Enlightened European control of the Middle East, for them,

14

IMPERIAL
PIETY

THE LIBERTY STATUE WOULD BECOME A HALLMARK FOR Americans as would the verse inscribed on its pedestal: "Give me your tired, your poor, your huddled masses yearning to breathe free." Those words, from the second stanza of "The New Colossus," were penned by Emma Lazarus, an American Jewish poet from New York, an unreserved patriot who initially displayed little interest in religion and none whatsoever in the Middle East.

That indifference vanished for Lazarus in 1881, when czarist-approved pogroms ravaged Jewish villages in Russia, killing thousands. The atrocities coincided with the pinnacle of the thirty-three-year-old poet's career. She had been writing verse since age seventeen, but only now had her work finally gleaned praise from the general public as well as from the age's literary mandarins—Emerson, Henry James, and Walt Whitman.

Swarthy and pert, with the prominent nose and aristocratic mien of her Sephardic ancestors, Lazarus had never denied her heritage, but neither did she celebrate it. News of the atrocities in Russia, however, and the world's indifference toward them, suddenly spurred her to reexamine her roots and to seek out a solution to what was then called the "Jewish problem." The answer, she concluded, lay in the creation of "a home for the homeless, a goal for the wanderer, an asylum for the persecuted, a nation for the denationalized," in Palestine. Suddenly Lazarus was writing a different type of poem, one that exhorted her people to "Recall today the glorious Maccabean rage," and "Wake, Israel, wake!"

The Lamp and the Golden Door

Lazarus was not the only Jew to undergo a nationalist transformation in the 1880s. Zionism, or the belief in the Jewish people's right to a recognized polity in *Eretz Yisrael*—Hebrew for the Land of Israel—was just then taking root among the Jews of Eastern Europe. Small groups of Zionists had even immigrated to Palestine and settled on its parched and inhospitable terrain. In contrast to the 26,000 Jews already residing in the country, most of them urban-based rabbis or tradesmen, the new colonists tried to reintroduce the Jews to agrarian life—the same objective sought by American evangelists like Clorinda Minor and George Adams—in order to prepare them for sovereignty.

Enthusiasm for Zionism remained largely limited to Europe, however, and was virtually nonexistent among American Jews. The decade of the 1880s inaugurated the period of mass Jewish immigration to the United States. Over two and a half million Eastern European Jews would enter the country, many of them sailing past Lady Liberty en route to *de goldene medine*, as they called it in Yiddish, the "land paved with gold." Though generally more traditional than the German Jews who had settled in America earlier in the century, these newcomers were too preoccupied with integrating into their new Promised Land to contemplate relocating to the old one. American Jews contributed generously to maintaining their coreligionists in Palestine. Judah Touro, the renowned New Orleans philanthropist, funded construction of the first modern neighborhoods in Jerusalem, and Macy's co-owner Nathan Straus bought the land on which the Israel city named for him, Netanya, still stands. But most members of the American Jewish community were unwilling to devote their lives to Zionism, preferring the tenements and sweat-shops of urban America to Palestine's deserts and swamps.

American Jews' indifference to Zionism did not, however, daunt Emma Lazarus. Palestine, she maintained, would serve as a refuge for oppressed European Jews, not for the freedom-blessed Jews of the United States. These would continue to reside in the major American cities or, better yet, "renew their youth amid the pastoral plains of Texas and the golden valleys of the Sierras." Even without an American contingent, Lazarus was sure that new state would serve as an "organic center" for the entire Jewish people, providing it with "a defense in the court of nations," and humanity with an example of neutrality and peace. "The world will gain as Israel gains," she wrote.

But Lazarus's assurances brought little comfort to American Jews who, ever wary of anti-Semitism, feared that supporting Zionism would cast doubts on their loyalty to the United States. "We consider ourselves no longer a nation, but a religious community," stipulated the Union of Reform Congregations in 1885. "[We] expect therefore neither a return to Palestine nor a restoration of . . . the Jewish state." The conservative Jewish scholar Abram S. Isaacs lectured Lazarus that it was "unwise to advocate a separate nationality . . . at a time when anti-Semites are creating the impression that Jews . . . are only Palestinians, Semites, [and] Orientals." He reminded her that Zionism was not unrelated to restorationism, a Christian doctrine that aspired to convert all the Jews.

Unfazed by these barbs, Lazarus mounted a one-woman struggle for the right of Jews to work as "artisans, warriors and farmers" in their own sovereign polity. She established the Society for the Improvement and Emigration of East European Jews and promulgated Zionism through her prose and fiery verse. The idea of Jewish statehood, she told a friend, "opens up such enormous vistas in the past & future, & is so palpitatingly alive at the moment, that it has about driven out of my thoughts all other subjects." A proponent of enlightened imperialism, Lazarus looked forward to Europe's anticipated conquest of the Middle East, relieving the United States of the burden of liberating the Holy Land. She persisted in believing that American Jews would eventually surmount their hesitations and join her in lifting the lamp—to paraphrase the last line of "The New Colossus"—above "the golden door" of Palestine.

Lazarus's optimism was misplaced. She remained largely alone in her campaign for a Jewish Palestine and her society, lacking membership and funds, dissolved. In September 1887, the poet fell ill, apparently with cancer, and died two months later.

Lazarus's Zionist legacy appeared to have perished with her. The movement had failed to claim the respect, much less the allegiance, of even a segment of American Jews. Of the nearly two hundred delegates to the First Zionist Congress, held in Basel, Switzerland in 1897—a gathering then likened to the Constitutional Convention in Philadelphia and the landing on Plymouth Rock—only four hailed from North America.[1] The dream of renewed Jewish sovereignty in Palestine had yet to grip America's Jews, but millions of their countrymen remained seized by it. Love for the Jewish people was still their primary motivation, not as an end in itself, but rather as a means for hastening Christ's return.

Forgotten Memorials

Christianity in the United States had, by the 1890s, reached the apex of "the Protestant century," a term coined by scholars to describe the period in which religion pervaded all aspects of society. The neighborhood church and its varied activities—services, social gatherings, and Sunday school—became the linchpin of American life. Congregations rallied to raise funds for foreign missions and to welcome itinerant preachers. Beyond its provincial dimensions, though, religion in America was attaining a broader national scope. With the aid of a vigorous press, prominent theologians could now reach millions of readers weekly, if not daily, syndicating their sermons and tracts.

One of the most popular and revered of these "pulpit princes" was T. De Witt Talmage, a Levitical figure with deep-set eyes, a determined mouth, and a nose of exacting angularity. As pastor of the famed Brooklyn Tabernacle and spiritual adviser to President Grover Cleveland, Talmage commanded a vast audience for his pronouncements. These ranged from the connections between musculature and spirituality to the temptations of a summer vacation. Yet no subject possessed him more intensely—indeed obsessed him—than Palestine. "I have read about it, and talked about it, and preached about it, and sung about it, and prayed about it, and dreamed about it until my expectations were piled up into something like Himalayan proportions."

Talmage satisfied his Holy Land yearnings, finally, on December 1, 1889, when he stepped from a steamer onto the Jaffa shore. He came, like most Christian clergymen of his day, with an abiding hatred of "that curse of nations, that old hag of centuries," the Ottoman Empire, and of Islam, which he denounced as antithetical to Western civilization. But Talmage, an ardent restorationist, was concerned less with Palestine's present situation under the Muslims than with its future as the state of the Jews. "All the fingers of Providence now-a-days are pointing to that resumption of Palestine by the Israelites," he attested, and prophesied that the repatriated Jews would transform the country from a wasteland into a cultural and economic Eden.

Though primarily concerned with precipitating redemption, Talmage's concept of Jewish statehood was similar to Emma Lazarus's. He, too, recognized the urgency of finding shelter for the Jewish refugees from Russia and Eastern Europe where, he predicted, displays of anti-Semitism would soon "quadruple and centuple." He agreed with Lazarus that the Jews of the United States would not be expected to emigrate. "They would be foolish to leave their prosperities in our American cities where they are among our best citizens, and cross two seas to begin life over again in a strange land." Rather, American Jews would ally with their Christian countrymen in an ecumenical effort to influence govenment policies toward the Middle East. In this respect, at least, he differed from Lazarus. While the poet assumed that Europe would pry Palestine from the Ottomans, the preacher believed that America should lead the world in wresting the Holy Land from Islam.[2]

The proposition that the United States could spearhead an international effort to free Palestine from Muslim rule and to settle the land with Jews would have surely sounded delusional in the Civil War or antebellum periods. But America in the final decades of the

nineteenth century was a much altered country, an industrial juggernaut with a valid claim to global status. Quite naturally, then, in pursuing his dream of an American-emancipated Palestine, Talmage
would join forces with one of the yielders of this booming financial
clout, a real estate magnate named William Eugene Blackstone.

Born in Adams, New York, in 1841, self-educated and self-made,
Blackstone by age thirty had amassed a real estate empire and, with
it, the time to pursue his true, evangelical passions. In 1878, he
attended the Niagara Conference, dedicated to the Jews' return to
Palestine, and emerged a diehard restorationist. The result was *Jesus
Is Coming*, a book in which Blackstone departed from the traditional creed by absolving the Jews of the need to convert to Christianity before or after their ingathering. "Shall we Christians
condemn the Jews for not accepting the cumulative evidence that
Jesus is the Messiah; and ourselves refuse this other cumulative evidence that His second coming is near?" The volume, later translated
into thirty-six languages with nearly a million copies in print,
became one of the age's most popular disquisitions. But literary
accomplishments meant little to Blackstone. Deceivingly avuncular-
looking with his balding pate and muttonchops, he had grander
plans, and upon completing a tour of Palestine in 1888, he put them
into motion.

"We believe this is an appropriate time for all nations, and especially the Christian nations of Europe, to show kindness to Israel,"
stated the "memorial" that Blackstone submitted to President Benjamin Harrison and Secretary of State James G. Blaine on March 5,
1891. Some "2,000,000" Russian Jews, Blackstone explained, were
"piteously appealing to our sympathy, justice, and humanity," and
desperate for shelter in Palestine. Just as Europe had succeeded in
detaching Bulgaria and Serbia from the Ottoman Empire, so, too,
the United States could now secure Palestine's freedom for the Jews.
The president had merely to summon an international conference of
leaders, including the emperors of Germany and Austria-Hungary
and Britain's Queen Victoria, to decide the best means of achieving
this goal. "Not . . . since the days of Cyrus, King of Persia, has there
been offered to any mortal such a privilege opportunity to further
the purposes of God concerning His ancient people."

As anticipated, Talmage swiftly affixed his signature to the memorial, but, less expectedly, so did more than four hundred noteworthy individuals—clergymen, businessmen, journalists, and politicians. These figures were neither controversial nor peripheral, but representatives, rather, of America's financial, political, and cultural elite: John D. Rockefeller, Charles Scribner, J. Pierpont Morgan, Supreme Court Chief Justice Melville W. Fuller, and Congressman William McKinley. Several dozen Jews also signed the petition, marking the first time that personages of the two faiths cooperated on staking the Jewish claim to Palestine.[3]

Though radical in its recommendations, the Blackstone Memorial was in spirit consonant with long-standing American policy. For nearly a decade, since the outbreak of the 1881 Russian pogroms, Washington had been urging the Porte to open Palestine to Jewish immigration. The State Department instructed America's ambassador in Istanbul, Lew Wallace, to take the issue up personally with Sultan Abdul Hamid II. An avowed restorationist, Wallace showed no hesitation in pressing for the resettlement of Jewish refugees in Palestine. His successors, Oscar Straus and Solomon Hirsch, though both anti-Zionist Jews, also pursued the matter. None of their efforts prevailed. Justifiably fearful of Zionism and any effort to disassemble their empire, the Ottomans placed increasingly draconian strictures on all Jewish immigration to Palestine. American diplomats denounced these measures as "inquisitorial" and "utterly repugnant to . . . our Constitution," but again without effect. The European powers, for their part, showed no inclination to intervene on the refugees' behalf or to follow America's lead on Palestine.

With the Europeans withholding support for Blackstone's memorial and the Ottomans vehemently opposed to it, Harrison refrained from taking any dramatic action on the issue of Palestine. Blackstone continued to lobby for American leadership in the campaign for Jewish statehood, but neither Harrison nor the next presidents, Cleveland and McKinley, ever yielded. As often happened in America's Middle Eastern experience, one man's faith proved to be another's fantasy, while policy was determined by power.[4]

The refusal of successive administrations to endorse the creation of a Jewish state did not, however, discourage great numbers of

American Christians from continuing to cherish the idea. Some, like Blackstone, even began describing themselves as Zionists. Among the general public, however, explicit enthusiasm for restorationism was diminishing. The once dissident Methodist and Presbyterian churches were gravitating toward the mainstream and leaving many of their millenarian doctrines—restorationism included—behind. American Protestantism in general was moving away from the revivalist fervor that had animated it since the late eighteenth century and reverting to more conventional practices. Though the renewal of Jewish sovereignty in Palestine remained a dream for many Americans, the urge to achieve it had waned.

The mellowing of restorationist zeal and the transition from evangelical to more traditional forms of worship, was illustrated by the last attempt to create an American colony in Palestine. The saga revolved around the Spafford family and its followers and around an American diplomat, Selah Merrill, who became their inveterate foe.

It Is Well with My Soul

The Spaffords, Horatio and Anna, were a respected, churchgoing Chicago couple, close friends of William Blackstone. Having survived the Great Fire of 1871, Anna and four of her daughters embarked on a pleasure cruise to Britain, but the ship sank when it struck another vessel, and the four daughters were lost. Shortly thereafter, the couple's only son died of scarlet fever. "When sorrows like sea-billows roll, whatever my lot," the devastated but still devout Horatio wrote, "Thou hast taught me to say: 'It is well, it is well with my soul' "—a hymn that is still sung by many Protestants. Resolving to transform their personal tragedy into a spiritual force, the Spaffords founded a new sect, the Overcomers, and decided to move to Jerusalem.

A full decade would pass, however, before the family, together with twelve of their followers, landed at Jaffa. The group proceeded immediately to Jerusalem, riding in "American-made spring wagons" that had once belonged to the ill-fated Adams settlement. The failure of that venture fifteen years earlier did not deter the Spafford group from attempting to establish its own colony in Jerusalem. The pilgrims rented a large house outside of the Old City walls and set to work making textiles, cabinets, and bricks. Soon, too, they opened a girls' school and a shop selling Holy Land souvenirs. The new American Colony, as it was known, quickly became a tourist site. Visitors included such luminaries as the British general Charles "Chinese" Gordon, then en route to the Sudan, where Muslim warriors would later kill him. "He taught me [how] to swear," one of the Spaffords remembered.

Like earlier American settlers in Palestine, the Overcomers sought to emulate the life of Jesus, the "Man of Sorrows" who suffered immensely on earth but who later gained heavenly glory. They also longed for the fulfillment of biblical prophecies, in particular those predicting the Jews' return to their native land. Unlike their predecessors, though, the Spafford group felt no compulsion to help prepare the Jews for their ingathering, no injunction to teach them how to farm. They were content merely to climb each day up the Mount of Olives, equipped only with tea and cake "hoping," they professed, "to be the first to offer refreshment to the Messiah."[5]

The American Colony was also unique in that it was spared the fate of the previous farms and was never ravaged by famine, disease, or bandits. Though the settlement's construction coincided with the anti-Western reign of Abdul Hamid II, the Overcomers enjoyed excellent relations with the Ottoman governor of Jerusalem, as well as with the city's more established religious communities. The colonists faced only one serious adversary—ironically, an American.

As a doctor of theology and the chaplain of an African American battalion during the Civil War, Selah Merrill appeared to have much in common with the Overcomers and their tolerance, piety, and courage. He also shared their love of Palestine. Starting in 1882, he served several terms as America's consul in Jerusalem, and over the course of the next quarter-century authored numerous books on the history, topography, and archaeology of the Holy Land. Yet Merrill, whose kindly, fatherly face, studious glasses, and patriarchal beard disguised a curmudgeonly disposition, saw no room in that land for the American Colony or for its subversive communal ideas.

Merrill denounced the Spaffordites, as he called them, as

swindlers and heretics, accusing them of kidnapping and brainwashing young people and, on at least one occasion, of assaulting him with intent to kill. He urged Jerusalem residents not to purchase goods made by settlers and told tourists to avoid the colony's shop. "They hate the United States Government . . . and all of the . . . American residents of Jerusalem outside their own circle." The consul also submitted depositions from former colony residents testifying to various "lewd practices" that the Spaffords encouraged, including isolating unmarried couples in dark rooms and later forcing them to confess their transgressions.

Tensions boiled over when Merrill, an amateur archaeologist, decided to excavate a historical area outside of the Old City Wall that also happened to contain the American Colony cemetery. Though he later claimed that he had conscientiously relocated the graves, the horrified Spafford family complained of finding Horatio Spafford's bones unearthed and wantonly scattered. Hounded by protests from the colony's American supporters and suffering from throat cancer, Merrill ultimately resigned. By that time, however, the community had merged with a Swedish group and lost its distinctive American identity. The house was refitted as a hotel and a restaurant that, a century later, still served as a favorite purlieu of foreign journalists. All of Merrill's vindictiveness was futile.

Merrill's malice toward the American Colony was outdone only by his rancor toward Jews and their nascent Zionist movement. Again, as a former professor of Hebrew at Andover and a man whose first name derived from the Jewish liturgy, Merrill might have been expected to empathize with Jewish refugees and with efforts to build them a state. But the Jews, according to Merrill, were to blame for much of their own suffering. Their "character," their lack of "cleanly habits and civilized modes of life," had provoked the Russian pogroms and anti-Jewish outbursts elsewhere. "The Jew needs . . . less flattery," he averred; "the Jew needs to learn his place in the world." Asked by the State Department to submit his opinions on the Blackstone Memorial, Merrill dismissed the document as "one of the wildest schemes that was ever brought before the public." Retarded by "trifling observances" and interested only in money, most Jews would never settle in an inhospitable, unprofitable Palestine, he predicted, even if given the chance. The consul concluded by urging the United States to avoid any contact with Zionism and eschew all sympathy for the Jews. "[They are] a race of weaklings of whom neither soldiers, colonists nor enterprising citizens can be made."[6]

IN HIS contempt for the Spaffords' millenarianism and his antipathy toward Zionism, Selah Merrill reflected some of the views that were gaining prominence among mainstream American Protestants. Yet revivalist forms of worship were still immensely popular in the United States and anti-Semitism, even if privately condoned, was still publicly frowned upon. Support for the idea of restoring Jewish sovereignty in Palestine, though less exuberant, nevertheless remained widespread. Public opinion on such issues was reflected less by Merrill than by America's favorite everyman, Mark Twain. Although he often lampooned evangelicals in prose, Twain also retained an inbred respect for the "old time religion," and while his writings sometimes revealed an anti-Jewish bias, he disavowed any animus toward Jews. Twain's attitude toward Zionism was unknown, however, before 1897, when he began a two-year sojourn in Vienna. It was during that period that Twain was himself mistaken for a Jew. He also came into contact with outstanding Jewish figures, among them Theodor Herzl, journalist, playwright, and father of the Zionist movement.

Twain's arrival in Vienna coincided with the denouement of the infamous Dreyfus affair. A French army captain falsely accused of spying for Germany and a highly assimilated Jew who considered himself more French than Jewish, Alfred Dreyfus became the focus of an anti-Semitic onslaught unleashed by the military, the Catholic Church, and other conservative elements. The impact of the Dreyfus trial reverberated across Europe, and especially in Austria, where anti-Semitism had gained legitimacy as a journalistic motif as well as a political platform.

Irrespective of his misgivings about Jews, Twain was scandalized by the libel against Dreyfus. He had come to Vienna to accompany his daughter, Clara, a musician married to an Austrian Jew, and through her was able to meet many of the city's leading Jewish intellectuals, including the struggling philosopher-therapist Sigmund Freud. Consequently, Twain learned the perversions of anti-Semitism, though never so profoundly as when he personally became its target. The Viennese press, noting that his original first name, Samuel, was a favorite among Jews, and that his nose was rather large and crooked, dubbed him *der Jude Mark Twain.*

Twain struck back with a characteristically stinging essay, "Concerning the Jews," in which he assailed the fact that so few Christians had publicly stood up for their spiritual cousins. The Dreyfus trial was especially disgusting. "It is un-English; it is un-American; it is French." Twain nearly defeated his purpose by mentioning the Jews' alleged love of money and their reluctance to serve their country in war—he later apologized for these slurs—but redeemed himself by praising the Jewish intellect. "The difference between the brain of the average Christian and that of the average Jew—certainly in Europe—is about the difference between a tadpole's and an Archbishop's," he reckoned. "It's a marvelous race—by long odds the most marvelous the world has produced, I suppose."

Twain's newfound affinity for the Jews was further illustrated by his interest in Herzl. While covering the Dreyfus trial for a Viennese paper, Herzl became convinced that the Jews could never integrate into Europe, but rather had to emigrate and found their own independent nation. He subsequently convened the First Zionist Congress and published his vision of a future polity, *The Jewish State.* Herzl and Twain had already met once, briefly, at a reception in Paris in 1894. Herzl was disappointed to behold "a short, spare man . . . a bit shaky . . . [with] a blank look [and] shabby cheeks," rather than the barrel-chested comic he had imagined. He even managed to misidentify the creator of Tom Sawyer and Huckleberry Finn as an Englishman.

Their next meeting, four years later in Vienna, proved more satisfying, and not only for Herzl. Twain, too, was apparently impressed with the charismatic reporter turned visionary whose intense ebony eyes and thick square beard often evoked Michelangelo's statue of Moses. After attending the opening of Herzl's play *The New Ghetto,* the story of an assimilated Jew named Samuel who is rejected by Christian society, Twain offered to translate the drama for the New

York stage. He also evinced a gritty regard for the movement Herzl had founded. In his idiosyncratic, satirical fashion, Twain conveyed support for the proposed creation of a Jewish state by appearing to oppose it. "If that concentration [in Palestine] of the cunningest brains in the world were going to be made on a free country (bar Scotland), I think it would be politic to stop it," he counseled. "It will not be well to let that [Jewish] race find out its strength. If the horses knew theirs, we should not ride anymore."[7]

Twain never got around to translating *The New Ghetto*. Instead, he turned his attention to criticizing America's suppression of the nationalist revolt in the Philippines and to denouncing imperialism. But Twain did not regard Zionist colonization of Palestine as a form of imperialism, nor did he condemn French and British incursions elsewhere in the Middle East. In this respect, too, his opinions were typical of turn-of-the-century Americans. Whether pro- or anti-imperialist, most of them still looked forward to the day when the Middle East would be freed from despotic rule and made to resemble the United States. That transformation did not have to take place through conquest, however, but rather through philanthropy and the dedicated work of preachers, educators, and physicians. The Protestant century may have been ending, but great numbers of Americans still supported the missions.

Apostles to Islam

In the single decade between 1885 and 1895, the budget for missionary institutions in the Middle East expanded sevenfold. In addition to over four hundred schools and nine colleges with a total enrollment of 20,000, the money also paid for nine hospitals and ten dispensaries treating an estimated 40,000 patients annually. Along with journals, newspapers, and Bibles in five Middle Eastern languages, American presses rolled out some four million textbooks on topics ranging from astronomy to dentistry, lithography to moral philosophy.

The missionaries' contributions to the ethical and educational uplifting of the Middle East became a wellspring of pride for Americans and a yardstick for measuring their altruism against Europe's imperialist avarice. "Too high praise cannot be given to the faithful men and women of our country, who . . . do their duty so . . . fearlessly here amid arid sands and burning sun," one of those Americans, Simon Wolf, reported from his consulate in Cairo. "The mention of the United States or 'I am an American' serves at once as a passport to their [the Egyptians'] kindness and confidence." One of Wolf's successors, Lewis Idding, further pressed the claim by positing that "Americans occupy Egypt as fully as does England." Though Britain had developed the country economically, Idding explained, the United States had molded its people into citizens.[8]

The missionaries, too, reveled in these achievements, but their failure to realize their original goal—salvation—still stung. "In the war against Islam we are only yet putting on the armor and not by any means ready to wave the ensigns of victory," confessed Henry Jessup, the doyen of American evangelists in Lebanon. Jessup was alluding to the fact that, despite the establishment of over nearly one hundred churches and the work of over two hundred missionaries throughout the Ottoman Empire, the total number of converts remained negligible. Many of these, moreover, later immigrated to the United States—so many that the Syrian Protestant College, lacking Arabic-speaking professors, changed its language of instruction to English.

Uniquely in the Middle East, no amount of cultural or material inducement proved effective in luring local populations away from their traditional rites in favor of those of Protestant America. In contrast to the Far East, where the services provided by American missionaries gave them a well-oiled conduit to conversion, Middle Eastern peoples saw no contradiction between receiving instruction and medical care from evangelists while maintaining their original faith. "No man ever came into a mission hospital who needed his hernia mended one-half so badly as he needed to learn about Jesus Christ," one exasperated doctor complained.

The missionaries' failure was illustrated by the case of Alexander Russell Webb. A former New Yorker and consul to the Philippines, Webb converted from Presbyterianism to Islam in 1888. He returned to his native city five years later, stout, bearded, and turbaned, and proceeded to establish one of the nation's first mosques and Muslim newspapers. Webb's efforts to Islamicize the United States were scarcely less successful than the missionaries' attempts to Christianize the Middle East, but his campaign underscored the challenges Protestants faced from a proud, equally proselytizing Islam.

Stymied by this opposition, some Americans resolved to become "modern missionaries," a term invented by Howard Bliss, who had succeeded his father as president of the Syrian Protestant College. The objective was now to preach a "Social Gospel," introducing Christ whenever and however possible "with or without [a] resulting change in . . . ecclesiastical affiliation." For Bliss and his circle of comfortably ensconced clerics in Beirut, the new definition of the missionary's role meant that medical and educational institutions could continue to expand, even at the expense of purely evangelistic activities. The Middle East might one day reflect America politically and intellectually, but spiritually speaking the mirror would remain Muslim.

Not all missionaries were prepared to adopt this modern, social calling, however, and to abandon their quest for converts. Many were still willing to strike out, Bibles in hand, to the remotest areas of the region, braving brigands and disease.[9] Indeed, the closing decades of the nineteenth century saw redoubled efforts by American missionaries to establish stations in eastern Anatolia, Persia, and the Sudan.

No evangelist, however, had ever set foot in the Arabian Peninsula. A waterless and sun-seared landmass roughly the size of the United States west of the Mississippi, the area today includes Yemen, Saudi Arabia, and the independent emirates of the Persian Gulf. In the 1890s, though, Arabia was nominally part of the Ottoman Empire. The Islamic heartland, home to the Holy Cities of Mecca and Medina, the peninsula was also the cradle of the extremist Islamic sect known as the Wahhabis. The movement formed an alliance with the Saudi family, which mobilized Wahhabi warriors in its battles with other desert tribes. Such an environment was unlikely to accommodate an American intent on transforming Muslims into born-again disciples of Christ. Yet that was precisely the aspiration of Samuel Marinus Zwemer, a twenty-three-year-old missionary from Vriesland, Michigan.

One of thirteen children of a Reformed Dutch minister, Zwemer believed from the earliest age that he was destined for overseas evangelizing. At seminary school, he stared for hours at the metronome his teacher had placed before the class, ticking every time a soul died unsaved in Asia. Zwemer consequently resolved to fulfill the biblical injunction "Oh, that Ishmael might live before Thee" (Genesis 17:18), and to preach throughout Arabia. The region had long been recognized as an exclusive Dutch domain, but the church, convinced that the Arabs could never be saved, refused to finance a mission. Zwemer had to obtain his own funds for the journey. He also acquired a rudimentary knowledge of map reading, medicine, and Arabic. Fully equipped, at last, in June 1890, Zwemer set off for "the very heart of Islam."

Zwemer's journey took him first to Cairo and then across the Red Sea to Jidda. He traveled light, equipped with little more than the two volumes of Charles M. Doughty's *Travels in Arabia Deserta*, both of which he later sold to a young British officer named T. E. Lawrence. Trekking southward, Zwemer claimed to be the first Westerner ever to enter the Yemeni city of San'a—a feat for which he was made a fellow of the Royal Geographical Society. He then rounded the tip of the Arabian Peninsula and sailed north through the Persian Gulf to Basra, where, reuniting with an old seminary friend, James Cantine, he founded his first station.

Preaching in the middle of Muslim Mesopotamia could prove precarious, the Americans quickly learned. A hefty six-footer with blond hair and chiseled Nordic looks, Zwemer was singled out by Ottoman authorities, placed under house arrest, and forbidden to preach. Nevertheless, "a steam engine in breeches," as one colleague called him, Zwemer managed to flee Basra and relocate to Muscat (Oman) and the island of Bahrain. His memoirs tell of bizarre encounters with lizard-eating boatmen armed with Civil War surplus muskets and with an American prospector in search of Persian gold. Over the course of his travels, Zwemer was robbed, threatened with beheading, and dehydrated by 107-degree heat. "Pioneer journeys in Topsy Turvy Land are not without difficulty," he allowed. In time, though, Zwemer was joined by his younger brother, Peter, by Kamil Aetany, one of the few Muslim converts from Beirut, and by the British missionary Amy

Wilkes, who became Mrs. Samuel Zwemer and the mother of his six children. Together, they distributed Bibles, tended to the sick, and sheltered fugitive slaves. They also found time to erect Muscat's first windmill, imported in sections from Waupun, Wisconsin.

Such services, both secular and sacerdotal, had been an American missionary tradition in the Middle East since the 1820s, but rendering them invariably exacted a price. Two of the Zwemers' daughters succumbed to illnesses, as did Zwemer's brother Peter. Kamil Aetany also died, poisoned, Zwemer's associates thought, by his own father. Finally, after sacrificing all of their lives, and devoting twenty years of his own to the effort, Zwemer had to confront the ineluctable truth: the Arabs could not easily be converted.

Zwemer consequently fell back on the practice well known to missionaries throughout the Middle East: he began to open schools. "A country [without] . . . such schools cannot progress," he reasoned. "Some day education in Arabia will be what it is now in America." Clinics followed and a full-time physician, Paul Harrison, was brought in from Baltimore. "All the missionary can do is to give to those who care for it a picture of the Christian life and an opportunity to follow," Harrison later recalled. The fact that none of those patients was ever baptized undoubtedly challenged Harrison's—and Zwemer's—faith, but never broke it.

Respectfully nicknamed "the Apostle to Islam," Samuel Zwemer would also fulfill another traditional missionary function by interpreting the Middle East to Americans. He authored dozens of books on the Muslim world—its mores, outlooks, and beliefs. Returning from Arabia, he taught at Princeton and helped build the university's Department of Near Eastern Studies. Generations of students, many of them the sons and daughters of missionaries, would study there and go on to become State Department Arabists and executives with American corporations operating in the Middle East. "American religious-philanthropic organizations in the Near East have a tendency to combine religious, educational and medical services with business investments," observed one prominent financier of the missions.[10] Arabian leaders would remember those services early in the next century, when choosing between American and British oil contractors.

Though apostolic in its initial intent, Zwemer's mission would have vast ramifications for the economic and strategic interests of the United States. The modest efforts to disseminate American religious beliefs in Arabia would ultimately produce an efflorescence of American might.

Soldiers of the American Crusade

The symbiosis of faith and power in America's Middle East involvement became increasingly pronounced toward the end of the nineteenth century. Pro-imperialist American leaders routinely marshaled religion to justify their policies, while prominent clerics hailed imperialism as a weapon in the war for global redemption. "America is to become God's right arm in his battle with the world's ignorance and oppression and sin," proclaimed Josiah Strong, the Congregationalist minister and radical social Darwinist. "[T]his land of ours . . . must take the lead in the final conflicts of Christianity for possession of the world." Embarked on a common crusade, missionaries, soldiers, and statesmen could unreservedly collaborate with one another, and not only in Arabia but throughout the Middle East.

THIS BLENDING of foreign policy and evangelical zeal was especially manifest in Persia. American missionaries had long been active in Urmia, Hamadan, and Tabriz, but these areas held little attraction for the State Department. A commercial treaty signed by the United States in Persia in 1856 had never been activated, nor had the two nations ever exchanged ambassadors. The situation changed in 1883, however, when Persia's Qajar rulers appealed to Washington for help in resisting British and Russian attempts to dominate the country. The Chester Arthur administration responded positively, not out of sympathy for Persia but rather from fear for the missionaries' safety during a period of domestic and international unrest.

The head of America's first official mission to Persia was, fittingly, the son of missionaries, Samuel Green Wheeler Benjamin, a forty-six-year-old painter and art historian. Approaching Teheran,

Wheeler was greeted by a royal entourage that included six governors and a thousand horsemen arrayed, he wrote, in "the most brilliant European uniforms, with some . . . touches of Oriental splendor." With his artist's eye, Wheeler noted the details of Persian decor and dress, especially those of the shah, Naser ad-Din, whose coat was buttoned with diamonds "fully the size of pigeons' eggs." Yet, like a competent diplomat, the envoy also listed the products—"iron, coal, copper, sulphur . . . wheat, maize, sugar-cane, tobacco, rice . . . tropical and semi-tropical fruits"—that Persia proposed to exchange for advanced American weaponry, especially Gatling guns. But the United States balked at the offer. Apart from the security of the missions, Washington disavowed any interests, economic or strategic, in the Persian Gulf.[11]

Nevertheless, the burgeoning missionary presence in the Middle East, and the growing willingness of missionaries to defy Muslim authorities, compelled the United States to adopt a more muscular policy toward the region. The death of twenty-four-year-old Howard Baskerville, a Presbyterian missionary who was killed defending rebellious peasants in Tabriz, elicited stern diplomatic protests from Washington. The trend was not confined to Persia. In Turkey, too, the United States abandoned the policy established by David Porter in the 1830s of withholding protection from those missionaries who antagonized local rulers. "The wayward Turks are accused of having roasted . . . a stray missionary . . . over his rosy kitchen fire and we are supposed to . . . wring satisfaction from the Sultan," wrote Lieutenant Charles Sperry in February 1885 as his cruiser demonstrated along the Anatolian coast. The distinction between church and state, so jealously guarded at home, was steadily blurring for Americans in the Middle East. Lieutenant Sperry was also detailed to accompany Ambassador Lew Wallace on a tour of Christian sites throughout the eastern Mediterranean. Wallace's "pilgrimage," Sperry noted was undertaken entirely at the public's expense.

The line between religious and governmental activities in the Middle East was further effaced by the emergence of missionary dynasties capable of exerting far-reaching influence over America's foreign relations. The descendants of the original missionaries to the region—the Blisses and the Birds, the Dodges and the Dwights—now presided over its premier cultural institutions. They maintained intimate connections with leading American universities, most notably Princeton, and with preeminent American families such as the Rockefellers, the Morgans, and the Roosevelts. The primary supporters of the missionary effort circulated in the same social milieu as the country's political elite, sent their children to the same schools, and allied with them through ties of marriage. Through their personal connections with decision makers, the missionaries and their backers could place evangelism and its advocates at the head of America's overseas priorities, particularly in the Middle East. One consul in the area calculated that nine-tenths of his time, at least, was devoted to dealing with the missions and their multifarious concerns. "Even the head of our State Department used to quake when the head of a Bible society walked in."[12]

Americans might celebrate the empowerment of their missionaries in the Middle East, but the joy was scarcely shared by the region's rulers. With growing intensity, the Ottomans complained about the evangelists' insolence and about the presence of U.S. warships along their coasts. Tensions between Washington and the Porte were then brought to the breaking point, starting in the mid-1890s, by the mass execution of Armenians.

THE DESCENDANTS of an ancient people that flourished on the scraggy terrain between the Caspian and the Black Seas, and between the Caucasus and the Taurus Mountains, the Armenians were early converts to Christianity who remained a formally protected, but often persecuted, minority under Ottoman rule. Resented for their relatively higher levels of education and professional success, the Armenians were also suspected by the Turks of owing allegiance to the Christian powers, and to Russia especially, which were plotting to dismantle the empire. The buildup of Ottoman oppression and Armenian anger erupted finally in the spring of 1894, when Turkish troops set out to crush a local rebellion, but then went on to raze entire villages and slaughter all of their inhabitants. "All the Armenians in sight were killed and their houses and stores robbed," reported an appalled American consul in Trebizond. "Dead bodies were scattered over the streets all bearing fearful evidence of their cruel deaths." Some 200,000 Armenians died—20 pecent of the population—and a million homes were ransacked.

"Armenian holocaust," cried a *New York Times* headline in September 1895, employing the word that would later become synonymous with genocide. The American press was virtually unanimous in calling for urgent action to save the Armenians and to remove, "if not by political action than by resort to the knife," the "fever spot of the Turkish Empire." Clergymen, too, stood united in their concern for Armenians, even though most of them followed Eastern Orthodox rites. "Not all the perfume of Arabia can wash the hand of Turkey clean enough to be suffered any longer to hold the reins of power over one inch of Christian territory," fumed the *Catholic World*, while the Reverend De Witt Talmage urged "the warships of the western powers [to] ride up as close as possible to the palaces of Constantinople and blow that accursed government to atoms." The ecumenical furor, meanwhile, was matched by bipartisan outrage in Congress. Newton Blanchard, a Democratic senator from Louisiana, demanded American intervention to erase this "blot upon civilization of the age." His Republican colleague from Illinois, Shelby Cullom, declared, "The demon of damnable and fanatical hate has spread ruin, desolation, and death." In his presidential platform for 1896, William McKinley listed saving the Armenians, along with annexing Hawaii and securing Cuba's independence from Spain, as his foreign affairs priority.[13]

The American reaction to the Armenian massacres—the first of many such atrocities soon to blot the Middle East—had multiple sources. There was the deeply entrenched aversion that Americans felt toward Islam and their no less rooted empathy for the Christians straining under Muslim rule. Popular opinion in the United States also tended to identify with the hardworking and family-oriented Armenians and to see them as "the Yankees of the Orient." Finally, the Armenians were linked in the American mind with the mission schools from which many of them had graduated and which were seen as extensions of the United States. Some of these institutions had been extensively damaged in the pogroms, spurring demands for restitution not only for the Armenians but equally for the evangelists who served them.

"The policy of the United States Government in this world crisis has been one of impotence as far as the cause of humanity is concerned, contemptible from the standpoint of national honor, and suicidal as regards American interests," exclaimed the veteran evangelist Frederick Davis Greene in his popular monograph, *Armenian Massacres; or, The Sword of Mohammed*. To remedy these failings, the missionaries exploited their privileged access to the Congress and the McKinley White House. The president of Robert College, George Washburn, petitioned Secretary of State John Hay, his cousin, to confront the Turks openly. At the same time, James B. Angell, a headstrong Congregationalist who served as America's ambassador to the Porte, urged the legislature to approve military action against Turkey. A fleet of gunboats must be dispatched at once, Angell argued, to "rattle the Sultan's windows."

Pressure from Washburn and Angell proved persuasive, and in December 1900 the USS *Kentucky* steamed toward Turkey. Exactly one hundred years after the *George Washington* exemplified America's impotence in the Middle East by conveying Algerian tribute to Istanbul, the newly christened *Kentucky* arrived in Smyrna bristling with more than fifty guns. The *Kentucky*'s captain, the ruddy-faced "Red Bill" Kirkland, bluntly warned Smyrna's governor, "If these massacres continue I'll be swuzzled if I won't someday forget my orders . . . and find some pretext to hammer a few Turkish towns. . . . I'd keel-haul every blithering mother's son of a Turk that wears hair." Though softened by the translator and conveyed with a smile, Kirkland's message penetrated. The sultan paid $83,000 in compensation to the missionaries and even placed an order for an American-made destroyer.[14]

Still, muscle was not the only means through which Americans expressed their concern for Armenia. No sooner had news of the massacres reached North America than societies for the support of their victims sprang up in virtually every major city. In Boston, Julia Ward Howe, whose husband had volunteered to fight in the Greek war of independence in 1825 and whose fame as author of the

Union's favorite hymn proved to be an asset in fundraising, organized the United Friends of Armenia. New York's chamber of commerce formed the National Armenian Relief Committee, an elite group whose backers included Supreme Court Justice David Josiah Brewer, the American Jewish philanthropist Jacob Schiff, and the railroad executive Chauncey Depew. John D. Rockefeller contributed hundreds of thousands of dollars to the effort, while less moneyed people donated blankets, clothing, and foodstuffs. American women were especially active in the drive, spurred by reports of the rape and enslavement of thousands of Armenian girls.

Contributions poured in, but the problem remained of how to transport them to the victims. For a solution, the relief committee turned neither to the State Department nor to the missions nor even to the U.S. Navy but rather to a seventy-four-year-old woman, one of the most extraordinary Americans of her day.

Born on Christmas in the presidency of James Monroe, Clara Barton was raised on a Massachusetts farm, but later took up a teaching position in Washington. The Civil War, though, furnished her with a new profession. Tending to the Union wounded, spearheading supply drives, and distributing provisions among the troops, Barton attained a legendary status, the Angel of the Battlefield. After the war, she befriended Frederick Douglass and Susan B. Anthony, joining their struggles for racial equality and women's suffrage, and volunteered for the newly created Red Cross in Europe. She returned to the United States determined to establish a national branch of the organization and realized her vision in 1881 by establishing the American Red Cross.

Fifteen years later, Clara Barton was well past retirement age, a petite, wizened woman whose indefatigable smile made permanent mounds of her cheeks. That smile would often be her only protection as she confronted the terrors of Ottoman bureaucracy. Denied permission to display the symbol of the cross, Barton had to present her mission as a private initiative to aid all Ottoman subjects, irrespective of creed. She also had to manage her affairs from Istanbul, under the army's eyes. "I shall never counsel nor permit a sly or underhand action with your government," she promised the Ottoman foreign minister. "I shall expect the same treatment in return."

Barton succeeded in obtaining the authorities' full cooperation and in directing a series of food- and medicine-laden expeditions deep into the Armenian hinterland. Though members of the National Armenian Relief Committee resented the exclusive credit she received, and some Armenians protested the assistance she lent to distressed Turkish minorities in their districts, Barton solidified her reputation as "perhaps the most perfect incarnation of mercy the modern world has known." Even the Ottomans honored her with a medal.

America's aid to the Armenians remained a collaborative effort of the members of all faiths and parties, an unparalleled pooling of religious and political resources. It represented the continuation of decades of American solicitude for downtrodden Middle Eastern minorities, including Jews, Bahais, and Orthodox Christians. While many Americans believed that they were fated to dominate large sections of the world, they also insisted on saving that world from oppression. The Reverend Strong praised America as "the representative . . . of the largest liberty, the purest Christianity, [and] the highest civilization," destined to "impress its institutions upon mankind." Barton, by contrast, vowed to "defy the tyranny of precedent" by liberating subject peoples and alleviating their plight. Not just in the 1890s but for many decades to come, America's interaction with the Middle East would waver between these impulses, the imperialist and the humanist, between the Strongs and the Clara Bartons.[15]

This dynamic relationship between strength and conviction in America's relationship with the region seemed to leave little role for the element of fantasy. Yet, in fact, romantic notions continued to color Americans' perceptions of the area and to govern their actions toward it. Indeed, as the century drew to close, myths about "Oriental" sensuality and exoticism attained renewed poignancy in many American minds. Such illusions would be fostered not by reading novels and memoirs about the Middle East or even by traveling to it, but rather by a single visit to America's own heartland, the Midwest.

15

IMPERIAL
MYTHS

VISITING CHICAGO IN THE SUMMER OF 1893, A RECENTLY married couple from Stockton, California, or a retired schoolteacher from Paterson, New Jersey, could have beheld the most spectacular sight ever displayed by Americans on their own continent. Covering over six hundred acres, replete with Japanese gardens, flower-lined waterways, and restaurants with seating for seven thousand, the World's Columbian Exposition hosted an unfathomable 65,000 displays. The fairgrounds, according to the *Century* magazine, "flamed with the human energy that handed the torch of civilization across an ocean" and "touched the romantic sense of the whole wide world."

Ostensibly, the exposition commemorated the four hundredth anniversary of Columbus's discovery of the New World, yet it also tacitly celebrated America's transition from a mainly agricultural society to an industrial powerhouse, and provided a diversion for the innumerable laborers who had been displaced or benumbed by that process. The exposition's planners sought to endow all Americans with a sense of their common fate and pride in their global ascendancy. Eager to be feted, distracted, and inspired, Americans flocked to Chicago, and not only from California and New Jersey but from forty-three territories and states, a total of 27.5 million attendees.

Arriving, as did most visitors, via elevated train, the Stockton couple and Paterson's erstwhile schoolmarm could proceed eastward into the magnificent White City with its two hundred buildings and Beaux-Arts halls, the tallest of which was topped only by the engineer George Ferris's 264-foot-high wheel. From there, they could stroll through pavilions dedicated to progress in transportation, manufacturing, and electricity, while others showcased the cultures of twenty-three foreign countries and the accomplishments of American women. They could thrill at the sight of a map of the United States made entirely of pickles or at the statue of a knight inventively sculpted from prunes. They could peep at moving pictures through Thomas Edison's newfangled kinetiscope, shrink before Krupp's quarter-million-pound cannon—the world's largest—or gape at the latest innovation in "humane" capital punishment, the electric chair. Relaxing on the banks of a willow-shaded lagoon or on the classical colonnade overlooking Lake Michigan, they could delight in the latest American snacks: Cracker Jacks and Shredded Wheat, hamburgers and Aunt Jemima's pancakes. Later, after sunset, they could gaze in wonderment as some 200,000 incandescent bulbs, powered by 127 dynamos, encased the White City in light.

Instead of heading into the fairgrounds proper, the tourists could veer north toward an elongated park known as the Midway Plaisance. Here, more prosaic forms of entertainment awaited, such as carnival games, freak shows, and a Wild West extravaganza starring Buffalo Bill Cody, the sharpshooter Anne Oakley, and over two hundred U.S. cavalrymen and Indians.[1] Further along the Midway lay the most sensational attraction of all. Bypassing the balloon rides, the reproductions of St. Peter's Basilica and Blarney Castle, ignoring the barkers and the hawkers, the Californians and the New Jerseyan would enter—in downtown Chicago—the Middle East.

Horatio Algeria

More than a few Americans in 1893 recalled with enchantment the Egyptian and Moroccan pavilions at the Centennial Exhibition in Philadelphia sixteen years earlier. Many would have welcomed the chance to view them again, to reexperience that mystique and frisson. But for Sol Bloom, who was only a child in 1876, the inspiration for bringing the Middle East to America sprang not from Philadelphia's fair but from an Algerian revue in Paris.

The youngest of six children born to Orthodox Jewish immigrants from Poland, Bloom was raised in San Francisco and received almost no formal education. At age seven he started working in a brush factory, but soon branched out into other occupations—advertising, real estate, and, most prosperously, the theater. By nineteen, he was already a wealthy man, and decided to take a European tour, his very first vacation. Visiting the French capital in 1889, Bloom wandered open-mouthed through the International Exhibition, the largest fair ever mounted, with its displays of technological and natural marvels. None of these wonders impressed him more, however, than those supposedly imported from the Middle East. French engineers had meticulously re-created Cairo streets—even the buildings were painted to look dirty—and a labyrinthine Algerian Village. Bloom was awestruck. "I came to realize that a tall, skinny chap from Arabia with a talent for swallowing swords expressed a culture which to me was on a higher plane than the one demonstrated by a group of earnest Swiss peasants who passed their days making cheese and milk chocolate," he recalled some sixty years later. "The spiritual intensity of the performance exceeded the emotional power of a pre-Renaissance tapestry."

The experience tweaked not only Bloom's intellect but also his commercial instincts. "I knew that nothing like these dancers, acrobats, glass-eaters, and scorpion swallowers had ever been seen in the Western Hemisphere, and I was sure that I could make a fortune with them in the United States." At five feet six, a nonimposing figure whose oversized smile and nose seemed to compress his squinty eyes, unknown and utterly ignorant of French, Bloom seemed unlikely to succeed in fin-de-siècle Paris. Yet the same persuasive powers that had made him rich in America enabled him to secure a two-year exclusive option on the Algerian Village for a mere one thousand dollars. The contract provided for a world tour, but Bloom had no intention of exploiting it. "The rest of the globe would have to wait until I had brought the Algerian Village to America."

Inducing the French to part with the Algerians proved less difficult for Bloom than persuading the august heads of the Chicago exposition to host them. The organizers saw the Midway Plaisance as a cultural promenade, not a carnival arcade, and entrusted its development to a Harvard ethnologist. "To have made this unhappy gentleman responsible for . . . entertainment," remembered Bloom, "was about as intelligent a decision as . . . to make Albert Einstein manager of the Ringling Brothers and Barnum & Bailey Circus." Nevertheless, after his appointment as the fair's entertainment director, Bloom was well placed to convince the overseers that the village could be both edifying and profitable. He further proposed that not only Algerians be exhibited but also Egyptians, Moroccans, Tunisians, Sudanese, and Turks. These would all be showcased in a "Mohammedan world" situated in the Midway's center, just a short distance from the Ferris wheel.[2]

Over the course of eighty years, beginning with Mordecai Noah's appointment as consul in Tunis and Edwin De Leon's in Egypt, through the recent ambassadorships of Oscar Straus and Solomon Hirsch to the Porte, the United States had viewed its Jewish citizens as a natural bridge to the Middle East. Now, though his sole impetus was commercial, another American Jew was fulfilling a similar purpose. In contrast to his coreligionists serving abroad, Bloom had no interest in projecting his country's power into the Middle East or in safeguarding the agents of American faith. His objective, rather, lay in making the cultures and wonders of the Middle East available to vast numbers of Americans, enabling them to access their dreams.

The Midway's Middle East

The exposition formally opened, to international acclaim, on May 1, 1893, with an inaugurating speech by Grover Cleveland. Many of the fair's structures had yet to be completed, but the Middle Eastern section of the Midway was already teeming. At the Algerian Village, the president was greeted by dozens of young women in brazenly diaphanous pantaloons and brightly embroidered vests, who lowered their veils as he passed. "I doubt very much whether anything resembling it was ever seen in Algeria," he later confessed, "but I was not at the time concerned with trifles." Neither were the bulk of Americans who swiftly flooded the site. Indifferent to the real Middle East, their main concern lay in confirming their myths about the region, the illusions spawned by *A Thousand and One Arabian Nights* and the images painted by Irving, Melville, and Twain.

In Chicago, on the Midway, those myths fabulously leapt to life. Approaching the concourse, our California newlyweds and New Jersey retiree would already glimpse the tips of minarets, silken pennants, and multicolored tents and hear what one disdainful visitor from Virginia, a Reverend Eggleston, called "the strange music of a foreign tambourine, and the hideous yelling (music, so-called) of non-American girls." Soon they would encounter a scene similar to that first described by John Ledyard more than a hundred years earlier: meandering streets teeming with exotically dressed Levantines—Arabs, Copts, Armenians, and Jews—all yammering in guttural tongues. Shopkeepers in white turbans and gilded shoes hawked carpets, swords, and other "authentic" mementos, while hooded women balanced water jugs on their heads. "Memories of childhood stories trooped before us, of Joseph and his brethren, of Pharaoh's daughter and her maids bending over the babe Moses," wrote a tourist who referred to herself only as Mrs. Mark Stevens. "With a little stretch of the imagination our dream of the Orient was realized."

Spellbound, Mrs. Stevens felt little compulsion to investigate how many of these natives in fact hailed from the Middle East and how many were merely actors culled from Chicago's ethnic communities. The *Century* correspondent Gustave Kobbe was not so complacent, however, asserting that "the Midway Plaisance is probably the greatest collection of fakes the world has ever seen." One berobed figure in particular, Kobbe claimed, was the "greatest fakir [a Muslim mystic]" of them all. "I am proud to say he was an American."

Some exhibits did, in fact, employ Middle Easterners, such as the sixty-five women, men, and children recruited from various Ottoman provinces to populate the Turkish Pavilion. They, along with an array of kiosks, mosques, and quaint Istanbul-style houses, helped generate an otherworldly, Oriental atmosphere through which Americans could wander, gawking at a sultaness's solid silver bed or a "Wild East show" staged by Bedouin lancers on steeds. Alternatively, they could browse through the forty souvenir shops at the Grand Bazaar, take in a medieval Turkish play with simultaneous English translation, or smoke a water pipe at a *café chantant* while sipping Mecca coffee or "Turkish Temperance Drinks," such as orange juice and lemonade.

The Turkish Pavilion, produced by another Jewish entrepreneur, Joseph Levy, proved immensely popular. So did the Moorish Palace, with its hall of mirrors and its wax museum of horrors, the Persian Tent, and the Kabyle (North African tribal) House. More alluring than all of these curios, though, was Cairo Street. Like its Parisian predecessor, this exhibit was reconstructed in painstaking detail, though not by Frenchmen but by a Hungarian, Max Herz, the Egyptian khedive's personal architect. It featured latticed windows and closed wooden balconies, scalloped water fountains and a souk with sixty booths, a replica of the Qayt Bey Mosque, and the house of one Gamal El Din El Yahbi, a fictitious Egyptian merchant. Real Egyptians were also brought in to reenact scenes from daily life—180 of them dressed up as dervishes, tent makers, beggars, and fortune-tellers. Donkeys, too, were imported, as well as dogs, monkeys, and, of course, camels. The latter, for fifty cents, could be ridden. "Such a jaunt was honey for lovers, but gall and wormwood for prudes and fat people," recounted one rider who had straddled the hump.

For those with less adventurous inclinations, Cairo Street also offered ornate Egyptian temples from the pharaonic age, copies of ancient tombs, and even mummies. The cumulative effect was hypnotic. "Cairo was strikingly resplendent when bathed in the golden rays of the departing sun," Mrs. Stevens swooned. "[W]hen . . . the cold, gray moonlight shone upon its quaint architecture and grave-looking people, the visitors felt they were indeed in Egypt."[3]

The "Mohammedan world" exhibits also spurred another, more invidious type of revelry, one that Western men had long derived from the Middle East. Both Cairo Street and the Algerian Village were equipped with sumptuous theaters, and the Persian Tent had its Palace of Eros, in which women clothed in so-called Oriental dress—translucent skirts, bare midriffs, a profusion of bracelets and beads—performed snake and candle dances to the rataplan of tom-

toms and flutes. "This high art dancing of the Nile consisted of distorting and knotting the muscles, reminding us of a cat in a fit," Mrs. Stevens wrote, recalling how one of the dancers "flew into a rage at the audience . . . threatening the musicians and also the audience." Yet the violence these entertainers contrived paled before the wantonness of the belly dancers or, as Sol Bloom continentally called them, *danseuses de ventre*.

Since these shows appealed mostly to men, the California groom would separate from his now irritated bride, leaving her, together with the indignant schoolteacher, outside of the theater. Within, he could ogle "splendid specimens of oriental beauty" executing suggestive contortions of their sporadically clad bodies. "It is the coarse animal passion of the East, not the chaste sentiment of Christian lands," remarked one onlooker, after viewing the "Dance of Love," a solo. "Every motion of her body is in the illustration of her animalism." And of the performers few were as feral as the Syrian-born Fahred Mahzar, the coquettishly nicknamed Little Egypt, whose "genuine native muscle dance" was said to "deprive [a man] of a peaceful night's rest for years to come." Accompanied by a minor-key ditty that Bloom fingered out on a piano—later replayed by countless cartoon snake charmers—Little Egypt would mesmerize her male audiences with her sinuous, sensuous gyrations. As another breathless spectator observed:

> Now she revolves and turns, her face assuming a dreamy smile, her painted eyes half closed, her white teeth showing between lips made redder and fuller by art. . . . [H]er movements are snake-like and vulgar, and she sinks lower and lower, wriggling, twisting, jerking, her face half veiled with her handkerchief, until she almost touches the stage.

Not all the spectators were similarly titillated, however. Anthony Comstock, the plump and fulsomely whiskered founder of the Society for the Suppression of Vice, the congressionally sanctioned burner of *A Thousand and One Arabian Nights* and hundreds of similarly "obscene" books, demanded that such performances be outlawed. The aged Julia Ward Howe denounced the belly dance as "simply horrid" and as a "most deforming movement of the whole abdominal and lumbar region," and concluded, "We thought it indecent." Yet, the majority of fairgoers found nothing objectionable about Little Egypt and preferred to fault her detractors' prudishness. Poking fun at Howe, the *Chicago Tribune* wondered "whether the apprehensions of the good ladies were due to infringements of morality or to the anticipation that the performers may bring on an attack of peritonitis if they persist in their contortions."[4]

THE MIDDLE EASTERN pavilions proved to be the most popular attraction of the fair, drawing more than 60 percent more admissions than its next highest moneymaker, the Ferris wheel. Approximately 2.5 million people ambled down Cairo Street, and, according to the exposition's *Final Official Report*, nearly fifty thousand of them rode on camels. For many of those tourists, this proved to be a culturally stimulating—and comfortingly sterile—experience. "The denizens of the Midway . . . give the observer an opportunity to investigate these barbarous and semi-civilized people without the unpleasant accompaniments of travel through their countries and contact with them," New York's senator Chauncey M. Depew harrumphed. For others, such as the effusive Mrs. Stevens, the Midway was "the model of the New Jerusalem," curative and spiritually uplifting. For most Americans, however, presumably including our exemplary teacher and reunited husband and wife, the encounter with Chicago's Middle East was simply, unequivocally fun. "We were all knocked silly," John Hay, the usually saturnine secretary of state, tittered. "It beats the brag so far out of sight that even Chicago is dumb."

Sol Bloom had every reason to exult. "The crowds poured in," he exulted. "I had a gold mine." Building on his Chicago-earned reputation, Bloom would soon move to New York, become a congressman, and, in that capacity, play a prominent role in America's relations with the Middle East. Looking back, Bloom regretted only that the belly dance, which he considered "a masterpiece of rhythm and beauty," later degenerated into burlesque and that he failed to copyright the snake charmer's song. He also missed the company of the Algerian who served as his personal bodyguard during the fair, a swarthy giant named Archie.

The Chicago exposition lasted only six months, but Bloom's recreation of the Middle East—"Haroun al-Raschid's new capital," the *Century* now called it—would resonate for decades. The *dance de ventre*, renamed and further eroticized as the "hoochy koochy," became a Vaudeville standard, and Little Egypt an off-color sensation, giving rise to dozens of imposters and several high society scandals. A generation of Americans danced to the "Cairo Street Waltz" or sang "She Never Saw the Streets of Cairo," while children, appropriating Bloom's "Oriental" tune, sniggered, "There's a place in France where the ladies wear no pants." Encouraged by the Midway's success, future world's fairs would also feature Middle Eastern pavilions, and the Ringling Brothers and Barnum and Bailey Circus presented pageants with such seductive names as "Persia—The Most Gorgeous Oriental Display Ever Seen in Any Land" and "Orientally Splendid and Weirdly Romantic Spectacular Pilgrimage to Mecca."[5] For perpetuating Middle Eastern illusions, a visit to any of these attractions could easily rival a reading of *A Thousand and One Arabian Nights*, further imprinting those myths on America's imagination.

MYTHMAKING MAY have been the Midway's major accomplishment, but the fair's organizers never lost sight of their original, educational goal. Along with more mundane amusements, they sponsored nearly six thousand lectures on an ambitious range of economic, social, ethical, and religious topics. Many of the nation's foremost speakers participated, including the Reverned T. De Witt Talmage and a young Princeton professor, Woodrow Wilson, who addressed the need for university reform. William Blackstone also attended, circulating his memorial in favor of a Jewish state in Palestine as well as his newest proposal for resolving international disputes through arbitration. Mark Twain was invited to talk about his fiction, but was confined to his bed with a stomach ailment. Ultimately, the series' most significant lecture had nothing to do with education, or even with fantasy and faith, but rather with the course of American power.

"He would be a rash prophet who should assert that the expansive character of American life has now entirely ceased," declared Frederick Jackson Turner, a thirty-two-year-old historian from Harvard. Rather, the "restless, nervous energy" that had driven Americans to conquer their own frontier, "that coarseness and strength combined with acuteness and inquisitiveness," would spur them to subdue even vaster territories overseas. Though slight, almost boyish looking, Turner sounded brawny in his call for an aggressive, unambivalent imperialism. That injunction clashed directly with the appeals of Twain and the members of his Anti-Imperialist League, who kept urging the United States to distinguish itself from rapacious Europe and pursue more enlightened, altruistic policies. Yet, as the country crossed into the new, twentieth century and sought to extend its influence throughout the Middle East and other areas, Turner's voice, not Twain's, would accompany it. "American energy," it proclaimed, "will continually demand a wider field for its exercise."[6]

16

A REGION RENAMED
AND REORDERED

THE TERM "MIDDLE EAST" APPEARED FOR THE FIRST TIME in the September 1902 edition of the *National Review*, published in London, in an article entitled "The Persian Gulf in International Relations." The journal originated in Great Britain, but the author was a citizen of the United States. As a young officer on the USS *Iroquois* in 1867, Alfred Thayer Mahan had sailed around the Arabian Peninsula and been impressed with the area's value as the crossroads of three continents. For centuries, Westerners had referred to the Muslim-ruled lands between Fez and Kabul, Baghdad and Belgrade, as the Orient or, more simply, the East. Now, with the opening of Japan and China to the West and the escalation of imperialist struggles in Asia and the Pacific, the need arose to distinguish between the Far East and the Near East, and between the Near East of Bulgaria and the Balkans and the regions of Arabia, Persia, and the Gulf.

Mahan not only fulfilled that need but created an entirely new strategic concept. Trading in the quarterdeck for the classroom, he became the most venerated naval theorist of his day. In his classic book *Sea Power and America* (1897), he emphasized the connection between great-power status and the control of international trade by massive navies. To sustain the communications and supply routes between East and West, Mahan argued, the powers had to govern "the neck of land which joins Africa and Asia," including "Asiatic Turkey, Persia, Egypt, the basin of the Mediterranean Eastern," an area he called the Middle East. The nation that succeeded in controlling this Middle East—its canal, coastlines, and coaling stations— would capture the race for the more distant and lucrative Far East, and consequently dominate the world.[1]

Mahan's recommendations were directed at Britain, still the regnant naval power, but they also had growing relevance for America. As the new century dawned, the United States surpassed Europe in energy consumption and in total manufactured output and was gaining on Britain in foreign trade. Its population of 64 million, second only to Russia's, mined more coal, iron, gold, and silver, cut more timber, than any other country in the world and produced more steel than Britain and Germany combined. With no major enemies abroad and led by presidents endowed with far-reaching authority in foreign policy, the American people were poised to challenge Europeans for primacy in the Far East and in the newly demarcated Middle East as well.[2]

One barometer of rising American influence in the region was the steady expansion in the volume and variety of trade. The same United States that would conclude the twentieth century as one of the world's largest consumers of Middle Eastern oil was, in 1900, supplying much of the region with petroleum and kerosene. No less ironic, the country once famous for its fine tobaccos began importing Turkish blends for America's first national brand of cigarettes, emblazoned with the image of a camel. Still, American exports to the Middle East exceeded imports by a ratio of fourteen to one. "The newspapers of . . . England, Germany, and Austria are sharply calling attention . . . to the fact that a new and dangerous commercial rival has entered the field," reported Britain's consul in Istanbul, Charles M. Dickinson. Among the products available at the American Oriental Agency, he claimed, were "house and office furniture . . . electro-plated goods, machinery of various kinds, [and] typewriters . . . all displayed in a very attractive manner."

Just as the growth of missionary activity necessitated a more prominent American naval presence in the Middle East, so, too, booming trade required greater protection from American warships. While battleships such as the *Kentucky* and the *George Washington* paid occasional visits to Ottoman ports, the cruisers *Marblehead* and *San Francisco* routinely patrolled the coast of the eastern Mediterranean. As if acting on instructions from Mahan, the U.S. Navy had begun constructing the sixteen battleships that would eventually form the Great White Fleet, America's first global fighting force.

The power of this Great White Fleet and its impact on the Middle East, was already anticipated by the Irish-British playwright George Bernard Shaw. In his 1899 comedy, *Captain Brassbound's Conversion*, set in Morocco, Shaw introduced Hamlin Kearney, "a robustly built western American . . . with all the nations of the old world at war in his veins." Kearney, a Navy captain, demands the immediate release of two British subjects who he believes have been taken hostage by a fanatically anti-Christian sheikh. He cavalierly informs the sultan, "As the search will be conducted with machine guns, the prompt return of the travelers . . . will save much trouble to all parties." The ultimatum succeeds, and the pair is promptly released. Shaw concludes with some wistful musing about Kearney: "The world, pondering on the great part of its own future which is in his hands, contemplates him with wonder as to what the devil he will evolve into in another century or two."[3]

Shaw would not have to wait anywhere near that long in order to encounter a real-life embodiment of his Captain Kearney. When, in September 1901, an anarchist gunman assassinated William McKinley, his pugnacious vice president, Theodore Roosevelt, assumed office.

A Man for All Vocations

Lover of nature. Valiant leader. Ranchman and hunter. Intrepid explorer. Author and ardent observer. All of these designations decorate the Roosevelt Memorial at the American Museum of Natural History in New York. The careers, interests, and accomplishments of the twenty-sixth president indeed seemed beyond the grasp of a normal human being, and certainly of one who began life as pampered and ailing. Still, the roster might be lengthened to include yet another appellation: Middle East expert. That proficiency could be traced to November 1872, when the precocious fourteen-year-old—then nick-named Teedie—embarked with his family for Egypt, Syria, and Palestine.

Like so many American travelers before him, Roosevelt was enthralled with the idea of the Middle East. "How I gazed upon it!" he told his diary of his first sight of the Egyptian coast. "It was Egypt, the land of my dreams. . . . A land that was old when Rome was bright, was old when Troy was taken! It was a sight to awaken a thousand thoughts, and it did." The teenager's descriptions of Alexandria closely resembled those of American visitors to the city throughout the nineteenth century—the chaos, the cavalcade of ethnicities and dress. Typically, too, Roosevelt saw "a glimpse of the ineffable, of the unutterable" in Egypt's ancient relics. "I *felt* a great deal but I *said* nothing. You can not express yourself on such an occasion."

The family took the obligatory cruise up the Nile, rendezvoused and shared a picnic lunch with Ralph Waldo Emerson, and indulged in the American tradition of slaughtering the river's wildlife. Teedie shot and stuffed a warbler, the first specimen in what would become a vast and scientifically valuable collection. Exhibiting the bargaining skills that would someday serve him in diplomacy, he haggled for quails in the souk. "The Arabs always talk a great deal," he gloated. Later, he followed in Mark Twain's tracks by crossing Syria and Palestine on horseback. As might be expected of a regular attendant at his Dutch Reformed Sunday school, the young Roosevelt was deeply stirred by the holy places he saw, not only the Christian ones but also the Mosque of Omar and the Wailing Wall. Yet, like Twain, he found Jerusalem "remarkably small" and the Jordan disappointingly narrow, "what we should call a small creek in America."

Roosevelt returned from the trip sickened with asthma, but more determined than ever to build up his physical strength and endurance. He also brought back a sharpened sense of the Middle East, one which, over time, blended with his interests in myth and religion and colored his strategic thinking. "Spain and Turkey are the two powers I would rather smash than any in the world," he revealed as a bullish assistant naval secretary in 1898, before volunteering for combat in Cuba.

A friend to both Alfred Thayer Mahan and the Reverend Josiah Strong, Roosevelt harbored an almost mystical belief in the virtues of naval power and in America's inviolate right to wield it. Nations, in his worldview, were like individuals, some weak and others stalwart, and the latter were obliged to defend the former. Some "barbarous and semi-barbarous peoples" were "so utterly incompetent either to protect the rights of foreigners against their own citizens, or to protect their own citizens against foreigners," that "honorable and upright" states were morally impelled to police them. Accordingly, Roosevelt praised Britain for avenging the death of General Chinese Gordon by Islamic forces in the Sudan in 1898 and for defeating those who practiced "bigotry, tyranny, and cruel religious intolerance." The United States, in his view, was similarly bound to intercede on behalf of the Armenians and other Middle Eastern peoples threatened by the "dreadful scourge of the Turk."[4]

Before entering the White House, Roosevelt had focused primarily on South America and the Far East, to the near exclusion of the Middle East. This region, for him, remained peripheral to American interests, a source of few valuable commodities and an exclusive European purview. Paradoxically, the first real test of Roosevelt's foreign affairs philosophy came from the Ottoman Empire, the very entity he longed to destroy, and only a few days after he assumed the presidency.

Bulgarian bandits, Roosevelt learned, had kidnapped an American missionary named Ellen Stone, together with Katerina Tsilka, the pregnant wife of a mission school graduate. The abductors, though "dressed like Turks and talking bad Turkish," were in fact local Christians trying to finance their rebellion against Turkey. Forgetting America's earlier contributions to Bulgaria's struggle for independence, they demanded $100,000 in gold from the United States and gave the government eighteen days to pay.

The incident unsettled Roosevelt's sense of noblesse oblige, forcing him to cooperate with the "uncivilized" Ottomans against freedom-seeking Bulgarians. Beyond declaring that "the people of

the United States are thrilled with horror" by the women's abduction, there was little he could do to secure their release. Roosevelt
considered sending gunboats to the area, and even landing troops,
but it was unclear how the American people would react to a military intervention so soon after McKinley's murder. There was also
the danger that the kidnappers, suspecting a rescue attempt, would
promptly kill their prisoners. The president could not even appropriate money for ransoming Tsilka and Stone—a prerogative reserved
for Congress. Like George Washington, who in the 1790s found
himself powerless to redeem American captives in Algiers, Roosevelt
could only sit passively and let the public raise the funds.

Fortunately, the donations poured in. Stirred by press depictions
of Stone as a delicate ingenue—she was, in fact, dull, middle-aged,
and schoolmarmish—Americans generously contributed to her
redemption. George Washburn, the president of Robert College,
made contact with the kidnappers and persuaded them to extend the
deadline. News of the prisoners' release on March 1, 1902, was
greeted tumultuously by well-wishers throughout the United States,
but privately the president seethed. "Women have no earthly business to go out as missionaries into these wild countries," he grumbled, and pledged never to become so hamstrung again.[5]

Just over a year passed before Roosevelt's resolve was again challenged and once more in the Middle East. On August 27, 1903, word
reached Washington that the American vice consul in Beirut had
been assassinated. The presumed victim was William Magelssen, a
thirty-year-old preacher's son from Bratsberg, Minnesota, who had
purportedly protested renewed Turkish attacks against Armenians
and the American missionaries who tried to defend them. The president no longer hesitated; the next day, he ordered the USS *San Francisco*, the *Brooklyn*, and the *Machias* to proceed at full speed to
Lebanon. The intention was to demand the immediate arrest and
punishment of the diplomat's murderers and so demonstrate the end
of Roosevelt's patience with the Porte. Before the ships could arrive,
though, the White House learned that Magelssen was very much
alive. A bullet fired by celebrants at an Arab wedding had whizzed
past the diplomat's ear, but mercifully left him unharmed.

Roosevelt, though, was not so easily mollified. Even if Magelssen was safe, he contended, the missionaries remained endangered. Consequently, the cruisers took up position in Beirut harbor, trained their searchlights on the city, and threatened to impose a blockade until the Turks guaranteed the safety of all the American missionaries working in Syria. Some five hundred Marines were armed and readied for landing, in case the Porte refused.

Learning of the impending attack, Chekib Bey, the Ottoman ambassador in Washington, burst unannounced into the office of Secretary of State Hay. "We have allowed the missionaries great liberties, and with what result?" Chekib protested. Rather than expressing gratitude, the missions had plotted to "wipe [his] country off the map," by inciting the Armenians to rebellion. "Suppose I should establish . . . a school for [American] Negroes, and my teachers should tell the Negroes . . . that they ought not to submit to lynching and should rebel?" the diplomat asked. "Do you think I would remain in this country long or that my school would flourish?"

Chekib's remonstrations failed to dissuade Roosevelt. American battleships anchored for several weeks near Beirut and the following year returned to the Middle East, this time to Smyrna. The president ordered them to remain on permanent patrol off the Turkish coast, a reminder of America's commitment to protect all of its citizens residing in the Middle East.[6]

The Stone and Magelssen affairs, though certainly discomfiting for Roosevelt, were merely rehearsals for the direst challenge to his prestige in the region and the boldest display of his gunboat diplomacy. The drama commenced in Tangier on the evening of May 18, 1904, when a band of two hundred armed tribesmen raided the home of Ion Perdicaris, sixty-four, a convivial businessman described by the U.S. consul as the city's "most prominent American citizen." The intruders beat Perdicaris's servants and took him and his stepson hostage, riding with them into the almost inaccessible Riff Mountains. They were now the prisoners of a diminutive but charismatic Berber chief known locally as Ahmad ben Muhammad al-Rasul li-llah (Messenger of God) and in America, more succinctly, as Raisuli.

Swearing by "all we hold sacred" that no harm would befall his captives if they refrained from trying to escape, Raisuli told Perdicaris that he sought nothing from the United States, but only justice from Morocco's sultan, 'Abd al-'Aziz, who had long oppressed the Riffian Berbers. Raisuli wanted an end to the depredations, as well as compensation for past offenses in the form of a generous ransom. Not surprisingly, the sultan disregarded these demands, forcing Raisuli to change his position. Perdicaris would not be released, he now stated, until Washington exacted the concessions from Morocco.

Secretary of State John Hay, renowned for his stalwart handling of the Boxer Rebellion in China in 1900 and his demand for an "Open Door" for American trade in the Far East, had scant patience with a lone upstart such as Raisuli. He dismissed the chieftain's terms with a single word—"Preposterous!"—and instructed the American consul in Tangier to avoid "anything which may be regarded as an encouragement to . . . blackmail." Roosevelt, too, insisted that the United States not "surrender to the demands of those Moroccan brigands" and invited Britain and France to join him in an armed coalition to free Perdicaris. The British rejected the offer, though, as did the French, who took the additional step of reinforcing the defenses of Tangier against the possibility of an American attack.

Livid, Roosevelt thundered, "I had much rather be a real President for three years and a half than a figurehead for seven years and a half." Yet his grandiloquence softened somewhat when he learned that Perdicaris had left the United States during the Civil War, apparently to dodge military service, and was no longer even an American citizen. That fact, if publicized, would not only weaken Roosevelt's leverage on Raisuli but might prove particularly embarrassing in an election year. Such pitfalls might have deterred a different president, but this one responded by ordering a task force of seven warships to steam toward the Moroccan coast.

On the morning of May 30, the gleaming white bow of the battleship *Brooklyn* was sighted off the shores of Tangier. Soon, a detachment of Marines landed in the port to guard the American consulate, while an additional twelve hundred leathernecks prepared to occupy Tangier, if necessary. For the fourth time in less than a century (in the Barbary Wars, during the Civil War, and in the course of Britain's invasion of Egypt), American troops were intervening in the Middle

East. But the move was merely an admonishment, as Roosevelt made clear in a telegram to the sultan:

PRESIDENT WISHES EVERYTHING POSSIBLE DONE TO SECURE THE RELEASE OF PERDICARIS. HE WISHES IT CLEARLY UNDERSTOOD THAT IF PERDICARIS IS MURDERED, THIS GOVERNMENT WILL DEMAND THE LIFE OF THE MURDERER.
WE WANT PEDICARIS ALIVE OR RAISULI DEAD.

From a hampered Washington, Roosevelt had transformed into an activist Jefferson pursuing an "erect and independent attitude" toward the Middle East. The Moroccan government subsequently relented to Roosevelt's pressure and paid Raisuli his ransom. On June 23, Ion Perdicaris was freed. Apart from a dislocated thighbone he suffered while falling from his horse, the former hostage was otherwise unhurt and full of praise for his captor, "one of the most interesting and attractive personalities I have ever encountered." His warmest admiration, though, went to the country he had willfully abandoned, to "that flag, and that people—aye, and that President, behind those frigates, thousands of miles away, who have had me dug out."[7]

The saga of Roosevelt's intervention in Morocco, replete with images of scimitar-slashing horsemen, defenseless captives, and Marines dashing to the rescue, once again stimulated America's fantasies of the Middle East, inspiring a number of dime store romances and, many years later, a Hollywood movie. But in addition to stoking imaginations at home, the episode tempered the impression of American power internationally. Though some of Roosevelt's domestic critics claimed that the administration had gone too far in naval spending and in flexing its muscles overseas, the president remained obdurate. "Do they object to the fact that American warships appeared promptly at the port of Beirut when an effort had been made to assassinate an American official, and in the port of Tangier when an American citizen had been abducted, and that in each case the wrong complained of was righted and expiated?" he wondered. Did they complain, Roosevelt asked, when "the visit of an American squadron to Smyrna was followed by the long-delayed concession of the just rights" of American missionaries in Turkey?

The Middle East would again give Roosevelt a chance to respond to his detractors—once more in Morocco, where a contest for primacy between Germany and France was dragging all of Europe into war. Wanting to stay clear of that downslide, the United States had declared its neutrality in the Moroccan dispute. Roosevelt, though, fresh from his Nobel Prize–winning mediation of the Russo-Japanese War, believed that he could perform the same peacemaking role for the French and Germans. Thus, the United States, which had never participated in the great-power conferences on the Middle East, became a cosponsor of the international deliberations on Morocco that convened in Algeciras, Spain, in January 1906.

The instructions issued to America's delegates at the talks were precise: do not "side with either of the groups," but rather "remain an onlooker," showing "no concern beyond a kindly desire that harmony may prevail." Roosevelt, however, maneuvered dexterously behind the scenes. Though he personally liked the buffoonish Kaiser Wilhelm II, the president worked to "stand him [Wilhelm] on his head" by advancing the interests of Britain and France, which he felt were closer to America's. The result was an arrangement that gave France and Spain the right to police Morocco jointly, but virtually excluded Berlin. "It would be enormously to the benefit of the people of Morocco if the French took hold of them and did for them what they have done in Algiers," Roosevelt explained. Yet the president had more than Moroccan interests in mind. In the process of negotiating a multilateral agreement at Algeciras, he also secured his country's customary concerns in the area, protecting North African Jews from oppression and American merchants from unfair restrictions and fees.

At Algeciras, Roosevelt took the first step toward involving the United States in the Eastern Question. The principles he reaffirmed at the conference—support for the Anglo-French alliance, preserving minority rights and freedom for American trade—would remain the cornerstones of American diplomacy in the region for much of the next fifty years. Americans, Roosevelt proved, had not only invented the name "Middle East" but had played a pivotal role in refashioning the region geopolitically.[8]

Ambivalence Redux

America's status as a great power, almost universally acknowledged by the end of Roosevelt's presidency, was celebrated by a 45,000-mile, around-the-world voyage of the Great White Fleet. Twenty-one ships and fourteen thousand servicemen crossed the Arabian Sea and curved into the Gulf of Suez—the most massive American force ever to have entered the Middle East. It was also the largest single flotilla ever to have traversed the Suez Canal, closing the waterway to all other traffic during the first three days of 1909. While their ships coaled at Port Sa'id, the crews went on leave to Cairo, donned crimson fezzes, and photographed one another posing before the pyramids (see front cover) and careering on donkey-back through the souk. "We gave Cairo such a shaking up as it had not had for a long time," one of the sailors regaled. Others had a less amusing experience. "About us swarmed porters, guides, beggars, and impostors of every nation under the sun. . . . [B]lack men, white men, brown men, yellow men, some with long flowing robes, some almost naked, all forced themselves upon us, having heard, no doubt, of the 'easy American.' " The fleet's Middle Eastern debut nevertheless ended on a more amicable note, with hundreds of Americans and Arabs together laboring to dislodge the USS *Georgia* from a bank of Suez mud.[9]

The passage of the Great White Fleet through Egypt was followed, one year later, by that of Roosevelt himself. Over the course of the four decades since his last visit, the land of the Nile had been profoundly transformed. The limited military occupation that Britain once touted as temporary had sprawled into a permanent civil administration, recognized by a treaty with the French, and permeating every aspect of Egyptian life. But the occupation also fueled the rise of Egyptian nationalism, which had blossomed since 'Urabi's time into a nationwide movement of officers, students, intellectuals, and religious leaders. Demanding immediate independence for Egypt, protesters frequently clashed with British troops. Nationalist and sectarian friction peaked on February 21, 1910, when a Muslim shot and killed Egypt's prime minister, Butros Ghali—grandfather of the future UN secretary-general—a Coptic Christian. Five months later, Theodore Roosevelt arrived.

Though he was no longer president, he still drew throngs of well-wishers, eager to hear his insights on ethics and international affairs. In Egypt, though, his remarks only disappointed them. While stressing the country's need to embrace the principles of democracy, hard work, free enterprise, Roosevelt predicted, "It will be years, perhaps generations, before Egypt is ready to govern itself." He advised the university students to cooperate with the British authorities and told army officers to stay out of politics entirely. Were Britain to leave Egypt, Roosevelt warned, women would be denied the most basic rights and many more Christians would be murdered. "Many of the noisy leaders of the Nationalist movement were merely . . . emotional, rather decadent, quite hopeless as material on which to build," he confided to the British statesman George Otto Trevelyan, a historian of the American Revolution. The West had nothing to fear from these "Levantines in European clothes," Roosevelt averred, but only from their followers, "the mass of . . . bigoted Moslems" committed to "driving out the foreigner, plundering and slaying the local Christian, and return[ing] to all the violence and corruption which festered under the old-style Moslem rule."

Roosevelt was probably unaware that many of those "noisy nationalists leaders" had been educated at the Syrian Protestant College in Beirut and that some of the senior Egyptian officers had studied at the schools established by Civil War veterans. The yearning for freedom they expressed was, partially at least, forged by the United States. Hundreds of those nationalists subsequently gathered outside the former president's hotel for the first major anti-American demonstration ever in the Middle East. "Down with Roosevelt," they shouted, and "Down with the Occupation." Ali Yousuff, a venerated editor and al-Azhar-trained sheikh, assailed Roosevelt for impugning Egypt's readiness for self-government while praising the power that prevented Egypt from proving itself. Such effrontery, he foretold, would reverberate throughout the region and beyond, for "when Egypt is insulted every Mohammedan on the face of this world feels the insult." Unlike Roosevelt, Sheikh Yousuff recalled America's contributions to the struggle for Middle Eastern liberty. "We believe that Americans are still . . . the friends of freedom," he declared. "The friends of nations that are governed against their will."

Such exhortations had negligible impact on the leader who had refused to buckle to Raisuli, to the Ottoman sultan or Germany's kaiser. Retracing his childhood journey up the Nile, Roosevelt persisted in extolling the "intelligence, ability and . . . lofty sense of duty" with which the British strove to "raise the seventh century so as to bring it somewhere within touching distance of the twentieth." This "mighty task," he maintained, was a "high and honorable thing," one that "only a great and powerful nation could attempt." Still, he wondered whether the British in Egypt, or the French in North Africa, could ultimately succeed in their mission. He even fantasized about taking over the job once the Europeans had failed. "I should have things moving in fine order first." In Roosevelt's mind, at least, the ambivalence that some Americans had shown to Western conquests in the Middle East—indeed, to imperialism in general—was banished.[10]

IN THE European mind, meanwhile, the imperialist urge only burgeoned. In October 1911, Italian troops invaded Tripoli and Darna and inaugurated a bloody twenty-year campaign to subjugate Libya. The following year, France exploited the concessions it secured with Roosevelt's help at Algeciras and seized control of Morocco. The entire Middle East from the Atlantic coast to the Suez Canal was now under foreign occupation, with various powers already competing for hegemony in Syria, Palestine, and the Gulf. Germany had accomplished a subtler but more extensive penetration, providing weapons and military advisers to the Turkish army and laying troop-transporting railway systems across the Ottoman Empire. The Middle East, as Mahan had defined it, was now recognized as a distinct region bound not only by geography but also by communalities of language, religion, and culture. Yet it was linked, as well, by a nexus of colonies, protectorates, and trusteeships, all under European rule.

Though now a great power in its own right, the United States viewed most of these events with a remoteness approaching dispassion. The administration of President William Howard Taft was more concerned with America's standing in the Far East and South America than in the brutal takeovers of Libya and Morocco, and too focused on foreign commerce to fret over the Turko-German axis. While Washington did welcome the successful coup staged by a band of modernizing Young Turks in 1908 and the struggle for constitutional reform in Persia, its enthusiasm for these developments was less reflective of republican sympathy than of hopes for improved trade. Indeed, when the Ottomans beseeched Taft to follow Roosevelt's example and help mediate the disputes that had deprived them of 400,000 square miles of their empire, the obese, phlegmatic president swore to maintain "an attitude of absolute neutrality and of complete political disinterestedness." Congress even refused to allocate funds for building an official U.S. embassy in Istanbul. Ambassador John Leishman personally financed the project and received reimbursement only after he defeated the House Speaker, Joseph Cannon, in poker.

America's turn toward isolationism in its attitudes toward the Middle East was illustrated in 1909 when the State Department created the Division of Near Eastern Affairs (NEA). Though educated people in the region had begun to refer to themselves as Middle Easterners, American diplomats insisted on retaining the region's traditional name and included Greece, Italy, Abyssinia, and the Balkans within its boundaries. None of the NEA's original staff, moreover, could speak a Middle Eastern language or produce a contemporary map of the area. Rather than recommend policies for addressing the vast upheavals rocking the Ottoman Empire, the division watched over the special interests of American churchmen and entrepreneurs. At the request of one group of American investors, the NEA investigated the possibility of purchasing the Hill of the Beatitudes, in the Galilean section of Palestine, the scene of Jesus' Sermon on the Mount.

Individual Americans did, in fact, strive for a more substantive interaction with the Middle East, only to find their approaches stymied by Europe. Tenders submitted by the Ottoman-American Company, formed in 1913 with the intention of building railways across Syria and Anatolia, were quashed by German counselors to the sultan. Similarly, the Russians secured the banishment of a young and idealistic American lawyer named W. Morgan Shuster, who tried to reform Persia's political system. "It was a monumental error to bring Americans to this country," crowed one Russian official following Shuster's expulsion. "I know for what they stand . . . and you can't make them 'fit.' " Neither the White House nor the State Department took pains to protect these initiatives or to protest their annulment. Assistant Secretary of State Francis Huntington Wilson concluded that "it would be the veriest folly to irritate any government over the Persian question," though the reluctance to intervene typified America's attitude toward the Middle East in general. "[I]t's no place for us to waste ammunition."[11]

More than thirty years had passed since that July dawn when the silhouettes of British battleships had appeared off the Egyptian coast. Throughout that period, Americans debated the advantages and liabilities of imperialism—its material and spiritual benefits versus its ethical drawbacks. Though most, like Theodore Roosevelt, continued to endorse imperialism as a legitimate, if not divinely ordained, boon to American influence, others sided with Mark Twain in denouncing the policy as disreputable and un-American. The debate might have dragged on indefinitely but for the intrusion of global events. As the world careened toward war, Americans would again have to engage with the Middle East, to choose between their loyalty to the West and their sympathy for native peoples as well as between evangelism and rationalism, Zionism and Arab nationalism. While a calamity of incalculable dimensions descended on the region, the dictates of American faith would once more clash with the exigencies of power, and fantasy would be all but eclipsed.

Part Five

America,
the Middle East,
and the
Great War

17

SPECTATORS OF CATASTROPHE

"HISTORY," WROTE THE NOVELIST PHILIP ROTH, IS "WHERE everything unexpected in its own time is chronicled on the page as inevitable." Few observers in the summer of 1914 anticipated that Austria-Hungary's declaration of war against Serbia would spark an ineluctable chain reaction in which Russia dashed to Serbia's defense and Germany ran to Austria's, or that France would rally to its Russian allies while Britain sided with the French. Fewer still predicted that Turkey would fail in its efforts to stay clear of the fracas and be driven into an alliance with Germany and Austro-Hungary—the Central Powers—against the Triple Entente of Russia, Britain, and France. The shockingly unexpected, however, happened. World War I, the cataclysm that would last four unspeakable years, bring about the fall of empires and irrevocably transform the Middle East, had started. "The terror of the unforeseen is what the science of history hides," Roth concluded, "turning a disaster into an epic."

Americans watched this inadvertent slide into war with a rapt, but ultimately detached, fascination. They, too, had been surprised by the unforeseen chain of events leading to catastrophe, but, in contrast to the Europeans and the Turks, Americans bore none of the consequences for their shortsightedness. Evoking America's traditional disdain for foreign entanglements, President Woodrow Wilson vowed to maintain absolute neutrality between the combatants and to preserve proper, if not cordial, relations with each.

Maintaining amicability with Turkey would prove complicated, however, because ties between the United States and the Porte had long been frayed. The perennial source of friction was the oppression of Armenian Christians. Though a band of modernizing Young Turks, many of them graduates of Roberts College, had achieved power in Istanbul in 1908 and promised equal rights for all of the empire's citizens, barely a year passed before the slaughter of Armenians resumed. Some thirty thousand of them were butchered by Turkish troops in south-central Anatolia. "The only difference between Young and Old Turks is that the Young Turks are more energetic and thorough in their massacring," Helen Davenport Gibbons, the wife of the *New York Herald* correspondent in Tarsus, commented. Soon even the semblance of republican rule in Turkey collapsed and in 1911 the government was seized by a military junta. The United States responded with abhorrence to these events and, to register its protest, sent the battleships *Montana* and *North Carolina* to demonstrate near the Turkish coast.[1]

Outrage over the Armenian massacres might have caused a rupture in America's relations with Turkey but for the substantive rise in Turco-American trade. Economic cooperation between the United States and the Ottoman Empire had expanded vigorously since the turn of the century and by 1914 America accounted for 23 percent of all Turkish exports. Along with tobacco, figs, and licorice (some fifty thousand tons of it annually, for use in making candy and chewing gum), Americans were procuring a new Middle Eastern commodity: oil. Though the United States remained a major producer of petroleum—and an exporter of its derivatives to the Middle East— domestic wells could no longer satisfy the fuel demands of American industry, automobile owners, and the military. Acting on evidence of sizable Middle Eastern deposits, the Standard Oil Company of New Jersey started prospecting in Mesopotamia in 1910. Three years later, Standard of New York acquired rights to drill in Syria, Palestine, and parts of Asia Minor. Infrastructure for the oil rigs had already been constructed and drilling had begun when the global conflagration erupted.

Oil eventually became an obsession in America's policymaking toward the Middle East, but on the eve of World War I the country's principal interest in the region remained philanthropic. The number of American missionary institutions had multiplied prodigiously throughout the prewar period and now included world-class hospitals and colleges and well over four hundred schools. These establishments were deeply integrated into Ottoman society, serving not only local Christian populations but also the Turkish elite. "I am much gratified to learn of arrangements made for education of the [Turkish] war minister's brother and sons at Robert College," wrote Secretary of State William Jennings Bryan to his ambassador in Istanbul in October 1914. "It is an excellent sign." By receiving an American education, Bryan hoped, Turks might also learn to tolerate Armenians and other Middle Eastern minorities and restore their country to its former democratic course.[2]

The outbreak of war, however, only strengthened the military's primacy in Istanbul and threatened the safety of American institutions. The Wilson administration, acting "in the interest of humanity and from no political consideration," accordingly urged Turkey to declare its neutrality in the conflict. The Turks, American diplomats warned, were no match for the Allies, who dominated the Mediterranean and could swiftly capture its coastal cities, from Smyrna to Jaffa. But this advice went unheeded. No sooner had Turkey enlisted in the Central Powers than it initiated a campaign to expel all French and British citizens from the empire. The capitulations that for centuries provided extraterritorial privileges to Westerners in the Ottoman Empire were rescinded and English was outlawed as an "enemy language." Already precarious, the situation of Americans in the Middle East grew imperiled when the Turkish government proclaimed a holy war—jihad—against all Allied Christians.[3]

Panicked by the specter of frenzied Muslim pogroms, the missionaries implored Washington for help. The Syrian Protestant College president Daniel Bliss impressed on Secretary of State Bryan the "grave immediate necessity for the protection of American life and property" and urged him to send American warships to Beirut and Smyrna at once. Similar appeals came from Jaffa and from Jerusalem, which reported a mass seizure of supplies by Turkish troops and a "reign of military terrorism." In reply, Wilson dispatched the USS *North Carolina* and the *Tennessee* to deliver vital foodstuffs and money to the missionaries. America's fears were then heightened when Turkish shells, fired from Smyrna, whistled over the *Tennessee*'s prow. On December 12, Wilson approved a measure advising all Americans to leave the Middle East "wherever . . . it would be unsafe for them to remain."

Friction, meanwhile, intensified on the diplomatic level, in progressively acrimonious exchanges between the two governments. "Should organized massacres occur, the Turkish government would lose the good opinion of the United States," Washington cautioned, and further warned that "any loss of life or property of missionaries" would elicit a stern American response. Djemal Pasha, the notorious military governor of Syria, in turn swore, "For each Mussulman killed by the bombardment of an open town we will shoot three British or French subjects," and disavowed responsibility "if the bombardment . . . provokes a massacre of the Christians." The American press replied with furious attacks against Turkey and calls for an Anglo-French takeover of the Middle East. In a volcanic letter to the *Washington Star*, Ambassador Ahmet Rustem Bey accused the United States of hypocrisy for condemning Turkey while condoning the Russians, "who gave the world not one but twenty pogroms against an innocent [Jewish] race," the French, "who smoke to death in caverns the Algerians fighting for independence," and the British, "whose punishment of the 'rebels' in the Indian mutiny was to blow them off with guns." Rustem also reminded Americans of the "daily" lynching of blacks in their own country and the torture of Filipino insurgents. Rustem was consequently declared persona non grata and forced to leave the country.

Turco-American relations were close to rupturing in the fall of 1914, when suddenly and markedly they improved. Afraid to alienate an important noncombatant Western state, senior officials in Istanbul insisted that they "never doubted America's sincere friendship for Turkey" and that the United States remained "the only great power with no ulterior motive toward them." They reaffirmed the privileged status of American businessmen and apologized for any unpleasantness toward the missionaries. Though English was still outlawed, citizens of the United States were henceforth permitted to correspond in the "American" language. Washington, for its part, canceled plans for evacuating the Middle East and instead offered to send thirteen mobile Red Cross hospitals to care for Turkey's sick and wounded. The forty-eight U.S. consuls serving in Turkey stayed in their posts, as did the Turkish representatives stationed in San Francisco, Chicago, Boston, and New York. As the year ended and the Allies prepared to launch their mass landing on Turkey's Gallipoli Peninsula—a fiasco that would cost them a quarter of a million dead and prolong the Middle Eastern fighting for years—Americans seemed content to remain on the sidelines, uninvolved.[4]

Americans could not remain detached, however, indefinitely. War-stirred turmoil in the Middle East would soon engulf the United States and compel it to act on a multiplicity of levels—diplomatic, humanitarian, and even military. Religious and strategic considerations would once again vie for dominance in the making of America's policies toward the region, while popular illusions about the Middle East, obscured by massacres and famine, would vanish.

The Most Horrible Crime in Human History

The first reports, from December 1914, told of anti-Christian pogroms in Bitlis, in eastern Turkey, and the hanging of hundreds of Armenians in the streets of Erzerum. Armenian men between the ages of twenty and sixty were being conscripted into forced-labor battalions, building roads, and hauling supplies for the Turkish army. The following month, after their defeat by Russian forces in the Caucasus, Turkish troops salved their humiliation by pillaging Armenian towns and executing their Armenian laborers. In the early spring, Turkish soldiers laid siege to the Armenian city of Van, in eastern Anatolia, and began the first of innumerable mass deportations. The slaughter then raged westward to Istanbul, where, on April 24, security forces arrested and hanged some 250 Armenian leaders and torched Armenian neighborhoods. Interior Minister Talaat Pasha informed the Armenian patriach that "there was no room for Christians in Turkey" and advised him and his parishioners "to clear out of the country."[5]

The threat was anything but empty, as confirmed by eyewitness American accounts. "The Mohammedans in their fanaticism seemed determined not only to exterminate the Christian population but to remove all traces of their religion and . . . civilization," attested Leslie Davis, a Cornell-educated consul in Harput, eastern Anatolia, early in 1915. Davis's counterpart in Aleppo, Syria, Jesse B. Jackson, described a seemingly endless procession of railway cars crammed with Armenian deportees and estimated that no more than 15 percent were liable to survive the journey. Another American witness of these trains, Anna Harlowe Birge, remembered seeing "old men and old women, young mothers with tiny babies . . . and children, all huddled together like so many sheep or pigs—human beings treated worse than cattle." In Urmia, the Presbyterian missionary William Shedd described the execution of 800 villagers, mostly old people and young women, by the governor, Jevdet Bey, who purportedly delighted in nailing horseshoes to his victims' feet. The third-generation missionary Henry Riggs cataloged the tortures—"beating and starvation, extraction of teeth, branding with hot irons, stabbing in the face with sharp irons, burning of hair and beard"—to which the Armenians of southwestern Turkey were subjected. Reporting from the Caucasus, Dr. Richard Hill saw "children . . . dying by the hundreds" whose "frenzied mothers would . . . fling them . . . into the fields, so as not to see the[ir] dying agonies."

Turkey's leaders at the time insisted—and their present-day successors still do—that the suffering of Armenians was a by-product of the brutality that prevailed along all First World War fronts. They also claim that the Armenians were actively sympathetic to the Allies and collaborated with the invading Russians. The bulk of the massacres in fact occurred nowhere near the fighting, while the overwhelming majority of Armenians remained loyal to the Turkish state. Most contemporary observers agree that the massacres were scarcely connected to the war, but rather represented a systematically planned and executed program to eliminate an entire people. Indeed, foreshadowing the Nazi genocide of the Jews twenty-five years later, Turkish soldiers herded entire Armenian villages into freezing rivers, incinerated them in burning churches, or simply marched them into the deserts and abandoned them to die of thirst. "The Government . . . has decided to destroy completely all the indicated [Armenian] persons living in Turkey," Talaat Pasha wrote in a September 1915 dispatch. "An end must be put to their existence . . . and no regard must be paid to either age or sex, or to conscientious scruples." By the end of summer, an estimated 800,000 Armenians had been killed and countless others forcibly converted to Islam.[6]

In contrast to earlier atrocities committed in Ottoman lands, the details of which had been slow in emerging, information about the ethnic cleansing of Armenians was now relayed by telegraph and telephone lines and rapidly reached the West. Descriptions of Turkish brutality, together with photographs of its victims, were published widely. Compelled by these revelations, Britain, France, and Russia released a joint statement on May 24 pledging to hold Turkish leaders, as well as their collaborators, "personally responsible for such massacres." But with their forces bogged down in static warfare and their citizens banished from the Middle East, the Allies were powerless to intervene either militarily or philanthropically. Not even an appeal from Pope Benedict XV, sent directly to Sultan Muhammad V, managed to evoke mercy for the Armenians.

Among the few Westerners still capable of responding to the catastrophe were the Americans who had long been ministering to Armenia. In Harput, the missionary couple Tack and Henry Akinson emulated earlier American abolitionists by running an underground railway that smuggled Armenians into Kurdistan. At the same time, in Van, Dr. Clarence and Elizabeth Ussher and the nurses Grisell McLareen and Myrtle O. Shane worked indefatigably to care for the hundreds of gravely wounded and disease-stricken patients who overwhelmed their clinics and for the many Armenians who fled, "weary, starving, wailing like lost and hungry children," into Russia. Elizabeth Ussher died of typhus and her husband nearly succumbed to the epidemic as well. He managed to send off a desperate message to the State Department warning that "American lives [were] in danger" and urging immediate action by the United States.

The United States, however, had no intention of interposing between Turks and Armenians. Though the American press gave front-page coverage to the massacres—"State Department Shows Quarter of a Million Women Violated," a typical headline exclaimed—and while anti-Turkish rallies were staged in New York, the government reacted guardedly to the massacres. The Wilson administration assumed that overt criticism of Turkey was liable to provoke reprisals against American citizens and establishments throughout the Middle East, destroying a century of determined work. There was also the fear that the public, agitated by reports of atrocities, might press for a more active American role in the war. Secretary of State Bryan quietly asked the German government to help protect "non-combatants [and] non-Moslem foreigners" from "an outburst of fanaticism among the Moslems," but refrained from protesting formally to the Porte.[7]

The danger of being dragged into the war indirectly, through the rear door of the Middle East, now had to be weighed against the moral hazards of passively witnessing genocide. The value of American missionary schools and clinics had to be compared with that of the lives of the very people those institutions aspired to benefit.

An Evangelist of Americanism

One American, Henry Morgenthau, was determined to try to reconcile those interests and to resolve the conflicts in his country's policies toward the Middle East. His qualifications for doing so were far from exceptional, though. He had no diplomatic experience and had never worked in the region. His religion, moreover, put him at a marked disadvantage in dealing not only with Muslim rulers but also with many officials in the United States. Yet no adversity had ever proven insurmountable to Morgenthau, a German-born Jew who, at age twelve in 1870, immigrated to New York with his parents and eleven siblings, not knowing a word of English.

Two years later, however, Morgenthau entered New York's City College and swiftly went on to graduate from Columbia Law. A meteoric success as an attorney and businessman, he became a leader of New York's Reform Jewish community and an unsparing benefactor of the Democratic Party. By middle age, affecting a clipped white beard and silver pince-nez, Morgenthau had acquired a patriarchal look and was fond of citing the Bible. He was especially enamored of the prophets, with their emphasis on charity and social justice, and of the Quaker principles of moderation, fairness, and hard work. Morgenthau claimed that "conscience" rather than "pride" animated his actions and that his "true religion was to serve democracy."

An early supporter of Wilson, Morgenthau assumed he would be named to a cabinet-level position after the Democratic victory in 1912, but the president-elect had other plans for him. Like the prominent American Jews Oscar Straus and Solomon Hirsch before him, Morgenthau was to be posted as America's ambassador to Turkey. Unlike his predecessors, however, who were deeply flattered by their appointments, the assumption that Jews represented a natural bridge between Muslim Turks and Christian Americans merely rankled Morgenthau. "Would prominent Methodists or Baptists be told there is a 'Position' [for them], go find one of your faith to fill it?" Wilson, in reply, assured Morgenthau that Istanbul "was the point at which the interest of American Jews in the welfare of the Jews of Palestine is focused, and it is almost indispensable that I have a Jew at that post."[8] Though no Zionist himself, Morgenthau cared fervidly about the plight of his coreligionists and, eager to please his president, he accepted.

Replicating the experience of so many American envoys to the Middle East, Morgenthau at first found the Ottoman capital "dazzling" and "decadent," a scene out of *A Thousand and One Arabian Nights*. "This is undoubtedly going to prove an intensely interesting experience for me," he wrote. A year, however, sufficed to leave him disillusioned with the political machinations of the Turks and their addiction to "intrigue, intimidation, and assassination." But just as his image of Turkey had changed, so had his preconception of the American evangelists working in the Middle East. "I had hitherto had a hazy notion that missionaries were sort of over-zealous advance agents of sectarian religion," he recalled. "They were, I discovered, in reality advance agents of civilization," the exemplars of "the American spirit at its best." The ambassador was soon surprised to find himself acting as the missionaries' representative to the Porte, helping to spread their "gospel of Americanism." The Armenians, too, changed in Morgenthau's eyes, from a "few rug merchants" he had known in New York, to a people very much like the Jews, unshakably committed to their religion and infused with cultural pride.

Turkish officials, American missionaries, and Armenians together formed the complex and deadly triangle around which Morgenthau would have to maneuver. "Here was I, a Jew, representing the greatest Christian nation of the world at the capital of the chief Mohammedan nation . . . which was soon, because of its strategic position, to become one of the . . . centres of world diplomacy. Here was a worn-out empire, which in its death agony clutched other peoples . . . within its fatal embrace." Meeting such challenges would have proved inestimably difficult for Morgenthau even under peaceful circumstances. Once war broke out and as the evidence of butchery mounted, the task became gargantuan.

Daily at first and then almost hourly, the reports reached Morgenthau's desk. Consul Davis informed him of the closing of missionary schools in Harput and Jackson described a "gigantic plundering scheme" against the Armenian population of Aleppo. Consuls Oscar Heizer in Trebizond and W. Peter in Samsun told of mass deportations, of shootings, and of barges departing for the nearby Black Sea packed with Armenians but returning empty. Lewis Einstein, an American Jewish diplomat attached to the Istanbul embassy, saw a Turkish woman borrow an officer's pistol and, for sport, shoot a passing Armenian refugee in the head. Many more accounts of atrocities were deleted by the Turkish censor and Talaat dismissed the rest as mere rumors or isolated cases of "mob violence." German officials alternately denied that any massacres were occurring and absolved themselves of any responsibility for them. By July, however, the flood of dispatches from the field and the stream of Armenian survivors who staggered into his office persuaded Morgenthau that the Turkish government had embarked on a deliberate policy of "race extermination." Writing to the new secretary of state, Robert Lansing, Morgenthau listed the "terrible tortures, whole-sale expulsions and deportations," and "frequent instances of rape, pillage, and . . . massacre," designed to eradicate the Armenian people. "Untold misery, disease, starvation, and loss of life will go on unchecked," he warned, unless America interceded.[10]

Washington reacted to Morgenthau's cable with alarm, but little else. Though Wilson reportedly told a missionary friend, "You may be sure that we have been doing everything that is diplomatically possible to check the terrible business," America's policy remained one of noninterference. Lansing, severe and unimaginative, even expressed sympathy for the Turks' wartime concerns and distaste for the Armenians' "well-known disloyalty to the Ottoman Government." At most, the administration was willing to inform the Porte that the atrocities had "aroused strong sentiment among the American people" and that their continuation would "tend to jeopardize the good feeling . . . of the United States toward . . . Turkey." The statement failed to convey the moral gravity that Morgenthau needed. "Nothing short of actual force . . . would adequately meet the situation," he concluded, and determined to act on his own.

"Our people will never forget these massacres," Morgenthau now admonished Talaat. "You are defying all ideas of justice as we understand the term in our country." But the interior minister scarcely reacted. He no longer attempted to conceal the indiscriminate murder of Armenians or even his delight at its pace. "I have accomplished more toward solving the Armenian problem in three months than [Sultan] Abdul Hamid accomplished in thirty years!" Talaat questioned Morgenthau why he, a Jew, would worry about the treatment of Christians. Morgenthau explained that he was acting "not . . . as a Jew but as the American Ambassador, not . . . in the name of any race or religion but merely as human being." But Talaat was less interested in Morgenthau's motives than in the American insurance policies that many Armenians allegedly held. "They are all dead now," the minister maintained, "and the Government is the beneficiary."[11]

Such cold-bloodedness brought Morgenthau to the verge of eruption. "It is difficult to restrain myself," he wrote. Still, as the representative of a friendly country, forbidden to interfere in the affairs of a sovereign state, his venues for expressing that rage were few. At best, he could try to alleviate the Armenians' plight by soliciting the help of James Barton, secretary of the American Board of Commissioners for Foreign Missions, and of the philanthropist Cleveland H. Dodge. Morgenthau proposed to create a massive fund for purchasing food, clothing, and temporary shelter for those who managed to survive the massacres. Both Barton and Dodge responded enthusiastically and recruited their influential acquaintances to form the Committee on Armenian Atrocities. Its board brought together the Episcopal bishop David H. Greer with the Jewish leaders Oscar Straus and Isaac Seligman, and placed the American Zionist leader Rabbi Stephen Wise beside Charles Crane, a champion of Arab nationalism. In response to their country's political impotence, Americans rallied with unprecedented ecumenicalism and unparalleled largesse. The organization, later incorporated by Congress as Near East Relief, would ultimately raise $100 million, the equivalent of $1 billion today.

And yet Morgenthau did not stop at merely raising money. Through his friendship with the *New York Times* publisher Adolph Ochs, he ensured that the massacres continued to receive prominent coverage—145 articles in 1915 alone. He also offered one million dollars of his own money to resettle over 500,000 of the refugees in the American West. "The United States might be the Moses to lead the Armenian people out of bondage," Morgenthau, perhaps recalling his own immigrant experience, surmised. "They are a clean, industrious, intelligent race, the best class for immigrants, farmers and laborers." Turkey, though, and not the United States, ultimately vetoed the plan.[12]

The eradication of Armenians, meanwhile, accelerated. A pogrom of Turkish peasants in Marsovan devastated the American college and girls' school; many of the one thousand pupils were placed before ditches and shot. "One group of our college boys asked permission to sing before they died and they sang 'Nearer, My God, to Thee,' then they were struck down," recounted the Reverend George E. White, the school's Iowa-born president. With the flair acquired in his former profession as a journalist, Leslie Davis described the road to Lake Göeljük, a source of the Tigris, lined with "arms or legs or even the heads sticking out the ground. Most of them had been partially eaten by dogs." Visible beneath the water's surface, he noticed, were "hundreds of bodies and many bones," and strewn on the shores, an estimated ten thousand corpses. To conserve ammunition, the Turks were increasingly resorting to bayonets, swords, and pickaxes to eliminate their victims. Survivors recalled seeing rows of young women nailed naked to crosses and others dismembered for sport. "Women [who] escaped came back to beg at our doors," recalled Myrtle Shane in Bitlis, "fingers off, hands off, faces and bodies mutilated."[13]

The inescapability of these nightmarish scenes often became too much for their observers to bear. Walter M. Geddes, a licorice-purchasing agent for a New York confection firm, was in Aleppo for business and saw thousands of Armenian deportees die of exposure and starvation. He returned to Smyrna, filed a statement on his experience, and shot himself in the head. An American missionary named F. H. Leslie, who doubled as the consul for the southeastern city of Urfa, became physically and mentally debilitated by his futile efforts to save Armenian children and women. Arrested for attempting to help the refugees and tortured, Leslie committed suicide in prison.

For Morgenthau, too, the anguish was becoming insufferable. Turkish officials bragged to him of the new methods of torture they devised for the Armenians, some of them culled from records of the Spanish Inquisition. Enver Pasha claimed that American aid was only encouraging the Armenians to revolt and he strove to stem the flow of contributions. "The whole history of the human race contains no such horrible episode as this," the exasperated ambassador wrote. The once alluring Turkey had become "a place of horror" for him. "I had reached the end of my resources," he conceded. "I found intolerable my further daily association with men, however gracious and accommodating . . . who were still reeking with the blood of nearly a million human beings." Sickened and worn out by his twenty-six months of struggling, Henry Morgenthau resigned.[14]

The massacres continued, unabated. Abram Elkus, another Jewish lawyer from New York who replaced Morgenthau as ambassador, informed the State Department that the Turks were pursuing an "unchecked policy of extermination through starvation, exhaustion, and brutality of treatment hardly surpassed even in Turkish history." In all, as many as 1.5 million Armenians were killed in a genocide that the Turkish government would never acknowledge, much less regret. But Elkus also had other catastrophes to monitor, including the mounting Turkish attacks against the Greek population of Smyrna and western Anatolia and the displacement of Arabs from border lands. "Turkish authorities appear to be pursuing [a] policy of Turkifying Syria and adjacent Arabic-speaking countries," one State Department memorandum asserted, and estimated that 250,000 Arab families were slated to be removed and supplanted by Turks.

If such atrocities were not sufficiently horrifying, a famine of biblical dimensions struck the Middle East. An estimated 200,000 people perished in Istanbul alone and several times that number in the provinces from Egypt to Syria. "The air was filled with the sound of bells tolling for funerals and children crying for a crust to eat," wrote Cleveland Dodge's son, Bayard, the president of the Syrian Protestant College in Beirut. American philanthropists again mobilized to address the disaster and procured the use of the USS *Des Moines* and *Caesar* to deliver emergency supplies—another example of power in the service of faith. For hundreds of thousands of civilians, the arrival of these ships represented the difference between survival and almost inescapable death from starvation and disease. "The whole country was literally living on expectation," Margaret McGilvary, a young volunteer with the American Mission Press in Lebanon, recounted, adding, "In Syria we were fighting our share in the World-War just as truly as were our compatriots on the Western Front." Turkey, however, continued to deny the existence of any human emergency in its empire and often blocked delivery of the supplies. An American consular report confirmed, "In spite of the best efforts of the [American relief] committees, the number dying . . . is being augmented with terrible rapidity."[15]

For all their attempts to detach themselves from the conflict and its consequences, Americans had been caught up in the worst waves of bloodshed ever to ravage the Middle East, witnessing acts of inhumanity that, even by Great War standards, were appalling. The enormity of those horrors was to some degree diminished by the unflagging efforts of relief workers and missionaries, but the ability of Americans to alleviate Middle Eastern suffering would remain limited as long as the United States stayed aloof from the war.

18

ACTION OR
NONACTION?

ACROSS THE FRIGID NORTH ATLANTIC, ON THE NIGHT OF February 25, 1917, the *Laconia* steamed toward Liverpool. The Cunard liner carried some eighteen thousand tons of provisions and war matériel, 216 crew members, and seventy-three passengers, six of whom were Americans. All those on board understood that the voyage was potentially hazardous. Germany had recently resolved to launch unrestricted submarine attacks against American merchant vessels—the direst threat to the country's shipping since the Barbary Wars. At 10:30, just off the Irish coast, two German torpedoes smashed through the *Laconia*'s hull, puncturing the stern and exploding in the engine room. "It was bedlam and nightmare," recalled the Chicago *Herald Tribune* reporter Floyd Gibbons, who described the frantic rush for the lifeboats as the captain ordered the ship abandoned. Forty minutes later the *Laconia* was gone. "The ship sank rapidly at the stern until at last its nose stood straight in the air," read Gibbons's log. "Then it slid silently down and out of sight like a piece of disappearing scenery in a panorama spectacle." Of the twenty-two people killed in the attack, two were Americans, a mother and her daughter.

Five weeks later, on April 2, President Wilson, who had recently been reelected on a platform of continued American neutrality, asked

Congress for a declaration of war. Denouncing the "wanton and wholesale destruction of the lives of noncombatants, men, women, and children," he accused Germany of conducting "warfare against mankind" and of committing "wrongs which . . . cut to the very roots of human life." Wilson denied that the United States had any territorial or material ambitions in the war; it aspired only to uphold universal rights, preserve democracy, and assure the future peace through a concert of democratic nations. "America is privileged to spend her blood and her might for the principles that gave her birth and happiness and the peace which she has treasured," Wilson ended.

According to international custom, and in keeping with the pattern of World War I, when one country declared war against another, it also went to war against its enemy's allies. For America, this would have meant proclaiming a state of belligerency with all of the Central Powers, including Bulgaria, Austro-Hungary, and Turkey. But the president in his speech expressly denied harboring any animosity toward Germany's allies and omitted all mention of Turkey. Rather, he decreed, "We enter this war only where we are clearly forced into it because there are no other means of defending our rights." His meaning was precise: American troops had been forced to fight in the trenches of Europe, but not on the deserts and beaches of the Middle East.

Though couched in abstract principles, America's decision not to go to war against Turkey was, in fact, the product of a painful weighing of realities. Wilson was unconvinced that the United States had grounds for declaring such a war. "They [the Turks] do not yet stand in the direct path of necessary action," he said. On the other hand, the president and other members of his administration believed that Istanbul took its orders directly from Berlin and that any attempt to distinguish between the two was artificial. "The Central Empire runs from the Baltic to the Dardanelles," Wilson's chief foreign policy adviser, Colonel Edward Mandell House, averred. "Anything coming from a Turkish Cabinet official is under the suspicion of being dictated by Germany." That assumption appeared to be verified when, in response to America's declaration of war against Germany, Turkey severed relations with the United States.

Yet, even as they were evicting America's ambassador from their capital, the Turks made conspicuous gestures to appease the United States. "What can we expect to gain if we take part in a war against the United States?" Djavid Pasha, the finance minister, asked. "Absolutely nothing." He recalled that America, alone among the powers, had never coveted Turkish territory, and that it remained "Turkey's only hope" for postwar reconstruction. Talaat Pasha insisted that the Turkish-American friendship would continue irrespective of American involvement in the war and ordered all anti-American sentiment excised from the state-controlled press. "Our relations with Turkey remain normal and perhaps more friendly than for some time past," Ambassador Elkus concluded. "Turkey will not declare war against America."[1]

Even if Turkey did display hostility toward the United States, and if its alliance with Germany could no longer be overlooked, it was still unclear how American troops would enter the Middle Eastern war. Elkus was confident that Turkey's major cities could be easily bombarded from the sea and the empire swiftly invaded. "Turkey is the weakest link in the chain of the Central Powers, and . . . is on the verge of a breakdown," he essayed. "The people of Turkey only want some such excuse . . . to compel [them to sign] a separate peace." Some senior American generals agreed, stressing the many political and military advantages the country would achieve by contributing forces to the Middle Eastern theater.

From Wilson's perspective, however, the task of intervening in the Middle East seemed far less facile. The army was utterly unprepared to fight on any front, much less one twice as far from home as Europe's and in a less familiar environment. Supply and communications lines would be agonizingly long and exposed to submarine harassment. And even if the troops could be landed successfully in the Middle East, what guarantee was there that their intervention would lead to victory? Though the Allies had scored some crucial victories in 1917, including the capture of Baghdad, the Turkish army was far from defeated. Confronted with a new American threat, the Turks would likely seek a more active intervention by Germany and mount a joint and highly formidable resistance. If Wilson could see the potential for an eventual Anglo-American victory in the region, he could also envisage the possibility that hundreds of thousands of American soldiers would lie buried beside their British brethren beneath Middle Eastern sands.

In view of the technical complexities involved in attacking Turkey, and the lack of explicit Turkish aggression, the most compelling basis for American military intervention in the Middle East was humanitarian. The Turks had slaughtered as many as a million human beings in cold blood and seemed fixed on killing myriads more. The bloodshed would only stop, argued Cornelius Van H. Engert, a veteran American diplomat in the Middle East, when the United States intervened massively. "Nothing but a vigorous and sustained attack in Palestine and Mesopotamia will bring about this desired result." Writing to Wilson from Adana, the Congregationalist missionary William Nesbitt Chambers wished that "such a power as the United States should become so strong on land and sea that . . . Turkey would never dare to commit such a horrible crime," and that America with "a great gun . . . in one hand [and] the Gospel in the other" would come to the Armenians' rescue. Most bellicose of all was the former New York City College president John H. Finley, head of the wartime Red Cross in Palestine. "America!" he urged. "You must send not only the Red Cross to this front. You must send that which Christ said he came to bring—a sword . . . [and] make common cause with the forces of justice against the demons of cruelty."

The call to wage a war of conscience against Turkey was not, however, confined to Americans serving in the area. Members of both houses of Congress, Democrats and Republicans, were also calling on the president to act. "I should be sorry as an American . . . if when this war ends . . . we should appear at the great council of nations as still the friend of Turkey," declared Henry Cabot Lodge, the chairman of the powerful Senate Foreign Relations Committee. House Speaker James Beauchamp Clark, a Republican, announced, "The present anomalous situation . . . is perfectly demoralizing. It is ridiculous to fight one half of the enemy and not the other half." Minority Leader Frederick Gillette said, "Turkey's course during the war has been so contemptible that I do not think we should hesitate . . . in declaring war against her." The *New York Times* speculated that there was scarcely a single congressman or senator in favor of maintaining peace with the Turks.

Even more outspoken than the congressmen in his criticism of American neutrality was the contentious ex-president Theodore Roosevelt. "We ought to declare war on Turkey without an hour's delay," he bellowed. Asserting that the Turkish empire had "surpassed the iniquity of Germany herself by what she has done to her Christian subjects in Asia," Roosevelt warned that the motto "making the world safe for democracy" would be reduced to empty rhetoric by American inaction in the Middle East. "We have the only chance that has ever been offered to us to interfere by force of arms in an entirely disinterested fashion for the oppressed nationalities that are ground under Turkish rule," he reasoned. "It will be a lasting disgrace to our nation if we persist in this failure."[2]

The recommendations of Lodge, Roosevelt, and others for war were rebuffed by an American who, before the war, had prayed for the Ottoman Empire's demise. "I hesitate to butt in on matters of State," began a letter to Wilson from his loyal friend, political patron, and Princeton classmate, Cleveland Dodge. After apologizing for his impertinence, Dodge urged against going to war with Turkey, warning of large-scale retribution against the Americans working there and the accelerated massacre of the peoples they were struggling to protect. "A declaration of war . . . would be fatal to our interests," the philanthropist contended, adding, "From all accounts the Turks are treating our people with great & actually friendly consideration." Dodge stressed that his opinions were formed without concern for the welfare of his daughter, who was teaching at Robert College, or his son, who was working in Beirut. His sole interest lay in preserving the "great educational, missionary and relief work in the Turkish Empire."

Wilson replied with sympathy for "every word" of Dodge's letter. "I have thought more than once of your dear ones in Turkey with a pang of apprehension that was very deep . . . and my heart is with you." But other Americans dismissed the fears raised by Dodge and bitterly dissented from Wilson's response. "We are guilty of a peculiarly odious form of hypocrisy when we profess friendship for Armenia and the downtrodden races of Turkey, but don't go to war with Turkey," countered Roosevelt, who went on to assert, "The Armenian massacre was the greatest crime of the war, and failure to act against Turkey is to condone it." The ex–commander in chief who more than once sent American warships to the Middle East to safeguard missionaries and rescue hostages now accused church and relief workers of a "grave moral dereliction" for failing to leave the region while they could and frustrating American intervention. "The presence of our missionaries . . . did not prevent the Turks from massacring between half a million and a million Armenians, Syrians, Greeks and Jews," he lectured Dodge. "Our declaration of war now will certainly not do one one-hundredth part of the damage already done by our failure to go to war in the past."

Dodge and Roosevelt were quarreling over the best way to oppose despotism and preserve minority rights, over how best to uphold the tenets of American faith by preserving its primary agents, the missionaries. Traditional considerations of power such as oil, trade routes, and spheres of influence that impelled the European powers to wage war against Turkey and strive to conquer its territories scarcely entered the internal American debate. For Americans, the pivotal question was simple: how can the United States act most humanely?

In the end, Wilson sided with Dodge. The son of a Presbyterian minister, an intensely principled man whose global outlook was forged in the missionary milieu, the president could not bring himself to abandon those Americans who were risking their lives for the values he honored. Nor could he countenance the almost certain result of that abandonment—the deaths of the many thousands of people who were now dependent on American relief for food, shelter, and medical care. While the president did seek and obtain a war declaration against Austro-Hungary in December 1917, and seriously considered making war against Bulgaria, he never wavered from the status quo with Turkey.

The decision confounded the British and the French, who failed to understand how the United States had benefited from its neutrality, either militarily or politically, and why it would not assist them in defeating so despicable an enemy. The region needed American arms, they insisted, not American aid. Roosevelt could not have agreed more. "It is rather bitter to think that the cold selfishness and utter lack of all ethical qualities in Wilson made us onlookers at the . . .

smashing of the Turkish Empire, instead of . . . valiant co-warriors," he complained. Wilson, however, remained firm. To Cleveland, he pledged to do his utmost to restrain Congress from "following its inclination" to make war on Turkey. "I hope with all my heart that I can succeed."[3]

Wilson did indeed succeed, overcoming robust opposition from the press, both houses of Congress, his own military commanders, and a popular former president. America never went to war against Turkey. Concern for the missionary institutions and the many populations they served had trumped all other strategic considerations in Wilson's thinking. Yet, in deciding to forgo the use of force in the Middle East, the president would significantly diminish America's status in the region and circumscribe his ability to influence its future.

AT PRECISELY the time that Wilson was deciding not to make war against Turkey, the Allied Powers were conspiring to divide Ottoman lands among them. In a series of secret agreements that began with the Sykes-Picot treaty of May 1916, Britain laid claim to immense territories between the Jordan River and the Persian Gulf. France arrogated control over Syria and Mosul, and Russia and Italy staked eastern and southwest Anatolia, respectively. Together, these agreements assured that at the war's end not only the Ottoman Empire but Turkey itself would vanish.

As a nonbelligerent in the Middle Eastern war, the United States lacked the qualifications for participating in these talks. Moreover, deeply opposed to the allocation of Middle Eastern territories irrespective of their inhabitants' wishes, the United States might well have boycotted the discussion anyway. But the absence of American input in planning for the postwar Middle East meant that Wilson could not effectively apply his principles of freedom and democracy to the region. He was undoubtedly earnest in pledging to protect "the rights and liberties of small nations" and "make the world itself free at last," but without going to war against Turkey, he could scarcely defend the rights of those small Middle Eastern states that he ranked among the world's least liberated.

A Chimerical Peace

The impact of America's refusal to go to war in the Middle East was demonstrated by the futility of its one effort to attain peace. The initiative came in the late spring of 1917 in response to reports of growing resentment over German imperiousness in Istanbul and of Turkey's desire to pursue an independent foreign policy. One source even intimated that Turkish officials might be induced to allow Allied submarines to pass through the Dardanelles and destroy German battleships anchored in the Bosphorus.

These communications were eagerly welcomed by Henry Morgenthau. Though Turkey, in his eyes, "was the cancer in the life of the world," and one that must be "properly treated," he always believed that the treatment would be diplomatic and not military. Now, convinced that the Turks were "heartily sick of their German masters," Morgenthau proposed to undertake a secret mediation mission. In return for receiving guarantees for its continued sovereignty over Anatolia and the Straits, Turkey would withdraw its forces from the war. Lansing expressed doubt whether the plan would work, yet he told Wilson that if "there was one chance in fifty of success" he would "not leave any stone unturned which will lessen the power of Germany." The president, too, was skeptical, but he saw no danger in offering America's good offices. "If it succeeds it would be a decisive factor in the war," he hypothesized. "If it failed, we would be no worse off than before."

Morgenthau left the United States on June 21, 1917, in what was billed as an effort to investigate the plight of Palestinian Jews. To reinforce that alibi, Morgenthau was accompanied by the prominent Zionist Felix Frankfurter. A blunt and brilliant professor at Harvard Law, an adviser to Wilson's War Department, Frankfurter had a low opinion of Morgenthau, finding him fulsome and inflated with "hot air impressions" of Turkey. The jurist's main objective was to ensure that Morgenthau not succeed in allowing Turkey to exit from the war with its control over Palestine intact. The Holy Land, the Zionists hoped, would soon be conquered by the British, who would then work to transform it into a Jewish national home.

Frankfurter's brief was closely coordinated with the most preeminent Zionist leader of the day, the Russian-born but naturalized British chemist Chaim Weizmann. Bald-headed and hooked-nose, endowed with an immense moral stature and charm, Weizmann had forged a close alliance with the British foreign secretary, Arthur Balfour. Like many British restorationists, Balfour combined zealous religious beliefs with a firm sense of realpolitik; Palestine, if given to the Jews, would not only summon Christ but also serve British imperial interests. Balfour consequently shared the Zionists' concern that Turkey would abandon the war before British troops could reach Jerusalem, and appointed Weizmann Britain's emissary to Morgenthau. "Talk to Morgenthau," the secretary told the scientist, "and keep on talking until you've talked him out of his mission."

Weizmann rendezvoused with Morgenthau and Frankfurter on the Rock of Gibraltar. Also present was Arshag K. Schmavonian, an Armenian who had served as an adviser to the U.S. embassy in Turkey. Weizmann bluffly informed Morgenthau that his effort was premature, that the Central Powers would merely interpret it as a sign of Allied weakness and redouble their commitment to fight. He also pressed Morgenthau for assurances that "on no account would the Zionist organization be in any way identified or mixed up with even the faintest attempts to secure a separate peace." Peace would come, Weizmann, conveying the British line, ventured, but only after Turkey's defeat and its concession of Armenia, Syria, and Palestine.

Weizmann's remarks mortified Morgenthau, though not so keenly as the message borne by Schmavonian. The Turks, he said, were furious over an interview in which Morgenthau alleged that the Porte was willing to sell Palestine to the Jews. They also accused him of bragging about his supposedly secret mission and of provoking harsh reactions in the Western press. "Is then the Young Turk clique to be trusted again with the matters of the Armenians, Arabs, and Zionist Jews?" a spokesman for the Armenians had protested. As a result, Morgenthau was now considered unwelcomed in Istanbul, which, in any case, had no intention of severing its alliance with Germany.

In light of these devastating discussions, Morgenthau saw little sense in continuing his mission. "Time is not ripe to enter into negotiations," he cabled Washington. "It is useless therefore to proceed to Turkey." The State Department agreed and ordered him to leave Gibraltar at once. For Frankfurter, the entire experience had been "a wild goose chase," and Wilson also regretted the effort, dismissing it as "chimerical and of questionable advantage, even if it could be accomplished." In its major debut at Middle East peacemaking, the United States had shown itself to be naïve and clumsy. Morgenthau, the frustrated savior of the Armenian people, had proved to be a disappointment as a negotiator as well, a gullible, tragic figure. A humbled Colonel House told his diary, "Morgenthau's trip has turned out to be a fiasco."

The failure of the Morgenthau mission sealed U.S. policy toward Turkey for the remainder of World War I and solidified America's neutral status in the Middle East. The Turks remained appreciative of that impartiality, as their troops retreated before the Allied onslaught. The British, too, were pleased not to have to share the glory with America when their forces entered Jerusalem in December 1917. Most delighted of all, perhaps, were the American missionaries and relief workers who, thanks in part to American neutrality, survived the war and were now thriving under a sympathetic occupation. In their view, the collapse of Ottoman rule throughout the Middle East, and in particular in the Holy Land, appeared to augur redemption. "We have been in the seventh heaven these past days over the news from . . . Palestine," Cleveland Dodge giddily informed Wilson. "I am . . . grateful to you for your wise and patient course of action—or nonaction."[4]

American missionaries and their backers were not alone in hailing the outcome of the war. Zionists, too, were ecstatic. But if, in the past, missionaries and Zionists would have rejoiced for the same reasons—the opportunity to restore Palestine to the Jews—they now celebrated on different and ultimately irreconcilable grounds. Having abandoned their original restorationist goal in favor of Arab nationalism, the missionaries saw the war's end as the advent of liberation for all Arab lands, including Palestine. The Zionists, by con-

19

An American
Movement Is Born

THE TRANSFORMATION OF LARGE NUMBERS OF AMERICAN
Jews into American Zionists would be a slow and often turbulent
process. The reasons for this tortuousness had virtually nothing to
do with the presence of another people in Palestine, but rather with
reasons peculiar to the Jewish community. Fearful of provoking the
anti-Semitism that lurked beneath the surface of American society,
the majority of Jews still viewed the idea of re-creating Jewish statehood as anachronistic, if not dangerous. Zionism, warned the celebrated Reform rabbi Rudolf Grossman in 1897 strikes "a fatal blow
at the patriotism and loyalty of the Jew to the country under whose
protection he lives." Congressman Julius Kahn of California, also a
member of a Reform congregation, feared that Zionism would
expose the American Jew to charges "of merely being a sojourner in
the United States, using the benefits . . . that he get by residence here
with the ultimate object of becoming a Palestinian and a resident of
the Jewish State."

Anti-Zionism was not confined to Reform Jews. Orthodox Jews
also opposed the movement—not because of its emphasis on Jewish
nationhood but rather because of its secularism. Zionists represented
"the most formidable enemy ever to have arisen among the Jewish

people," according to the Orthodox association Agudath Israel. "Their entire desire . . . is to remove the burden of Torah . . . and to uphold only their nationalism," claimed Shalom Dov Ber Schneerson, the revered Lubavitcher rebbe. For the broadening ranks of socialist Jews who saw themselves not as members of a distinct people but as workers in an international proletariat, Zionism was also anathema. Indeed, antipathy to the Zionist idea was one of the few positions around which, in the early 1900s, most of American Jewry could rally.

Earthshaking events were required to detach even a small portion of that community from its anti-Zionist stance. The Russian pogroms of the 1880s, taking tens of thousands of Jewish lives, convinced American Jews of the need for concerted action, while the Dreyfus trial in 1890s France reminded them that anti-Semitism continued to fester even in presumably enlightened Europe. With Western Europe looking increasingly inhospitable and American cities already bursting with immigrants, American Jewish leaders began to consider alternative havens. One possible shelter was Palestine, climatically harsh and politically problematic though it seemed. "I am in favor of any . . . outlet for any portion of our Russian coreligionists," wrote Oscar Straus, the former ambassador in Istanbul, to the former American consul in Alexandria, Simon Wolf. "No failure, however great, can result in a condition comparable with the Russian condition." But supporting the resettlement of Russian Jews in the Holy Land was one thing; converting that land into a Jewish state—a move that both Straus and Wolf opposed—remained distinctly another. The same Adolph Ochs who gave front-page coverage to the Armenian massacres in the *New York Times* sought to squelch all articles on Zionism.

Zionism nevertheless gained adherents, especially among the recently arrived Eastern European Jews, and in 1897 the Federation of American Zionists was formed. In contrast to Zionist unions in Russia and Poland, which urged their members to relocate to Palestine, the American organization never promoted Jewish emigration from the United States. Zionism, rather, remained as it was in Emma Lazarus's conception, a refuge for Europe's downtrodden Jews. "We believe that such a home can only naturally . . . be found in the land of their fathers," posited Richard J. H. Gottheil, the Columbia Semitics professor who served as the first president of the Zionist Federation. But, the scholar added, "we hold that this does not mean that all Jews must return to Palestine." Gottheil's dynamic student Stephen S. Wise, one of the few Reform rabbis to promote the creation of "a little Jewish principality within . . . Palestine," also specified that the American Jew "longed for no Palestine," but rather "gives his allegiance to this land which alone can satisfy his very passion for liberty." Those Jews who did leave the United States for Palestine—among them Golda Meyerson (later Meir) and Henrietta Szold, both profiled in a later chapter—were rarities.[1]

In spite of its success in redefining itself in distinctly American terms, the Zionist idea of reviving Jewish statehood appealed to only a fraction of the country's Jews. Of the approximately three million Jews living in the United States in 1914, only fifteen thousand paid dues to the Zionist Federation, whose budget barely exceeded $12,000. Zionism remained an overwhelmingly European movement, with its headquarters situated in Berlin. The question posed by Zionism's founder Theodor Herzl, "Will the Jews of America . . . in their own happiness in the glorious land of freedom, forget the heavy bondage of their brethren?" seemed fated to remain unanswered.

Though statistically minuscule, American Zionists nevertheless wielded influence greatly disproportionate to their numbers. Talented and articulate leaders such as Gottheil, Wise, and Felix Frankfurter enjoyed access to American policymakers and to Jewish philanthropists who, even if opposed to statehood, were willing to cooperate with the Zionists in rescuing Jews. Unlike the marginalized Jews in Europe for whom Zionism presented a solution for deepening insecurities, these assimilated American Jews viewed Zionism as an expression of the growing confidence they felt as citizens of the United States. The same processes of secularization and modernization that were alienating American Christians from the restorationist idea were freeing and emboldening many American Jews to embrace it. Overcoming anti-Semitism, university quotas, and social restrictions, they had succeeded in breaching the bastions of Protestant power to become respected—if not yet fully accepted— members of the American elite. And like other minorities that had successfully integrated into the country, they saw no contradiction between pride in their ethnicity and allegiance to their flag. "Is the German-American considered less of an American because he cultivates the German language and is interested in his fellow Germans at home?" Professor Gottheil asked. "Is the Irish-American less of an American because he gathers money to help his struggling brethren in the Green Isle?"[2]

Of this emerging breed of superbly educated and connected Americanized Jews, none would prove more effective in wedding Zionist goals with those of the United States than Louis Dembitz Brandeis. Named for an uncle who had helped nominate Lincoln for president in 1860 and born in the American heartland of Kentucky, Brandeis had almost no contact with Jewish customs or religion, considering himself thoroughly American. "Sanity, soundness, clarity, nobleness, all were his," Wise later wrote of Brandeis. "I never see him without thanking God for him." He was also handsome, blessed with sharp, chiseled features, and stunningly brilliant. Graduating from high school at age fourteen, he finished first in his class at Harvard Law a mere six years later. Success came naturally to Brandeis, both as a law professor and as a litigator. By middle age, he had established his reputation as a debonair, if sometimes domineering, figure with a headstrong devotion to the principles of racial and social equality and to America's role in liberating the world.

These convictions, Brandeis came to believe, fully accorded with Zionism. He initially encountered the idea at Harvard, where, in spite of almost impenetrable restrictions against the admission of Jews, a Zionist society had been formed and was even encouraged by several restorationist-minded professors. The young attorney saw parallels between the hardworking frontiersmen of colonial America and the Zionist pioneers in Palestine—"Jewish Pilgrim Fathers" with whom "the descendants of the [American] Pilgrim fathers should not find it hard to understand and sympathize." While arbitrating an end to a strike by Jewish garment workers in New York in 1910, Brandeis was for the first time exposed to his people's traditions and outlooks. The Jews, he deduced, were natural democrats, "possessed . . . of a deep moral feeling [and] . . . a deep sense of the brotherhood of man," and worthy of national preservation. Two years later, while conversing with Jacob de Haas, an old colleague of Herzl's and now editor of a Zionist paper in Boston, Brandeis heard about a Zionist experimental farm that the U.S. Department of Agriculture had helped establish near Haifa and about the Jewish nationalism of his own uncle, Dembitz. Excited by the goals of "these so-called dreamers," he joined the Zionist Federation and, in 1914, at age fifty-eight, was unanimously elected its chairman.

On matters of Jewish nationalism, Brandeis was hardly an original thinker. "There is no inconsistency between loyalty to America and loyalty to Jewry," he posited, closely echoing Wise and Gottheil. "Every American Jew who aids in advancing the Jewish settlement in Palestine, though . . . neither he nor his descendants will ever live there, will likewise be a better man and a better American for doing so." The European Zionists, who preferred unglamorous settlement building to abstract ideas, found Brandeis overly attached to his theories and unwilling to be dissuaded by facts.[3] But while Europeans might supply picks and shovels to those settlements, Brandeis, the quintessential American Zionist, supplied the movement with the one commodity it needed most: power. A close adviser to Wilson and soon to become the first Jewish justice on the Supreme Court, Brandeis had access to the most senior levels of American governance. With the transfer of the World Zionist headquarters from belligerent Berlin to neutral New York, that entrée would become crucial not just to the economic well-being of Palestine's Jews but, in many cases, to their physical survival as well.

The New Zion Rescues the Old

Palestinian Jewry had long lived under precarious circumstances, distrusted and often oppressed. The Turkish authorities made no distinction between the old *Yishuv*, or community, of religious and largely indigent Jews, and the new *Yishuv* of Zionist farmers. Rather, they suspected all Jews of plotting to create an independent state and secede from the Ottoman Empire. The Porte consequently sought to limit Jewish immigration and land purchases in Palestine—policies that the United States considered discriminatory. Anti-Jewish measures nevertheless persisted in Palestine in the years leading up to 1914 and intensified during the war. Like the Armenians, the Jews were accused of acting as a fifth column for the Allies, and threatened with a similar fate. While warning of the dangers to those French, British, and Russian Christians who remained in Palestine, Lansing predicted "a general massacre of all Jews."

Events in Palestine indeed seemed to be hurtling toward calamity. The Reverend Otis Glazebrook, the American consul in Jerusalem, detailed large-scale depredations against the area's Jews, the confiscation of their property, and the closing of their banks. Turkish authorities had stripped Jewish settlements of their defensive weapons, while arming the neighboring Arab tribes and encouraging them to wage holy war against the infidels. Though not an "Allied" language, Hebrew, too, was proscribed, including the Hebrew-language stamps and bills that served as the *Yishuv*'s internal tender. Most devastating, though, was the planned expulsion of some fifty thousand Russian Jews—three-quarters of the entire community— whom the Turks now considered enemy aliens. The destruction of the Zionist project appeared imminent, warned Glazebrook, a former pastor from Georgia and a Princeton Seminary professor whom Wilson had personally appointed. "A great blow," he feared, was soon to be dealt "to the religious aspirations of the Jews throughout the world" and to the "message of hope . . . that has let them to once more feel the national spirit."

With the other Western states either aligned or at war with Turkey and European Jewry divided by battlefields and preoccupied with its own survival, there remained only one power to which the Palestinian Jews could turn. "In name of [the] Holy Land, in name of [the] book whose language we revived [and] whose spirit we endeavour to realize," they pleaded, "we implore [the] noble powerful American nation to use [its] influence and save [the] Jewish colonization work in Palestine."

Answering that call could prove complicated for the United States, a neutral nation with little justification for intervening in any Ottoman territory, much less in Palestine. In contrast to their long-standing missionary, medical, and cultural work in other Middle Eastern areas, Americans had only a limited presence in Palestine.

The mere absence of institutions, however, would not deter a president with strong religious ties to the Holy Land and to the chosen people he associated with it. Nor could Wilson, who was not only spiritually attuned but also politically shrewd, miss the opportunity to court the increasingly consequential American Jewish vote. "If ever I have the occasion to help in the restoration of the Jewish People to Palestine I shall surely do so," he went on record saying, at the height of his 1912 campaign.[4]

The pledge, Wilson proved shortly after his election, was not empty. "Anything you can do to improve the lot of your coreligionists will reflect credit upon America," he told Morgenthau. "And you may count on the full power of the Administration to back you up." That backing proved crucial after affluent American Jews raised hundreds of thousands of dollars for emergency medical and alimentary relief in Palestine, but were prevented from delivering it by the Allied blockade and by Turkish resistance to Zionism. With Wilson's approval, Brandeis activated America's foreign relations machinery—its legations, communications systems, and ciphers—into service for the Zionist cause. Turkish officials were alternately assured of the Zionists' "unqualified loyalty" and warned that the American people would hold them personally "responsible for [the] lives and property of Jews and Christians in case of massacre or looting." The British and the French were promised that the food, gold, and gasoline supplied to the Jews would not be diverted to the Turkish war effort. With all sides conciliated, the supplies were loaded onto U.S. Navy vessels and transported to Jaffa for distribution. Some of those same ships were then steeved with the products of Zionist settlements—oranges and Carmel wines—for export.

Complicated though it proved, getting cargoes in and out of Palestine was less onerous than evacuating those "enemy alien" Jews with Russian or other Allied passports. Through Morgenthau's intervention, these Jews were given one month to renounce their original citizenship and become Ottoman subjects. Many accepted that option, but others either preferred banishment to Turkification or could not afford the ten-dollar naturalization fee. Brandeis and the American Zionists again intervened and arranged for the transport of these endangered Jews to British-controlled Egypt. Four U.S. Navy cruisers, along with several neutral-flag ships, were involved in the dramatic rescue, ferrying for seven months through the war-torn waters between Jaffa and Alexandria. In August 1915, a committee representing the six thousand Jews saved by the USS *Tennessee* presented its captain with a silver tablet—a testimonial, they said, for an act that "would long remain in the minds of the Jewish people." Captain Benton Decker responded by pronouncing Zionism "undoubtedly one of the great movements of the world," and he accepted the gift in the name of the American people "who stood, in this time of great turmoil and upheaval, for the interests of humanity."

After picking up Jews in Jaffa, the cruisers often proceeded northward to Beirut, to take on scores of missionaries, pilgrims, and professors from the Syrian Protestant College. Thus, on warships—symbols of American might—the descendants of the nineteenth-century Christian proponents of restorationism met the twentieth-century Jews who were now perpetuating that quest. Among the latter were Alexander and Rivka Aaronsohn, a brother and sister from the Zionist experimental farm, who had been implicated in a pro-British spy ring. Forced to flee to Lebanon, they were sheltered by the Bliss family until they finally managed to board the USS *Des Moines*. "A great cry of farewell arose from the refugees," Alexander recalled, as the cruiser steamed out of port. "A cry in which was mingled the relief of being free . . . [and] fear and hope for the future." The ship hoisted its colors, and its ecumenical passengers, "moved by a powerful instinct of love and respect," silently stood.

Sanctions against Palestinian Jews persisted, however, and worsened as the war progressed. Retreating before the advancing British forces, Turkish soldiers ravaged the already denuded Jewish farms and ejected the few remaining Jews from Jaffa. That the *Yishuv* survived at all owed much to America's intervention and to Turkey's fears of antagonizing the United States. A 1921 Zionist Organization report acknowledged that "America was . . . the one country which . . . was able to save Palestine from permanently going under."[5] The United States had not only preserved the economic and social foundations of the future Jewish state but had rescued many of its most dynamic leaders, including a young labor activist named David Ben-Gurion.

The Son of the Manse and the Jews

America's motive in aiding Palestinian Jewry was principally human-itarian rather than political. The United States treated the Jews' plight much as it had the Armenians', as an atrocity inflicted on a people closely associated with American philanthropic and religious interests in an especially cherished area of the world. Just as the Wil-son administration extended assistance to the Armenians irrespective of their political aspirations, so did it relieve the *Yishuv* without ever taking a position on Zionism. But as American doughboys marched to the front in Europe, and as European statesmen secretly drafted maps of the postwar Middle East, Washington found that it could no longer remain nonpartisan on Palestine.

American Zionists, more than any single factor, were responsible for shaking the White House out of its complacency. Representatives of a rapidly expanding constituency, Zionist leaders by 1917 were pressing the White House to officially sanction their cause. "The Jews from every tribe have descended in force," Colonel House informed Wilson, "and they seem determined to break in with a jimmy if they are not let in." But American Jews were not alone in exerting such pressure; restorationist Protestants also demanded a presidential endorsement of Zionism. "The Zionist movement of recent years has impressed profoundly many students of the scrip-tures . . . as the beginning of the fulfillment for that great line of prophecies," declared the Wheaton College president Charles Blan-chard. William Blackstone, author of the 1891 memorial in support of Jewish statehood, joined with a number of evangelical ministers in circulating a new pro-Zionist petition. Their efforts won the backing of important public figures, including Norman Hapgood, a defender of women's rights and editor of *Harper's Weekly*, and former president William Taft. "It seems to me that it is entirely proper to start a Zion-ist State around Jerusalem," wrote Teddy Roosevelt, who also asserted that "there can be no peace worth having" until Armenian and Arabs are granted independence "and the Jews given control of Palestine."

Pressure on Wilson to go public with his support of Zionism came not only from domestic quarters but also from the pro-Zionist government of Great Britain. Though he had secretly agreed with France to place Palestine under an international regime, Foreign Secretary Balfour hoped that the United States would administer the Holy Land, either alone or in conjunction with Britain. The plan had the double benefit of affording greater protection to the Suez Canal while formally associating America with the effort to create a Jewish national home. Yet Balfour had other, less rational reasons to seek an Anglo-American declaration on Zionism. Such a proclamation would, he believed, persuade influential American Jews, many of them still tied culturally to Germany, to sanction America's involvement in the war. It would also dissuade Russia's increasingly powerful Communists, a sizable number of whom seemed to be Jews, from seeking a separate peace.

In pursuit of these goals—concrete and illusory—Balfour arrived in the United States in April 1917. He intended to present his ideas on Palestine in a "man to man" talk with Wilson about the secret Allied agreements on the Middle East. Born at the height of British imperial power, in 1848, and deeply conservative in his views, the stately Balfour was schooled in the white-man's-burden approach to foreign relationships. That attitude had always evoked ambivalence in Washington, striking both Anglo-Saxon supremacist and anticolonialist chords. Colonel House, though, displayed no such uncertainty. "It is all bad and I told Balfour so," he wrote after learning of the foreign secretary's plans. "They are making [the Middle East] a breeding place for future war." Particularly offensive to House was the proposed American stewardship over Palestine. "The English naturally want the road to Egypt and India blocked, and . . . [are] not above using us to further this plan," he surmised.

The choice might have been more difficult for Wilson, a longtime admirer of Britain, but he, too, reacted negatively. The Sykes-Picot treaty, the secret European agreement for carving up the Ottoman Empire, sounded to him like some brand of tea. "[It's] a fine example of the old diplomacy," Wilson grumbled, and one which was liable to "cool [America's] ardour" for the war. "Our people and Congress will not fight for any selfish aim on the part of any belligerent . . . least of all for divisions of territory such as have been contemplated in Asia Minor." America, he said, opposed all clandestine attempts to partition the Middle East, including British proposals on Palestine.[6]

Snubbed by the administration, Balfour turned to Brandeis. "I have heard much of you and I want to have a talk with you," Balfour accordingly greeted the justice, the man he would call "probably the most remarkable" American he had ever met. In fact, Balfour learned little from Brandeis that he did not already know. Though American Zionists preferred to build the Jewish national home under Anglo-American auspices, they were certain that the United States would never approve of British imperial aims or assume a colonial role in Palestine. Brandeis did, however, believe that Wilson would endorse a broadly worded British declaration in support of Zionist aims. "The vast mass of Christian opinion in this country, particularly of course the Protestant Churches, supports our idea," he asserted. Balfour was delighted. By working through Brandeis, he would obtain indirect but official American approval for Britain's Middle East ambitions. "I am a Zionist," Balfour proclaimed.

The close alliance between Britain and Zionism confronted Wilson with a fundamental dilemma—how to oppose colonialism while simultaneously supporting the Jewish national home? The decision was further complicated by Wilson's divided feelings toward Jews and Zionism. Though he esteemed accomplished Jews like Brandeis and Frankfurter, Wilson also subscribed to popular anti-Semitic canards about Jewish power and moneygrubbing. But he also believed that returning Palestine to the Jews had divine, and not just political, ramifications and that he, Woodrow Wilson, was destined to facilitate that reunion. "To think," he once told Rabbi Wise, "that I the son of the manse (parsonage) should be able to help restore the Holy Land to its people." Reconciling his two minds about Jews and Zionism, and Zionism with the need to chart a principled foreign policy independent of Europe's, would rank among Wilson's weightiest challenges throughout the war and its aftermath.

The difficulty of surmounting that challenge was evident on May 9, 1917, during the forty-five minute interview Wilson afforded Brandeis. The president expressed his admiration for the Zionist movement and its goal of establishing "a publicly assured, legally secured homeland for the Jewish people in Palestine." He pledged to someday publicize those sentiments, but, in view of the fact that the United States was not at war with Turkey and that various Allies had other plans for the Middle East, Wilson thought it best to keep quiet. He did, however, promise Brandeis that he could draft the presidential statement on Zionism when the time indeed came to proclaim it.

Other figures in the administration, however, above all Secretary of State Robert Lansing, were opposed to making any pronouncement on Zionism, ever. Colonel House warned Wilson of the "many dangers lurking in" issuing such a statement. The result was a series of mixed messages from the White House, at first resistant and then favorably disposed to a British-sponsored Jewish homeland. In either case, though, Wilson demanded that no mention be made of his role in the deliberations surrounding the document. But Brandeis seemed unperturbed by this reticence and continued to assure Zionist leaders that the president was in "entire sympathy" with their cause. His communications, according to Weizmann, became "one of the most important individual factors in . . . deciding the British Government to issue its declaration [on Zionism]."

Balfour was indeed encouraged by what he believed to be Wilson's implicit backing and proceeded to finalize a text. Thus, on November 2, 1917, the British cabinet published what would become one of the century's most influential, and controversial, documents. The Balfour Declaration, as it would be called—actually a letter from Balfour to the Zionist financier Lionel Walter Rothschild—was distinguished as much by the obligations it made as by those it managed to sidestep. The British government "viewed with favor" the establishment of a Jewish national home in Palestine, but did not pledge to transform Palestine into a sovereign Jewish state. Moreover, in concessions to both the Foreign Office and the non-Zionist Jews, British leaders pledged that the national home's creation would not impinge on the "civil and religious rights of existing non-Jewish communities in Palestine" or the "status enjoyed by Jews in any other country."[7]

In spite of its ambiguities and disclaimers, the Balfour Declaration was widely interpreted as a commitment to ensure Jewish statehood and as an unqualified triumph for Zionism. Jews throughout the world believed that it could not have been formulated without Wilson's consent. A crowd of 100,000 Jews reportedly danced in gratitude outside the U.S. consulate in Odessa, with smaller demonstrations occurring in front of legations in Greece, China, and Australia. Telegrams of thanks billowed into the White House.

Perhaps the most concrete expression of Wilson's approval of the Balfour Declaration came in the form of American support for the Jewish Legion. A unit of the British army, the legion was organized by the headstrong Zionist leader Vladimir Jabotinsky and composed of Jews from various countries. Though federal law forbade foreign armies from recruiting on American soil, the Wilson administration raised no objection when Jabotinsky began to enlist American Jews. Together with Ben-Gurion and other Palestinian exiles who had found refuge in the United States, some 1,720 American Jews—the largest national contingent in the force—volunteered. In New York, Baltimore, and Boston, the inductees sang the Zionist anthem, "*Hatikvah*," (the Hope), as they marched past brass bands, orating politicians, and throngs of gift-giving Hadassah women en route to the ships that bore them to boot camp in Canada. Constituted as the Thirty-ninth Battalion of the Royal Fusiliers, the unit saw action only in September 1918, fording the Jordan near Jericho under fire, a month before the armistice. Nevertheless, the mere existence of a Jewish combat force—the first in nearly two thousand years—bearing Star of David flags and insignia provided a major fillip to the hard-pressed *Yishuv* and a model for later Zionist defense organizations. The Americans, in particular, gained a reputation for fortitude and élan. "The Americans brought with them a strong, often feverish interest in Palestine and everything Palestinian," commented Jabotinsky. Among the legion's American veterans were the sculptor Jacob Epstein, the future Jerusalem mayor Gershon Agron (Agronsky), and Nehemia Rabin, whose son, Yitzhak, would one day lead the Jewish army and state.[8]

Some Americans, however, were less elated by the impression that the declaration had originated in Washington, rather than in London. Lansing, for one, urged that the United States keep its distance from the policy and do nothing publicly to endorse it. America was in danger of becoming party to the theft of Turkish territory and of allying with the minority of Jews who were Zionists against the anti-Zionist majority. As a final word of caution, Lansing warned that "many Christian sects and individuals would undoubtedly resent turning the Holy Land over to the absolute control of the race credited with the death of Christ."

Lansing's reservations about Zionism were shared by other American diplomats. Samuel Edelman, head of the State Department's Near East Intelligence Unit and himself a Jew of German extraction, depicted Zionism as the product of pedestrian eastern European Jews who would have a "polluting and intolerable" effect on Palestine. America's ambassador to Britain, Walter Hines Page, considered Zionism "sentimental, religious . . . unnatural and fantastic" and recommended that the United States give it no further consideration. Henry Morgenthau, too, subscribed to Lansing's caveats. Never an advocate of Zionism and scarcely endeared to the movement by its opposition to his peacemaking efforts with Turkey, Morgenthau now claimed that any attempt to grant Palestine to the Jews would spur "400 million Christians" to revolt.

Few Foreign Service officials were more outspoken in their opposition to Zionism than William Yale. A thirty-year-old graduate of the university of the same name, a strapping self-described "playboy" who traveled with a pair of "brass knucks" in his pocket, Yale had roamed the Middle East as a representative for Standard Oil. In 1917, however, he left the petroleum business to become the State Department's special agent, attached to the British army in Palestine and Syria. The appointment coincided with the issuance of the Balfour Declaration, and Yale's estimations of the document's impact were rife with both prejudice and prescience. He described the anger of the "younger and more hot-headed among the Moslems" whose "plans . . . bode no good for the peace of Palestine," and the arrogance of "young, hot-headed Jews" representing the "disagreeable . . . type of their race . . . in many cases dishonest and ignorant adventurers." But Yale also foresaw a worldwide Muslim backlash against both Britain and the United States in retaliation for their support for Zionism. "Religious fanaticism and national intolerance," both Arab and Jewish, would generate "fierce antagonisms" in virtually every social and political sphere. Balefully, Yale predicted, "If a Jewish State is to be created in Palestine it will have to be done by force of arms and maintained by force of arms amid an overwhelmingly hostile population."

Such fervent admonitions could scarcely go unnoticed by Wilson. "Very unwillingly," he told Lansing, he was "forced to agree" about the dangers of outright support for Zionism. Chief among these was the possibility that the Turks would seek vengeance against American missionaries and relief workers—the very fear that had deterred the United States from joining the Middle Eastern war. But Wilson also believed that the Balfour Declaration had been promulgated partly on the strength of his approval and that, in time, he would have to go public with that consent.

The moment came on September 6, 1918, the eve of the Jewish New Year. The war in the Middle East was nearing its end, and the threat to American missionaries and relief workers had faded. Wilson now felt free to fulfill his promise to Brandeis. In wishing Jewish citizens a pleasant holiday—itself a groundbreaking gesture—Wilson expressed the "satisfaction" he felt "in the progress of the Zionist Movement" in his own country and "of Great Britain's approval of the establishment in Palestine of a national home for the Jewish people."[9] Though he pledged to preserve the "civil and religious rights" of the non-Jews in Palestine and the status of those Jews remaining in the Diaspora, the president had officially identified Zionism with the foreign policy of the United States.

FROM ITS tiny beginnings at the turn of the century, Zionism, by the end of World War I, had registered impressive gains. The Zionist Federation of America now claimed over two hundred thousand members and a multimillion-dollar budget. Wilson had given his imprimatur to the movement as had other influential non-Jewish figures in the United States, along with some of the most revered figures in American Jewry.

Much of the credit for this achievement was due to the man who had spent the bulk of his life estranged from all aspects of Jewish life. Louis Brandeis would nevertheless be remembered as the father of American Zionism, the Harvard grandee who bestowed legitimacy and prestige on what was originally perceived as a marginal, if not dubious, movement. Brandeis would remain an activist for Zionist causes until his death, in 1941, and a communal settlement—*Ein*

HaShofet, the Spring of the Judge—would later be named for him in Palestine. Only during World War I, however, did his contributions prove crucial. Thereafter, the goals of Zionism changed. Brandeis's vision of creating an amorphous Jewish homeland bound by economic and cultural ties would gradually be superseded by the struggle for an independent polity defined by citizenship and borders. New Zionist leaders would emerge who sought not only a shelter for refugees in the Land of Israel but an empowered, sovereign state.

Zionism was changing and so were the challenges it confronted. The most formidable of these was the impediment most conveniently and astonishingly overlooked by Brandeis and his generation. "The Arabs in Palestine . . . do not present a serious obstacle," Brandeis, on his sole visit to the country in 1919, conjectured. "The Arab question, if properly handled by us, will in my opinion settle itself."[10] Other Americans—Lansing, Edelman, and Yale—were already taking issue with that assumption. So, too, were expanding numbers of Arabs.

20

ARISE, O ARABS, AND AWAKE!

ON UNIVERSITY CAMPUSES AND ON TEEMING URBAN STREETS, on the pages of newspapers and in the minutes of literary clubs, the idea slowly took root. An Arab nation had always existed and, through a combination of domestic revolt and international diplomacy, would soon reassert itself in the form of a unified, independent state. The concept of Arabism, it will be recalled, originated in the nationalist ideologies of the West and penetrated the Middle East with the help of mission schools and colleges, many of them American. "I know why the Turks are hated in this country," Djemal Pasha, the governor of Syria, reproved the American consul in Damascus. "The Syrian Protestant College . . . breeds contempt for the Turk [and] . . . the very books used in the institution . . . breathe this spirit." Arab Christians, numbers of whom attended those schools, naturally became adherents of nationalism and worked to forge a common bond with the surrounding Muslim majority.

Arab Muslims, however, having long rejected the missionaries' religious teachings, felt little affection for their secular Western ideas. They already possessed a nation—the Islamic nation (*Umma*), as embodied by the Ottoman state. Few among them sought a common identity with Christians, much less a chance to join them in impugning Ottoman rule. Rather than secede from the empire, they preferred to attain additional rights within it and to achieve unity not through an alien philosophy but by returning to their native Islam. Rarely defining themselves as Arabs, they remained, first and foremost, Muslims. By contrast, those residents of the Middle East who saw themselves as Arabs primarily, irrespective of their religious affiliation, and who longed for a separate state, remained a tiny minority. It consisted of small groups of Western-educated intellectuals, mostly Christians, in Syria, and Arab expatriates in Europe. The cry "Arise, O Arabs, and awake," raised by the Syrian Protestant College graduate Ibrahim al-Yaziji in 1868, was, by the turn of the century, still unheeded.[1]

That is, until the Young Turk revolution in 1908. The Ottoman Empire, for centuries the bastion of Islam and the protector of Arabic language and culture, was suddenly transformed into a vehicle for imposing secular Turkish identity. The revolution served to strengthen the nationalist inclinations of Arab Christians and, for the first time, forced Arab Muslims to question their allegiance to Istanbul. In secret societies in Cairo, Damascus, and Baghdad, Muslim philosophers such as Abdullah al-Nadim and the young officer Nuri al-Sa'id joined with their Christian countrymen and discussed the possibility of Arab independence from the Porte. The same year saw mass demonstrations against British rule in Egypt and, in Palestine, the first stirrings of Arab resistance to Zionism.

Though they had profited from the enhanced trade and employment opportunities generated by the new Jewish settlements, Palestinian Arabs had grown increasingly concerned about the rise of Jewish immigration and land purchases. Resentment surfaced in March 1908, when a public celebration of the Jewish holiday of Purim provoked a scuffle with Arab onlookers in Jaffa. At the same time, in Haifa, the editor Najib Nassar founded a new journal, *al-Karmil*, dedicated to exposing the Zionist threat. Like Nassar, a recent convert from Greek Orthodoxy to Protestantism, most of the early Arab opponents to Zionism were Christian. Not a few of them had acquired their nationalism at American schools and the Syrian Protestant College. They warned of the dangers Zionism posed not only to the Arabs of Palestine but to the Arab nation as a whole.

But Muslim Arabs were also becoming wary of the Zionist challenge. In Palestine, especially, the centuries-old Muslim community feared being cut off from the broader Islamic nation and finding itself a second-class minority in a Jewish state. "The Jews' . . . right [to Palestine] died with the passage of time; our right is alive and unshakeable," wrote one of them, Khalil al-Sakakini, from Jerusalem in 1914. "What will the Jews do if the national feeling of the Arab nation is aroused; how will they be able to stand up to [the Arabs]?"

The future of Palestine—and of the Arab Middle East in general—would preoccupy Arab nationalist thinkers as war raged through the region. Arab Muslims in general responded zealously to the Porte's call for holy war and many thousands of them served in Turkish ranks. While the British managed to spark an Arab revolt against Turkey and to rally many nationalists to its cause, the rebellion was in fact spurred less by Arabism than by the desire to revive a purified Arab caliphate independent of the Westernized Turks. The uprising's leader, Sharif Husayn, the head of the Hashemite clan and guardian of Mecca, believed that the Arabs could unite only under Islam and not beneath some racial or cultural banner.[2]

Arab nationalism, though destined to become a tectonic force in the Middle East, remained in an inchoate stage in the years leading up to World War I. The movement was largely confined to the margins of Arab society and ruthlessly suppressed by the Turks. The war, however, helped prepare the ground for a dramatic flowering of Arab nationalism. And while most of these preparations took place in the Middle East, a significant number were also undertaken in the United States by inspired groups of Arab Americans.

Of Prophets and Judges

Between 1880 and 1914, approximately 100,000 Arabic-speakers arrived in the United States, settling mainly in the Northeast but also founding smaller communities in every state in the Union. They emigrated from Syria, mostly, but also from southern Anatolia, Palestine, and Egypt, seeking freedom from religious persecution and from famine. Roughly 90 percent of them were Christians, large numbers of whom worked as peddlers, bearing domestic necessities—utensils, thread, matchboxes, candles—to America's far-flung cities and homesteads. They traveled far, forming notions of their new homeland as romantic as those which Americans traditionally harbored toward the Middle East. "The land of hope . . . the land of contentment . . . the land of liberty . . . where the dreams of men come true," one of them, Salom Rizk, recalled. "I could see America . . . looming out of my ignorance, thrusting its huge continental shores . . . out of the fog that was in me."

The immigrants may have been happy to leave the troubled Middle East for the peace and opportunities of America, but they remained committed to their native language and culture. Many of these Arab Americans had been educated at missionary schools that emphasized Arabic instruction or else had benefited from the Arabic-language textbooks and dictionaries that the missionaries had produced. As early as 1892, New York had its first Arabic newspaper—*Kawkab Amerika* (The Star of America)—and by the end of World War I, nine Arabic journals were circulating. Literary societies, meanwhile, sprang up in several American cities and served as laboratories for avant-garde Arab poets, essayists, and playwrights.

Of these, the best known was Gibran Khalil Gibran. Quiet and slight, a mustachioed Maronite from northern Lebanon, Gibran settled in Boston's impoverished South End in 1895. After returning to Lebanon to complete his Arabic education, Gibran sailed back to the United States during the war and became an activist for Arab liberation. He called on Arab Christians and Muslims to unite in armed struggle against Turkish rule, wondering, "How long are the Cross and the Crescent to remain apart before the eyes of God?" Yet it was his poetry, rather than his politics, that made Gibran famous in his adopted land. Boston society feted him, convinced that his abstract imagery contained poignant insights on love, nature, and God. In searching for his esoteric meanings, though, readers often overlooked the themes of national identity and longing for independence that ran subtly through his verse. "Freedom when it loses its fetters becomes itself the fetter of a greater freedom," Gibran declared in his epic classic, *The Prophet*.[3]

Gibran's close friend and occasional literary collaborator,

Ameen Rihani, may have been less acclaimed artistically but proved far more politically influential. Like Gibran, he was a Lebanese Maronite who, at age twelve, moved with his family to the United States but briefly returned to Beirut to complete his Arabic education. Moved by Washington Irving's *Alhambra*, with its mystical evocation of Muslim Spain, Rihani aspired to create a literature of fusion between Arab and Western cultures. "Carry to the East some of the western vigor and bring to the West some Eastern repose," he exhorted ships departing and entering New York harbor. "Deliver to Egypt and Syria an abundance of your engineering sciences and bring over a heap of its noble Arab traits." Also like Gibran, Rihani was passionate about freedom, in particular the "American spirit of freedom" inculcated by the Syrian Protestant College. "Of all the other educational institutions of Syria that encourage this lofty spiritual view . . . the American College at Beirut stands foremost."

Dark complexioned and dapper, an orator of spellbinding charm, Rihani proclaimed his love of his New World liberties before Arab American audiences, urging them to help achieve those freedoms for their Middle Eastern homeland. "In a land where . . . the freedom of the citizen has not yet been realized, one can better serve one's country from a safe distance," he explained. Yet it was not safety that Rihani sought, for with America's entry into World War I, he exhorted all Middle Eastern immigrants to volunteer for combat. "Our first duty is toward our adopted country, whose political ideals will yet be the ideals of every nation in the world," he proclaimed in a letter to Teddy Roosevelt, adding, "I have never been so proud of being an American citizen as I am to-day." Rihani's pride sometimes proved effusive, though, and dangerous. While trying to recruit Syrian and Lebanese immigrants in Mexico to join the American army, the writer was arrested and expelled.

Rihani's love for the United States was inextricable from his adoration for the Arab world, yet he could also be merciless in criticizing that world's shortcomings. Ignorance, sectarian factiousness, and religious fanaticism were, in his view, just some of the ills endemic to the Middle East. "It was unfortunate that you should allude to some of the defects in Islam at a time when the best people are trying to draw together in the interest of . . . the Empire," Howard Bliss, after listening to one of Rihani's critiques, reproached him. But Rihani's criticism merely targeted those aspects of Arab society that he felt were in need of radical reform. Such changes would be effected by indigenous movements—one of which, curiously, was Wahhabism, cited by Rihani as "proof of the aptitude of the Arab's spirit, its liberal aspirations, and the elastic quality of its religious fibre"—as well as by a beneficent United States. "The voice of America . . . is destined to become the voice of the world."

The transformation of the Arab people that Rihani envisioned would encounter innumerable obstacles. Among the most trying of these was the release of the Balfour Declaration in November 1917. "The Land of Promise had indeed become a too much promised land," he chortled. Rihani distinguished between the "native Jews" of Palestine, whom he considered Arabs, and the European Zionists, who were essentially reactionaries, "harking back . . . to pre-Roman days." Instead of to Palestine, he suggested that Jewish refugees from Russia move to Texas, a far larger and emptier area, where they could be resettled—so Rihani quipped—"without prejudicing the civil and religious rights of existing non-Jewish communities."

The following month brought a no less devastating shock. As one of its first acts after seizing power in Moscow and signing a separate armistice with Germany, the Bolshevik government published the Allies' secret agreements on the Ottoman Empire. The world suddenly learned that the powers planned to reapportion the Middle East and that Britain's beguiling promise to create an independent Arab state—the quid pro quo for the Arabs' revolt—was baseless. The revelation was devastating for Arab nationalists throughout the Middle East and searingly painful for Rihani. His vision of a strong and united Arab state had been abruptly replaced by a "dream of empire . . . supported with American money and English bayonets." Rihani warned of disastrous consequences if the Arabs were denied their liberty—of rebellions and wars into which the United States, torn between domestic political pressures and its expanding Middle East interests, might be dragged.[4]

Rihani was the Arab answer to Brandeis, a dynamic intellectual who marshaled America's moral force to advance his nationalist arguments. Similarly secular in outlook, both men were committed to spreading America's civic faith in the Middle East. Neither saw a contradiction between his loyalty to the United States and advocacy of his people's independence. Unlike Brandeis, however, with his political connections, strong organizational base, and a possible pool of several million American Jews, Rihani had little access to power and few followers, actual or potential. Nonetheless, Arab nationalism had begun to attract influential sympathizers in the United States, both within and outside of government.

"I have a kindly feeling for the Arabs and my influence will be thrown in their direction whenever they are right," Colonel House confessed to his diary. Yet the president's adviser was scarcely alone in viewing Arab political goals sympathetically. A small but politically potent group of industrialists—oilmen, in particular—fearful of Anglo-French competition, also sought a mutually lucrative alliance between the United States and Arab nationalism. State Department careerists, many of them the descendants of the American missionaries who had promulgated Arab nationalism, now joined with the evangelists working in the Middle East to portray Arabism as a long-term American interest. This new and increasingly influential fusion of business, diplomatic, and religious interest was exemplified by Charles Crane, the entrepreneur and philanthropist who became the Arabs' outstanding champion in America.

Born in Chicago in 1888, the son of a bathroom fixture magnate, Crane quickly tired of the family business and instead cultivated a lifelong fascination with Asia. He was also a religious man, a devoted member of the Presbyterian Church. These two interests converged for Crane in the Middle East, where he served on the boards of Robert College and the Constantinople Women's College and helped to finance new missions. Cherub-faced but introspective—a *Time* magazine portrait showed him thoughtfully engaged in Solitaire—Crane was in fact politically shrewd. He supported Taft, a Republican, for president in 1909 and, four years later, became one of Wilson's most generous contributors. His son Richard served as Robert Lansing's private secretary.

Crane was also an early advocate of Arab independence and in 1914 sponsored a series of lectures on Arab history and culture at select American universities. If Brandeis saw Zionists as avatars of the hardworking Pilgrim colonists, then Crane subscribed to the popular American image of the Arabs as lovers of liberty and revilers of radicalism, the "Unitarians of the desert." He served as the patron to several Arab intellectuals, Muslim as well as Christian, including George Antonius, the eminent historian. Antonius would dedicate his seminal study of the Arab nationalist movement, *The Arab Awakening*, to "Charles R. Crane, aptly nicknamed Harun al-Rashid"—a reference to the illustrious caliph of *A Thousand and One Arabian Nights.*

Crane's admiration for the Arabs was rivaled only by his antipathy toward Zionism and Jews. In contrast to the nineteenth-century patrons of American missions, Crane had no ardor for restorationism and nothing but disdain for what he deemed "the menace . . . [of] the modern, pushy Jew." A defender of the czar's anti-Jewish pogroms and an admirer of Henry Ford's rampages against the "international Jew," Crane considered the term "anti-Semite" to be a "title of honor." Though named America's ambassador to China, Crane was so flagrant in his Jew hatred that President Taft was compelled to rescind the appointment.[5]

Anti-Semitism did not, however, figure prominently in Arab nationalist thought of this period. On the contrary, activists in the movement often went out of their way to express fraternity with the Jews of the Middle East and, on occasion, even a willingness to coexist with the Zionists. At least one hundred Jews from Baghdad fought with the Arab Revolt and shared in the jubilation when, on October 30, 1918, Turkey finally surrendered.

One month later, World War I came to a close, leaving American policymakers with a welter of postwar conundrums. Among the thorniest of these were the questions relating to the Middle East. Arab nationalism, once insignificant as a political force, could no longer be disregarded, but neither could Zionism. America's allies Britain and France, whose cooperation was vital for establishing the new world order, also had demands in the Middle East—far-reaching demands. Reconciling all of these concurrent and often conflicting ambitions while maintaining America's principles and interests was the herculean challenge awaiting Wilson at the international peace conference in Paris. Other Americans would join him there—Brandeis and Frankfurter, Rihani and Crane—a procession of judges and prophets, each aiming to reshape the region in accordance with his party's goals. Ultimate decisions, however, would continue to reside with Wilson, a president who also saw himself in the Old Testament mode, meting out justice and wrath.

21

THE FIRST MIDDLE EAST
PEACE PROCESS

MANY OF THE WARS AND REVOLUTIONS THAT HAVE CON-
vulsed the contemporary Middle East, as well as the dreams and disappointments of its inhabitants, can be traced to the Paris Peace
Conference of 1919 and to its most inspired, and ultimately deluded,
participant.

Woodrow Wilson came to Paris not only with his presidential
brief but also with much personal, theological, and ideological baggage. He once reflected how "a boy never gets over his boyhood and
never can change those subtle influences which have become a part
of him." Wilson's early years were spent amid the ruins and depriva-
tions of the post–Civil War South. The memory left him permanently
hateful of war and its ravages and determined to preserve peace
whenever possible. His father and his grandfather, meanwhile, both
of them Presbyterian ministers, instilled in him a belief in the need
for Christian fellowship between individuals as well as among
nations and a sense of his own destiny to achieve it. Later in his youth,
during his travels through Great Britain, Wilson became enamored
of Anglo-Saxon civilization and its ability to "do the thinking of the
world." His confidence in the righteousness of the United States led
him, as president of Princeton and governor of New Jersey, to advo-

cate an activist foreign policy based on fundamental republican ideals. America's mission, Wilson held, was to "go to the ends of the earth carrying conscience and the principles that make for good conduct," to bring democracy and stability to the world.[1]

These ideas impacted Wilson's concept of the postwar order, especially as it applied to the Middle East. He sympathized with the peoples of the region who had suffered so poignantly during the fighting and he recognized their need for dignity and independence. To assist them in achieving those goals and to safeguard peace worldwide, Wilson envisaged the creation of a League of Nations, an international assemblage in which Anglo-Saxon values would predominate. Out of the ashes of famine and genocide, the Middle East would emerge as a constellation of free and westward-looking nations, modeled on the United States and championed by its twenty-eighth president.

But Wilson brought more than ideals to Paris; he also brought his prejudices. He despised all forms of European imperialism, Britain's included, and displayed a particular distaste for the Turks. As early as 1889, he characterized the Ottoman Empire as "abnormal" and as "a belated example of those crude forms of politics which the rest of Europe has outgrown." The Turks were a "docile people," he thought, who ought to be "cleared out" of the Balkans and western Thrace. Wilson assured Colonel House in 1912 that, should the world go to war, "there ain't going to be no Turkey."

Guided by rarefied principles, repelled both by imperialism and by some of imperialism's victims, Wilson came to Paris with a lofty but often muddled mind. On the one hand, he looked forward to the dissolution of the Ottoman Empire and the establishment of independent states on its pieces. Point Twelve of his Fourteen Points plan, presented to Congress in January 1918, promised "an undoubted security of life and an absolutely unmolested opportunity of autonomous development" to "nationalities which are now under Turkish rule." Less than a year later, however, Wilson told the State Department that "America believes in helping the whole of the Turkish Empire to obtain good government and the advantages of modern civilization" and that "this is an unassailable position." The president, moreover, never specified which of the multifarious peoples of the Middle East were deserving of self-determination and how that right would be realized. He knew little of the region's geography, cultures, and traditions, beyond what he had read in the Bible.[2]

Wilson's confusion regarding the future of the Middle East became apparent to Walter Lippmann, a former *New Republic* editor who was serving as the assistant secretary of war, six months before the Paris conference. In an internal memo of May 1918, Lippmann warned that America was liable "to win a war and lose the peace" unless it found the "sheer, startling genius" necessary to reconcile Wilson's conflicting plans for the Middle East. Heeding his caveat, the government established a secret task force, headquartered in the New York Public Library and code-named The Inquiry. More than one hundred scholars were enlisted in the group, leaders in fields as diverse as engineering, Egyptology, and Native American cultures. None of them, however, were specialists on the Middle East. Rather, The Inquiry's "experts" consulted encyclopedias, travel books, and missionary manuals—everything but Arabic and Turkish texts—in formulating their plans for the region. Others pursued personal agendas. The American Board secretary James Barton, for example, proposed that the entire Ottoman Empire be placed under America's aegis, with spiritual and ethical guidance provided by missionary schools and colleges.

The Inquiry nevertheless devised many of the concepts that were later implemented in the Middle East. Most of these emanated from the project's Western Asian Division, under the diligent leadership of William L. Westermann, a distinguished professor of ancient history at the University of Wisconsin. Westermann believed that Europe's secret plans for the Middle East should "be thrown in the waste paper basket" and that the United States should take the lead in reorganizing the entire region. Thus, Turkish Anatolia would be maintained as an independent entity, with international administrations arranged for Istanbul, the Dardanelles Strait, and a newly created state of Armenia. Foreign tutelage would also be necessary to bind the tribal peoples of Syria and Mesopotamia into cohesive nations and to guarantee religious freedom. Palestine would be reserved for the Jews. "It was the cradle and home of their vital race, which has made large spiritual contributions to mankind, and is the only land in which they can hope to find a home of their own." Recognizing, however, the need to ensure the rights of the area's non-Jewish population, and the potential for "fanaticism and bitter religious differences," The Inquiry proposed that Palestine too, be placed under Western supervision, preferably Britain's.[3]

The Inquiry's recommendations for the Middle East were assembled in a report, "Just and Practical Boundaries for the Turkish Empire," in November 1918, the month the armistice was signed. Wilson, though, chose not to share them with his Allies. The result was to thicken the curtain of uncertainty surrounding the president's policies. To Britain and France, these seemed concerned less with punishing Turkish aggression than with denying the victors their hard-earned spoils of war. Lansing, too, who had long ago fallen out with his president, and Colonel House, who would also grow estranged from him, had at best an indistinct comprehension of Wilson's plan for applying the self-determination principle. "Will not the Mohammedans of Syria and Palestine and possibly of Morocco and Tripoli rely on it?" the secretary of state ruminated. "How can it be harmonized with Zionism, to which the President is practically committed."

The peoples of the region, on the other hand—Arabs, Jews, Armenians, Kurds, and even the Turks—were ecstatic about the Fourteen Points and profoundly grateful to their author. "No people . . . has felt [more] strongly the joyous emotion of the birth of a new era which, thanks to your virile action, is soon . . . to spread everywhere the benefits of peace," the Egyptian nationalist leader Said Zaghlul saluted Wilson.[4] Regarded by large parts of the West as a potentially dangerous dreamer and by much of the Middle East as a savior, Wilson, looking neither dreamy nor messianic but ecclesiastical—tophatted, bespectacled, and stiff—set out for the peace talks in Paris.

The Great Loot of the War

He arrived on December 12, 1918, the first president to journey outside the Western Hemisphere during his term in office, to a lavish welcome. The throngs that greeted Wilson, though, merely camouflaged the multiple hazards awaiting him at the talks. Although France and Britain had publicly committed themselves to "the complete and definite emancipation of the peoples so long oppressed by the Turks," and to the "establishment of national governments . . . deriving their authority from the . . . free choice of the indigenous populations," the two powers still had secret, imperialist plans for the Middle East. Prime Minister Lloyd George of Britain was eager to extend his country's empire from Egypt to the Persian Gulf and to use the United States as a bulwark against French and Russian encroachments. His French counterpart, the wily and vengeful Georges Clemenceau, was determined to keep Syria for France and to place Palestine under an international regime. Both leaders favored the partition of Anatolia, with sectors reserved for the Italians and Greeks, and no role whatsoever for the Turks. "Is it not better that the Allies should determine the fate of . . . the former Ottoman Empire without the encumbrance of negotiations with that Empire?" Jean Jusserand, a senior French diplomat, asked Lansing. The British also objected to any discussion on Persia, a country that the United States considered neutral but that Britain included in its exclusive sphere of interest, or on the British protectorate in Egypt. For most of the conference's participants, the Middle East remained, in Professor Westermann's words, "the great loot of the war."

Wilson, though, came determined to oppose any mass purloining of the Middle East. "The United States intends to completely ignore these [European] agreements," read one of his guidelines, "unless by chance, they happen to contain certain provisions which we consider to be just and proper." The president was also determined to preserve America's economic and cultural interests in the region, but without taking on additional political and military responsibilities.

His ability to achieve these goals seemed, at first glance, formidable. Wilson's was the only country to emerge unexhausted from the war, with an intact million-man army. But that edge was blunted in the Middle East, which, apart from the few hundred volunteers in the Jewish Legion, was devoid of American troops. "Not having declared war upon Turkey," Westermann recalled, "we were always . . . outsiders, impotent to affect the actual course of the negotiations or put our own stamp upon the decisions taken." By contrast, some 200,000 British soldiers now occupied the strategic cities of the Middle East, from Baghdad to Damascus, and dominated western Anatolia. "The other governments had only put in a few nigger policemen to see that we did not steal the Holy Sepulcher!" boasted the impish-looking but unscrupulous Lloyd George. By joining the war, Wilson had hoped to gain admittance to the peace conference and not have to "call through a crack in the door," but in the Middle East, where he chose to protect American missionaries rather than project American power, the door remained frustratingly closed.[5]

America revealed its relatively weak hand in Middle Eastern matters on January 30, 1919, when the conference finally took up the subject of the Ottoman Empire. The European Allies refused to apply Wilson's understanding of self-determination to the area and to relinquish their claims to colossal swaths of territory. Wilson accused the powers of seeking to annex the Middle East and, by so doing, undermine his envisioned League of Nations. "In spite of . . . [the] propaganda in regard to the liberation of oppressed races," carped William Yale, now serving as one of Wilson's advisers, "the British and the French are . . . working only for their own interests in the Near East." The former French colonial minister Gaston Domergue willingly confirmed this charge, exclaiming, "The obstacle is America!"

The logjam was opportunely broken when Jan Smuts, a lean and leathern South African statesman (and the inventor of the words "holistic" and "apartheid") devised the concept of "mandates." According to this, the League of Nations would bestow control over former enemy territories to various powers, which would prepare their populations for self-rule. The idea dovetailed closely with The Inquiry's recommendations for the future of the Middle East and appealed to European officials eager to acquire colonies under an enlightened and internationally sanctioned guise.

A council of representatives from ten Allied nations consequently voted to create mandates for Armenia, Syria, Mesopotamia, Palestine, and Arabia. Little thought, however, was given to how these mandates would be apportioned and even less to whether the native populations wanted them. The British, still anxious to keep the

French away from the Suez Canal and the new Soviet regime out of the Middle East entirely, wanted the United States to become the mandatory authority in Syria and Armenia. "We ought to play self-determination for all it is worth," counseled Lord Curzon, Britain's newly appointed foreign secretary, "knowing in the bottom of our hearts that we are more likely to benefit from it than is anybody else." His cynicism was shared by General Tasker Bliss, the Army general, linguist, and accomplished diplomat who served as Wilson's chief military adviser. "Wherever a mandate covered oil wells and gold mines Great Britain would get it," he reckoned, "and the United States would be asked to take a mandate over all of the rock-piles and sand-heaps that might be left."

For Wilson, though, the question of American mandates was moot. Though he personally warmed to the suggestion of administering Armenia, where Americans had considerable cultural investments, he doubted whether the majority of his countrymen agreed. "I can think of nothing the people of the United States would be less inclined to accept than military responsibility in Asia," he explained. The decision whether or not to embark on such an immense undertaking could not be made by one man, not even the president, Wilson explained, but only by the Senate. The Allies nevertheless continued to press Wilson on the issue, if only to contrast America's reluctance to accept mandatory burdens in the Middle East with Europe's willingness to shoulder them.[6]

While grappling with the Allies' demands, Wilson was subjected to intense lobbying efforts by religious and ethnic interest groups from the United States. The best organized of these were the Zionists, who kept up a robust flow of information in support of what they now called a "Jewish Commonwealth" in Palestine—still less than a state but more than a mere national home. Augmented by the influx of eighty thousand Jewish immigrants annually, this commonwealth, the Zionists reasoned, would soon represent the majority of Palestine's inhabitants and thus fill the Wilsonian criteria for self-determination.

The argument persuaded many participants at the conference, including, however improbably, Feisal, the son of Sherif Husayn and commander of the Arab Revolt. Visiting the emir, or prince, at his villa outside of Paris, Felix Frankfurter assured Feisal that the Jews had no desire to deprive the Arabs of their national rights and that the two movements could coexist peacefully to their mutual advantage. "Here was little me meeting this Arab prince," the diminutive Frankfurter recalled, noting how that same prince graciously served him coffee. Already delighted by this display of Arab hospitality, Frankfurter was further thrilled as Feisal praised the Jews as "cousins in race" and wished them "a hearty welcome home." He expressed his "deepest sympathy" for Zionist aspirations, which he described as "moderate and proper" and "national and not imperialistic." Syria was large enough to accommodate Zionism and Arab nationalism, the emir concluded. "Indeed I think that neither can be a real success without the other."

Feisal later denied making these statements, but his contribution to the Zionist case was irrevocable. Yet that same Feisal, solemnfaced and regal in his traditional Arab robes, was also revered by American supporters of the Arab position at Paris. Listening to this "ancient seer and . . . Moslem paladin," whose demeanor "suggested the calmness and peace of the desert," the habitually tight-lipped Lansing swooned into a reverie long known to American travelers to the Middle East. "His voice seemed to breathe the perfume of frankincense and to suggest the presence of richly colored divans, green turbans and the glitter of gold and jewels." Feisal claimed that 100,000 Arabs had taken part in his revolt—Yale put the number closer to 2,000—and predicted that Arab villagers would one day erect statues in honor of the United States. Hyperbole, however, only fortified the charm that the Hashemite prince managed to exude toward Americans. Edith Wilson, the First Lady, remarked on the prince's "startling resemblance to . . . pictures of the Christ," and even William Westermann, The Inquiry's Nordic and notoriously staid academic, was struck. "Great is Feisal," the historian exclaimed. "I am a convert."

Lansing and Westermann provided redoubtable counterweights to the Zionist influence at Paris, but their voices were hardly lone. The American delegation was deluged with letters decrying the creation of a Jewish commonwealth, and not only from American Arabs but also from American Jews, Orthodox and Reform alike. Henry Morgenthau submitted a petition signed by 299 "prominent American Jews" that denounced Zionism as an attempt to impugn their allegiance to the United States. The severest blow to the Zionist campaign, though, came from the segment of the American public formerly most enamored of the Jewish state idea. "The opposition of the Moslems and Christians to granting any exceptional privilege to the Jews in Palestine is real, intense and universal," warned Otis Glazebrook, the Jerusalem reverend and consul who expressed empathy for Jews at the beginning of the war but whose words now evoked those of his anti-Zionist predecessor, Selah Merrill. Glazebrook predicted that Russian Jews would bring Bolshevism to Palestine and that Yiddish-speaking Jews were pro-German. "Jerusalem will be quickly inflamed—Nablous and Hebron are the danger points."

Glazebrook belonged to the generations of missionaries, the followers of Henry Jessup and Daniel Bliss, who ventured to the Middle East in order to convert the Arabs, but were eventually converted to Arabism. As the goals of Arab nationalism became separate from, and antithetical to, those of Zionism, the final break between missionaries and Zionists grew inexorable. The most dramatic display of that schism occurred on February 13, as Howard Bliss appeared before the Council of Ten.

A monument of a man, tall, thin, and yoke-shouldered with a silver corona of hair, the sixty-nine-year-old Bliss entreated passionately for the Arabs. "They are intelligent, able, hospitable and lovable, but with the sure defects of a long oppressed race; timidity, love of flattery, indirectness," Bliss asserted, but then assured his listeners that the Arab inhabitants of Syria would, with time and guidance, "grow into capacity for self-determination and independence." He urged the delegates to ask the Arabs what they favored, foreign rule or self-government. Their preference, Bliss ventured, would be for a free Syria, including Palestine, safeguarded by the United States.[7]

Wilson did not have time to consider Bliss's proposal, though. The next day, with a draft covenant for his League of Nations in hand, the would-be peacemaker departed for the United States. Awaiting him there was a powerful block of senators opposed to America's membership in the League. Henry Cabot Lodge and many of the same senators who had once insisted that the United States intervene in the war against Turkey now wanted the United States to recoil from any involvement in that conflict's resolution. The League, Lodge and his colleagues feared, would curtail American's sovereignty and mortgage its security to blocs of small, nondemocratic principalities.

Opposition to Wilson was particularly keen on Middle Eastern issues. Years of press reports on the Armenian massacres and other atrocities had hardened the public's traditional animosity toward Turkey and the Islamic religion. "So long as the Koran makes murder a part of the Mohammedan religion, the Moslem must not be permitted to rule over Christians or Jews," raged Henry Morgenthau. The esteemed and aristocratic novelist Edith Wharton also visited the Middle East during the war and published scathing reports. "Nothing endures in Islam, except what human inertia has left standing," she wrote, charging that the entire Middle East, "from Persia to Morocco," was predicated on "slavery, polygamy and the segregation of women." The air of enmity further dissuaded Congress from endorsing those parts of the postwar settlement dealing with the Middle East or from accepting any mandatory responsibilities there. "I cannot imagine how these gentlemen can live and not live in the atmosphere of the world," Wilson protested. "America is the only nation . . . that can undertake that mandate and have the rest of the world believe that it is undertaken in good faith and that we do not mean to stay there."

On March 20, 1919, the president returned to Paris and to yet another maelstrom. Backed by the British, Feisal was demanding independence for all of Arabia, with the exception of parts of Lebanon and Palestine, with a possible American mandate over Syria. France produced Syrian representatives of its own who testified in support of French control of their country—Lansing sketched caricatures as they spoke, and Wilson gazed disinterestedly out of a window. "The Turkish Empire at the present time was as much in solution as though it were made of quicksilver," he recorded, ruing the fluidity of the Middle East. "Austria . . . had been broken into pieces . . . but the Turkish Empire was in complete solution." In order to conquer Syria, Wilson said, the French would have to crush

Fesial's 100,000-man army and risk a clash with Britain as well. Colonel House warned of "widespread trouble of a religious and racial character" about to erupt in Syria and Palestine.[8]

To avoid this "scrap," as he called it, Wilson took up Howard Bliss's proposal for sending an international fact-finding mission to Syria to ascertain its inhabitants' desires. France and Britain consented, though only on the condition that the investigators covered not only Syria but also all other territories slated for mandates. Wilson accepted this proviso, but then Clemenceau refused to participate in the project as long as British soldiers occupied Syria, and Lloyd George said that if France boycotted the commission, Britain would, too. Such were the machinations at Paris that what began as a multilateral effort was soon reduced to an exclusively American plan.

To implement it, Wilson appointed two individuals who, he claimed, "knew nothing about" the Middle East and therefore could render objective opinions. Such assurances were scarcely ingenuous. The first commissioner, Dr. Henry Churchill King, though currently the president of Oberlin College, was by training a Congregationalist minister and former YMCA official who had traveled extensively in the Holy Land. The second was the exponent of Arab nationalism and self-described anti-Semite Charles Crane, "a very experienced and cosmopolitan man," according to Wilson. Attached to the delegation staff were William Yale, whose reservations about Zionism and European designs on the Middle East were well documented, and Albert Lybyer, a professor from Robert College.

The appointment of a commission so obviously predisposed against European and Zionist objectives in the Middle East was a curious move for Wilson, who, in spite of many misgivings, had formerly supported the mandate system and the Balfour Declaration. But the missionaries were now against Zionism and opposed to British imperialism, and their influence on Wilson once again proved paramount. "Our [Allied] governments . . . have undertaken a commitment toward the Jews to establish something which resembles an Israelite state in Palestine, to which the Arabs are very much opposed," the president now admitted. The same faith-guided mindset that had prevented Wilson from making war on Turkey now led him to side with Bliss in seeking to create a unified Arab Syria, including Palestine, possibly under an American mandate.

The commission, accordingly, terrified the Zionists. "A crazy idea," Frankfurter called it, and a plot "to cheat Jewry of Palestine." The French, too, were furious, insisting that Americans "were too honest to deal with the Orientals." Only Feisal was elated. Bliss, he said, was "the root of all good in the Near East" and America, with its twenty-eight states, would serve as the protector and model of the future Arab federation. "I am confident that when the Commission visits Syria, it will find a country united in its love and gratitude to America," he guaranteed Wilson. Toasting to the commission's imminent success, the Arab prince for the first time tasted champagne.[9]

America's Commissions Eclipsed

Feisal's optimism, however, was unfounded. Wrangling over guidelines repeatedly delayed the commission's departure, as did inter-Allied squabbles over the fate of western Anatolia. In an effort to stake their claim to the area, the Italians in April began landing troops near Antalya, on the Mediterranean coast, spurring the Greeks to follow suit. Wilson, evoking America's old Philhellenic traditions and the rights of Smyrna's Greeks to self-determination, joined with Lloyd George and Clemenceau in backing Greece's demand for the city. An Allied armada that included the USS *Arizona* and four Navy destroyers accompanied the Greek invasion force that swiftly occupied Smyrna, but then turned on its Turkish minority. "Old men, unarmed, and other unoffending civilian Turks were . . . killed by stabbing with knives or bayonets, and then . . . having their valuables and clothing stripped . . . were thrown into the sea," remembered John D. McDonald, the *Arizona*'s captain. Turkish soldiers, surrendering after a spirited fight, were paraded before the public and shot. American residents of the city were forced to take shelter aboard the destroyers, while U.S. Marines once again charged ashore to safeguard American institutions.

The war that began with attempts by individual Americans to prevent the slaughter of Christians by Muslims concluded with the massacre of Muslims by Christians—an atrocity facilitated, however unintentionally, by the United States. Members of the American delegation were indeed disgusted by this crime, but French and British ministers welcomed the opportunity to divert America's attention away from the Arab lands questions and focus it on Turkey. Clemenceau and Lloyd George exploited the moment by reopening the issue of an American mandate for Armenia and parts of Asia Minor. Wilson still wished "with all [his] heart that . . . the country could assent to our assuming the trusteeship for Armenia," but asked to delay a final discussion on the subject until June 27, assuring the Senate sufficient time to decide.

With the conference's attention fixed on Turkey, the Allies proceeded to split the Middle East into areas of Occupied Enemy Territory that conformed to their anticipated mandatory borders. France conceded Palestine, including present-day Israel and Jordan, to Britain, along with Mosul in what became Iraq, in exchange for a free hand in Syria. "I, myself, have never been able to see by what right France and Great Britain gave this country away to anyone," Wilson protested, and vowed not to recognize the spheres. Apart from such rhetoric, however, the United States had still done little to contest the powers' claims to the Middle East or to ascertain its inhabitants' preferences. Dr. King complained that "it was something of a scandal" that he and the other Americans appointed to investigate the situation in Syria and other Arab provinces had yet to leave Paris.[10] Wilson, at last, agreed, and on May 29, over three months after its creation, the American Section of the Inter-Allied Commission on Mandates departed the Gare de Lyon for Bucharest, en route to the Middle East.

Over the course of the next forty days, the commissioners visited some sixty towns and villages in Syria and Palestine. In canvassing public opinion, they employed no formal methodology—no questionnaires or formula for assembling statistics. King, a slight and compact scholar with a notable military mien, packed several books "for atmosphere," including the *Rubayait* of the medieval Persian poet Omar Khayyam, *The Talisman*—Sir Walter Scott's saga of the Crusades—and *A Thousand and One Arabian Nights*. These, and the impressions gleaned from hundreds of interviews with residents, would serve as the basis for the commission's extensive conclusions, which proved to be remarkably clear-cut.

"The people of the area declared themselves almost unanimously for United Syria, for its complete independence," Crane and King discovered. With the exception of the Maronites and their centuries-long loyalty to France, all the peoples consulted, including Sunnis, Druze, Orthodox and Protestant Christians, and Jews, preferred to live under a British or an American mandate and expressed unqualified distaste for the French. Feisal, for his part, clearly preferred an American administration for Arabia. "A real great lover of Christians," he allegedly offered to permit the opening of a missionary-style women's school in Mecca and impressed the commissioners as a malleable politician who, "given proper sympathy," would take "no . . . big step without Anglo-Saxon approval."

Whether under British or under American auspices, the Arabs fully expected to attain their freedom as solemnly promised to them by the Allies and by Wilson's Fourteen Points. The world could not ignore that desire, nor could it overlook the fact that Syria and Palestine, "the birthplace of the three great religions [and] contain[ing] places sacred to all three," were "a center of interest . . . for the whole civilized world." Any solution that failed to recognize that truth, the commissioners warned, or that addressed the needs of only one ethnic group, was doomed to fail. And no policy was more likely to elude success—and perhaps trigger large-scale violence—than the "extreme Zionist Program for . . . making Palestine [into] a distinctly Jewish State."

Zionism would serve as the commission's principal, if not overriding, focus. The authors claimed that they had begun their study "with deep sense of sympathy for the Jewish cause" and "with minds predisposed in its favor," but had been "driven" by their findings to strenuously oppose the idea. The "civil and religious rights" of the Arabs who constituted the vast bulk of Palestine's population could not, as stipulated by the Balfour Declaration, be safeguarded by a Jewish movement that planned to dispossess that population through immigration and land purchases. Nor could a Jewish "right" to Palestine, based on an occupation two thousand years ago, "be seriously considered." Moreover, the commissioners expressed doubts whether the Jews could ever be seen as trustworthy custodians of the Holy Land and its abundant sacred sites. "It is simply impossible . . . for Moslems and Christians to feel satisfied to have these places in Jewish hands." Arab rejection of Zionism was "intense," the commissioners found. They concurred with the numerous British officers they interviewed that "a force of not less than fifty thousand soldiers would be required even to initiate" the Jewish national home.

Though adamant, the commission's conclusions on Zionism were not unanimous. "Whereas injustice may be done to individuals who inhabit Palestine an injustice is not being done to a nation," submitted William Yale in an astonishing volte-face of views, "[but] the wishes and desires of 14,000,000 Jews who have a national history, national traditions, and a strong national feeling must be taken into consideration." Astounded by the commission's lack of scientific method and impressed by the Jewish settlements he visited, the same Yale who had earlier seen Zionism as the source of unending bloodshed now insisted that the Allies honor their pledges to Zionism and "suppress with a strong hand any . . . demonstrations against the Jews." The special agent extolled the potential contributions that "Jewish energy, Jewish genius, and Jewish finance" could make to the Middle East, and the advantages of establishing an "outpost" of "western culture" in the region. For the United States, especially, Yale now believed, the creation of a Jewish state imbued with "American ideals and American civilization" would have untold strategic and educational benefits.

Yale's arguments, though fervidly pressed, could not divert Crane and King from reaching their unequivocal conclusion. "On account of her large and influential Jewish population," which would demand the realization of Zionism, and in view of Anglo-French resistance and the reluctance of its own people to take on overseas burdens, the United States should not assume the mandate over Syria. That role, the commissioners averred, would best be fulfilled by Britain, which would oversee an Arab government under Feisal. America, meanwhile, would concentrate on areas outside of the Arabic-speaking Middle East. "No other Power could come into

Asia Minor, with hands so free to give impartial justice to all the peoples concerned." The commission also recommended the foundation of an independent Armenia and the preservation of Turkey as sovereign entity."[11]

The King-Crane Commission anticipated many of the central themes of American policy toward the Middle East in the period after World War I: sympathy for Arab nationalism, antipathy toward European imperialism, and a keen divergence of opinion, for and against, Zionism. Identifying these motifs did little to affect America's position at the peace conference, however. After gathering for a "true oriental affair" at Feisal's Damascus palace, complete with Arabic music, sword dances, and Bedouin costumes for all the American guests, the commissioners drafted their final report.

It arrived in Paris in the last week of August 1919 after the signing of the Treaty of Versailles. Rather than peace, many observers thought, the Paris conference had merely imposed impossible strictures on Germany and possibly laid the groundwork for future war. On Middle Eastern matters, too, the conference seemed to generate, rather than ameliorate, conflict. Enraged by British attempts to edge France out of Anatolia, Clemenceau hollered "Lloyd George is a cheat!" and challenged the prime minister to a duel. But while European leaders accused one another of subterfuge in the Middle East, they assailed Wilson for his ignorance of the region, his pedantry, and his self-righteousness. "God himself was content with ten commandments," Clemenceau groused. "Wilson . . . inflicted . . . on us . . . fourteen commandments of the most empty theory!"[12]

Already obscured by these tensions, the findings of Crane and King were further eclipsed by the controversies surrounding the proposed American mandates over Asia Minor, Armenia, and Istanbul. Lansing, evoking the isolationist element in American foreign policy, denounced the plan as a "perfectly useless proposition" that would merely embroil the United States in Europe's relentless conflicts and make it an occupier of native peoples. Frank Polk, America's first undersecretary of state, agreed and advised Wilson to get out of the "whole disgusting scramble" for the Middle East. Even the senior American official in charge of Armenian relief, the future president Herbert Hoover, rejected the mandate scheme on the grounds that it would cost American taxpayers at least $100 million to finance and require 100,000 troops to sustain. In Istanbul, by contrast, where American relief ships were anchored alongside the battleships of Britain and France, Turkish bakers were adorning their loaves with miniature Stars and Stripes and the sultan was imploring the United States to assume control of the city. Turkey's pioneering feminist writer Halide Edip reasoned that only "America, which knows how . . . a people's government is constituted . . . can create . . . a new Turkey in which every individual . . . will carry true independence in his head as well as in his pocket."

Torn between these pro- and anti-mandate poles, the Wilson administration sent yet another investigating mission to the Middle East. Headed by U.S. Army Chief of Staff General James G. Harbord, a team of experts in August set out to tour the Armenian areas of eastern Anatolia and the Black Sea coast. Harbord's report listed thirteen reasons for not accepting the mandates (the costs, for example, and the dangers of foreign entanglements) and thirteen in favor (humanitarianism, the need to protect American institutions in the area). For a fourteenth argument in favor, however, the team could find no counter. "Here is a man's job that the world says can be better done by Americans than by any other," determined the square-jawed and by-the-book Harbord. "If we refuse to assume it . . . we shall be considered by many millions of people as having left unfinished the task for which we entered the war, and as having betrayed their hopes."[13]

Ideals and principles had once again trumped strategic considerations in the conception of American policy toward the Middle East, but for the last time during Wilson's presidency. Harbord's report reached Paris, but Wilson had again left the city, embarking on a United States tour whose scope—eight thousand miles and twenty-nine cities in three weeks—dwarfed those of the King-Crane and Harbord commissions. His overriding objective was to rally public support for American membership in the League of Nations. While he asked Cleveland Dodge and other evangelical leaders to back his effort, Wilson scarcely mentioned the Middle East. His opponents, however, exploited the mandate controversy as a means of attacking Wilson's platform on the League. The Republican National Convention of 1920 thus denounced him for seeking an American mandate over Armenia, and Henry Cabot Lodge assailed the notion that Americans had any "obligation to preserve the territorial integrity or political independence of any country." Lansing predicted that "the President will have to abandon any plan . . . to assume guardianship over Armenia or Constantinople," noting that not only Republicans but also "many Democrats . . . feel the same way."

The argument over the mandates soon proved immaterial. Wilson had just finished reminding a crowd in Pueblo, Colorado, that "the American people always . . . extend their hand to . . . the truth of justice and of liberty and of peace," on September 25, when he suffered a nearly fatal stroke.[14] Though his wife managed to hide the fact from the public, Wilson was subsequently incapacitated, unable to continue his campaign for the League and his advocacy of the mandates. The Senate on November 19 voted against American participation in the League of Nations and effectively declined to play a prominent role in reshaping the Middle East.

Postwar Postmortem

The work of reassembling the region continued, however, first at Paris and then, in April 1920, at San Remo, on the Italian Riviera. Deliberating on the sparkling waterfront, delegates finalized the British mandates over Palestine and Mesopotamia—now renamed Iraq—and the French mandate of Syria, from which Feisal's forces would soon be expelled and another country, Lebanon, cleaved. Control of the Dardanelles Strait was placed under an international commission, Smyrna and eastern Thrace went to Greece, and France and Italy received territories in southern Anatolia. In the east, the Allies decided on independence for an Armenian state and autonomy for the Kurdish regions. The Ottoman Empire, the forbidding and exotic polity that, for centuries, had dominated the crossroads of the world, alternately terrorizing and enchanting Westerners—Americans included—was demolished.

But not Turkey. A forty-year-old general named Mustapha Kemal, the hero of Gallipoli, refused to accept the San Remo dictate and rallied the army against it. Three years later, Kemal—later to take the title Ataturk (Father of the Turks)—had succeeded in driving all foreign troops from the Anatolian homeland. Collaborating with the Soviets, Kemal crushed the Armenian independence movement and suppressed Kurdish separatists. In the Smyrna area, tens of thousands of Armenians and Greeks were killed and 250,000 people expelled as Turkish troops sacked and burned the city. The Marines again landed to protect American institutions, which now included the offices of Standard Oil, and help evacuate hundreds of refugees. Countless more, however, were stranded on the docks, exposed to the approaching flames. "I'll never forget the screams," Melvin Johnson, a sailor aboard one of the two U.S. destroyers that aided in the evacuation, testified. "A lot of 'em were jumping in, committing suicide." For George Horton, the best-selling novelist, literary critic, and Chicago *Herald* correspondent who also served as America's consul in Smyrna, the massacre represented the culmination of seven years of indescribable brutality, "a fittingly lurid and Satanic finale to the whole dreadful tragedy."

THOUGH ONCE again appalled by Turkish cruelty, the British and the French were also intimidated by the Turks' ferocity and the Soviets' proximity to the Straits and duly sued for peace. The historic treaty was signed on July 24, 1923, in the Swiss city of Lausanne. As a result, the Republic of Turkey arose out of the decimated Ottoman heartland and a modern city, Izmir, on the ruins of Smyrna. The whirlwind unleashed by World War I in the Middle East had subsided, but not before etching new borders into the region, carving out new identities, and exposing the fault lines of innumerable future upheavals.

The majority of Americans watched these events much as they had observed the earlier stages of the war, from the side. The United States sent an observer to San Remo—the acclaimed poet and novelist Robert Underwood Johnson, who spent most of the conference in a courtyard, reading the newspaper—and to Lausanne. America's goals at these summits were, modestly enough, ensuring an open door to the Middle East for American businesses and maintaining

American schools and hospitals. There remained a vague impulse to "find [the] means to wipe away at once the causes for this waste of human life and human suffering"—a vestige of Wilson's world-view—and to work for the creation of an "Armenian National Home." Lacking a military presence in the area, however, or even a seat at the postwar conferences, the United States had little or negligible leverage. Warren Harding, the lackluster, laissez-faire Republican who won a landslide victory in the 1920 presidential election, a contest billed as a "solemn referendum" on the decision to abstain from the League of Nations, finally acknowledged this fact. Soberly, he wrote, "The most ardent supporters of the Armenians in America would hesitate to sanction armed warfare in order to establish a separate territory for the Armenians."[15]

THE ASSESSMENTS of this first Middle East peace process varied between bad and execrable. Clemenceau came away feeling he had been duped by Lloyd George, and Lloyd George resented Wilson for letting him down on the Armenian mandate. Within the region, many people wondered why they had been denied Wilson's promise of self-determination and why Middle Eastern nations from Morocco to Egypt had been left languishing under colonial rule. Americans, too, were bitter. "When boldness, confidence in the strength of our own political integrity, and active support of a new political ideal might have saved Armenia and with it the Near East, we held back," Professor Westermann lamented. "Where we might have led at the zero hour of political opportunity, we faltered and refused to go over." The ever dour Lansing prophesied that "the seeds of discontent and hatred have been sown in fertile soil" and that, in time, "those seeds . . . [will] germinate and . . . bear the bitter fruit of conflict." Most astringently, General Bliss wished "there never had been a war—or else that it lasted longer—for peace seems to be worse than the war."

Many historians of the period would agree that the effort to construct a new and viable Middle East from the debris of World War I was an unqualified failure—and the cause of much consequent bloodshed. The conclusions of the Harbord Commission, they note, were never implemented and those of King-Crane remained unpublished until 1922. The idea of endowing all of the Middle East's peoples with an inviolable right of self-determination was not even partially realized. The very institutions that Wilson hoped to protect—the churches, schools, and hospitals—and for whose sake he refrained from warring against Turkey, were largely closed by the war's end. A large percentage of the missionaries had been banished or killed.

The harsh judgment of America's performance in the diplomacy of World War I nevertheless overlooks several impressive and long-lasting achievements. In accordance with The Inquiry's recommendations, the Ottoman Empire was dismantled, but Turkey's sovereignty was preserved. The foundations of the future Jewish state were laid in British-administered Palestine and in mandates provided for Syria and Iraq. Presently, Britain would designate a separate Arab emirate east of the Jordan River—Transjordan—and the French would detach Maronite-dominated Lebanon from Syria, granting each of those areas the potential for self-determination. (See map on page xiii.) The right of Armenians to independence, though not realized for another seventy years, was for the first time universally recognized.

Though greatly restricted during the war, missionary activity resumed in peacetime and flourished. In 1919, evangelists established the American University of Cairo, dedicated to the cultural enrichment and modernization of Egypt. In the following year, the Syrian Protestant College changed its name to the American University of Beirut and became the first Middle Eastern university to admit women. "It is not possible for an American to realize . . . the respect, faith and affection with which our Country is regarded throughout that region," wrote one postwar visitor to Syria. "[The] impartial missionary and educational influence exerted for a century . . . is the one faith which is held alike by Christian and Moslem, by Jew and Gentile, by prince and peasant in the Near East."

None of these accomplishments, not even the award of the Nobel Prize for his contributions to peace, could console Woodrow Wilson. He had dreamed of creating a different world, unsullied by avaricious empires, secret treaties, and wars. Yet, in many ways, the new global order that emerged from the Great War's killing fields seemed virtually indistinguishable from the old one that triggered that cataclysm. Wilson's disappointment was especially acute in the Middle East, which he longed to illuminate with America's democratic and civically virtuous light. Now, rather than enjoying a period of peaceful development and amiable relations between states, the region would be gripped by relentless domestic and international turmoil. As a testament to his failure and a warning to those future presidents who would claim to be his heirs, Wilson hung a portrait of a young Armenian refugee over the mantel of his Washington home. Her haunting, hunger-widened eyes would continue to beseech visitors, reminding them of America's unrealized vision for the peoples of the Middle East.[16]

22

FANTASIES
REVIVED

ALMOST AN ENTIRE GENERATION OF EUROPEAN MEN HAD been butchered and those who survived were maimed, physically or emotionally or both. An estimated 10 million civilians died as well, victims of hunger and disease, rapine and genocide. Though American troops entered the fighting a mere half year before the armistice, over 53,000 of them were killed—almost as many as in the entire decade of the Vietnam War—and some 320,000 wounded. In spite of the talk of "hallowed dead" and "sacrifices for democracy," there seemed little or nothing ennobling about the carnage. The great modern age that had given birth to the automobile, the aircraft, and moving pictures also produced tanks, warplanes, and machine guns. The same Flanders fields that were once mellifluous with lavender and poppies now lay sodden, a morass of shell holes and trenches, barbed wire and body parts, a landscape as hellish as any painted by Hieronymus Bosch.

But then, just as World War I threatened to leave the human imagination as indelibly scarred as those battlefields, another image arose—dashing, masculine, principled, and, above all, premodern. Instead of limping in mire-encrusted fatigues, he seemed to flow in spotless robes, with a gold-plated kaffiyeh rather than a helmet on his head and a dagger in his belt in place of a pistol. He rode out of the Middle East, a region renowned for its saviors, and with a face that was pale and boyish, intensely blue-eyed and flaxen-haired—a visage that many Westerners associated with Christ's. They could not have picked a more unlikely candidate for messiah.

Thomas Edward Lawrence was the illegitimate son of a minor British aristocrat and a descendant of Sir Walter Raleigh. Immature and sometimes described as effeminate, short (five feet, four inches), with an overlarge head and a high-pitched voice, he hardly seemed the swashbuckling type. Yet he was determined to remake himself into one and, to that end, spent untold hours testing his endurance and building his physique, mastering riflery and Arabic. "As other men lust for power or wealth or women," the historian David Fromkin wrote of him, "he craved to be noticed and remembered."

In 1916, the twenty-eight-year-old Lawrence was sent to Cairo as an army cartographer and intelligence officer, but soon found himself attached to Prince Feisal and the pro-British Arab Revolt against the Turks. If politically valuable in muffling the Ottomans' call for jihad, the rebellion had proved incapable of dislodging the Turks from any part of the Arabian Peninsula. Lawrence also produced no victories, but with the help of insurgent Bedouin tribes he did manage to capture the Red Sea port of Aqaba. British ships were consequently able to transport Feisal's forces from Arabia to Transjordan, where they could harass the enemy's supply lines to Damascus. The British hoped that Feisal would liberate the city, declare a pro-British Arab kingdom, and deny control of Syria to the French. But even that plan went awry when Australian troops reached Damascus first. The British dream of ruling Syria through Feisal was finally dashed at the peace conference, where the French succeeded in realizing their demand for a mandate. Lawrence, who played a double game of publicly encouraging Arab independence while manipulating Feisal for Britain, ultimately failed at both.

A success neither as a military commander nor as a statesman, Lawrence might well have slipped into obscurity. But the world at that funereal moment was desperate for heroes and the nonconformist colonel who wore a green silken scarf and an Arab headdress to the Paris talks seemed ripe to fill that need. "The younger successor of Mohammed," Professor James Shotwell, an adviser to Wilson, called him, "the most interesting Briton alive." Lawrence quickly became a focus of public attention, a favorite of the press, and the friend of outstanding literary figures such as Robert Graves and George Bernard Shaw, who likened him to a prima ballerina followed by "the limelight of history." He made no effort to deflect this attention; on the contrary, he cultivated it, with increasingly embellished versions of his exploits. "On the whole I prefer lies to truth, particularly when they concern me," he admitted. "History is but a series of accepted lies."

Proof of that preference was furnished in *Seven Pillars of Wisdom* (1922), Lawrence's highly literate account of the Arab Revolt, in which historical facts served as launching pads for flights of personal fantasy. The many setbacks of the desert war were all but forgotten amid the exhilarating descriptions of camel charges, spying missions, and Turkish trains blown skyward by tulip mines planted by the valorous author.[1] The book was ebulliently received, yet for all of his gifts at self-promotion, T. E. Lawrence could not have metamorphosed into the mythic Lawrence of Arabia without the help of a hype-wise American journalist.

Lowell Thomas, a specialist in manufacturing legends, was himself rather larger than life. Raised in Cripple Creek, Colorado, he worked as a gold miner and a cook before getting hired as a reporter for the *Chicago Journal*. Lanky and rakish-looking with a thick black pompadour and pencil-thin mustache, he procured a name for slickness and innovation, experimenting with slide shows about faraway places like Alaska. He next moved to Princeton University, where he studied and taught oratory, and where President Wilson found him in 1917 and asked him to make propaganda films favorable to the war. Thomas, camera in hand, departed for Europe, but the trenches and no-man's lands proved too dismal a subject. In search of a more inspiring story, he continued eastward to Palestine, to document the British advance under General Allenby.

Traveling first to Jerusalem, Thomas stayed with the Spafford family at the American Colony and wandered through the Old City's alleyways. On one of these jaunts, while rounding a corner, Thomas suddenly glimpsed the nobly robed colonel. "He walked rapidly with his hands folded, his blue eyes oblivious to his surroundings, . . . wrapped in some inner contemplation. . . . My first thought . . . was that he might be one of the younger apostles returned to life." Gripped by the "power of . . . [this] fantasy," Thomas requested permission to visit Lawrence and his rebel Bedouin and to accompany them on some of their raids.

Thomas spent a mere two days in the desert, yet they sufficed to produce a hefty memoir, *With Lawrence in Arabia*, published in 1924. Though he probably never saw Lawrence in actual combat, Thomas nevertheless painted him as utterly fearless under fire, capable of picking off "400 Turks" with a "heavy American frontier model weapon," but also of showing compassion toward his prisoners. Lawrence, for Thomas, was a character culled from *A Thousand and One Arabian Nights*, a "reincarnation of a prophet of old" and "one of the most picturesque personalities of modern times" who was destined to be "blazoned on the romantic pages of history." Most crucially for the hustling American journalist, Lawrence was "a great scoop."

Dissatisfied with merely creating a hero, however, Thomas managed to transform his thoroughly English subject into an American-style champion. Thus, the same Lawrence who assured his superiors that the Arab Revolt would "break up the Islamic 'bloc' " and render the Middle East "a tissue of small jealous principalities incapable of cohesion" became, in Thomas's telling, a freedom fighter who "united the wandering tribes of the desert" and persuaded them to "die willingly for the liberation of the whole Arab world from Ottoman oppression." The same Lawrence who chided the missionary schools that "quite without intention . . . taught revolution" to their Arab pupils, and who "chuckled in the desert" upon hearing of Wilson's Fourteen Points, was portrayed as the "George Washington of Arabia," struggling to forge a United States of the Middle East founded on constitutional ideals. From a lapsed Anglican with little patience for his own religion and even less for that of the Jews, Thomas refashioned Lawrence into a modern-day crusader for the Holy Land and an enthusiast for Zionism.

With Lawrence in Arabia met with prompt commercial success, but the former prospector from Colorado knew when he struck a lode. With the aid of projectors and magic lanterns, he mounted an early version of the sound-and-light show based on his book. "Come with me to lands of history, mystery, and romance," Thomas began, offstage, to the strains of Arabic music. "What you are about to see is an untold story, part of it as old as time, and part history in the making." Then, stepping into the spotlight, he narrated the Lawrence tale as only he, Thomas, had witnessed it—the passion and the blood. In London alone a million people saw the show, but it was in the United States that the Lawrence fad became a national frenzy. The performance packed the largest theaters in New York and San Francisco and even drew huge audiences in remote midwestern towns. Not since the belly dancers and camel rides at the Chicago exposition thirty years before had so many Americans been exposed to the gossamer charms of the Middle East, to the same alluring aura that had surrounded Feisal in Paris.

Of all the myriad viewers of Thomas's act, only one was notably dissatisfied. "I saw your show last night and thank God the lights were out," Lawrence wrote to Thomas, rebuking him for his flagrant exaggerations and lies. The peculiar cipher who became a master of self-invention could not abide his fabrication by anyone else. "I don't bear him [Thomas] any grudge," he confessed to an old army friend. "He has invented some silly phantom thing, a sort of matinee idol in fancy dress, that does silly things and is dubbed 'romantic.' "

Unrepentant, Thomas continued staging his Lawrence of Arabia extravaganza to full houses for nearly a decade. He would go on to write an astonishing fifty-five books and to gain celebrity as a correspondent for CBS News, a position he held for almost half a century. Lawrence, on the contrary, sought anonymity, joining first the Tank Corps and then the Royal Air Force as a simple soldier, each time changing his name. He died in 1935, the victim of a motorcycle accident and a refugee from the fiction on which he had partly collaborated.

The Lawrence myth had by that time taken on a life of its own, particularly in that part of the United States most adept at mythmaking. As early as 1915, the Hollywood screenwriter and director Cecil B. DeMille produced *The Arab*, a tawdry melodrama about the love between a Bedouin herdsman and an American missionary girl. The tale drew on the popular nineteenth-century perception of the Middle East as a realm of the senses and of the Arab as a manly paragon. The plot appeared to be less titillating for twentieth-century audiences, however, who judged the movie a flop. But then came Lowell Thomas and the Lawrence craze, and suddenly Americans were reawakened to the urge for Arabian romances. Consequently, *The Sheikh*, made in 1921 with essentially the same story line—sensual nomad seizes innocent Western lass—became an overnight bonanza and catapulted its leading man, Rudolph Valentino, to stardom. Hollywood rushed to capitalize on the success, churning out *The Sheik of Araby*, the *Son of the Sheikh*, and *The Thief of Baghdad*, each with its profusion of harem girls, defenseless maidens, and cruel but lascivious Arabs.[2]

The Orientalist trend started by Lawrence soon permeated many areas of American culture, not just the movies. In her 1918 classic, *My Ántonia*, the novelist Willa Cather described one character, festooned with fraternal pins, as "more inscribed than an Egyptian obelisk," and another with "the beard of an Arabian sheik." The fad was further animated by the discovery, in 1922, of the treasure-packed tomb of Tutankhamen—King Tut. Flappers suddenly started sporting Cleopatra-like hairstyles and public buildings were adorned with Egyptian deco. And when not giving vent to Middle Eastern fantasies in their fiction, fashion, and art, Americans indulged them in song:

I'm the Sheik of Araby,
Your love belongs to me.
At night where you're asleep
into your tent I'll creep.[3]

Films and recordings had, by the 1920s, replaced travel literature as the principal media for conveying impressions of the Middle East to Americans. And in contrast to Europeans, so many of whom were disillusioned by the war, Americans could still dream. Over the coming decades, myths surrounding the Middle East would continue to excite and even inflame the American mind, coloring public opinion and influencing policymakers. The country's material investments in

Part Six

OIL, WAR, AND ASCENDANCY

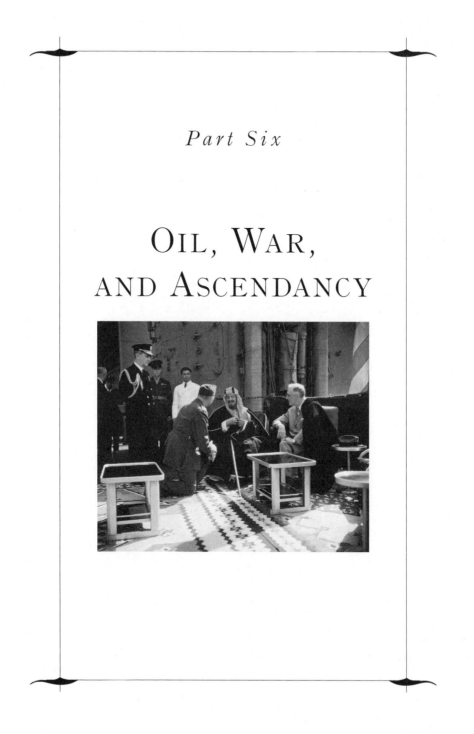

23

FROM BIBLES TO
DRILL BITS

THE POSTWAR SETTLEMENT IN THE MIDDLE EAST DID NOT, as its architects intended, bring concord and stability to the region, but only endemic conflict. The 1920s were a time of mounting resistance to European rule in the region, with anti-British revolts breaking out in Egypt and Iraq, and a rebellion raging against French rule in Syria. Palestine would become a perennial center of bloodshed. Safely removed from this upheaval, the Arabian Peninsula was virtually forgotten by the colonial powers as well as by the nationalists who sought to oust them. A wasteland of flinty sand, salt flats, and rock, the area seemed devoid of the most basic natural resources. Its principal source of income was the Muslim pilgrimage to the holy cities of Mecca and Medina, both located in the western Hejaz district. The British were content to let their Hashemite allies rule the Hejaz and to ignore the rest of the peninsula. The French were utterly indifferent.

No less than the Europeans, the United States was consistently uninterested in Arabia. The State Department scarcely reacted when, in 1923, a coalition of tribes led by 'Abd al-'Aziz ibn Saud (1880–1953) and backed by the militant Wahhabi movement conquered the holy cities and ousted the Hashemites. The region "is of little commercial importance," remarked one expert at the Division of Near Eastern Affairs, while another felt that the Saudis' warlike behavior "demonstrated that the Arabs . . . have not progressed from where they were 13 centuries ago." Ibn Saud subsequently declared himself king over a new country, Saudi Arabia, but the United States withheld formal recognition and refused to accord it an ambassador.

But the State Department's insouciance toward Arabia was not shared by all Americans. Missionaries remained keenly engaged in the area. Before the turn of the century, it may be recalled, the American missionary Samuel Zwemer established the peninsula's first modern medical clinic and imported an American physician, Paul Harrison, to head it. A dashing, Valentino-like figure with a penchant for Bedouin garb, Harrison in fact had little affinity for the natives' culture. "Not even their religion has ever been able to unite them for any long period into a stable state," he attested, and listed the succession of "intrigue and assassination, revolt and riot, and wars great and small" that had haunted Arab history. Such shortcomings could not, however, deflect Harrison from ministering to the medical needs of the natives or from seeking to save their souls. "We want them to become Christians," he admitted, "but in Arabia that is an extremely slow process."

To expedite the procedure, Harrison expanded his medical services in the years before World War I and established branch clinics in Kuwait, Oman, and Bahrain. New doctors were added to the staff, among them several American women. Eleanor Calverly recounted her serendipitous arrival in Arabia in 1912, remarking, "What had, until that moment, seemed a tragic sacrifice instantaneously became the only thing in the world I wanted to do. . . . Never had I felt such joy!" Another physician, Mary Allison, found that landing in the Hejazi port of Jidda was "like being born anew," a rapt experience both spiritually and sensuously. "I knew what ecstasy felt like—to reach the place of my dreams."

Allison's experience was hardly unique. Drawn to Arabia by their religious convictions, many missionaries would become enchanted with the desert's immutable beauty and the romance of its perambulant tribes. And few aspects of Arabia were more mesmerizing for Americans than that of its king, ibn Saud. Towering at over six feet, four inches, in flowing robes and braided hair, with his teeth gleaming and an ebony glint in his eyes, the monarch overwhelmed the missionaries. "Every line of him . . . told of intelligence, energy, determination, and reserves of compelling power," one of them recalled. The fact that ibn Saud had 125 wives, was accompanied by machine-gun-toting guards, and maintained an alliance with the infidel-hating Wahhabis failed to disillusion the spellbound evangelists.

Ibn Saud was less concerned with enthralling Westerners, though, than with obtaining effective medical care. He first heard of the American doctors in 1911, when missionary physicians in Bahrain tended to ten of his men who had been shot in a pearl-fishing dispute. In 1914, ibn Saud sent some of his malaria-stricken kin for treatment at the American clinic in Kuwait, and three years later he invited Harrison to Riyadh. "I know you are a Christian," the monarch greeted him, "but honorable men are friends though they differ in religion." Finally, stricken by a swollen facial cellulitis in November 1923, the king summoned another American doctor, Louis Dame, from Kuwait. With his dark, fleshy features and trim black beard, Dame blended well into the local population and passed for a Bedouin sheikh as he rode nearly forty hours by camel to Riyadh. He cured ibn Saud within a week. Over the course of a quarter century, Dame, Harrison, and the other missionary doctors treated some 300,000 inhabitants of Arabia, among them many grateful Saudis.[1]

That indebtedness would soon prove pivotal in ibn Saud's choice of a Western ally. Resentful of the British who prevented further expansion of his realm into Transjordan and southern Iraq and inherently distrustful of the French, he would turn to the nation whose citizens had worked so selflessly for his people's welfare. When the possibility arose that his country contained not only rock and sand but also the wellsprings of the world's most sought-after fluid, the king would remember Harrison and Dame.

In Search of "Liquid Muck"

While American missionaries were laboring in the parched Arabian desert, their countrymen back home were acutely thirsting for oil. By the early 1920s, accelerated industrialization, the mass production of automobiles, and electrification of households had propelled the demand for petroleum in the United States well beyond its production capacity. American oil companies were forced to search desperately for overseas reservoirs, with much of their hopes fixed on the Middle East. But beyond the technical difficulty of locating the oil in this remote and inaccessible region lay numerous political obstacles to American exploration. Iran had the largest proven deposits, but Britain's national oil company already had a monopoly over the southern part of the country, while the recently established Soviet Union dominated the north. In Syria, Iraq, and Palestine, where American prospectors had looked for oil before World War I, Britain and France now claimed that the mandatory powers granted them by the League of Nations—an organization boycotted by the United States—endowed them with exclusive drilling rights. "The Anglo-French combination is determined to keep American companies out of the new oil fields of the Near East," America's ambassador in Paris, Hugh Wallace, complained. Wallace's attempts to remind the former Allies that, without America's intervention in the trenches of Europe, there would have been neither a League nor any mandates proved unpersuasive.

Eager to break the European monopoly over Middle Eastern oil, the U.S. government for the first time became actively involved in the oil business. In 1921, Secretary of Commerce Herbert Hoover, a seasoned manager of international relief efforts, rallied the seven leading American petroleum companies—New Jersey (later Esso/Exxon), Texas (later Texaco), Sinclair, Mexican, Atlantic, Gulf, and New York (SOCONY, later Mobil)—into a potent consortium. Assailed by this united front, the European companies relented and invited the Americans to join them in forming a new cartel, the Iraq Petroleum Company (IPC). In return for forfeiting their right to explore for oil outside of the IPC framework (the so-called self-denial clause), the Americans received 23.75 percent of all the petroleum extracted from the Middle East. The formula, which satisfied the escalating energy needs of the United States without saddling it with political responsibilities in the Middle East, marked a victory for American diplomacy and a potential bonanza for American oil.

The vastness of the riches hidden beneath Iraqi sands was partially revealed in October 1927, when prospectors in the northern city of Kirkurk unleashed a geyser so powerful it killed two of them.

Questions nevertheless persisted regarding the geographical scope of the IPC contract and the exact borders of the Middle East. Did the agreement cover only Iraq, Syria, and Palestine, for example, or did it apply to the Arabian Peninsula as well? To resolve these issues, the heads of the cartel solicited the advice of the Armenian-born businessman, sybarite, and financial genius Calouste S. Gulbenkian, who had managed to procure for himself a full 5 percent of the IPC's shares. In a meeting with IPC executives in July 1928, Mr. Five Percent, as the Americans admiringly called him, unfurled a map of the Middle East and, with a bright red pencil, encircled Turkey, Arabia, and the mandated areas. "That was the old Ottoman Empire which I knew in 1914," the squat, potbellied Gulbenkian explained. "And I ought to know, I was born in it, lived in it, and served in it."

This Red Line Agreement essentially excluded all but IPC members from exploring for Middle Eastern oil. This was devastating news for ibn Saud. A sudden drop in the numbers of Muslims making pilgrimage to the holy cities had left the ruler desperately short of funds, yet he hesitated to let IPC's British engineers survey his kingdom for oil and other minerals. He preferred to work with countries that would respect Saudi Arabia's sovereignty and with professionals like Harrison and Dame, who seemed free of European imperialist agendas.

A solution to ibn Saud's dilemma was provided in February 1931 by his chief adviser, Harry St. John Philby. A brilliant but unconventional British explorer who had converted to Islam and become a peevish critic of Britain's Middle East policies, Philby was alert to the king's needs and fears as well to the possibilities of personal gain. Already he had obtained the exclusive right to sell Ford automobiles in the kingdom, augmenting his wealth and connecting him to American industry. Now, addressing the country's deepening economic crisis, Philby suggested that ibn Saud turn to the United States for help and to the American most closely identified with Islam and the Arab world.

Charles Crane, the philanthropist and long-standing advocate of

Arab nationalism, had not been discouraged by the failure of world leaders to implement the recommendations that he, together with Henry King, had made for reordering the postwar Middle East. Throughout the 1920s, he continued to fund Middle Eastern studies programs in the United States and to act as a goodwill emissary between America and the rulers of Iraq, Transjordan, and Yemen. While journeying across the Arabian desert in 1929, Crane was attacked by Wahhabi bandits and his traveling companion, the Reverend Henry Bilkert, was killed. While recovering from the trauma, Crane received a letter from ibn Saud expressing regret that "the friend of the Arabs should have been attacked in Arabian lands," and inviting him to visit Riyadh.

The visit was an extravagant success. For four days, Crane was feted with Bedouin feasts, horse and camel races, and reviews of the royal guard. At one point, purportedly, ibn Saud asked his guest to remain in Arabia, to become a Muslim, and serve as the chief muezzin of Mecca. The real purpose of the meeting was not revelry, though, but business, Would Crane fund a geological study of the country, the king finally asked Crane, to be conducted by American engineers? The reply was unreservedly positive. Crane left Riyadh on March 3 with a pair of the king's prize stallions and permission to launch the first American survey of Arabia.[2]

To lead that expedition, Crane chose an engineer who had previously worked for him in Yemen, a quiet Vermonter named Karl S. Twitchell. Though fated to be the progenitor of Saudi-American relations, Twitchell, spare and sad-eyed, was hardly a patriarchal type. His outstanding assets, it seemed, were an unflagging esteem for ibn Saud, "a man of wisdom and righteousness . . . of justice, generosity and hospitality . . . [who] ranks among the foremost figures of this age," and a no less unwavering faith in Arabia's economic potential. From his Yemen experience, he knew that even the harshest deserts could mask artesian springs and profitable mineral deposits.

To prove his hunch, Twitchell set out from the Red Sea port of Jidda in February 1932 and trudged over four hundred miles inland. On the outskirts of Medina, he succeeded in identifying an ancient gold mine, which he then reactivated and restored to profitable production. But the proceeds from the mine could not compensate the Saudis for the loss of pilgrimage revenue and the kingdom still faced insolvency. Twitchell continued his search, journeying an additional six hundred miles to the Persian Gulf, without finding a single resource of worth, not even water. The situation appeared irremediable when, on June 1 of that year, engineers from the Standard Oil Company of California (SOCOL) suddenly struck oil on the barren Gulf island of Bahrain.[3]

The discovery augured a windfall for Twitchell. Located a mere twelve miles from the Saudi mainland, Bahrain was geographically linked to the Arabia Peninsula, and it was reasonable to assume that if the island contained oil, so, too, would the adjacent coast. Acting on this premise, Twitchell returned to the United States and met with the representatives of the IPC. The American companies, however, bound by the Red Line Agreement to work collectively in Arabia, refused to take on projects independently. "Some of these firms think that 'Hejaz' is the name of a new drink," Twitchell complained. Only SOCOL, a non-IPC member, was prepared to take the risk. Accompanied by SOCOL's attorney, Lloyd Hamilton, Twitchell arrived back in Jidda in February 1933 and immediately sought a royal concession for prospecting in the al-Hasa region, on the shoreline opposite Bahrain.

Not since the Jackson administration's secret negotiations with the Ottomans in 1830 had Americans engaged in such intense and direct discussions with a Middle Eastern government, and the talks once again proved convoluted. No sooner had Hamilton and Twitchell opened discussions with ibn Saud's shrewd and unflappable finance minister, Abdullah Suleiman, than Suleiman began negotiating with lawyers from the IPC. A bidding war ensued in which the two sides offered increasingly stratospheric sums, which the Saudis then coyly rejected. The Americans ultimately triumphed, however, thanks to their willingness to pay in gold (the IPC offered rupees) and to provide Philby, who had served as SOCOL's consultant, with a thousand-pound annuity. Even then, the entire deal nearly collapsed when, in response to the currency crisis triggered by the Great Depression, the U.S. government banned all gold exports.

The bullion was only secured at the last moment—ironically—from a British bank. In Jidda on August 25, under Suleiman's scrutinizing gaze, Twitchell counted out 35,000 gold sovereigns—the equivalent of $15.5 million today—and offered the Saudis loans totaling many millions more.[4]

The agreement with ibn Saud represented a turning point in America's relations with Arabia and indeed with the entire Middle East. Penetrating a region formerly regarded as an exclusive British sphere, Americans had entered into a binding bilateral relationship with a respected Arab monarch and laid the groundwork for enduring economic ties. But the strategic and financial value of that treaty was still far from guaranteed. Without roads, aerial surveillance, or access to the most basic supplies, American engineers had to survey an area of 320,000 square miles of virtually uncharted desert.

The first of Twitchell's team, Schuyler Henry and Bert Miller, arrived in September 1933, both of them veterans of the Bahrain explorations the preceding year. Dozens eventually followed—not only engineers, but drillers, rig builders, mechanics, bureaucrats, and cooks. Initially living in camel-hair tents near the port of Jubail, they eventually built blockhouses and imported American luxuries such as air-conditioning, radios, and even a swimming pool. Several workers also brought over their wives. With a fusion of fascination and contempt, Philby wrote of Americans "descending from the skies on their flying carpets with strange devices for probing the bowels of the earth in search of the liquid muck for which the world clamors to keep its insatiable machines alive." Yet life in the Arabian desert, plagued by sandstorms, brackish water, corrupt local officials, and 120-degree heat, was rarely romantic for these Americans. Deep cultural clefts divided them from the native population, which took umbrage at some of their coarser habits, such as cursing. The revulsion was often mutual. The engineer Thomas Barger, formerly of North Dakota and future oil company president, recoiled from the age-old Bedouin practice of eating locusts. "They boil them, dry them in the sun, pound them in mortar and make a sort of locust mush," he reported. "I think I'll stick to oatmeal."

No challenge, however, environmental or cultural, was as daunting as that of choosing one site in the barren vastness and boring through thousands of feet of sand and bedrock in search of a Jurassic lake. From their Bahrain experience, the engineers knew to look for the mesa or hill—*jabal*, in Arabic—under which hydrocarbons sometimes collected. The most promising of these was a dome-shaped protrusion not far from Jubail, at Dammam. Starting in 1935, six wells were dug at the dome, and while some of them struck oil, none produced the hundreds of barrels a day necessary to register a profit. The executives of SOCOL, who, in their optimism, had changed their corporate name to CASOC (California Arabian Standard Oil Company, later Chevron), were growing panicky. Immense sums of money had been spent, at the height of the Depression, on a project that appeared to be stillborn. CASOC's demise and the collapse of the inchoate relations between Saudi Arabia and the Americans seemed imminent.

Yet, almost in defiance of these dangers, one last well was dug—number 7. Drilling began at the end of December 1937 and three months later, at a depth of more than one-half mile, the bit at last touched oil. A bounteous 3,690 barrels were pumped out in a single day, March 4, and similar quantities were found at comparable depths at numbers 2 and 4. By the year's end, Saudi wells were producing a phenomenal one-half million tons of oil—so much oil, in fact, that a new pipeline had to be laid to the coastal oasis of al-Khobar, where the crude could be pumped to American tankers offshore.

The honor of turning the valve at al-Khobar was reserved for ibn Saud, who arrived at the site together with his five-hundred-car, two-thousand-man retinue. Exceedingly pleased with the Americans' achievements, he indicated his readiness to negotiate for the rights to survey the rest of the peninsula. Once again CASOC found itself competing against the IPC, as well as with the Fascist governments of Germany and Japan, which needed fuel for their expanding military machines. A combination of goodwill and gold—$900,000 in grants and "rental fees"—ultimately secured another victory for the Americans. They now possessed permission to scour an additional 120,000 square miles along Arabia's southern and northern borders for a period of sixty years.[5]

Ebb and Flow

Saudi oil and Saudi contracts together infused fresh vitality into an American industry long wearied by massive unemployment and economic depression. The reaction of the U.S. government, however, remained stolid. "We should let matters stand as they now are until such a time as American interests in Saudi Arabia have made further developments," the State Department, rejecting yet another proposal for establishing diplomatic ties with the kingdom, concluded in May 1937. Americans were still investing more in mission schools and churches (roughly $4.5 million per year) than in Middle Eastern rigs. The department continued to balk at the notion of impinging in an area it still considered a British bailiwick, and of opening a consulate solely to serve the employees of a single American corporation.

Yet not even the State Department's obduracy could conceal the fact that the output of Persian Gulf wells had increased 900 percent since 1920 and that the United States now received 14 percent of its petroleum from the Middle East. Oil in economic quantities had also been discovered in Kuwait—a joint Anglo-American venture—and evidence pointed to the existence of plenteous reserves in another Persian Gulf emirate, Qatar. Oil company officials persistently reminded American policymakers of the immense economic potential of Arabia and the Gulf and stressed the many affinities, cultural as well as political, between the people of the region and those of the United States.

"Though outwardly autocratic in several respects," Karl Twitchell submitted, "the [Saudi] government . . . shows certain aspects of democracy." Twitchell was only one of the many Americans who, in the 1930s, returned from working stints in Saudi Arabia brimming with praise for its tolerant, freedom-loving, and inveterately pro-American king and his subjects. And few Americans were more admiring of these purported Saudi traits than Charles Crane. Now in the last years of his life—he died in 1939—and deeply enamored of the leader he called "the real bulwark of Christian culture," Adolf Hitler, Crane also remained a fierce advocate for close ties between the United States and Saudi Arabia, and an unstinting devotee of its king. "Ibn Saud," he assured President Roosevelt, "is the most important man who has appeared in Arabia since the time of Mohammed," thirteen hundred years earlier.

Many of these glowing assessments of ibn Saud and his kingdom were, partly or wholly, mythic. There was no democracy in Saudi Arabia and only provisional tolerance for non-Muslims. "We Muslims have the one, true faith," ibn Saud matter-of-factly informed one American diplomat. "We will use your iron, but leave our faith alone." And while generally loyal to the United States, ibn Saud displayed no reservations about negotiating with Britain and France in order to extract higher contract fees from the Americans. Indeed, when asked by American negotiators why he favored the United States over the Europeans, ibn Saud candidly replied, "You are very far away!"

And yet, in spite of its less savory realities, Arabia continued to evoke wonder among many of the Americans who worked there. These included representatives of a new amalgamated type of missionary, businessman, and diplomat. In need of executives familiar with the Middle East and conversant in its languages, oil companies were keen to employ missionaries and their descendants. Louis Dame, for example, left his mission clinic to become the company doctor for CASOC. That led to a highly symbiotic relationship between the oil industry and evangelism. "Saudi Arabia is presumably the only country in the world whose development of oil and mining resulted from purely philanthropic sentiment," wrote Twitchell, who, when not surveying, helped supply notebooks and footballs to the missionary schools. The State Department also sought to make missionaries into diplomats in the Middle East and the oil companies, in turn, recruited executives from the diplomatic corps. William Eddy, the scion of a missionary dynasty in Lebanon, served as America's ambassador to Riyadh and later as an oil company consultant.

The melding of these three factors—romance, religion, and economics—in the making of America's image of Saudi Arabia was lionized by the Pulitzer Prize–winning novelist Wallace Stegner. Commissioned by the oil industry in 1955 to write a history of the search for Arabian crude, Stegner compared the Saudi desert to the chaparrals of the Old West and wildcats like Twitchell and Barger to the early American preachers and pioneers: "If utter faith in a way of life . . . constitute[d] the essential elements in missionary fervor," he wrote, "these men were missionaries as surely as were Dr. Harrison's Christians over on Bahrain."[6]

By 1939, Saudi wells were spewing an impressive five million barrels per year and had become a tangible, indisputable American interest. That investment was suddenly jeopardized, however, in September of that year, with the outbreak of World War II. Though avowedly neutral in that conflict, the Saudi government was reported to be "appreciative" of "German ruthlessness" and sympathetic to the Axis. Nazi agents had allegedly made contact with ibn Saud and were offering him competitive sums for his oil. American petroleum companies consequently grew anxious over the fate of their Saudi operations and redoubled their pressure on the State Department to formalize relations with Riyadh. The department relented, finally, and extended the responsibilities of its ambassador in Cairo, Bert Fish, to Saudi Arabia as well. Fish visited the country only once, but the experience impressed him indelibly. "It can easily be said that American economic interests in Saudi Arabia now surpass those of any [Middle Eastern] country," he wrote.[7]

Nevertheless, neither the rumor of German blandishments to ibn Saud nor the enthusiasm of Fish's report produced a change in official American policy toward Saudi Arabia. Reeling from economic setbacks caused by the war, ibn Saud in 1941 appealed to Washington for an emergency lend-lease loan of $10 million. Oil company executives warned that, without such support, the Saudi kingdom and perhaps the entire Arab world would be thrown into chaos and ultimately into the arms of the Axis. The Roosevelt administration, however, responded that lend-lease aid was specifically designed to bolster freedom from tyranny and that "extending financial assistance to a backward, corrupt and non-democratic society like Saudi Arabia" was not in the national interest. The State Department continued to view Arabia as a British, rather than an American, responsibility, and bankrolling the king as Britain's exclusive obligation.

America's rejection of ibn Saud's request for financial assistance deeply offended the king. But monetary disagreements would not remain the principal source of Saudi-American tensions. Looming in the years ahead was the incendiary issue that would generate unprecedented friction between the White House and the king—and between the United States and Arab governments in general. "[The] Jews had been hostile to Arabs from time of Prophet Mohamed," ibn Saud lectured the State Department. "[B]ecause of the vast wealth at their disposal and their influence in Britain and the United States, [the] Jews are steadily encroaching on the Arabs." The alleged aggression took place in Palestine, a land for which the king, "as the leading Arab and Moslem," claimed an eminent responsibility.[8]

Over the course of the past twenty years, since the end of the Paris Peace Conference, relations between the Jews and Arabs in Palestine, and between both communities and the ruling British authorities, had steadily deteriorated. The corrosion occurred as a result of a spiraling pattern in which Jewish immigration to the country sparked Arab antagonism and Arab resistance drove Britain from its pledges to the Jews. America's attitude toward this roiling conflict was one of strict neutrality. But as Britain recoiled from its commitments in Palestine, the United States would find itself becoming irresistibly dragged, against its will and contrary to its stated policies, into the Arab-Jewish morass.

24

AN INSOLUBLE CONFLICT
EVOLVES

IN SPITE OF SPORADIC TENSIONS, ARABS AND JEWS IN Palestine managed to avoid major internecine clashes in the period before World War I. The Zionist community, or *Yishuv*, continued to expand, numbering 75,000 people by the war's end, many of them residing on communal (*kibbutz*) or cooperative (*moshav*) farms, or in modern history's first Jewish city, Tel Aviv. New national institutions were devised to assist in the settlement process, to develop infrastructure, and disseminate a resurgent Hebrew culture. The defeat of the Turks eliminated the last restrictions on Jewish immigration and land purchases. Large swaths of territory in Galilee and along the coast were consequently bought by Jews and rapidly settled. Diplomatically, too, the Zionist movement seemed to have achieved an irreversible momentum. The text of the Balfour Declaration, issued in 1917 and promising support for the establishment of a Jewish national home, was embedded in the League of Nations mandate through which Britain ruled Palestine. Herzl's dream of creating an independent Jewish State in *Eretz Yisrael*, the Land of Israel, appeared to be imminently coalescing.

But the half million Arabs of Palestine were scarcely included in Herzl's vision. They did not celebrate the blossoming of the *Yishuv* or the patronage the British afforded it. Though attracted to the economic benefits generated by Zionist settlement—an estimated 300,000 Arabs would eventually enter the country from neighboring Arab states—thousands of Palestinian fellaheen, or peasants, were displaced by Jewish land purchases while urban workers were marginalized by more technologically skilled Jewish laborers. With mounting anxiety Arabs watched as a Western-style, largely secular Jewish entity took root in the Islamic heartland. Inspired by the same nationalist ideas that were fueling anti-imperialist revolts in Egypt, Iraq, and Syria and influenced by revivalist Islamic views that were also gaining prominence in the region, the Arabs of Palestine began to rally against the Zionist project. Beginning in 1919, a series of national congresses convened to demand Arab independence in Palestine and to coordinate anti-Zionist action.

The awakening of an Arab nationalist consciousness in Palestine coincided with the outbreak of a new scourge of pogroms in southern Russia and Ukraine. Tens of thousands of Jews were impelled to seek refuge overseas. Previously, many of these victims would have found asylum in the United States, but stringent quotas enacted by Congress severely curtailed immigration and channeled the homeless to Palestine. The fresh influx of Jews was welcomed by the *Yishuv* but feared and resented by the Arabs. Twice, in March 1920 and again in May 1921, Arab vigilantes attacked Jewish neighborhoods and farms, killing and wounding dozens.

The intensity of the Arab reaction utterly shocked the British. The Jewish national home, they suddenly realized, could not be built without enraging the Arabs of the Middle East as well as millions of Muslims throughout the British Empire. In his White Paper report of 1922, Colonial Secretary Winston Churchill recommended reducing Jewish immigration into the country and assured the Arabs that the British had no intention of transforming Palestine into a Jewish state. To underscore their sincerity, the British named a young Palestinian notable, Hajj Muhammad Amin al-Husayni, a spry and forceful anti-Zionist who had been arrested for his role in the riots, to the specially created office of Grand Mufti.

The Jews denounced what they regarded as Britain's retreat from the Balfour Declaration and its conciliation of Arab violence. They lobbied tirelessly to remove immigration limits and secretly organized their own army, the Haganah (the Defense). Another segment of the Zionist community, the Revisionists under the obdurate leadership of Vladimir (Ze'ev) Jabotinsky objected to Britain's decision to separate Transjordan from Palestine and demanded the immediate creation of a Jewish state "on both banks of the Jordan." But in provoking the Jews, the British failed to placate the Arabs. The mufti insisted that all Jewish immigration cease immediately and that the mandate be dismantled to make way for an independent Arab state.

By the mid-1920s, the conflict in Palestine had fallen into an intractable pattern. Anti-Semitism in Europe spurred Jewish immigration into Palestine, which, in turn, triggered Arab resistance. Subsequent British attempts to mollify the Arabs succeeded only in embittering the Jews and encouraging the Arabs to press their demands for independence.

The pattern recurred in 1924, when another wave of pogroms sent 67,000 Polish Jews fleeing to Palestine. Alarmed by this deluge, the Arabs were further incensed by rumors, many of them spread by the mufti, that Jabotinsky and his Revisionist supporters were plotting to conquer Jerusalem's Haram al-Sharif (the Temple Mount), the third-holiest shrine in Islam. Arab mobs subsequently turned on Jewish communities around Jerusalem, as well as in Safed, Hebron, and Gaza. The Haganah fought back, and after a week of skirmishes, 133 Jews and 116 Arabs lay dead. The British responded to the carnage with yet another investigation and the issuance of another White Paper recommending restrictions on Jewish immigration and redoubled efforts to assuage Arab fears. The Jews protested acridly, while the mufti renewed his calls for an end to the Zionist enterprise and the elimination of the mandate. Out of this pattern evolved the century-long struggle between Zionism and the Arabs of the Middle East.[1]

The United States had neither the desire nor the intention of becoming embroiled in this conflict, but, on the contrary, was determined to remain impartial toward its parties. Though numerous Americans, Jews, and restorationist-minded Christians, still looked forward to the reestablishment of Jewish sovereignty in the Holy Land, the official policy of American administrations throughout the interwar period was one of unwavering neutrality toward Palestine. The issue, American leaders explained, fell under the purview of the League of Nations, which the United States had never joined, and of the mandatory power, Great Britain. Yet, in spite of its efforts to stay safely removed from the controversy, the United States found itself being drawn into the accelerating vortex of Arab-Jewish enmity and into the vacuum left by Britain's retreat.

Clinging to Neutrality

"To commit the Government to the support of Zionists at this particular moment would be especially unfortunate," advised the head of the Division of Near Eastern Affairs, Allen Dulles. The Princeton-educated grandson of a Presbyterian missionary, the nephew of Robert Lansing, Dulles was emblematic of the professional diplomats who, by the 1920s, had replaced American Jews as the country's intermediaries with the Middle East. Inheriting the missionaries' aversion to Zionism, they regarded the movement as pernicious and aggressive and little more than a communist front. "[The Zionists] would turn Trotsky if they do not get to Palestine," one American consul surmised. These careerists rapidly transformed the department into an exclusive club that, even by British Foreign Ministry standards, was "decidedly anti-Jewish in . . . [its] sentiments." In the absence of an Arab American counterpart to the American Zionist Federation, the State Department emerged in the post–World War I period as the most sophisticated and vocal force opposing the Jewish National Home. When two Americans, Jakov Tucker and Ze'ev Scharff, both of them Great War veterans, were killed resisting an Arab attack on the Jewish settlement of Tel Hai in March 1920, Foggy Bottom remained conspicuously mute.

This antipathy toward Zionism did not, however, translate into blanket advocacy for the Arabs. The same British report that deemed the department anti-Semitic also described it as "rather [more] anti-Zionist than pro-Arab." While many careerists internalized the missionaries' sympathy for Arab nationalism, they also acknowledged the traditional American fear of foreign entanglements. That trepi-dation had deepened since the war, prompting the administrations of Warren Harding, Calvin Coolidge, and Herbert Hoover to turn inward, shrinking from overseas commitments. Sensing this trend, the department recommended that the United States preserve its neu-trality toward Palestine. "[We] should avoid any action which would indicate official support of . . . either the Zionists, the anti-Zionists or the Arabs," said Dulles.

Isolationism also characterized Congress's stand on Palestine. In contrast to the State Department, whose nonelected officials claimed to represent American interests free of "domestic political influ-ences"—a euphemism for Jewish pressure—Congress was more sen-sitive to the Jewish vote and accordingly more solicitous of Zionism. "It is entirely . . . commendable that the Jewish people in all portions of the world should desire to have a national home . . . [in] the coun-try which was the cradle of their race," declared Senator Henry Cabot Lodge in support of a joint resolution that, in September 1922, reiterated Congress's approval of the Balfour Declaration. But the same Lodge who led the fight against the proposed American mandate in Armenia was not about to prod his nation into what he saw as another Middle Eastern trap. The Anglo-American Treaty on Palestine, ratified by Congress in 1925, provided protection for American business and philanthropic interests in the Holy Land, but otherwise ceded full authority to Great Britain.[2]

The 1929 riots, however, erupting on a far greater scale than any previous disturbance, threatened to shatter America's seclusion. Among the Jewish dead were eight Americans, mostly young reli-gious students. Descriptions of the atrocities recalled those which had recently occurred in Armenia. "[A] crowd of savage Arabs burst through the door," testified one American woman, a survivor of the massacre in Hebron, who continued:

> The first to get killed was the rabbi. After him came the young men who, unarmed and unable to protect themselves, recited the prayer for the dead. I saw some of my dearest friends killed right in front of my own eyes. Presently I was hit, too, and I fell unconscious. I was buried under a load of bodies.

Similar reports reached the State Department, along with numerous letters demanding American intervention in Palestine, and not only from American Jews. The Pro-Palestine Federation of America, composed of restorationist Christian clergy and intellectuals, united with Zionist groups in requesting assistance for Palestine's Jews. Congressman Hamilton Fish Jr., of New York, though an avid isolationist, pressed the government "to protect . . . the lives and property of American citizens endangered by fanatical and lawless mobs . . . by ordering the nearest American vessels to Palestine and by offering to land the marines." But the impact of these entreaties in favor of Jewish interests in Palestine was mitigated by the anti-Zionist voices raised by officials in the State Department and by none more stridently than Paul Knabenshue, the consul general in Jerusalem.

With a stout and humorless exterior that belied his sportier dimension—he organized baseball games every July 4 in Jerusalem—Knabenshue was uninterruptedly somber when it came to Zionism. He was archetypical of those State Department officials later known collectively—and often derisively—as Arabists, a diplomat who had spent many years in the Middle East, knew Arabic, and despised the Zionist movement. Dismissing that document as the product of "Jewish financial influence," Knabenshue further denied that the Western Wall was anything more than a late Roman ruin; he claimed that it had no connection whatsoever to the Jews. Nevertheless, through their "provocative acts," the Jews, Knabenshue claimed, had incited "ordinary law-abiding Arabs" to riot, much as they had precipitated the Russian pogroms. "The Jews are always responsible, for they generally bring their troubles upon themselves."

American Jewish leaders subsequently accused Knabenshue of anti-Semitism and insisted on his immediate recall. They also petitioned Secretary of State Henry L. Stimson to protest Britain's failure to safeguard Palestinian Jews and to adopt a more activist, pro-Zionist policy. Simpson responded by having Knabenshue transferred to Baghdad and by issuing a statement reaffirming American sympathy for Zionism, but his basic position remained unaltered.[3] Palestine, he reiterated, was the responsibility of Great Britain, not of the United States.

The dissonance between pro-Zionist Americans and State Department careerists like Knabenshue represented yet another clash between rival interpretations of faith. The former held that America's civic ideals, if not its religious heritage, mandated assistance to the Jewish national home, while the latter marshaled the same sources in opposing that project. Such tensions would later escalate in proportion to the rise of Arab-Jewish discord, but for much of the next decade, Americans would be gripped by other, internal ordeals. Four months after the 1929 disturbances, the stock market crashed and the economy was pitched into turmoil. For millions of Americans now preoccupied with securing their next meal, the future of Palestine became immaterial.

The Depression also diminished the ability of American Zionists to influence government policy toward Palestine. Jews, a high proportion of whom were investors and businessmen, were especially devastated by the crash and no longer able to engage in politics and philanthropy. They soon became targets of anti-Semites such as Henry Ford and Father Charles Coughlin, who accused "international Jewry" of engineering the Depression for its own ends and called on Christian Americans to rally against sinister Jewish influence. "Americans don't like Jews much better than do Nazis," observed *Fortune* magazine, referring to polls showing that over half of America's population held deep-seated anti-Jewish beliefs. Cowed by this prejudice, American Zionists were further hamstrung by the election of Franklin Delano Roosevelt to the presidency in 1933. Irrespective of his positions on Palestine, Roosevelt could count on the support of the traditionally liberal and Democratic American Jewish community and remained impervious to Zionist lobbying.

These three factors—American neutrality on Palestine, the State Department's opposition to Zionism, and the enfeeblement of American Jews—converged in April 1936, when violence again engulfed the Holy Land. Incensed by the arrival of 164,000 Jewish refugees from Nazi Germany, Palestinian Arabs once more demanded an end to Jewish immigration and land purchases. The mufti, now heading the multiparty Arab Higher Committee, called for a general protest strike, but passive measures soon gave way to armed raids against both British and Jewish targets. Charred and bullet-pocked vehicles—the victims of Arab ambushes—lined many of Palestine's

"Egypt Bringing Light to Asia," the original Lady Liberty intended by its creator, Frédéric Auguste Bartholdi, to grace the entrance to the Suez Canal.

"Wake, Israel, wake!" —Emma Lazarus, poet and proponent of American Zionism.

The American missionary to
Arabia in 1890 and father of
Saudi-American relations,
Samuel Marinus Zwemer.

"We were all knocked silly!" Middle East exhibits at Chicago's 1893
World's Columbian Exposition.

Angel of the Battlefield and founder of the American Red Cross, Clara Barton, who worked to save Turkey's Armenians in 1896.

Alfred Thayer Mahan, eminent naval historian and coiner of the term "Middle East."

Theodore Roosevelt, whose critique of "the mass of . . . bigoted moslems" earned him the ire of many Middle Easterners, visits Egypt in 1910.

"Our people will never forget these massacres" —Henry Morgenthau, American ambassador to the Porte during the Armenian genocide, 1914–15.

Louis Dembitz Brandeis, the first Jewish Supreme Court justice, wrote, "There is no inconsistency between loyalty to America and loyalty to Jewry."

Gibran Khalil Gibran, poet, author of *The Prophet*, and proponent of Arab nationalism.

Ameen Rihani, the voice of Arabism in America, who was determined to "bring to the West some Eastern repose."

American champion of Arabism, and arch anti-Zionist, Charles Crane.

Present at the creation. Wilson (right) and Balfour at the 1919 Paris Peace Conference and the birth of the modern Middle East.

The making of a Middle East myth, T. E. Lawrence (left) and Lowell Thomas.

"Every line of him . . . told of intelligence, energy, determination, and nerves of compelling power"— 'Abd al-'Aziz ibn Saud, the founder of Saudi Arabia and of the kingdom's complex alliance with the United States.

Golda Meir, the vice president of her junior class, in the Milwaukee State Normal School yearbook, *The Echo*, in 1917—"I was not fleeing from oppression [in America]. . . . I was leaving to participate in the setting up of independence for my own people."

GOLDIE MABOWETZ
Vice President

"Arab-Jewish relationships should have been the central point of our Zionist thinking"—the Hadassah founder, Henrietta Szold.

Judah Leib Magnes (hatted, in center), American Zionist leader and advocate of a binational Arab-Jewish state in Palestine.

The Zionist leader David Ben-Gurion in a Jewish Legion uniform shortly after his sojourn in New York. "The weight of our enterprise is in America."

The dapper State Department veteran Loy Henderson, avid Cold Warrior and opponent of the Jewish state.

The Palestine Pavilion at the New York World's Fair, 1939. Visitors were feted with "delicious Palestinian dishes," such as schnitzel, and greeted by "the most beautiful girl in Palestine," a member of the Haganah.

"A strange noise travels toward the pyramids"—American forces on duty in Egypt during World War II.

King ibn Saud and Franklin Delano Roosevelt aboard the USS *Quincy,* February 1945. "I learned more about the [Middle East] by talking with Ibn Saud for five minutes than I could have learned in the exchange of three dozen letters."

Liberty-loving Middle Nationalist or anti-American ally of communism? Mohammad Mossadegh of Iran.

Golda Meir and Henry Kissinger during shuttle diplomacy of 1974. "Oh, Mr. Secretary," she exclaimed, "I didn't know you kissed girls, too!"

The Camp David Accords: Egyptian President Anwar Sadat, President Jimmy Carter, and Israeli Prime Minister Menachem Begin (from left to right). The treaty, claimed Carter, "had now become almost like the Bible."

Middle Eastern fantasy seduces early Hollywood: Rudolph Valentino as the libertine, liberty-loving nomad and Vilma Banky as the Western naïf in the 1926 sensation *The Son of the Sheik*.

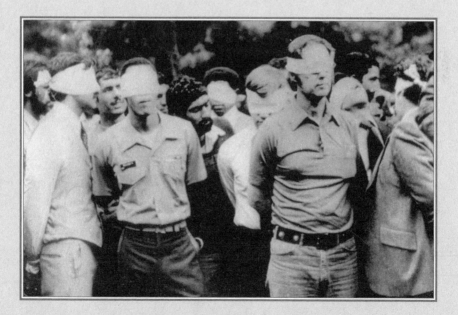

November 1979: American hostages in Teheran during their 444-day incarceration. "We will teach the CIA not to interfere with our country," the Iranians chanted. "We will teach you about God."

The bombing of the Marine headquarters in Beirut, December 1983, which claimed 241 American lives and introduced the United States to large-scale terror.

GIs in Kuwait. The Gulf War, 1991.

In search of the new world order, George H. W. Bush's Secretary of State James Baker at the Madrid peace conference in 1991.

"Shalom, salaam, peace. Go as peacemakers." From left to right, Israeli Prime Minister Yitzhak Rabin, President Bill Clinton, and PLO Chairman Yasser Arafat sign the Declaration of Principles, September 1993.

The attack on the USS *Cole*, October 2000. "We are at war," the CIA concluded, but the administration remained passive.

9/11: the day the fantasy died (photograph taken by the author's son, from Brooklyn Heights).

U.S. Marine Second Platoon Bravo
Company, First Recon Battalion,
photographed in Iraq during the
Second Gulf War. First Lieutenant
Nathaniel Fick stands second
row from the bottom.

roads, and fire-blackened fields and sabotaged pipelines littered the countryside. "Palestinian Jews who have lived for so many months in the shadow of terrorism . . . have seen members of their community stabbed in the city streets, shot in the fields or . . . killed even in their very homes," wrote George Wadsworth, the American consul in Jerusalem, an Arabist whose sympathies scarcely lay with the *Yishuv*. A total of 415 Jews were murdered.

Britain's reply to this Arab Revolt, as it came to be known, was to initiate another investigation, another report. A royal commission headed by Lord Peel recommended the establishment of an Arab state in most of Palestine, including Gaza and the West Bank, and a Jewish state in the coastal plain and Galilee. Britain would retain an enclave around Jerusalem and a corridor to Jaffa port. The commission also proposed that Jewish immigration be limited to twelve thousand per year. "It seems to me that the only thing to do will be to break the country up into two autonomous districts," wrote a precocious Harvard senior, John Fitzgerald Kennedy, in support of the plan. After traveling through Palestine and witnessing the violence firsthand, Kennedy became convinced that partition was the only way to reconcile the "arrogant attitude of the Jews" for "complete domination" of the country with Arab fears of Jewish "superiority" and conflicting British promises to both sides. "The whole situation [is] impossible."

That situation, however, only worsened as attacks against Jews in Central and Eastern Europe multiplied, climaxing in the notorious November 1938 pogrom known as Kristallnacht. Government-sponsored rampages throughout Germany, Austria, and the Sudetenland left nearly one hundred Jews dead and thousands injured. More than 1,000 synagogues and 7,500 Jewish businesses were destroyed, and 30,000 Jews were rounded up and deported to concentration camps. The United States emphatically condemned these outrages, but refrained from assisting its victims. Meeting in Evian, France, delegates from the United States and from thirty-two countries considered various options for relieving the misery of Europe's growing refugee population, but ultimately adopted none. With the doors to Palestine effectively bolted, European Jewry was doomed.

Terrified by the prospect of an entire people's destruction, many

American Jews—Zionists and non-Zionists together—cast off their Depression-era constraints and mobilized against Peel's recommendations. Letters went out to hundreds of congressmen, urging them to protest this "radical departure from, if not a complete reversal of, the policy of the Palestine Mandate" and preserve "the [Jewish] national home . . . as the primary avenue of hope" for Europe's victimized Jews. The results of the campaign at first seemed propitious. Congressman Donald O'Toole assured Stephen Wise, the Zionist leader, that, "as the descendent of Irishmen who fought for hundreds of years to establish a nation for themselves," he would "fight with whatever courage, intelligence and ability [he had] against the United States approving in any manner of this partition." Twelve senators petitioned President Roosevelt to deter Britain from unilaterally altering the mandate.

The government might well have acceded to these demands, but the Zionists were not alone in exerting pressure. The State Department showed no discomfort with the Peel report proposals and warned against showing undo sympathy for the Jews. "In America there is a growing Hitler complex . . . [but] among the Arabs there is growing a very ugly Roosevelt complex," confirmed Wallace Murray, another Near Eastern division head distinguished by his antipathy toward Zionism. European Jews, he proposed, should be diverted as far as possible from the Middle East, perhaps to Madagascar, Cameroon, or Angola. Missionary leaders also cautioned against adopting Zionist-leaning policies, as did the chairmen of oil companies. "Any disposition on the part of this Government to support Jewish claims in . . . Palestine might have serious repercussions on American oil interests in Saudi Arabia," one CASOC executive warned. "[It] might even result in their expulsion."[4]

The decision whether to intercede in this seemingly irresolvable conflict, and if so, on which side, ultimately fell not to Congress, the State Department, or big business. Rather, it remained solely with the president, who guided his nation's foreign affairs with a magisterial authority, even while wielding it from a wheelchair.

Disarming, in spite of his disability, with his patrician demeanor and ease-inducing charm, a cigarette holder cantilevered in his grin, Franklin Delano Roosevelt was also a politician of exceptional shrewdness, a statesman who understood the potential—and the limits—of power. Over the course of his public career, he wavered between a Wilsonian internationalism and a preoccupation with domestic issues, between the pursuit of American ideals and a hard-nosed realpolitik. "A chameleon on plaid," his predecessor, Herbert Hoover, called him, and on the Palestine issue, in particular, Roosevelt swayed.

American Zionists were convinced that the president firmly backed them and even senior officials believed he quietly favored a Jewish state. To Secretary of State Cordell Hull, Roosevelt expressed frustration with Britain's attempts to limit Jewish immigration into Palestine, swearing, "It is something that we cannot give approval to by the United States." Yet Roosevelt was also fearful of unleashing what he termed "a Holy Gehad" with the Arab world over Palestine and preferred that refugee Jews be settled elsewhere—in Paraguay or Ethiopia. "I would put a barbed wire around Palestine," he admitted to his treasury secretary, Henry Morgenthau Jr., an American Jew and son of the former ambassador to Turkey. "I would leave Jerusalem the way it is and have it run by the Orthodox Greek Catholic Church, the Protestants, and the Jews." Convinced that many Palestinian Arabs had even "less right there than the Jews," the president suggested that, "with a little baksheesh," hundreds of thousands of them might be induced to resettle in Iraq.

Yet Roosevelt was far too savvy a statesman to embroil his country in what appeared to be an inextricable conflict, especially when facing fiscal crises at home and a world teetering toward war. A member of the Episcopalian Church, which had never embraced restorationism, he saw little advantage in repatriating the Jews at the expense of alienating the Arabs. Though he would occasionally and in private express affinity for the idea of Jewish statehood, the president found few benefits—and manifold dangers—in endorsing it.[5]

The United States consequently responded to the Palestine crisis by once again clinging to neutrality. "Large sections of the American public have for many years taken a close interest in the development of the Jewish National Home in Palestine," Hull wrote to the British foreign secretary, Anthony Eden. He mentioned the deep concern that "influential Jewish circles in the United States" felt toward the immigration issue, but rather than stressing the need to admit more Jews into the country, Hull merely requested guarantees for the safety of the American nationals living there. Hull's conclusion, assuring Eden that he would not "of course presume to interfere in any way with the policy which Great Britain may adopt," underscored America's reserve.

The lack of a more robust American position was cause for relief among British officials. "[It] is hardly worth taking very seriously," wrote one Foreign Office official of Hull's correspondence, while also pointing out that "the Ancient Race"—the Jews—"are not especially popular in the United States" and were incapable of influencing policy. Yet satisfaction with American impartiality did not prevent the British from crushing the Arab rebellion, inflicting nearly 20,000 casualties, and banishing the mufti from Palestine to the Seychelles. But having suppressed Arab aspirations in Palestine, the British proceeded to obliterate those of the Jews. On May 17, 1939, His Majesty's government published a White Paper that virtually eliminated Jewish land purchases in Palestine, limited Jewish entries to 75,000 over a five-year period, and accorded the Arabs virtual veto power over additional immigration. The Haganah, which had aided the British military in defeating the Arabs' insurrection, was disarmed and outlawed for its attempts to smuggle refugees into Palestine. "The White Paper is a distinct victory for the Arabs," opined Consul Paul Knabenshue, approvingly, from Iraq. "The new British policy . . . makes impossible the creation of a Jewish state."

The White Paper again infuriated Zionism's supporters in the United States, but the government remained obstinately detached. Palestine was still a British problem, in Washington's perception, and European Jewry, the world's. The task of preventing Jewish refugees from reaching America's shores fell to Breckinridge Long, yet another Princeton graduate who pursued a career in the State Department and who considered Jews "the exponents of Communism and chaos." Arguing that many of the refugees were either Soviet or Nazi agents, Long managed to exclude all but small numbers of them from receiving visas. His policy raised few objections within the government—Roosevelt, Long claimed, "was 100% in accord with my ideas."[6] Afraid to assail a popular president at a time of mounting anti-Semitism in the United States and with national attention riveted on the global downslide toward war, American Jews believed themselves incapable of helping their coreligionists in either Palestine or Europe. Bereft of power, reluctant to rely solely on their faith, they turned instead to fantasy.

One of the most fashionable attractions of the New York world's fair, upstaging other Middle Eastern exhibits, was the Palestine Pavilion. Dedicated by the physicist Albert Einstein in the same month that the White Paper was published, the pavilion featured a Café Tel Aviv "specializing in delicious Palestinian dishes," a model of Solomon's Temple, and murals depicting Zionism's achievements in agriculture, science, and the arts. Visitors to the site were greeted by a young woman, a kibbutz worker and soldier in the Haganah, billed as "the most beautiful girl in Palestine." In addition to culinary and visual pleasures, though, the guests were also treated to a political message: "At this time, when our homeland is being used as a pawn in international machinations, the enlightenment which this pavilion provides on Jewish aims and aspirations in Eretz Israel is of the utmost significance."

By 1940, over three million Americans had toured the Palestine Pavilion, more than all the attendees of the "Oriental" shows at the 1893 Columbian Exposition. The mastermind behind those earlier extravaganzas, Sol Bloom, now a congressman from New York, helped obtain the permits for constructing the site. The *Yishuv*, Bloom claimed, was the reincarnation of the old American West, the embodiment of the pioneering spirit. Another visitor to the exhibit, New York's mayor, Fiorello La Guardia, was similarly reminded "of the resolute effort and sacrificial spirit the pioneer must have in order to succeed." Conspicuously absent from the pronouncements—indeed, from any of the pavilion's displays—was any reference to the Arabs or their determination to contest both Jewish claims and British pretensions to Palestine.

Neither the sensations of the Palestinian Pavilion nor the declarations of pro-Zionist politicians ultimately proved capable of jarring the United States from its fast-gripped neutrality. America was still watching passively when, four months after the White Paper's issuance, Germany invaded Poland with its Jewish population of more than three million. By denying these Jews their last possible refuge in Palestine, the British broke the pattern through which anti-Semitism in Europe led to surges in Jewish immigration and reactive Arab revolts. For the next six years, as a whirlwind enveloped the world from London to Singapore and Moscow to the South Seas, the sliver of the Middle East known as Palestine was largely forgotten. "Meanwhile the poor Holy Land," George Wadsworth cheerlessly observed in Jerusalem, "must remain a veritable hell for all those who are in it, be they Arab, Jew, or British."[7]

Profiles in Palestine

For most Americans in the interwar period, whether Zionists or State Department Arabists, Palestine remained an abstraction, a factor in domestic debates or a distant haven for refugees. But for the estimated nineteen hundred U.S. citizens residing temporarily or permanently in Palestine—more Americans, in fact, than in all other areas of the Middle East combined—the questions surrounding the country's future went far beyond politics and philanthropy. Rather, Palestine for these Americans was a matter of intense emotional and often physical commitment, of sacrifice, and of personal as well as national survival. Though insignificant in terms of their percentage in the overall population, Americans exercised a disproportionate influence on Palestine's educational, technological, and agricultural development and figured critically in the struggle for its final status.

Well over two-thirds of Palestine's Americans were Jews, most of them exceptionally motivated individuals who, like the Christian colonists of the preceding century, were willing to forfeit their New World comforts to work and settle the land. Some of them had served in the Jewish Legion and remained in Palestine at the end of World War I, while others had fled American ghettos in search of a more fulfilling and salubrious life. A surprising number of the immigrants were women, married and unmarried, who were eager to break from the bonds of tradition and seize the promise—not always redeemed—of Zionist egalitarianism. One of these women, a former seamstress and schoolteacher named Golda Mabovitz, was especially destined for prominence.

"New food, the baffling sounds of an entirely unfamiliar language," she recalled of her arrival from Kiev, as a child in 1906, in Milwaukee, Wisconsin. "I can still remember standing in the street and wondering who and where I was." Sharp-willed and precocious, effervescent behind her melancholy façade, she swiftly adapted to American life, participating in high school clubs while working to relieve the family's poverty. Like many urban Jewish communities of that time, Milwaukee's was a cauldron of competing ideological movements—Communist, Bundist, and Zionist. The last instantly appealed to Mabovitz and she became active in the mainstream Socialist Zionist wing. In 1921, after her marriage to Morris Meyerson, she left Wisconsin for Palestine.

"I owed America much," she later reminisced. "I was not fleeing from oppression and insecurity. . . . [Rather] I was leaving to participate in the setting up of independence and security for my own people." The journey, a monthlong ordeal aboard the unseaworthy and incongruously named *Pocahontas*, ended in Alexandria, Egypt. Meyerson's disenchantment with this, her first contact with the Middle East echoed that of generations of American travelers—"Crowds of beggars—men, women and children wrapped in filthy rags and covered with flies"—and she hastened to catch the train to Jaffa. Once there, however, encountering Zionist pioneers from Eastern Europe, she experienced a different kind of letdown. "They made it quite clear that we were 'soft,' spoiled immigrants from the United States . . . who would probably run away from Palestine after a few weeks." Later, in the Jezreel valley, as a member of Kibbutz Merhavia, a collection of shacks abutting swamplands, Meyerson suffered an impoverishment worse than any she had weathered in Milwaukee. "There was very little to eat, and what was available tasted dreadful." Nevertheless, working ten-hour shifts in the fields and the chicken coops generated immense contentment in this big-boned, strong-willed idealist, a sense of belonging and purpose. "I was profoundly happy."

Meyerson did not remain on the kibbutz, however. Her organiza-

434 / POWER, FAITH, AND FANTASY

tional skills and command of English soon led her to positions in the major Zionist labor union and to breakneck fundraising tours across the United States. "Look, Golda," the president of one sisterhood reproached her, "you speak very well, but . . . you talk like a man, and no one weeps." Divorcing her husband and often leaving behind their two children, Meyerson advanced to senior positions in the labor movement. Closely linked with Zionist leaders—several of whom purportedly became her lovers—she revealed herself to be a cunning politician, alternately quick-witted and coarse, and relentlessly ambitious. After the founding of the Jewish state, she Hebraicized her name and served as a competent foreign minister (1956–65) and as a more controversial prime minister (1969–74) before her death in 1978.[8] Today, a century after her landing in the United States, Golda Meir remains the Zionist figure most commonly recognized by Americans, the subject of a Hollywood movie and, more recently, a one-woman Broadway play.

Meir was not the only American Jewish woman to have left a tangible legacy in the Land of Israel. Refined, bourgeois, and well-educated, artless in politics and luckless in love—Henrietta Szold could hardly, however, have differed more thoroughly from Meir. She was born in Baltimore, the daughter of a well-established rabbi, and grew up in an environment of liberal Jewish and Quaker principles. While working as a teacher of history, botany, and European languages, she began writing a nationally syndicated column that attacked imperialism and lobbied for minority rights. Later, as head of the prestigious Jewish Publication Society, she lectured at the 1893 Chicago exposition. Her enchantment with Zionism began not like Meir's, with political activism, but like Emma Lazarus's, while providing humanitarian relief to Jewish refugees from Russia. "I eat, drink and sleep Russians," Szold wrote, but she also imbibed their unconventional ideas, especially Zionism. "I became a Zionist in 1891, five years before Herzl," Szold boasted, but twenty years would pass before she made her first visit to Palestine.

The experience proved to be as shocking as it was inspirational. Impressed by the dedication of Jewish settlers in Galilee, Szold was equally appalled by the squalid conditions in Palestine's cities, among Arabs as well as Jews, and the plight of women in particular.

"I think Zionism is a more difficult aim to fulfill than I ever did before," she admitted, but insisted, "I am more than ever convinced that if not Zionism, then nothing." She returned determined to relieve the suffering she had witnessed and, to this end, in New York on February 24, 1912, Szold convened a meeting of America's first Zionist women's group. Its maiden task was to fund the dispatch of two trained nurses to Jerusalem, but the organization grew rapidly and by World War I was furnishing Palestine with a team of forty-five medical personnel and four hundred tons of supplies. Like Clara Barton, Szold viewed modern health care as a uniquely American gift to the Middle East, and the name she initially gave her organization—the American Daughters of Zion—reflected this patriotic outlook. Szold subsequently adopted a more traditional title, though, taken from the original Hebrew name of Queen Esther, Hadassah.

Later to flourish as America's largest Zionist organization, Hadassah would engage in a variety of social and political activities, but its primary focus remained medicine and the Jerusalem hospital that bore its name. For Szold, though, Hadassah was merely a starting point. At age fifty-nine, heartbroken over her failed romance with a younger Bible scholar, she moved to Palestine permanently. She initiated efforts to absorb refugee children from Germany, meeting each boat as it docked in Haifa, and helped build the social services infrastructure of the embryonic Jewish state. Though never as politically astute as Golda Meir, Szold nonetheless matched her in doggedness and sheer physical endurance. She was, by her own admission, a "hard worker" equipped with "a strong constitution, a devotion to duty and a . . . pretty big capacity for righteous indignation." Few issues would arouse Szold's animus more than the escalating conflict within Palestine. "I have always held that Arab-Jewish relationships should have been the central point of our Zionist thinking," she averred.

In a further contrast to Meir, who, as a national leader, would gain notoriety by denying the existence of a Palestinian people, Szold believed that the country's Arabs did, in fact, constitute a separate nation with a legitimate demand for independence. She began campaigning for compulsory Arabic education in Jewish schools and, after the outbreak of the Arab Revolt, for a rapprochement between

Zionism and Arab nationalism. "Political scores are settled with bombs," she lamented. "Liberty and conscience and freedom of speech threaten to slip away from our guardianship." To avoid that tragedy, "the first lady of Palestine," as Szold was sometimes titled, proposed the creation of a binational state, one in which Jews and Arabs would have equal status and opportunity.[9] This position served to make Szold, always an outsider in *Yishuv* politics, increasingly isolated. She was not, however, alone.

No other Palestinian Jew struggled longer for binationalism and became more widely identified with it than Judah Leib Magnes. He, too, was born in the United States, in 1877, in Oakland, California, where he distinguished himself as editor of his high school journal and the starting pitcher for its baseball team. But it was to the rabbinate, rather than to literature and sports, that Magnes gravitated, and to Zionism.

With his finely etched features and resounding oratorical skills, Magnes rose swiftly to the head of the American Zionist Federation and to the pulpit of New York's premier Reform congregation of Emanu-El. Evoking the founding fathers, Magnes stressed the harmony between his faith in God and his commitment to democratic and pluralistic virtues: "I have learned from the Hebrew prophets how absolutely the religion of Israel meant for them their intervention in the political affairs of the nation." As chairman of the New York *Kehillah*, or organized Jewish community, he applied those principles to reconciling the city's disparate Jewish factions. But those same ideals inspired him to declare himself a pacifist during World War I and to distance himself from the majority of American Zionists who longed for independence in *Eretz Yisrael*. Instead, Magnes identified with the smaller, more elitist group that envisaged Palestine as a cultural and religious center for Jews, but not necessarily their state.

Leaving behind criticism of his political views, Magnes moved to Jerusalem in 1922 and became chancellor and later president of the newly dedicated Hebrew University. Though he associated with *B'rith Shalom* (Covenant of Peace), an intellectual movement that included Albert Einstein and the philosopher Martin Buber among its members, and which propounded binationalism as the solution for Palestine's strife, Magnes strove to keep himself—and the university—above politics. The riots of 1929, however, compelled him to intervene. A Jew, he wrote, "may have to live in other lands upon the support of bayonets, but . . . he should not . . . want a Jewish Home that can be maintained in the long run only against the violent opposition of the Arab and Moslem peoples." The uprising that Eastern European Zionists perceived as merely another pogrom appeared to Magnes to be an intercommunal conflict similar to those he had mediated in New York. The answer, he claimed, lay in creating an American-style Palestinian congress, with one house composed of delegates elected by party and another reserved for equal numbers of Arabs and Jews. "We can establish a Home here only if we are true to ourselves as democrats and internationalists," Magnes asserted. "[T]here is a better chance of averting . . . bloodshed if we make every possible effort . . . to work hand in hand—as teachers, helpers, friends—with this awakening Arab world."

Magnes proceeded to offer his hand, but found no one willing to take it. In secret conversations with the historian George Antonius, Iraqi premier Nuri al-Sa'id, and St. John Philby, the apostate Saudi adviser, Magnes presented his bicameral plan and discussed the possibility of creating an autonomous Jewish canton within a greater independent Arab state. Antonius and Nuri, however, insisted on preserving the Arab majority in Palestine by limiting Jewish immigration and demanded strict controls on land purchases. Philby offered to extend ibn Saud's protection to Palestinian Jews, but only in return for a £100,000 loan. None of Magnes's Arab interlocutors would espouse these ideas publicly or even acknowledge that the talks had taken place. The mufti and his protégés, meanwhile, denounced any semblance of compromise. "We all know that the land [has] no space for both of us," Jamal al-Husseini, chairman of the mufti's Palestine Arab party, declared. "We must drive them out or be driven [by] them."

Zionist leaders, for their part, saw Magnes as a self-righteous and naïve negotiator whose eagerness to concede the Jewish national home would only encourage more violence. "Just another little pogrom and we'll decamp—that's how the Arabs interpret our [Magnes's] advances," warned Weizmann. Magnes, however, complained that "the great drawback on the Arab side was the lack of moral courage" and that "the finger of scorn had been pointed at me because not even one Arab stood up." Ultimately, it was Arab fear, more than Jewish distrust, that frustrated Magnes.

In spite of these disappointments, Magnes never lost sight of his vision of "a country of two nations and three religions, all of them having equal rights," even as war descended on Palestine and the world.[10] He would persist in his campaign for binationalism, together with several noteworthy Jews, among them Henrietta Szold, who were drawn to his universalist convictions. For the bulk of Palestine Arabs and Jews, however, pitted in a desperate fight, that faith was beguiled by fantasies.

Palestine played host to other American dreamers, individuals who sought to allay the country's crisis not through mediating between its people but by scientifically cultivating its land. In the period between the two world wars, the United States supplied many of the technical experts who enabled the *Yishuv* to develop agriculturally and, in certain respects, to thrive. Unlike Meir, Magnes, and Szold, few of these specialists had any prior involvement with Zionism, nor did they regard Palestine as their home. Two of the most influential of them, in fact, were not even Jewish.

Best known as a pioneering hydrologist, chief engineer of the Hoover Dam, and creator of the Nevada lake later named for him, Elwood Mead probably never heard of Zionism growing up in Patriot, Indiana, or as a student at Iowa State and Purdue. His success in introducing modern irrigation techniques to California's Imperial Valley—an area geographically and climatically akin to Palestine—and his appointment as head of the Federal Reclamation Bureau, brought him to the attention of Zionist leaders. Twice, in 1923 and 1927, they invited Mead to Palestine in order to prove that the country could, contrary to British claims, absorb many millions of Jews.

Mead did not disappoint them. Much like George Perkins Marsh, the father of American conservationism, a century before, Mead was dismayed by the devastation of Palestine's countryside. Centuries of neglect and environmental abuse by indifferent Arab and Ottoman owners had deforested the land and drained it of vital resources, he felt. The sole remaining hope lay in the Zionist settlements, which, Mead predicted, "promise to be a replica of Southern California," and Tel Aviv, "[which] is as attractive and up-to-date as Los Angeles."

As obsessed with orderliness as he was fascinated with farming, dour in his gold-rimmed specs and distempered scowl, Mead furnished Zionist leaders with a rigorous plan for developing the Jezreel, Esdraelon, and Jordan valleys. He recommended that, rather than trying to construct numerous small settlements, the Zionists consolidate their farms into large, more efficient cooperatives, and he warned against oversubsidizing the farmers, lest they become "wards of the organization." The Zionist penchant for placing socialist ideals ahead of sound agrarian practice especially irritated Mead. "How are you going to determine what the work is worth unless you begin thinking that a day's work is worth a certain sum of money?" he asked. His concluding report, reminiscent of that filed by William Francis Lynch back in 1848, emphasized Palestine's immense agricultural potential and the progress that a modern Jewish state would stimulate throughout the Arab world. "The Zionist movement is in the hands of a group of exceptionally able and enlightened leaders," he asserted. "They can create along the shores of the Mediterranean spots that will rival Cannes and Nice."[11]

From Mead, the Zionist leadership received not only a blueprint for national development but, equally crucial in those contentious times, a powerful propaganda tool. That instrument was further honed by Dr. Walter Clay Lowdermilk, the Department of Agriculture's leading specialist on soil. A native North Carolinian and former Rhodes Scholar, Lowdermilk was an ardent Methodist who realized his life's dream when he first visited Palestine in 1938. His purpose, paradoxically, was not to apply America's expertise toward making the desert bloom but to comb the Middle East for clues on the origins of the Dust Bowl then dehydrating the American Midwest.

His first impressions of the area were essentially indistinguishable from Mead's. The Middle East, he found, that "morgue of civilizations," was the victim of "Moslem fanaticism, with its fatalistic belief that what happens is the 'Will of Allah.'" Depressed by this "general decadence," Lowdermilk was nevertheless buoyed by "the most remarkable devotion to reclamation of land that [he had] seen in any country of the New or Old World," the Jewish settlements of Palestine. Using modern methods of cultivation, soil renewal, and reforestation, the Zionist farmers had succeeded in restoring the land to what Lowdermilk believed was its biblical fertility. Still, the beefy, broad-cheeked agronomist found room for improvement. The Zionists needed a nationwide irrigation project and Lowdermilk had the perfect model.

The Tennessee Valley Authority, the agency established in 1933 to provide power and flood control to seven states, served as Lowdermilk's template for irrigating Galilee and the Jordan Valley with conduits from the Jordan River and its tributaries. Once watered, Palestine, he reckoned, could sustain a population of four million people and furnish "the lever that will lift the entire Near East from its present desolate condition to a dignified place in the free world." In his subsequent book, *Palestine: Land of Promise*, essentially a Zionist manifesto, Lowdermilk established a link not only between Jewish settlers and American frontiersmen but also between the *Yishuv* and Roosevelt's New Deal.[12]

Inspired by the Zionist enterprise and indifferent if not disdainful toward the Palestinian Arabs, Mead and Lowdermilk represented a channel between the Zionist leadership and the American government that bypassed the hostile State Department. They also helped convince Zionist leaders whose worldview was formed in the shadow of Britain's empire that the future of Palestine would not be determined in London alone but in the capital of an even more preeminent power. Chief among those leaders was David Ben-Gurion, one of Palestine's most outstanding Zionists, and the only one who was not a citizen of the United States.

He had, however, lived there. Born in Plonsk, Poland, in 1886, Ben-Gurion had devoted much of his youth to Zionist activism and, at age twenty, immigrated to Palestine. He soon rose to leadership in the labor federation, in the Jewish settlement and defense movements, cementing a reputation for foresight, resilience, and a political stature far above his bantam frame. After his evacuation from Palestine in 1915, Ben-Gurion sailed to the United States, teaching himself English en route, and arriving bedraggled, still sporting an Ottoman fez. New York's skyscrapers, when he first spotted them, seemed "absurd, resembling cages," yet the city, "bustling, industrious, materialistic," also bedazzled Ben-Gurion, electrifying him with the "pulsing modern life of the most developed and democratic of nations." Not unlike Lowdermilk and Mead, the Zionist firebrand saw similarities between the American frontiersmen of the Old West and the Middle East's Jewish pioneers. "We, who seek to build a new land amid ruins and desolation, must see how the persecuted exiles from England founded a rich and mighty country singular in its resources and creative powers," he stated.

Over the next three years, Ben-Gurion crisscrossed the United States in an effort to promote Labor Zionism and recruit for the Jewish Legion. When not on the road, he closeted himself in the New York Public Library and pored over books on democratic thought and the American political system. Drawn to these ideas, he was also attracted to American Zionist leaders, Brandeis in particular, who emphasized the movement's practical achievements and its break from the passive Jewish past. These Zionists, he maintained, could channel public opinion against America's pylonlike neutrality on Palestine, steadily dislodging it. Returning to Palestine in 1918 with his American bride, the former Paula Munweiss, Ben-Gurion also brought a new strategic orientation. Though "London has not ceased being the center of the world . . . she is not the center of *our* prospects," he asserted. "The weight of our enterprise [is] . . . in America."[13]

That direction ran counter to Jabotinsky's, grounded in Polish Jewry and, more critically, to the Anglocentric worldview of Chaim Weizmann. By 1935, however, Ben-Gurion had supplanted Weizmann as the foremost Zionist figure, emerging as the ascetic, nimbus-haired, indefatigably calculating "Old Man" who would dominate the movement's politics for decades. Four years later, with the outbreak of World War II and the issuance of Britain's White Paper, he swore to fight the Nazis as if there were no White Paper while fighting the White Paper as though there were no war. The answer to this conundrum lay in the country that, though still neutral toward Palestine as well as toward the unfolding global conflict, had nevertheless impressed him with its unbreached reservoirs of might. Ben-Gurion believed that the same United States that had given birth to the Zionism of Golda Meyerson and Henrietta Szold, of Magnes, Mead, and Lowdermilk, would midwife the Jewish state.

Decision at Biltmore

War, meanwhile, enveloped much of the world, including the Middle East. As Japanese forces rolled from triumph to humiliating triumph over Britain and its allies in Asia, Nazi Germany conquered most of Europe. The puppet Vichy regime, installed after France's fall in June 1940, controlled Morocco, Tunisia, and Algeria—a million square miles—as well as the mandates over Syria and Lebanon. Libya, too, became fascist-ruled territory, after Italy's entry into the war. The Arab world in large measure welcomed these developments. By the spring of 1941, a pro-Axis uprising, led in part by the exiled Grand Mufti Haj Amin al-Husseini, had all but overwhelmed British forces in Iraq. Rioters looted the partially American-owned facilities of the Iraq Petroleum Company and besieged the American consulate in Baghdad, where Paul Knabenshue, once a champion of Arab nationalism, contracted an infection and died. The mufti subsequently made a pact with Hitler, declaring his desire to "solve the [Jewish] problem . . . by the same method, that the question is now being settled in the Axis countries," and recruited Balkan Muslims for service with the Waffen SS. In Egypt, meanwhile, crowds cheered in support of Germany's Afrika Korps as it smashed through the Western Desert, aiming for the Suez Canal.

The threat to Jewish Palestine could not have been more acute, yet the outbreak of World War II wrought deep fissures in American Jewry—between Zionists and non-Zionists, and even among the Zionists themselves. The keenest schism separated mainstream Jewish leaders from a group of nine Palestinian Jews under the charismatic and innovative leadership of Hillel Kook, alias Peter Bergson. Members of Jabotinsky's Revisionist movement, Bergson and his team were sent to America in July 1940 to garner support for a Jewish fighting force to help in Palestine's defense. "An army with such a spirit can actually change the course of the war in Africa," Bergson claimed. "They can win it!" To this end, Bergson employed tactics that, though considered commonplace today, then appeared audacious. He took out some two hundred ads in American newspapers—"Jews Fight for the Right to Fight," declared one in the *New York Times*— built bipartisan congressional coalitions in favor of the Jewish army, and secured endorsements, by the war's end, from many Hollywood stars, including Frank Sinatra, Jerry Lewis, and Marlon Brando.

But Bergson's brazenness also intimidated American Jewish organizations. The non-Zionist heads of the American Jewish Committee resented the effort to pressure Roosevelt into abandoning his neutral position on Palestine, while the Zionist establishment under Rabbi Stephen Wise, closely allied with Labor Zionism, opposed this infringement from the Zionist right. "Mi samcha?" he assailed Bergson in Hebrew: *Who empowered you?* Members of Bergson's group subsequently found themselves under investigation by both the FBI and the Internal Revenue Service, which threatened to deport them.[14]

American Jews were quibbling still in June 1941 as German troops stormed into Soviet Russia and initiated the Final Solution. As many as 1.6 million Jews were rounded up by Nazi killing squads (*Einsatzgruppen*) and their local collaborators, forced to dig their own graves, and shot. Hundreds of thousands of others, herded into ghettos, died of hunger and disease pending their deportation to concentration camps. News of the massacres eventually reached the United States, but American Jewish leaders remained incredulous of the reports and the press relegated them to the back pages. Further rumors about the Holocaust were effectively drowned out in December by the drone of Japanese warplanes over Pearl Harbor and by Roosevelt's declaration of war. Suddenly, the struggle to rescue Jews and to secure them statehood was subordinated to America's all-encompassing effort to win.

The Zionists could nevertheless not overlook the fact that the United States was now the dominant Allied power, the determining factor in the war, and the presumed architect of its aftermath. "Right now there is no outside [assistance] other than America," Ben-Gurion explained. "The vast amount of help needed to set up an army, redeem the land, settle, and maintain our position can only come from . . . America." The need to save European Jewry while exploiting America's newfound status spurred Zionist leaders to overcome many of their differences and to decide on a revolutionary plan.

Convening in the art deco dining halls of New York's Biltmore Hotel in May 1942, Zionist representatives approved an eight-point plan that, for the first time, explicitly called for the creation of "a Jewish Commonwealth integrated in the structure of the new democratic world." Gone were the proposals for an amorphous Jewish national home in Palestine, for carving out Jewish cantons or delineating autonomous regions with an overarching Arab state. Similarly effaced was the long-standing Zionist assumption that Palestine's fate would be decided in London. Instead, the delegates agreed that the United States constituted the new Zionist "battleground" and that Washington would have the paramount say in the struggle for Jewish sovereignty. Henceforth the Zionist movement would strive for unqualified Jewish independence in Palestine, for a state with recognized borders, republican institutions, and a sovereign army, to be attained in cooperation with America.

Still, not all Zionists applauded these decisions. The pro-British Weizmann bristled at them and binationalists such as Szold and Magnes rejected them and broke off to establish their own party, *Ichud* (Unification), that advocated an Arab-Jewish federation. Opponents of the Biltmore program nevertheless represented a small portion the Zionist movement. The overwhelming majority of Zionists, Americans as well as Palestinians, voted in favor of the proposals for Jewish statehood. That plurality was no longer willing to watch passively while the Roosevelt administration ignored the genocide of European Jewry and remained neutral on Palestine. Employing tactics introduced and perfected by Peter Bergson, American Zionists would increasingly press their case in Congress and the media. A new stage in America's relationship with the Palestine issue had commenced.

Roosevelt, though, remained unresponsive, if not indifferent, to that change. American Zionists beseeched him to endorse the Biltmore program and State Department officials conversely urged him to disavow it. But the president made no statement either for or against Biltmore. "The more I think of it, the more I feel that we should say nothing about the Near East or Palestine or the Arabs at this time," he ruminated. "If we pat either group on the back, we automatically stir up trouble."[15]

While supporters and detractors of Jewish statehood grappled over the future of Palestine, Roosevelt's attention was fixed on an entirely different section of the Arab world. In November 1942, as Zionist representatives approved a final draft of the Biltmore resolutions, the largest seaborne invasion force assembled in modern times steamed toward North Africa's tawny coast. After a great many months of War and State Department skepticism, inter-Allied disputes, and White House indecision, the United States was at last entering the war in Europe, by way of the Middle East.

25

A TORCH FOR
THE MIDDLE EAST

WEIGHTED BY STEEL HELMETS AND BANDOLIERS OF AMMU-
nition, laden with lifejackets, backpacks, gas masks, entrenching
tools, and weapons, and weakened by three weeks at sea, the soldiers
could scarcely appreciate the approaching shoreline. There were
nearly 74,000 of them, the majority of them GIs, participating in the
first massive Allied landing of the war. Its destination was not
France, as the Russians and many American generals preferred, but
the Middle East. Soon, the sons of Kansas sorghum farmers and
short-order cooks from the Bronx would be fighting in the casbahs
of Casablanca, Oran, and Algiers and in the wind-scraped wadis of
Tunisia's desert.

Aware of the enormity of this contrast, the War Department in
Washington prepared a handbook designed to introduce Americans
to this "strange country." If disinclined to gaze at the picturesque
minarets and whitewashed dwellings looming larger on the coast, a
GI could flip through the pamphlet's fifty-odd pages and gain some
valuable, as well as some curious, insights about the Middle East. He
would learn, for example, that Muslims felt inherently superior to
Christians and Jews, but could lord their supremacy only over the
defenseless Middle Eastern Jews. But he would also be told that Mus-

lims, unlike his own racially segregated and hierarchical American army, "drew no color line," were kind to their servants, and "very democratic." The soldier was further informed that Arab men walking hand in hand were "not queer" and, when dancing, were "usually . . . a bit plastered." And if these insights proved insufficient, the infantryman was provided with a detailed list of do's and don'ts:

> If offered a drink by a native host, you should not refuse it or throw away any part of it. The polite thing is to accept three cups if they are offered, but under no circumstances to accept a fourth.
>
> Don't enter mosques. Don't give Moslems alcoholic drinks. . . . Don't refer to the people as heathen, they are very religious.
>
> Never stare at a Moslem woman. Never jostle her in a crowd. Never speak to her in public. Never try to remove the veil. This is most important.

The handbook represented an earnest, if offbeat, effort to ease American soldiers from their industrialized and largely middle-class society to that of the mostly premodern Middle East. But it also signaled an end to America's ambivalence toward entering the war in the region.

In the period before Pearl Harbor, American policymakers had watched querulously as Britain strove to protect its Middle Eastern interests by destroying the French fleet at Mers-el-Kebir in Algeria and occupying Vichy-controlled Syria and Lebanon. Churchill, now Britain's prime minister, warned the United States about the dangers of losing Middle Eastern oil and East–West communications through Suez, but some American leaders were skeptical. "We in the United States just simply do not understand your problem in the Middle East," Harry Hopkins, one of Roosevelt's closest aides, told Churchill. For all of its assets, he explained, the region did not merit the resources that Britain was investing in it. Better to let the Germans have the area, perilously stretching their supply lines while conveniently shortening Britain's. The president, for his part, gave priority to resupplying Britain during the dismal days of the Blitz. "We should not get bogged down in any of the side issues such as . . . sending all our mercantile marine to the Middle East," he deter-

mined. Many Americans, moreover, recoiled from associating with a
campaign whose real goal, they suspected, was not so much winning
the war as saving the British Empire. "Our reputation in the Arab
world is solidly established on confidence and good faith in our
motives," Wallace Murray observed. "This is an asset no longer possessed by the British."

Anglo-American disagreements over the Middle East were further
exacerbated by Roosevelt's insistence on maintaining formal relations with Vichy. Through his personal emissary, the wan and
middle-aged but seemingly inexhaustible Robert Murphy, the president agreed to meet North Africa's basic food and fuel needs, even
to help fund the colonial administration. In return, the Vichy authorities were expected to desist from collaborating with Germany and
to allow American spies to operate under consular protection.
According to one intercepted Nazi cable, "The vice consuls whom
Murphy directs represent a perfect picture of the mixture of races
and characteristics in that wild conglomeration called the United
States of America. . . . [T]he danger presented by their arrival in
North Africa may be considered as nil." In fact, the information
these agents furnished proved invaluable when American troops
finally charged onto North African soil.[1]

The Americans were content to keep France hors de combat in
North Africa and to monitor German activity in the area, even after
Pearl Harbor and Hitler's declaration of war against the United
States. Roosevelt continued to rebuff Churchill's requests for massive
American intervention in the Middle East, a region for which he
believed Britain bore sole responsibility. American troops would
enter the war through the western coast of France, not North Africa,
the president explained. The prime minister countered by asking,
"Why stick your head in the alligator's mouth at Brest when you can
go to the Mediterranean and rip his soft underbelly?" but with little
effect. The War Department still estimated that a Middle Eastern
campaign might serve Britain's imperial interests but only make, at
most, an "indirect contribution to the defeat of the Nazis."

That assessment changed radically, however, in June 1942, as German forces invaded the Soviet Union and drove the British army to
within sixty miles of Alexandria. Already in possession of Greece,

Yugoslavia, and Crete, the Axis was now poised to dominate the entire Mediterranean basin, blocking the supply routes to southern Russia and obstructing communications between the western and far eastern theaters. To relieve some of the pressure on the Soviets, the United States agreed to open a second front against the Germans, but its armed forces still lacked the immense transport necessary to cross the English Channel. Nor did Britain have time to wait. On July 30, Roosevelt informed his senior advisers that North Africa "was now our principal objective," to be attained "at the earliest possible date."

Operation Torch, as it was code-named, called for large-scale landings near the principal ports of Morocco and Algeria. From there, Allied forces would proceed eastward toward Tunisia, trapping the Afrika Korps between themselves and the British Eighth Army advancing from the west. This seemingly facile maneuver was vastly complicated by the Americans' lack of combat experience, by chronic disagreements between U.S. and Allied commanders, and by a terrain that was at best forbidding and, at worst, impassable. The difficulties encountered by Torch could not, however, alter the reality that the United States had now committed itself to the ground war against Germany, solidified its alliance with Great Britain, and begun to establish a lifeline to the beleaguered Soviet Union. Not since the Barbary Wars had Americans conducted such a decisive and all-consuming Middle Eastern campaign.

The connection between the Barbary Wars and the North African invasion was not lost on American observers. Some noted the participation of the USS *Philadelphia* in the Allied invasion fleet or the fact that the Eighth Army was following the trail—from Egypt to Darna—blazed by U.S. Marines in 1805. Major General George Patton, leading three divisions into Morocco, recalled how an ancestor of the current sultan had presented George Washington with America's longest-standing consular building in Tangiers. The most inspirational connection, however, was made by the War Department authors of the GI's guide to North Africa. "In the early days of the Republic, Americans fought over this same soil for their country's honor and on behalf of the principle of freedom of the seas," the handbook said. It reminded readers of Preble and Decatur and William Eaton, whose "scratch army . . . campaigned through the desert to win respect for the United States." It assured them that, though they now faced a "much mightier enemy," they were "defending the same principles." Americans had returned to the Middle East not for material gain or territorial conquest, the pamphlet decreed, but solely to ensure that "men will be free and humanity will have a chance for a decent existence."[2]

Balancing Strength and Fidelity

Militarily, at first, Torch indeed resembled America's early forays against Barbary. Murphy's negotiations with Vichy proved effective in softening French opposition to the landings, and limiting American casualties to 337 killed and 637 wounded. But just as initial successes against the pirates in 1801 misled Americans into believing that total victory would be swift, so did the ease of the North African invasion spawn a false sense of bravura. In fact, the untried American army had yet to clash with the battle-seasoned Wehrmacht. Though significantly outmanned and outgunned, still reeling from their recent defeat by the British at El Alamein in the Egyptian desert late in 1942, the Germans crushed American forces in Tunisia's Kasserine Pass, killing over six thousand of them. Rapidly, though, the GIs acquired the toughness and killer instinct necessary to pummel the Afrika Korps in successive engagements and to force its surrender in May 1943. If the Barbary Wars represented the first challenge to which Americans responded as a nation, then, as the historian Rick Atkinson wrote, "North Africa was . . . the place where the United States began to act like a great power—militarily, diplomatically, strategically, tactically."

But defeating the Germans was only the first hurdle that American forces would have to surmount in North Africa. There was, most frustratingly, the French, viscerally divided between Vichy loyalists and the Free French followers of General de Gaulle, and then the British, whose enmity toward the French often exceeded their anti-Nazism. "I was charged with . . . preventing a war against the French and getting on as rapidly as humanly possible with the war against the Axis," recounted General Mark Clark, Torch's deputy commander. "That meant I was trying to save American, British and French lives—a great many of them." Clark and his superior, General Dwight D. Eisenhower, managed to slalom around most of the Franco-American and Anglo-American obstacles. The North African landscape contained even thornier impediments for Americans, though, in their relationship with the native population.

While tens of thousands of GIs charged onto Middle Eastern shores, American planes dropped myriad leaflets over the interior. These contained an exhortation, in Arabic, to the "sons of the Mughreb," informing them that "the American Holy Warriors had arrived . . . to fight the great Jihad of freedom." Though undoubtedly shocking to twenty-first-century American readers, this use of Islamist imagery in 1942 had little impact on North Africa's twenty-five million Muslims. For them, the Second World War was merely another phase in the inter-Christian struggle over Islamic lands. The Allies had not come to free these territories but rather to restore them to French rule, while the Germans, for all their talk about liberating the Middle East, regarded its inhabitants as racially inferior. Native interest in the war was limited to watching firefights between Allied and Axis soldiers—one writer likened them to spectators at a tennis match, heads turning with each volley—and to pilfering provisions from both sides.

The Muslim perception of American policy proved accurate. While it was committed to aiding the local population materially, meeting nutritional and medical needs, the United States initially refrained from promoting the nationalist movements that had blossomed across North Africa. Such encouragement, Washington felt, would merely aggravate the French and hinder the fight against Germany. "I had constantly to reassure the French about the intentions of the United States," General Clark remembered. "I had to be careful . . . not to give native chieftains the false impression that the United States was going to help them get rid of the French."[3] But the twin tasks of assuaging the French while avoiding any insult to Muslims led the Americans to adopt some atypical, if not morally questionable, policies. The United States would preserve the pro-Vichy administration and, even more odiously, maintain the racist legislation against North Africa's Jews.

Some 350,000 Jews lived in the area, the descendants of communities that had settled in North Africa as early as a thousand years before Islam and that, since the Muslim invasion of the seventh century, had survived as a protected though periodically oppressed minority. Under European administrations, these Jews had attained equal rights only to have them revoked by the Vichy government and by the fascist forces in Libya and Tunisia. Jews were expelled from all government institutions and schools, herded into forced labor camps, and, in some cases, made to wear the Yellow Star. Many would have been exterminated had it not been for Torch, and for that reason the Jews greeted the Americans as liberators. The Muslim majority, though, failed to share that enthusiasm and violently resisted any attempt to rescind the anti-Jewish laws. Coming ashore in Algiers, the *New Yorker* correspondent A. J. Liebling reported that all signs of welcome for the GIs had been discouraged "as examples of Jewish bad taste" and that "there had been a wild competition . . . to gut the Jewish houses." The invasion also triggered pogroms in Casablanca, where, according to the *Nation*'s Kenneth Crawford, the Arabs mistook GIs driving jeeps emblazoned with American stars for "warriors fighting under the star of David" and had to be quelled by force.

The question of whether to restore the Jews to their antebellum status presented the United States with the first of the many moral dilemmas it would face as a Middle Eastern power, forcing it to prefer short-term strategic interests over its basic democratic ideals. "Arabs don't mind Christians, but they utterly despise Jews," Patton notified Eisenhower. "If we . . . favor the Jews we will precipitate trouble and possibly civil war." Murray at the State Department warned that undue consideration for the Jews would appear to confirm Nazi allegations that the Allies were aiming to impose Jewish rule over North Africa, inciting the natives to revolt. The French, too, rejected the notion of reinstating the Jews. "It would be a sad thing for the French to win the war merely to open the way for the Jews to control the professions and business world of North Africa," Morocco's resident general, Auguste Paul Noguès, rued to Roosevelt. The president agreed and ignobly suggested that large numbers of Jews be barred from the legal and medical professions to "eliminate . . . the understandable complaints which the Germans bore towards the Jews in Germany." Eisenhower, for his part, was convinced that Allied forces could not show justice to the Jews *and* win the war in the Middle East. "Many things done here that look queer are just to keep the Arabs from blazing up into revolt," the commander confided to his wife, Mamie. "We sit on a boiling kettle!" Though the United States saved North African Jews from deportation, it never restored their prewar rights.

The requisites of power had compelled the United States to abandon a faith-inspired policy it had followed since Lincoln's time, that of safeguarding North African Jews. Yet, just as the defeat of the Barbary States enabled the United States to focus on educational and medical work in the Middle East, so the retreat of Axis forces facilitated a return to a more principled American position. "[A] century of American missionary, educational and philanthropic efforts that have never been tarnished by any material motives or interests" had, according to Hull, generated "goodwill toward the United States" and a deep-seated conviction that America would guide the region to independence. Now, quietly at first, American military and civilian officials began to fulfill that expectation.

The change was especially evident in Roosevelt. When free to choose between the pro-imperialist policies of his cousin Theodore or the liberation ideals of his former boss Woodrow Wilson, the president consistently favored the latter. That preference was embodied in the Atlantic Charter which he framed, together with Churchill, in July 1941, and which protected all peoples from foreign conquest and promised them the right to self-government. Though Churchill applied these pledges solely to the occupied states of Europe, Roosevelt insisted that they held for all nations, including those of the Middle East.

Roosevelt lost no time acting on his interpretation of the Atlantic Charter. As early as January 1943, at the conference of Allied leaders at Casablanca, he invited Sultan Muhammad V to dinner. Crown Prince Hassan II also attended, as did Churchill, Noguès, and the president's son Elliott. This was the first time under French colonial rule that a Moroccan monarch had met with non-French heads of state and Noguès watched nervously as the sultan pressed Roosevelt on a number of political questions. How could Morocco retain its national wealth, he inquired, and so raise the health and educational level of its population? The American leader advised Morocco to adopt measures that prevented "French and British financiers" from "dredging [its] riches out" and intimated that America's prewar and postwar policies toward the colonial issue would "differ sharply." Churchill, already irritated by the absence of alcohol at the meal, coughed loudly and attempted to change the topic. But the sultan, slight but strong-willed, would not relent: what did the president mean by "differ sharply"? he asked. Inspecting his water glass, Roosevelt suggested that American firms might explore Morocco for oil, that Moroccan engineers could be trained in the United States, and that Congress, after the war, would provide substantial financial aid for Morocco. Muhammad V was jubilant. "A new future for my country!" he exclaimed. "Glowering, biting at his cigar," Churchill, according to Elliott, "snorted and tried not to listen."

Though concrete promises had not been made, the Moroccans were convinced that Roosevelt had guaranteed their independence. With diminishing discretion, Moroccan leaders such as the grand vizier, Si El Mokhri, and the nationalist activists Muhammad Lyazidi and Ahmed Balafrej now approached American officials and solicited their political assistance. In Algeria, too, the nationalist hero Ferhat Abbas extolled the role of the United States in securing his country's freedom and in Tunisia, crowds lined the roads to greet the advancing GIs. "Arab farmers by the hundreds . . . either saluted the soldiers or gave the V sign with their fingers," recalled the celebrated war correspondent Ernie Pyle. "In half a day's driving I got more V signs than I saw the whole time I was in England."[5] No longer indifferent to the American presence, North Africans now welcomed it as the first stage in their eventual liberation from France.

Roosevelt did little to discourage that perception, and in the period between Casablanca and the Allied conferences in Cairo and Teheran at the end of 1943, he ordered a low-profile survey of nationalist movements throughout the Middle East. Heading the study was Patrick J. Hurley, a brawny and gregarious Oklahoman fond of cowboy hats and boots, a general and former secretary of war who had risen from work in the mines to gain prominence as an attorney, diplomat, and defender of Native American rights. Lacking confidence in the State Department's ability to provide him with objective assessments of the Middle East, Roosevelt named Hurley as his personal emissary to the region. "My job," the general recalled, "was to winnow the truth from the facts." Completing a three-thousand-mile odyssey from North Africa to the Fertile Crescent and the Persian Gulf, Hurley indeed revealed much about the nationalist turmoil roiling beneath the Middle East's surface and much about the challenges America faced in balancing its military strength with fidelity to its principles.

"Our President, like the American people, acknowledges the moral leadership of Christ," Hurley told the Moroccan grand vizier, assuring him that the United States would stand with God-fearing Muslims against the threat of communist atheism. But he also informed Ben-Gurion that the United States would not cooperate in the eviction of one million Arabs—the inevitable outcome, he said, of creating a Jewish state—and that "America could not be bound . . . by Jewish interpretations of Old Testament verses." He made the same point even more emphatically to ibn Saud, promising him that his government would never support Jewish independence in Palestine and sharing his concern about "certain very rich, powerful, influential Jews who are using America's freedom of speech . . . to conduct a great propaganda drive." In a formal address to the king, bedecked for the occasion in the robes of an Arabian prince, Hurley expressed confidence that the Saudis would someday champion the establishment of a union of Arab states based "on principles similar to those embodied in the Constitution."

Hurley pursued his mission through Egypt, Lebanon, and Syria, fastidiously taking notes and submitting observations. His most assertive contributions, however, came in the largest non-Arab area he visited. Iran had traditionally been regarded with "friendly disinterest" by the United States, until August 1941, when it was occupied by Britain and the Soviet Union. Thereafter, Iran served as the "corridor" for transferring some five million tons of supplies and ammunition to the beleaguered eastern front, an effort involving thirty thousand American troops. Still, America's policy was to avoid entanglements in Iranian internal affairs. Roosevelt accordingly deflected appeals from Iranian leaders to help free them from foreign occupation. Arriving in the country in November 1943, he resided at the Soviet embassy rather than at the palace of Mohammad Reza Shah, a decision that generated much ill will locally. But Hurley experienced few difficulties with the Iranians or even with the Russians. Instead, he saw the British as the major threat to his mission and to the success of America's overall Middle East policy.

Though implacably conservative in his hatred of communism, Hurley also displayed a deep-seated liberal repugnance toward colonialism. Determining that "the economy of colonial imperialism is decadent, obsolete, and has failed as an economic system," he asked, "does the ambition, the greed, or the dire necessity of one nation ever justify the transgression of the rights of weaker nations?" Hurley could answer that question unequivocally, and enraged by the senior British officer who told him that "starvation was the easiest way to keep the Iranians subdued," he proceeded to map out a blueprint for Iranian independence. "It is the purpose of the United States to sustain Iran as a free . . . nation and to afford the Iranian people an opportunity to enjoy the rights of man as set forth in the Constitution . . . [and] the Atlantic Charter." To this end, Hurley proposed investing massively in industrial and transportation systems in Iran and sending American experts to help it erect democratic institutions. Once successful, Iran, Hurley believed, could serve as the model for America's postwar policy, promoting "free governments and free enterprise" and vanquishing "exploitation and imperialism" throughout the developing world.

Hurley's concept of "an unselfish American policy" found an eager advocate in Roosevelt. "The colonial system means war," he told his son Elliott. But the British, predictably, were less enthusiastic about the plan, and even the State Department dismissed it as "messianic globaloney."[6] Sobered by these responses, Roosevelt joined with Churchill and the Soviet leader, Joseph Stalin, in vaguely assuring Iranian independence, but otherwise abstained from adopting Hurley's program. For all of his discomfiture with imperialism in the Middle East and elsewhere, the president was a realist and the United States was still at war and still in need of its allies.

Yet, even as the United States displayed its military prowess in Western Europe and the Pacific, it continued to promote native independence in the Middle East. The Arabist and OSS officer Kermit "Kim" Roosevelt met with Egyptian nationalists and promised them a "New Deal" of liberation. "You will be the first ruler of a free Egypt in two thousand years," Roosevelt, the grandson of the president who had once praised Britain's occupation of Egypt, told King Farouk. In Tunisia, the American consul in Tunis, an aristocratic and white-haired careerist with the unlikely name of Hooker Doolittle, extended American protection over the Tunisian nationalist leader Habib Bourgiba, whom the French sought to arrest. The French persisted in their manhunt, and in March 1945 Doolittle helped Bourgiba fly to safety in Egypt and then secured him a U.S. visa to attend the opening of the United Nations in San Francisco.

The most explicit display of American support for Middle East liberation took place in Syria and Lebanon. Though the United States officially backed the Free French administration installed by Britain in 1941, the American University of Beirut remained, in the words of its president, Bayard Dodge, "the cradle of anti-French Arab nationalism." Mounting agitation for an end to the French mandate finally resonated with the Roosevelt administration, which, at the end of 1943, announced that the people of Lebanon and Syria were "prepared to make a good attempt at running their own show if given a chance." The French disagreed, however, and arrested the Lebanese leaders who had unilaterally declared their independence. Outraged, Roosevelt pressured de Gaulle to release the men immediately and later recognized Lebanon's sovereignty.[7]

In spite of the military and political pressures of wartime, the United States had bolstered independence-seeking movements throughout the Middle East, from Morocco to Iran. Americans could not devote their energy to Middle East liberation until victory in Europe was complete. In the interim, they strove to sustain the peoples of the Middle East through the most colossal development project ever implemented, and the finest equipoise of American idealism and strength.

Turning Swords into Plowshares

An area larger than that of the United States, four million square miles, stretching from Morocco to Arabia and the Sudanese desert to Iran, serving seventy million people—such was the monumental scope of the Middle East Supply Center. Britain created the center in the spring of 1941 to spare Middle Easterners from the disastrous famines of the Great War and to keep them dependent on Allied, rather than Axis, goods. The British administered the distribution, but the supplies—immeasurable tons of foodstuffs, textiles, farming equipment, and heavy machinery—were overwhelmingly American. In a presidential directive issued a few months before Pearl Harbor, Roosevelt authorized a massive increase in the provision of lend-lease materials to the region and the establishment of two bases, in Basra and Cairo, to supervise their delivery. Yet it was not until the following July that the United States sent an official representative to the center's headquarters in Egypt, arriving just in time to evacuate with British officers fleeing the German onslaught.

America's attitude toward Middle East supply, along with its policies on native nationalism, changed in the wake of Torch and the Afrika Korps' surrender. While the British continued to view the center as a framework for maintaining their regional hegemony, the United States gradually came to see it as an engine for generating Middle East development, self-sufficiency, and, ultimately, independence. Personifying this shift, and embodying America's emerging preeminence in the area, was James McCauley Landis, slated to become the center's first American director.

Typical of many Americans who served in the Middle East, Landis was the son of missionaries and a Princeton alumnus, distrustful of European imperialism and opposed to Zionist aims. In contrast to his State Department peers, though, many of whom had spent years in the region, Landis had no prior exposure to Middle Eastern politics, but rather had trained as a lawyer, a protégé, paradoxically, of Brandeis and Frankfurter. A brilliant attorney and dean of the Harvard Law School, he left law Cincinnatus-like to assume the chairmanship of the Securities and Exchange Commission and the Office of Civil Defense, and became a passionate New Dealer. Landis was a mandarin, dapper and voluptuary, full-mouthed and lofty-browed, with eyes that peered haughtily from photographs, but also a tireless worker for minority rights and social justice. "I've been called a Socialist and a Communist," he admitted, "but . . . my desire was to take this system of capitalism and make it live up to its pretensions."

Few sights upset his sense of noblesse oblige more than those of the Middle East. Assuming his post in October 1943, Landis was appalled by the scenes of squalor and disease he encountered in the capital cities of Cairo, Baghdad, and Damascus, and by evidence of widespread wastage in the supply center. "The trouble is that we do not have a policy in the Middle East," he complained. "The Middle East has been a stepchild of our foreign policy." The Arab world, he held, was ripe with "democratic aspirations," but rather than realizing them, the United States was helping imperialism to suppress them. "Are we going to stand supinely by and say, 'Fight your own fight'?" to the Arabs, Landis asked, "or are we going to help them realize their legitimate destinies?"

Answering categorically, he proceeded to overhaul the center, initiating far-reaching regional projects such as transporting Ethiopian grain to Saudi Arabia, controlling locust plagues in Egypt, and airlifting lifesaving medicines into Iran, while quietly encouraging nationalist movements. In Cairo, in particular, where Landis succeeded in befriending the plump, childlike King Farouk—the two enjoyed splashing one another with champagne—American economists managed to dissolve British monopolies and open markets to local entrepreneurs. "A diffusion of power and [the] breaking up of the unnecessary bureaucracies of the world" were essential to independence, Landis maintained.

Landis harbored great hopes for the Middle East, but he also learned of its hazards. On November 6, 1944, he politely refused the offer of a lift from Lord Moyne, the British minister in Egypt, who, shortly after entering his car, was gunned down by Revisionist Jewish extremists from Palestine. American relief operations in Iran were chronically impaired by British and Russian intrigues as well as by native graft and infighting. An American adviser to the Iranian government, the domineering and cantankerous Arthur C. Millspaugh tried to institute a comprehensive reform of the nation's monetary and tax systems, only to encounter blanket resistance from landowners, bureaucrats, and the nationalists led by a young lawyer, Muhammad Mossadegh. "The Persian government is a government of the corrupt, by the corrupt, for the corrupt," Millspaugh declared, shortly after tendering his resignation.[8]

Still, Landis and other Americans registered impressive progress, if not breakthroughs, in many areas of the Middle East. Palestine, for example, increased its imports from surrounding Arab producers by over 30 percent, while a law enforcement mission headed by Colonel H. Norman Schwarzkopf—the father of an American general who would also play a transformative role in the Middle East—modernized Iran's police force.[9] Some historians later credited the Middle East Supply Center with furnishing the model for future regional organizations, including the Arab League, which was founded in March 1945 with America's blessing.

"The time has come to turn our swords into plowshares," Landis, waxing biblical, declared toward the end of the war. Having contributed substantively to the economic development of the Middle East, policymakers in Washington turned their attention to safeguarding America's own interests in the area—above all, the colossal wartime demands for fuel. To move one hundred miles, for example, a battalion of American tanks required 17,000 gallons of oil, while the Fifth Fleet burned a colossal 3.8 billion gallons per year. The United States consequently mounted concerted efforts to purchase oil from Iran, only to be stymied by Russian, British, and nationalist opposition. That left only one proven reservoir in the region: Saudi Arabia.

Long recognized by American policymakers as one of the most influential kingdoms in the Muslim world, Saudi Arabia was also gaining renown as America's primary source of Middle Eastern oil. Though no longer threatened by the Axis, the country remained the focus of British petroleum companies seeking to monopolize its oil. Convinced now that "the oil of Saudi Arabia constitutes one of the world's greatest prizes" and that "a covert contest . . . [of] unpleasant proportions is prevailing upon the Middle East," Secretary of State Hull recommended far-reaching measures to bolster America's position in Riyadh. The task of coordinating those steps devolved onto the interior secretary, Harold Ickes, America's first energy czar.

A self-described curmudgeon and opponent of big business, Ickes nevertheless forged an intimate relationship with the American oil companies working in Arabia. Under his auspices, ARAMCO (the successor to CASOC) received permission to lay hundreds of miles of pipeline connecting Saudi refineries both to the Mediterranean and to Bahrain, and the U.S. military began building an airbase near the American oil entrepôt of Dhahran. Karl Twitchell, an architect of the U.S.-Saudi relationship, was called back into service to conduct an extensive water survey of the desert around Riyadh, and William Eddy received the appointment as America's first ambassador plenipotentiary in the city. Ickes's most tangible contribution, however, was securing approval for extending lend-lease assistance to Saudi Arabia. "Just how we could call that outfit a 'democracy' I don't know," Harry Hopkins fretted, but Ickes, together with State Department experts and the oil executives, prevailed.[10] Bound by influential business interests and powerful voices in government, cemented by millions of dollars in construction projects and financial aid, the alliance between the United States and Saudi Arabia was sealed.

Throughout the Middle East, the United States succeeded in refashioning armaments into agricultural tools and industrial infrastructure. Together with the encouragement, implicit and express, given to nationalist movements, America's boost to the economic and political development of the Middle East prepared the region to resist colonialism and to assume independence's burdens. Military might had combined with egalitarian ideals to ready native peoples to take on fresh responsibilities and cope with new realities. For a great many of the American servicemen and women on active duty in the area, however, the gulf between the idealized and the real Middle East remained yawning. Thousands of GIs had died on these dry, dust-strewn battlefields and so, too, had innumerable myths.

A Cross between the Bible and Hollywood

A cartoon published on the eve of World War II by the *New Yorker*'s Peter Arno shows a big American convertible racing through a Middle Eastern landscape of minarets and domes, past a bearded, hook-nosed Arab prostrate in prayer. Two Americans sit in the car—a woman in a stylish pillbox hat and her pith-helmeted husband, who, without braking, barks at the Arab, "Hey, Jack, which way to Mecca?" The drawing succeeds in being haughty and self-deprecating at once, employing popular and mostly mythic images of a region as props for showcasing American ignorance of its peoples and cultures. Scenes of a more genuine Middle East would soon be encountered by Americans driving not sedans but jeeps and half-tracks, their helmets now of steel. In the confusion of combat and in unfamiliar terrain, they, too, would seek the way to Mecca, and the roads to Tunis, Cairo, and Teheran as well.

Except for thrumming big-band hits like "Caravan" and "Night in Tunisia," misty romance films like *Casablanca* and Hollywood extravaganzas such as *Ali Baba and the Forty Thieves*, 1940s-era Americans had virtually no exposure to the Middle East. "You have seen moving pictures about the colorful life of the desert and the bazaars," a pamphlet prepared by the War Department cautioned GIs assigned to serve in Iraq. "[But when] you actually get there you will look in vain for things you have been led to expect. You will smell and feel a lot of things the movies didn't warn you about." Unaware of that reality, soldiers received their orders to ship out to the region with an almost childlike exuberance. The war correspondent Cecil Brown imagined being spirited to a world of "Aladdin and the Magic Carpet stuff," and Erasmus Kloman, a commander with the Office of Strategic Services (OSS), envisaged Egypt as "an extraordinary never-never land." Such reveries were indistinguishable from those of a genuine child, the ten-year-old Norman Schwarzkopf, who pictured his father traveling to a "magical, far-away place, the land of the Thousand and One Nights, where people wore long robes and carried knives in their belts and rode camels across the desert." Even so stony a personage as General Patton succumbed to romanticism at his first sight of Casablanca, "a city which combines Hollywood and the Bible."

Most of these dreamers, though, were doomed to repeat the experience of American travelers to the Middle East since the time of John Ledyard, to be brusquely awakened and cast down. Cairo, for the P-40 pilot Hal Marting was "certainly a dirty place" and the "last place [he] would ever want to live in." He complained acridly about the environment, the relentless heat, and the desert sand that gritted in his teeth day and night. "Even the beer tastes dusty." Colonel Schwarzkopf found neither magic nor legends in Iran, but only poverty, illiteracy, and wastefulness. "What are we doing over here in this filthy hell hole?" the men in Sergeant Ernest Whitehead's squad regularly asked. Their answer, Whitehead recalled, was usually to "save the asses" of British colonial troops.

Not all Americans saw their romantic preconceptions of the Middle East obliterated, however, and many even had them confirmed. General Clark was enchanted by the architecture of sultan's palace in Morocco, the colorful arches and mosaics "like illustrations from some long-forgotten dream of Aladdin." Eisenhower found Algiers to be "beautiful and picturesque," garlanded with palm and banana trees, flowerbeds and bougainvillea, "a very attractive layout." In terms of topography, the Middle East did not seem so alien to some soldiers, who found that, in fact, it looked much like the American West. "This is exactly the way it is around home," remarked Bill Phelps, a private from Twenty-nine Palms, California. "Only," he added, "we got no Ayrabs."[11]

"Arabs," in keeping with the American tradition, remained the collective GI term for all Middle Eastern peoples. The GI complaints about natives were also long established. "Scrofulous, unpicturesque, ophthalmic, lamentable," were the terms flung at them by one grumpy war correspondent, to which the Army's chief quartermaster added, "useless, worthless, illiterate, dishonest, and diseased." The local lack of hygiene proved especially unsavory for the Americans. Sergeant Whitehead was disgusted by the use of public gutters as bathrooms, while Jean Gordon Peltier, an officer with the First Infantry Division, bewailed how "the animals lived in the same room with the people." Though generally loath to fault-find, Eisenhower also lamented "that [the] Arabs . . . seem to have very little regard for personal cleanliness."

Like many American visitors to the Middle East since the time of Sarah Haight and John Lloyd Stephens, the troops were appalled by what they regarded as the mistreatment of native women. "The Arab men would come down the road, riding a jackass, and his 5 or 6 women would be carrying a load on their heads and backs," Whitehead recalled. "Our soldiers could never get used to it." Others were shocked by the sight of women walking in front of their donkey-riding husbands—a precaution, according to the Navy pilot K. Ray Marrs, against land mines. "The utter degradation of women," Patton thought, was "the outstanding cause for the arrested development of the Arab" and the principal reason that Muslims were stuck in the Middle Ages. But in addition to their alleged misogyny, the Arabs were also scorned by Americans for their lack of technical know-how, the crudeness of their agriculture, and the cruelty they showed toward their work animals. "The men spend two-thirds of the time beating . . . [them] and one third of the time guiding the plow," wrote Peltier. The deepest contempt, however, was aimed at the Arabs' penchant for thievery, for looting supply dumps and rifling American corpses. "Their long flowing wool robes could conceal a jeep if they were given enough time to work out the camouflage details," one GI complained while another griped, "If they could have carried it away, they'd have stolen the air out of tires."

The dearth of respect for the local population could sometimes lead to insults to their honor and even disregard for their lives. "I would rather be commanded by an Arab," Patton said of his British commander, General Anderson. "I think less than nothing of Arabs." In one emblematic incident that purportedly occurred at a roadblock outside of Cairo, an American military policeman stopped a black car containing a well-dressed Egyptian in a fez. The passenger identified himself as Nahas Pasha, Egypt's prime minister, but the MP refused him permission to pass, saying, "That may be so, mister, but to me, you are just another damn wog." Another GI was quoted as saying that he and his buddies had frequently shot at Arabs, that "they were open game, much as rabbits in the States during hunting season." The commander of Ensign Marrs told him that, given the choice between shooting an Arab or a donkey, "kill the Arab and spare the donkey." At the same time that the United States was earmarking millions of dollars to ensure the survival of North Africans, American bombers killed thousands of them in air attacks that missed their intended targets.

And yet American troops were not uniformly averse or indifferent to the native population. Some soldiers made an effort to understand the local culture, to communicate with these "Arabs," and occasionally even to befriend them. Memoirs from the war furnished affecting descriptions of Arab-American soldiers acting as ad hoc interpreters and of American Jewish soldiers trying—unsuccessfully—to converse with North African Jews in Yiddish. North African children, beneficiaries of the American largesse with chocolate bars and chewing gum, were especially drawn to the GIs. The soldiers, in turn, expressed admiration for the way that villagers could squat and talk politics for hours—"the morning edition of the daily news," one private called it—or could herd their goats heedlessly in the middle of shellfire. Departing from a long-standing American practice, a few troopers even developed a respect for Islam. Patton bristled at what he regarded as the Muslim mistreatment of women, but he also read the Quran and found it both inspirational and interesting. Less studiously, perhaps, Gunner Spike Milligan marveled at how "at sundown the Arabs turned towards Mecca to carry out their devotions," adding, "[That is] more than I could say for our lot, the only time *they* knelt was to pick up money."

After more than two years serving in the area, many Americans may have learned the direction of Mecca—contrary to Peter Arno's cartoon—and even to heed the do's and don'ts listed by the War Department handbook, but few seemed to have grown appreciative of the Middle East. Asked by the armed forces newspaper, *Stars and Stripes*, whether they had succeeded in mastering Arabic, Corporal Jesse Hillard of Haskell, Texas, responded that he had learned only one word, "sayeeda," which meant "hello, goodbye, and whatcha know, Joe," and the Illinois sergeant George Thompson claimed that "learning the language keeps your mind in the gutteral." Arab women also proved overly remote. Though Syrian women were "built like a brick latrine," in the estimate of Private Charles Hill, a Virginian, he never considered marrying one. "Their background, and habits, and traditions are too damn different," Hill explained. On the other hand, American soldiers seemed to think that they had contributed immensely to the Middle East, and not only in the form of food, roads, and factories, but—far more important in their eyes— with music. As *Stars and Stripes*, in a 1942 article entitled "Pharoah's Dancing Daughters Now Are Hep to Boogie-Woogie," reported:

> "Nobody ever taught the girls around here what real swing is," commented hep-cat T/Sgt William Bell of Detroit, Mich., "I knew right away then that us American soldiers had a big job on our hands." Now every night when the sun goes down and the moon comes up, a strange noise travels toward the Pyramids. . . . Because the girls of Egypt have caught on. It is no longer a novelty to hear an exotic little beauty with her hair hanging in her eyes and her feet beating in time, come up with something like, "Come on Jackson, give out with the jive."[12]

Sergeant Bell may have dreamed of dancing the jitterbug in the pyramids' shadows, but by the late winter of 1945, with the war in the Middle East long concluded and the conflict in Europe nearly won, such fantasies were growing pale. The United States was awakening to a new reality in the region, no longer an Arcadia of Aladdin-like palaces or of jiving, buxom girls, but rather an arena of great-power politics, intercommunal and religious rivalries, and intensified competition over oil. Aware of these changes—and of the influence that they exerted on America's postwar preeminence—Roosevelt returned to the Middle East.

A Scream on the Great Bitter Lake

Many burning issues were discussed at Yalta: the structure of the United Nations, the future of Germany and Eastern Europe, the question of reparations and war crimes. The Middle East, however, was not among them. Nevertheless, when the inter-Allied conference on the Crimean coast concluded on February 11, 1945, Roosevelt stunned both Churchill and Stalin by informing them of his plans to visit the region. The Middle East interested him, the president claimed, particularly the situation in Palestine, where, he now said, his sympathies were entirely with the Jews. The news evoked little interest in Stalin, but left Churchill, anxious about American designs on the British Empire, disquieted. Henry Hopkins was also taken aback, not least because Roosevelt had been diagnosed with advanced heart disease and advised not to attend Yalta, much less cruise the Mediterranean. The gaunt, high-strung Hopkins dismissed the entire idea as "horseplay," an attempt by Roosevelt "to thoroughly enjoy the colorful panoply of the sovereigns of this part of the world who thought that . . . the United States could probably cure all their troubles."

Hopkins, however, was unaware of the degree to which the Palestine conflict, having simmered throughout most of the war, was threatening to ignite America's precious new sources of oil. Beginning with Pearl Harbor and intensifying after Torch, the Roosevelt administration had labored to overlook the plight of European Jewry and the desire of its remnants to reach Palestine. In spite of his misgivings about the 1939 White Paper, the president sought to maintain a united front with Britain and the goodwill of the Arabs, in whose lands many thousands of Americans were serving. He assured Rabbi Stephen Wise and other Zionist leaders that the quickest way of saving European Jewry was to defeat Nazi Germany. "The mills of the gods grind slowly," he said, "but they grind exceedingly small."

For some American Jews, however, the milling process was proving too sluggish, while Roosevelt appeared less god-like. Overcoming opposition from the American Jewish establishment, Peter Bergson and his determined band of Palestinian Jews continued to agitate for government rescue efforts and unqualified support for Zionism, publishing more full-page newspaper ads, more congressional petitions, and a magazine bearing the logo "1776 is Palestine." Bergson also managed to stage a pro-Zionist musical, *We Will Never Die*, scripted by the Hollywood screenwriter Ben Hecht and directed by Moss Hart, with a score by Kurt Weill, which sold out

468 | P O W E R ,   F A I T H ,   A N D   F A N T A S Y

Madison Square Garden. These tactics helped mobilize an American Jewish community that, at least in its Eastern European grassroots, if not yet its German elite, had become staunchly pro-Zionist. As a result, by 1945, the Democratic and Republican parties had adopted pro-Zionist platforms, and both houses of Congress resolved that Palestine must be "opened for the free entry of Jews" and the country "reconstitute[d] . . . as a free and democratic Jewish commonwealth."

American Jewish activism also had its impact on Roosevelt. Reversing his early policy of postponing treatment of the refugee issue until after victory was achieved and maintaining neutrality on Palestine, the president created the War Refugee Board to plan for Jewish resettlement and also pledged his support for the Jewish commonwealth idea. But, once again, Zionism was not the only force acting on the White House. The State Department predicted that a presidential endorsement of the Jewish state would be ruinous for America's standing throughout the Middle East. "It would seriously prejudice our ability to afford protection to American interests, economic and commercial, cultural and philanthropic, throughout the area," warned Edward Stettinius, who replaced Cordell Hull as secretary of state in November 1944. Arab leaders confirmed these admonitions as, for the first time, they openly protested America's advocacy of Zionism. Prime Minister Sa'adallah al-Jabri of Syria described the "moral as well as material" damage the policy inflicted on America's image in his country, and King Abdullah spoke of the "economic concessions [that] might be withheld" in Transjordan. In a letter to Roosevelt, a society of prominent Arab intellectuals expressed disbelief that "Democratic America is capable of . . . discarding her friendship in the Arab world . . . for the sake of a race which is widely scattered and . . . which relies on the power of money for the realization of its designs."

Of all the American interests endangered by the Palestine dispute, none was more imperiled than oil and no Arab figure more incensed by America's Zionist drift than King ibn Saud. Early in the war, the administration had hoped the monarch would use his unequaled prestige in the Middle East to help squelch Arab remonstrations against Zionism. That expectation was dashed, however, in May

1943, by an enraged memorandum to Roosevelt. "Jews have no right to Palestine," ibn Saud insisted, and warned of harsh backlashes against American interests throughout the Middle East if, "God forbid . . . the Allies should, at the end of their struggle, crown their victory by evicting the Arabs from their home."

Roosevelt, in response, pledged that the United States would take no position on Palestine without first consulting ibn Saud and other Arab leaders, but the king was unassuaged. To save the strategically vital relationship between the United States and Saudi Arabia required nothing less than an extraordinary gesture. Roosevelt's voyage to the Middle East may have seemed like "horseplay" to Hopkins, but to the commander in chief it represented no less than a last-ditch effort to preserve America's economic and strategic status in the region.[13]

Aboard the nation's newest cruiser, the *Quincy*, Roosevelt crossed the eastern Mediterranean and entered the Suez Canal at Port Sa'id. The *Quincy* anchored in the Great Bitter Lake, where, over the next two days, Roosevelt received first Egypt's King Farouk and then Haile Selassie, the emperor of Ethiopia. Farouk, dressed in an admiral's uniform, listened politely as the president held forth on two topics of traditional American interest in Egypt—tourism and long-staple cotton. The former, the president predicted, would expand rapidly once the war ended, as would the world's textile demand. Farouk pledged to welcome all American visitors warmly and to produce more cotton, but the conversation ended without having addressed the most salient issue of all, namely, Egyptian independence. The diminutive emperor, clad in an oversized military coat and hat, fared somewhat better, obtaining Roosevelt's assurances against a restoration of Italian colonial rule in Ethiopia. Both leaders left the ship with sumptuous gifts—a twin-motored transport for Farouk and, for Haile Selassie, four reconnaissance cars.

These two meetings were merely rehearsals for the Valentine's Day summit with the Saudi king. Ashen and weak, Roosevelt awaited his guest under the *Quincy*'s forward guns, in an armchair with a large black cape draped over his shoulders. Ibn Saud, scarcely less ill, failed to make it up the gangplank of the USS *Murphy*, which had brought him from Jidda, and had to be winched onto the *Quincy* in a lifeboat. Assisting him, though, was an entourage of some sixty men, including his scimitar-wielding Nubian bodyguards, who, "lean and dark with murderous black eyes"—in one sailor's view— "looked as if they would get great enjoyment out of carving their initials on unfriendly anatomies." Total secrecy surrounded the event. This was the first time that ibn Saud had ever left his kingdom and, fearing a revolt in his absence, had departed incognito, with air raids sounding to keep the populace indoors. Roosevelt, too, worked to deflect publicity. He even managed to persuade his daughter, Anna, to leave the ship prior to the Saudi's arrival, telling her, "the Moslem will not permit women in his presence when he is talking to other men . . . [and] when he sees such a woman, he confiscates her."

Roosevelt greeted ibn Saud with a full honor guard and a panoply of snapping flags. In deference to his guest, he refrained from smoking while, in a traditional display of hospitality, the king served the president coffee. The discussion began amiably, with an animated Roosevelt describing the now long-established American vision of bringing modern technology to the Middle East, of transforming Arabia's deserts into luxuriant gardens. Ibn Saud graciously reminded Roosevelt that he was a warrior, not a farmer, and had no interest in altering his people's age-old ways of life.

The banter might have stagnated there, but for the spirited translation of William Eddy, America's ambassador in Jidda. Yet another Princeton-trained Arabist who was descended from missionaries in the Middle East, the forty-nine-year-old Eddy was also a decorated former Marine commander and OSS operations chief—an amalgam of faith and power. Though assigned simply to ascertain the "thoughts, wants, needs, and aspirations, both political and nonpolitical," of the Arabs, Eddy saw his role as strengthening the strategic ties between the United States and Saudi Arabia. Through its alliance with ibn Saud, Eddy believed, America could secure "the friendship, the good will, and the resources of the three hundred million Muslims" and safeguard the "most precious pearl" of the Middle East.

Protecting that jewel proved challenging for Eddy, though, as the topic of conversation on the *Quincy* switched from crops and electricity to Palestine. Roosevelt expressed sympathy for the Jewish survivors of Nazism and respect for the Jews who had fought against Hitler and who had struggled to make Palestine's deserts bloom. Would the Saudis agree, then, to admitting more Jews into Palestine? The king brusquely replied no. Millions of dollars from American and British capitalists had transformed the deserts, not Jewish farming, he said, and asked how such cultivation could serve the Arabs if "this prosperity will [only] be inherited by the Jews"? The king further alleged that Jewish soldiers were not fighting Germany in Europe, but rather the Arabs, and that instead of receiving Palestine, Jewish refugees should be granted the "choicest" German houses. "Make the enemy and the oppressor pay; that is how we Arabs wage war," he insisted. "Amends should be made by the criminal, not the innocent bystander." Roosevelt tried again and again to raise the refugee question, reminding ibn Saud that in Poland, alone, three million Jews had been murdered, but each time the king's response was more emphatic. If three million Jews had been killed in Poland, he countered, then there was ample room there for three million more.

While the atmosphere between Roosevelt and ibn Saud turned frigid, the air elsewhere on the ship was heating up. The king's servants had slaughtered some of the hundred sheep they had hoisted on board and were roasting them near the ammunition bins. Other members of the retinue delighted in test-firing the *Quincy*'s machine guns, raking the surrounding sea for thirty minutes before the captain determined that "serious damage could be done" and stopped them. Large sections of the deck were meanwhile covered with Persian carpets—the king's feet never alighted on steel—and a sheikh's tent erected, complete with silk cushions and gilded chairs. Never before had American military might and Middle Eastern myths so conspicuously and curiously merged. Missing only was the harem that Eddy had persuaded the king to leave behind, warning him that the ship's rolling might displace the ladies' veils.

The rapport between sailors and Saudis on the cruiser grew warmer, but then so, suddenly, did that between Roosevelt and the king. Roosevelt abruptly dropped his earlier request for cooperation on Palestine and instead promised ibn Saud never to assist the Jews at the Arabs' expense. He proffered assurances for Saudi Arabia's defense, and to do everything, "short of war," to strengthen Syrian and Lebanese independence. The president conceded that the American people were "misinformed" about the Middle East and later, at a press conference, stated that he had learned more about the region in five minutes with ibn Saud than he had through dozens of diplomatic exchanges.

The historic talk between the president and the Saudi king had ended on a positive and even amicable note, but that goodwill was nearly tainted by minor mishaps aboard ship. Invited to view the latest Hollywood comedy, two Saudi princes were shocked when its star, Lucille Ball, had her dress ripped off. No less stunned were the sailors detailed to swab sheep's blood from the deck and to clear from the forecastle the aftereffects of those Saudis who preferred the sea to naval privies. Ibn Saud was forced to flee, drenched, when his tent was struck by a wave and to seek shelter in the captain's stateroom. Ultimately, though, the occasion proved memorable for both visitors and hosts. The king presented Roosevelt with a set of Arabian robes and a diamond-studded sword, and doled out sabers, gold watches, and cash to officers and men alike. Ibn Saud returned to Jidda with a state-of-the-art wheelchair, which he pronounced "my most precious possession . . . the gift of my great friend, President Roosevelt, on whom Allah has had mercy."

Not everyone was equally delighted by this first Saudi-American summit, however. Hopkins thought that Roosevelt, perhaps because of his illness, had been "overly impressed" with ibn Saud and had too easily abandoned his proclivity for Zionism. The Zionists were, of course, devastated by the talks and incredulous of the administration's attempts to dismiss them as a "malicious misrepresentation" of its continued commitment to the Jewish commonwealth. By the same token, Arab leaders rejoiced over the meeting, their most significant achievement in Palestine since the 1939 White Paper. Legends arose regarding ibn Saud's bravura in his conversation with Roosevelt. Abdul Rahman Azzam, the Arab League secretary-general, quoted the king vowing to the president, "I will never rest until I and all my sons have been killed in the defense of Palestine," and then forcing him to "swear that you will never support the Zionists."

Many historians would later identify the Roosevelt–ibn Saud meeting as a landmark in America's ascent to Middle Eastern hegemony. Fewer would note that the leader of the world's most powerful democratic nation had in fact bowed to the dictates of an Arabian chieftain. For Roosevelt, though, the encounter seemed less a matter of strategic import than a source of exotic entertainment. "[The] Whole party," he wrote to his cousin Margaret Suckley, "was a scream!"[14]

Stridency, rather than applause, may indeed have been a more appropriate response to the talk between Roosevelt and ibn Saud. While the United States had consolidated its alliance with the Saudi kingdom, its position on Palestine, the region's most volatile issue, remained unclear and subject to opposing interpretations. That ambiguity would soon beset American leaders, pitting the Congress against the president and the president against the State Department, and ultimately dividing the White House itself. But Roosevelt would never know of those schisms. Two months after his chats aboard the *Quincy*, FDR died at his Warm Springs, Georgia, spa. Less than four weeks later, the war in Europe ended.

The legacy of America's involvement in the Middle East during the Second World War would prove to be both permanent and profound. In contrast to the previous global conflict, during which the United States proffered far-reaching benefits to the Middle East but in the end lacked the military presence and the domestic support to supply them, Americans in World War II promised positive change for the region and backed that pledge with troops and material assistance. With American encouragement, the states of North Africa embarked on the course that eventually led them to independence, and Syria and Lebanon freed themselves from French rule. The United States had also helped prepare Iran for eventual sovereignty and bolstered the nationalist movement in Egypt. Back in 1886, a statue originally designed for the Middle East had raised a beacon for millions of liberty-seeking immigrants to the United States, but Operation Torch, launched nearly sixty years later, had illuminated paths to freedom for many Middle Eastern peoples.

Less propitiously, however, Arabia and Palestine had become fused in America's strategic involvement in the Middle East. Every president after Roosevelt would have to grapple with that twinning

26

THE MIDDLE EAST AND THE MAN FROM MISSOURI

INELEGANT WITH A TWANGY DRAWL, LACKING A COLLEGE eduation, Harry S. Truman at first regarded the presidency as an insurmountable obstacle. "I felt like the moon, the stars, and all the planets had fallen on me," he told reporters. Inheriting the position from the almost universally admired, four times–elected Roosevelt, he entered office with little public support and confidence and with the reputation as a lackluster senator whose presence in the White House owed more to internal political machinations than to his leadership qualities or to expressions of popular will. Some of the fiercest criticism of Truman focused on his almost total inexperience in foreign affairs and on the fact that Roosevelt had never invited him into the White House Map Room, much less consulted him on world-impacting decisions. Describing Truman's succession as a "great, great tragedy," the Tennessee Valley Authority chief David Lilienthal conveyed the anguish it inflicted on many Americans, particularly those closest to the centers of power. "The country and the world don't deserve to be left this way," mourned Lilienthal. "God help us all."

The unspectacular appearance of this former farmer, bank clerk, and Kansas City haberdasher would, in fact, prove wildly deceiving.

His domestic accomplishments included groundbreaking efforts to relieve poverty, revamp the Social Security system, and integrate America's armed forces. But it was in the foreign policy field, the one in which he was least expected to succeed, that Truman truly excelled. In addition to overseeing the final defeat of Germany and Japan, he presided over the advent of the United Nations and the North Atlantic Treaty Organization, confronted communism in Berlin and South Korea, reconstructed war-shattered Europe, and, more controversially, introduced atomic weaponry to the world. He also altered the Middle East as no other American before him.

Truman's policymaking in the Middle East reflected the same blend of impetuosity and political shrewdness that he applied to other overseas issues. The lessons in resilience he had learned as an artillery officer on the front lines of World War I and the back corridors of the Democratic Party would influence his attitudes toward the region, as would his extensive reading on the historical roles of great men and women. More vividly, however, Truman's thinking on the Middle East was colored by his Baptist upbringing. Thoroughly versed in Scripture and its depictions of sacred landscapes, Truman, much like American presidents of an earlier time, possessed a detailed knowledge of Middle Eastern geography. "It wasn't just the Biblical part of Palestine that interested me," he recalled. "The whole history of that area of the world is just about the most complicated and most interesting of any anywhere." That fascination was on display in the Oval Office, where the president stunned General Eisenhower and Undersecretary of State Dean Acheson, both of whom thought him ignorant of the subject, by lecturing them on the strategic importance of the Middle East while referring to his personal, dog-eared map.

Belief, for Truman, meant not only confidence in God but also a commitment to the civic principles he perceived as God-given. Democracy, he maintained, was "a matter of faith—a faith in the soul of man, faith in human rights," and the United States was the product of divine providence. "God has created us and brought us to our present position of power . . . for some great purpose," he asserted. "It is given to us to defend the spiritual values . . . against the vast forces of evil that seek to destroy them." Fulfilling that task took precedence over all other considerations, Truman often stressed, whether it was courting votes or conciliating allies, or even safeguarding America's oil supply.[1]

An everyman in the manner of Mark Twain, imbued with the realism of Jefferson, Jackson, and Teddy Roosevelt, and Wilson-like in his ideals, Truman evinced many of the attitudes with which Americans had traditionally engaged the Middle East. Those approaches would be severely tested in the first years of Truman's presidency, as the man from Missouri grappled with consecutive Middle Eastern crises.

Rising Star in the East

The Middle East in April 1945 was a region of almost unremitting turmoil. French and British troops occupied Syria and forces from the United States, Britain, and France controlled North Africa. Palestine, Transjordan, and Iraq remained under exclusive British command, and Iran was divided between the British and the Soviets. It was a time of radical flux, of the waning of the French and British empires and their replacement by American and Soviet influence, and of rapidly shifting alliances. The Anglo-American-French-Soviet front that had successfully blocked German advances in the region was irreparably collapsing. The United States would confront Britain in some areas of the Middle East, in others ally with the British against the French, and in others still join with Britain and France in order to oppose the Russians. Truman was expected to manage this fluid situation, to respond to nationalist demands for freedom from European domination while maintaining a Western coalition against the mounting Soviet threat. Truman agreed with Loy Henderson, the new head of the State Department's Division of Near Eastern Affairs (NEA), that the peoples of the Middle East were "the most deserving . . . of the colonial world for post-war political independence." But the president also heeded the department's warning that the USSR was "determined to . . . sweep unimpeded across Turkey and . . . Iran and through the Persian Gulf into the Indian Ocean."

The first test of Truman's diplomatic dexterity began in Syria in early June 1945, a mere three weeks after V-E Day. Backing down on its pledges to respect Syrian independence, the French government refused to remove its garrisons from the country and, when protests broke out in Damascus, al-Hamma, and Aleppo, the French responded with artillery fire and warplanes. Ancient neighborhoods were leveled and their inhabitants strafed with machine-gun fire, leaving more than four hundred dead. "Your country has encouraged us in our stand to refuse special privileges to France or any other country," the Syrians remonstrated to Washington, "but . . . now the French are bombing us . . . with Lend-Leased munitions which were given for use against our common enemies." The protest struck home. State Department officials expressed remorse over America's failure to ensure Syria the freedoms promised by the Atlantic and UN charters, and consternation over the danger that Damascus would turn to Moscow for help. Henderson estimated, "Our refusal to meet the present Syrian request would be comparable, in its disillusioning . . . effect throughout the Near East, only to the retirement of the United States into isolationism after the First World War."

Truman, however, did not need to be prodded. He regarded Syria, which had declared war against the Axis in February 1945, as an American ally as well as a strategic asset, with vital oil pipelines spanning its interior. Joining with Churchill, the president sent a brutally worded cable to de Gaulle, warning of imminent intervention by British troops in the area on behalf of the embattled Syrians. "In order to avoid collision between British and French Forces, we request you immediately order the French troops to withdraw to their barracks and to cease fire thereafter except in self-defense."[2] Once again, de Gaulle relented and, under further pressure from the United States acting through the UN Security Council, he agreed to remove the last French soldier from Syria.

Truman had scarcely extinguished the flare-up in Syria when a larger conflagration confronted him in Libya. Liberated from its Italian Fascist colonizers, Libya was still occupied by British and French forces in July 1945, when Allied leaders met in Potsdam, Germany. Libyan nationalists, rallying behind their repatriated king, Idris, agitated for sovereignty, but the powers demurred. The country, they agreed, composed of three distinct districts—Tripolitania, Cyrenaica, and Fezzan—lacked the internal cohesion necessary for independence as well as the requisite natural resources. Indeed, Libya's largest source of income was selling the wrecks of World War II battle vehicles for scrap. The choice before the Allies was between restoring Libya to Italian rule or placing it under international supervision.

Truman, with his inbred distaste for imperialism, balked at returning Libya to Italy and would have preferred some form of international trusteeship. But then Stalin surprised him by demanding a Soviet mandate over Tripolitania. The arrangement would have furnished the Red Navy with its first warm water ports and denied the United States access to its strategically crucial Wheelus airbase, near Tripoli. The French also pressed for a section of Libya, as did the nationalists in Egypt—neither of them propitious options, in Truman's view. Clamped between his sympathy for North Africa liberation and his fears for the security of the Middle East, Truman chose a prudent but revolutionary road. Libya would be placed under the care of the newly created UN. The experiment succeeded and in December 1951—150 years after Tripoli declared war on the United States—America recognized Libya's independence.[3]

No sooner was the clash with Russia over Libya averted than a new and potentially more destructive collision loomed between the Soviets and the West in Iran. The United States and Britain in December 1945 began pulling their forces out of Iran, fulfilling their pledges to respect the country's sovereignty after the war. The Soviets, however, dallied. Through the pro-Communist Tudeh Party, they reinforced their influence in the Iranian government and promoted the secession of Soviet satellite republics in neighboring Kurdistan and Azerbaijan. Stalin was now poised to sever America's access to Iranian oil reserves and to threaten the petroleum fields of Saudi Arabia, Bahrain, and Kuwait. Reporting from Tabriz, the Associated Press correspondent Joseph C. Goodwin claimed he could scarcely hear his own shortwave radio for the thunder of passing Soviet tanks. Coinciding with the Soviet takeover of the Baltic states and Eastern Europe, the Iranian crisis appeared to constitute another front in the rapidly unfolding Cold War between the West and the Communist bloc. State Department experts, following the lead of the analyst George Kennan, advised the administration to meet the Soviet menace in Iran, as elsewhere, with a combination of assertive diplomacy and military muscle, known collectively as "containment."

Truman, agreeing, railed, "We ought to protest with all the vigor of which we are capable against the Russian program in Iran." He recalled Iran's pivotal contribution to the war effort and vowed with "an iron fist and strong language" to oust the Soviets from the Persian Gulf. Throughout the early months of 1946, American representatives pressed hard to secure UN censure of the Soviets' intransigence. The Kremlin, though, only dug in its heels, and soon Soviet troops were reportedly moving out of northeastern Iran in the directions of Teheran and the Iraqi border. "Now we'll give it to them with both barrels," swore James Byrnes, a secretary of state not otherwise renowned for truculence, slamming his first into his palm. Byrnes proposed dispatching an American fleet to the area, but just then, in April, the Soviets blinked. Wary of a condemnation in the Security Council and confident of obtaining exclusive oil concessions in Iraq, Stalin ordered his forces withdrawn. Without their support, the Kurdish and Azerbaijani republics swiftly collapsed. The Iranian assembly, or Majlis, subsequently voted to deny granting oil rights to Russia.[4]

Some of the first shots of the Cold War had been fired—metaphorically—in the Middle East, and in the Middle East Truman had for the first time tested the UN's crisis-management mechanism. The result was a clear-cut American victory. Unwilling to rest on that accomplishment, however, Truman dispatched the recently christened Naval Forces Mediterranean—later to be renamed the Sixth Fleet—to patrol the Eastern Mediterranean. Not since the days of Stephen Decatur in the early nineteenth century had the United States so massively and permanently projected its power into the Middle East.

But Soviet pressure on the so-called Northern Tier countries of Iran, Iraq, and Turkey did not abate and the UN proved incapable of relieving it. Soviet troops had scarcely completed their evacuation of Iran in August 1946 when they began massing along Turkey's border. Stalin, anxious to gain the naval access to the Mediterranean denied him in Libya, presented Turkish leaders with a demand for joint custody of the Dardanelles Strait. At the same time, communist-backed rebels in Greece threatened to topple the country's hard-line, but pro-Western, government. Though Britain bore responsibility for the defense of the Greco-Turkish front, its war-depleted economy could no longer finance that burden. There was only the United States.

"Greece and Turkey form the sole obstacle to Soviet domination of the Eastern Mediterranean which is an economic and strategic area of vital importance," a report filed by the NEA reminded the president. The State and War Departments agreed that the fall of the two countries would precipitate the communist conquest of the entire Middle East, together with its vast oil resources, and ultimately the collapse of Western Europe. But the danger was not only military. "There is, at the present point in world history, a conflict between two ways of life," an interdepartmental analysis explained, "between dictatorship and freedom; between servitude of the majority to a minority and freedom to seek progress." If Greece and Turkey surrendered, the Soviets could gain a global empire and isolate the United States.

In the last crisis involving Greece and Turkey, over a century earlier, President James Monroe had to choose between aiding Greece's rebellion against the Turks and seeking a lucrative treaty with Turkey—between fidelity to America's ideals and a commitment to its economic interests. For Truman, though, the question was not which side to support, the Greeks or the Turks, or whether to give precedence to ideology or finances, but rather whether the United States should assume the onus of Middle East defense. Truman was determined to show the Soviets "straight from the shoulder," as he phrased it, "where America stood," but to accomplish this he first had to convince the American people that the Middle East was worth defending. The task, arising in the wake of wartime sacrifices, shortages, and loss, was formidable. No less than Monroe before him, Truman needed a doctrine.

Addressing a joint session of Congress on March 12, 1947, Truman appealed for emergency aid for "democratic" Greece and "freedom-loving" Turkey. The integrity of the two countries, he said, was "essential to the preservation of order in the Middle East" and for the security of the West as a whole. To ensure the peoples of the

Middle East a "life free from coercion" and to bolster the United Nations, Truman requested congressional approval for far-reaching military and civilian assistance for Greece and Turkey, including training of their armed forces. "If we falter in our leadership, we may endanger the peace of the world," Truman warned, "and we shall surely endanger the welfare of our own nation."

By appealing to America's moral obligations as well as its strategic interests, Truman won over an initially skeptical public and Congress. Military assistance to Greece and Turkey subsequently surged, and the USS *Missouri*—the battleship named for Truman's home state and which had accepted Japan's surrender—sped toward the Aegean coast. "Our foreign policy is the same as it always has been from the day that the discerning Monroe first enunciated the principle of the Monroe Doctrine," the freshman congressman from Massachusetts, John F. Kennedy, said in praise of Truman's decision. "It merely means that time and space have brought a new interpretation to that historical document."

Two years had passed since Harry Truman proclaimed that the planets had fallen on him, a period of relentless upheaval, especially in the Middle East. The American people, which for generations had expressed ambivalence toward European colonialism in the region, now found itself saddled with many of the same imperial duties once borne by Britain and France and with the task of frustrating Russian designs. Some American officials had questioned the ability of the United States to shield this vast region from internal chaos and hostile incursions. They wondered whether the "star rising in the East," in Murray Wallace's words, would be Soviet or American.[5] Truman, however, assured that, for the near future at least, not only the stars but also the stripes of the United States would prevail in the Middle East. In contrast to the imperialist powers of the past, the United States had worked not to deny but rather to secure the independence of several Middle Eastern states and to immunize others against aggression.

Truman had thus far managed to harmonize America's strategic and ethical interests in his handling of the Middle East, to preserve the Western Alliance while uprooting French colonialism and blocking Soviet inroads. But maintaining that balance would prove nearly impossible in the wake of the region's next major crisis. Truman had deftly weathered upheavals in North Africa, Persia, and the Levant, but these were mere tremors compared with Palestine, the most volcanic controversy yet to shatter the Middle East.

The Sixty-Four-Dollar Question

For most Americans after the war, a far more harrowing image than that of Middle Eastern peoples straining under colonial rule or of Soviet troops descending toward the Bosphorus was the sight of tens of thousands of Jews languishing in displaced persons (DP) camps throughout liberated Europe. These survivors of the Holocaust's horrors had little desire to return to their former homes—for most, those homes no longer existed—and overwhelmingly preferred to leave Europe entirely. The refugees' plight increasingly seized public opinion in the United States and nightly haunted the president. "The American government could not stand idly by while the victims of Hitler's madness were not allowed to build new lives," he told himself. "The Jews needed some place where they could go."

But where? The most obvious destination, given the reluctance of almost all non-European states to absorb the refugees, was Palestine. The 1939 White Paper, however, remained in force, and no British leader, not even the avowedly pro-Zionist Churchill, was willing to risk inciting millions of Muslims by rescinding it. Instead, British gunboats intercepted Haganah ships crammed with Holocaust survivors trying to reach Palestine, sending them back to Germany or imprisoning them in exposed, makeshift jails on the island of Cyprus. "I cannot bear to think of the Jews of Europe who have spent so many years in concentration camps behind wire," wept Eleanor Roosevelt, the president's widow, but the State Department did not share her distress. Rather, Henderson and other specialists at the NEA agreed with Britain that by deluging Palestine with Jews, the West would sow instability throughout the Middle East, leading to the rise of Russian influence in the region and the loss of irreplaceable oil supplies.

The scenes of refugee suffering and the scenarios of Muslim rage presented Truman with the well-known American dilemma in the

Middle East between preserving interests and safeguarding ideals. Further complicating that decision, however, was Truman's own ambivalence toward Jews and Zionism. Much like Wilson and Roosevelt before him, he counted Jews among his closest associates, especially his old army friend and former haberdashery partner, Eddie Jacobson. As the descendant of farmers displaced by the Civil War and a target of southern racists who hated his liberal views, Truman could empathize with the uprooted victims of Nazism. "Everyone else who's been dragged from his country has someplace to go back to, but the Jews have no place to go," he said. His Bible reading had led him to accept the notion of Jewish restoration in the Holy Land and to join, in 1941, the Zionist-minded American Christian Palestine Committee. And yet, no less than his Democratic predecessors, Truman occasionally gave vent to anti-Semitic sentiments—the Jacobsons were never once invited to dine at the White House—and to fears of the mass immigration of Jews. He worried whether the future Jewish state would be a theocracy and whether American troops would be called upon to defend it. Conspicuously, when seventy-seven senators voted in favor of the Jewish commonwealth in 1944, Truman was not among them. "My sympathy is with the Jewish people," he explained, "[but] I don't want to throw any bricks to upset the applecart."

Truman, therefore, preferred "to make the whole world safe for Jews" and not necessarily resettle them in Palestine. But the thirty-third president always considered himself a politician first and a statesman only second. He could scarcely overlook congressional calls for Jewish statehood and the pro-Zionist telegrams that overwhelmed the White House at the end of the war with Japan. Arab leaders also went public with their views, opening an information office in Washington, and ibn Saud published the promises made to him by Roosevelt, but such measures had little effect on Truman. "I have to answer to hundreds of thousands who are anxious for the success of Zionism," he reasoned. "I do not have hundreds of thousands of Arabs in my constituents." In an effort to satisfy that demand, Truman asked Earl G. Harrison, dean of the University of Pennsylvania Law School, to investigate the refugee situation. A former immigration official with no previous ties to Zionism, Harrison was expected to file a terse, dispassionate report.

Harrison was unprepared, however, for the nightmarish scenes that greeted him on his arrival in Europe in July 1945. "We appear to be treating the Jews as the Nazis treated them," he wrote, "except that we do not exterminate them." Hefty and rugged, Harrison was nonetheless unnerved by the sight of destitute, physically and mentally devastated Jews still gazing through barbed wire, guarded by American troops. "One is led to wonder whether the German people, seeing this, are not supposing that we are . . . condoning Nazi policy." Such observations discomfited Truman, though not as deeply as Harrison's conclusions. The refugees did not want to be repatriated, Harrison confirmed, or, in most cases, to be admitted to the United States. They demanded, rather, the right to immigrate to Palestine. Driven in large part by "love for the country and devotion to the Zionist ideal," these Jews felt that only in Palestine would they "be welcomed and find peace and quiet and be given an opportunity to live and work."[6]

Harrison urged that Britain be asked to open Palestine to 100,000 Jews, about half the number that, with the aid of Zionist organizations, had reached the American zone of occupation. Clement Attlee, however, the urbane Labourite who replaced Churchill as prime minister in 1945, showed no inclination of altering British policy. The Jews should be treated as any other DP group, he coolly told Truman, and warned him that, by demanding their admission to Palestine, the United States would ignite a worldwide Muslim uprising, strengthen communism, and cause "grievous harm to relations between our two countries." Attlee's foreign minister, Ernest Bevin, a beefy former dockworker and union organizer, was less refined. He chided the Jews for pushing "to the head of the queue" for international assistance and the Americans for preferring to resettle Jews in Palestine "because they did not want too many of them in New York."

These responses served only to harden rather than mollify Truman's resolve. The American people, he told Attlee at the end of August, "firmly believe that immigration into Palestine should not be closed" and that "such action must not be delayed." Public criticism of Britain also stiffened, and visiting New York, Bevin found that the local stevedores refused to unload his luggage and that the crowd at Yankee Stadium rose to boo him. Anxious to deflect this obloquy, Attlee proposed creating an Anglo-American Committee of Inquiry to investigate the refugee issue and its possible implications for Palestine. Truman suspected that the commission would merely rubber-stamp the existing British policy, but lacking any alternative plan, he reluctantly endorsed it.[7]

The committee, made up of six American and six British delegates, began its work in January 1946, traveling widely through Europe and the Middle East and hearing testimony from a wide range of witnesses—relief workers and military officials, politicians and academics, Arabs and Jews. Judah Magnes, representing his *Ichud* movement, made his case for binationalism, while Ben-Gurion, Golda Meyerson, and Walter Lowdermilk argued fervidly for Jewish statehood. The Zionists assured the committee that 96.8 percent of the refugees preferred resettlement in Palestine, but Jamal al-Husseini insisted that the Arabs would resist Jewish immigration and fight to turn Palestine into an Arab state. "The position of Great Britain as Mandatory is not a happy one," the committee concluded, noting the rise in attacks by Jewish militias—not only the Revisionist groups but now also the Haganah—against British targets. Nevertheless, the delegates determined that "Palestine shall be neither an Arab nor a Jewish State" and recommended placing the country under a permanent UN trusteeship. To relieve the refugees' plight, meanwhile, the committee proposed admitting 100,000 Jews at once into Palestine and lifting the White Paper's limitations on Jewish land purchases.

The report, published in April, succeeded in infuriating all three of Palestine's antagonists. The Zionists accused the committee of sacrificing their political aspirations to philanthropy, and the Arabs assailed it for giving in on Jewish immigration and land purchases. The British, though satisfied with the provision for perpetuating the mandate, balked at the now sacrosanct figure of 100,000. Only Truman seemed pleased. He welcomed the abrogation of the White Paper and instructed the Pentagon to prepare an operation for transporting the refugees to Palestine. Also, to help assuage British fears, he appointed a career diplomat, Henry F. Grady, to meet with Herbert Morrison, the British official in charge of Palestinian affairs, to further explore the committee's recommendations.

The Morrison-Grady Plan was released on July 31, 1946, and instantly caused an uproar. Beyond providing for the entry of 100,000 Jews into Palestine, it envisaged the country's division into three autonomous provinces—a British district, including Jerusalem, accounting for almost half of the territory, a smaller Arab enclave, and a Jewish canton including less than 20 percent of the country. All three areas would be federated under a UN-British trusteeship. The Zionists, bitter over the curtailment of their canton and the denial of independence, totally rejected the proposal. "For the Jews of Europe it is now Palestine or death," exclaimed the voluble Rabbi Abba Hillel Silver, Stephen Wise's successor as the voice of American Zionism, "for the Jews of Palestine it is now liberty or death." The Arabs, for their part, refused even to consider the scheme. But Truman warmed to Morrison and Grady's suggestions, welcoming them as the best means of establishing "the promised Jewish homeland and easy access to it for the displaced Jews of Europe." A compromise, at last, seemed attainable.

Or so Truman thought. The Palestine issue, which, though volatile, at least appeared containable in the first year of the Truman presidency, exploded in 1947. American Zionists bitterly protested what they sensed was the administration's drift from its earlier support of statehood and once again flooded the White House with angry postcards and cables. The gathering confrontation between Truman and American Jewry pressed Eddie Jacobson, short, stocky, and bald, to the forefront, as Zionist leaders enlisted him in an effort to persuade the president to listen to their demands. "Harry, my people need help and I am appealing to you to help them," the retired haberdasher wrote. Touched by this appeal, Truman relented, but soon regretted his forbearance. Rabbi Silver stormed into the Oval Office protesting Truman's polices and pounded on the president's desk.

"Terror and Silver are the contributing causes of some, if not all, of our troubles," Truman grumbled. He refused to receive any more Zionist delegations and claimed to have burned an entire stack of telegrams from American Jews. "Jesus Christ couldn't please them when he was here on this earth," he pined, "so how would anyone expect that I would have any luck?"[8]

Not only Jews but also American Christians were hounding Truman. Chicago's Moody Bible Institute, for example, reminded the faithful that "the title deeds" granting Palestine to the Jews were "still extant in millions of Bibles the world around." Much of the press, even the *New York Times*, which had once excised most coverage of Zionism, was stirred by pity for the Holocaust's victims to support some form of Jewish independence in Palestine. Polls taken in 1947 found that Americans, by a ratio of two to one, were in favor of a Jewish state. Some of the most intense pressure on Truman originated not in the public sphere, however, but among Democratic leaders who warned that the failure to sanction Zionist goals would cost the party its majority in Congress, if not its hold on the White House.

Countervailing these influences were the ranks of senior diplomatic and defense officials predicting disastrous consequences for the United States if it followed a pro-Zionist course, and the supporters of philanthropic institutions in the Middle East who foresaw the "sacrificial labors of the generations of missionaries and educators" erased. Developments in the Arab world continued to corroborate these fears. Saudi officials threatened to retaliate economically against the United States and intimated the possibility of "underground guerrilla warfare against Americans throughout the Arab World." For the first time in the region's history, crowds in Egypt, Syria, and Iraq demonstrated against American policy and set fire to the U.S. information center in Beirut. Because of Palestine, recalled Acheson, the United States had replaced Britain as "the most disliked power in the Middle East."

Truman, the statesman, pledged to rise above partisan crosscurrents and Arab protests and to formulate his Palestine policy "not in the light of oil, but in the light of justice." As a politician, though, Truman could not act on principle alone. Following Wilson's precedent of addressing American Jewry on the eve of its holiest day, Yom Kippur, Truman on October 4 not only reiterated his call for admitting the 100,000 but also advocated creating "a viable Jewish state in an adequate area of Palestine."

The Yom Kippur statement represented the first time that an

American president had publicly sanctioned the Jewish demand for statehood and, as such, it antagonized all those in the United States and the Middle East who opposed it. But, by failing to define the term "adequate area," Truman also irked Zionist groups. The gesture, in the end, proved useless—the Democrats performed poorly in the 1946 congressional elections—leaving Truman embittered and riled. He fumed at the Jewish "crackpots," who, he claimed, "would turn the country [Palestine] over to Stalin if they had half a chance" and were plotting "to write the history of the U.S. or my history." Yet he also reserved vitriol for State Department careerists who seemed to him "more concerned about the Arab reaction than the suffering of the Jews" and often anti-Semitic.

Truman's rancor could not obscure the fact that the Palestine issue had alienated large segments of Congress and the American public from the foreign policy establishment. By the beginning of 1947, the schism had also begun to bifurcate the White House. Two of the president's most senior advisers, the elegant, articulate counsel Clark Clifford and the more reclusive and bookish David Niles, the first a Protestant and the second a Jew, urged Truman to adopt pro-Zionist views, on both political and ethical grounds. Opposing them was a formidable alignment led by James Forrestal, the depressive but strong-willed defense secretary, and by George Marshall, the Army's august former chief of staff, arguably the most respected figure in America. Basic democratic standards, Forrestal and Marshall maintained, mandated that Palestine be ruled by its Arab majority and that presidential policy be governed by strategic, rather than by domestic political, considerations.

The debate raged both within the White House and outside, while the situation in Palestine descended toward open war. Surmounting years of internecine feuding, the Revisionist underground and the mainstream Haganah allied in mounting attacks against British convoys, bridges, and trains. The British retaliated in June by combing the *Yishuv* for illegal arms and arresting twenty-five hundred Jews, including most of the Zionist leadership. On July 4, 1946, forty Jewish refugees were murdered in a pogrom in Kielce, Poland, further underscoring the impossibility of repatriation. The Jewish response to these events came less than three weeks later, when a bomb blew up the British headquarters in Jerusalem's King David Hotel. The attack, planned by the Haganah but carried out by the Revisionist *Irgun* militia, commanded by Menachem Begin, who claimed to have warned the British repeatedly, killed ninety-one people, including seventeen Jews. Buried beneath the hotel's smoldering rubble, it seemed, lay the last hopes of attaining some measure of reconciliation between Britain and Palestinian Jews, as well as of averting full-scale warfare between the Jews and the Palestinian Arabs.

This tide of violence threatened to overtake Truman's attempts to devise a coherent strategy on Palestine and to drown out the disagreements between his chief advisers over the country's future. As 1947 began, the direction that American policy would take toward the issue remained supremely uncertain, representing, in Truman's words, the "sixty-four dollar question."[9] The confusion was suddenly compounded in February when Britain, its troops exhausted and its economy spent, finally admitted that it could no longer administer Palestine. Responsibility for proposing a solution to this intractable conflict reverted to the United Nations.

Struggles over Partition and Recognition

The United Nations responded to Britain's decision by creating the Special Committee on Palestine—UNSCOP—composed of delegates from eleven member states. Beginning in May 1947, the committee traveled to the Middle East and conducted interviews with Arab and Jewish officials. The aged Zionist leader Chaim Weizmann spoke of "the thousands of years of martyrdom and wandering" of the Jewish people and of their yearning for one small state, while Ben-Gurion warned that the Jewish refugees were determined to reach Palestine, even if they had to sail there on "Dunkirk boats." As if to substantiate the claim, another Haganah ship, *Exodus 1947*, attempted to break the British blockade, but was stopped and its passengers sent back to Europe. The delegates were treated to a first-hand view of bayonet-wielding British troops herding more than forty-five hundred physically devastated but emotionally defiant survivors of Nazi death camps onto a boat back to Hamburg, Germany.

The Arabs, by contrast, officially boycotted UNSCOP. In informal conversations with the committee's staff, though, Arab rulers reiterated their opposition to a "Zionist beachhead" in the Middle East and their insistence on establishing a unitary Arab state in Palestine.

UNSCOP's experience in Palestine deeply influenced its findings, submitted on September 1. Though three of its delegates recommended that Palestine become a federated binational state, the majority of eight called for partitioning the country into separate Arab and Jewish states, with an international regime for Jerusalem. The two states were to achieve independence in two years and be linked by an economic union. (See map on page xiv.)

The plan left the Jewish state with convoluted borders and, before the arrival of Jewish immigrants, with an Arab majority, but the Zionists embraced partition as the realization of a two-thousand-year-old dream. The Arabs, both within Palestine and throughout the Middle East, denounced the scheme as the latest Western attempt to steal Arab land and colonize it with foreigners. The Arab League, after consulting with the mufti, now in exile in Egypt, pledged support for a "relentless war" by the Palestinian Arabs against partition and to supply it with "men, money and ammunition."

Though supportive of the Harrison, Anglo-American, and Morrison-Grady reports, Truman was troubled by UNSCOP's findings. The United States, he feared, might be drawn into implementing the partition—or worse, that the Soviet Union would also demand a role, gaining in Palestine the Middle Eastern foothold it was denied in Turkey, Libya, and Iran. The president also fretted over whether the *Yishuv*, famous for its communal farms and ultra-leftist politics, would emerge as a pro-Soviet state or whether the Arabs, despairing finally of the West, would strike an alliance with Moscow. Most daunting for Truman, however, was the prospect that Arab forces would overpower the Haganah and that, to prevent a second Holocaust, the United States would have to intercede militarily in Palestine. As many as 200,000 troops would be needed to enforce partition, the Pentagon estimated, leaving none to defend Greece and Turkey, much less Western Europe.

In light of these trepidations, Truman temporized, neither embracing nor rebuffing partition. He had "stuck his neck out once before"

on Palestine "and did not intend to do so again." But events converged to compel him to adopt a more definitive stand. Though traditionally antagonistic to the creation of a Jewish national home, the
Soviet Union suddenly realized it had less to gain by denouncing
"Zionist hooligans" than by ousting the British from the strategic
heartland of the Middle East. On October 13, the Kremlin
announced its support for partition. Less than a month later, the
enervated British government decided that it would not be capable
of maintaining order in Palestine during the two-year transition
period and would therefore withdraw its troops in May 1948.[10] With
the Soviets now expressly siding with the Zionists and the end of the
mandate pending, Truman had neither the diplomatic latitude nor
the luxury of remaining ambiguous about partition.

Zionist pressures on the president, meanwhile, mounted. Once
again, the White House was inundated with thousands of letters urging it to adopt a patently pro-partition stance. "The Jews, I find are
very, very selfish," Truman divulged to his diary, "neither Hitler nor
Stalin has anything on them for cruelty or mistreatment to the under
dog." Yet he managed to keep these ravings to himself and publicly
to endorse the UNSCOP's conclusions. "Get busy and get all the
votes you can," Truman instructed his UN delegation, as partition
came before the General Assembly in November.

Then situated on Long Island's Lake Success, the United Nations
became the scene of intense lobbying, even arm-twisting, by the
Zionists. Those states that seemed likely to oppose or abstain on the
decision—Cuba, for example, Haiti, and Ethiopia—were threatened
with a loss of American financial and political backing if they failed
to approve the resolution. Ten senators purportedly united to pressure the Philippines and thirty-one leaned on Greece. The president
of Liberia received a message from Harvey Firestone, telling him to
support partition or risk losing valuable rubber contracts, and an
importuning phone call from Congressman Sol Bloom. Arab countries also labored to persuade wavering delegates to vote against partition, though less effectively than the Zionists. Few of these efforts,
whether Zionist or Arab, succeeded in altering the delegates' positions. Convening on November 29, the General Assembly approved
Resolution 181 by a majority of thirty-three to thirteen, with ten

abstentions. Two independent states, one Arab and one Jewish, would emerge in Palestine, with the UN's approval and the imprimatur of the United States.[11]

Having placed his administration squarely behind the partition plan, Truman might have expected to move on to other global issues, but the UN vote only exacerbated the crisis. Angry mobs vandalized the U.S. embassy in Damascus and Islamic radical cells bombed the American consulate in Jerusalem. Elsewhere in the city, Arab snipers fired on an ambulance as it climbed Mount Scopus to the Hadassah Hospital, while in the north, nine hundred Arab irregulars crossed the Syrian border to assault Kfar Szold, the settlement named for Hadassah's founder. The State Department, together with the Joint Chiefs of Staff and the incipient Central Intelligence Agency, pointed to these incidents as proof that partition was "unworkable" and that order in the country could be restored only by the intervention of American *and* Soviet troops—the bleakest outcome imaginable.

Zionist pressure on the White House also intensified, rather than subsided, after the UN vote, as a safeguard against any presidential backsliding on partition. Such heavy-handed measures merely succeeded in further alienating Truman from the Zionists, to the point that he refused to speak with any of their leaders. Instead, in December, the administration announced the suspension of all American arms sales to the Middle East. The embargo had little impact on the Arab forces, which were traditionally equipped with European weapons, but deprived the *Yishuv* of a vital arms supplier. The Zionist leadership subsequently embarked on a global campaign to procure weaponry of all types. The Viennese-born Teddy Kollek, a future Jerusalem mayor, headed the operation in the United States, soliciting funds from underworld figures such as Bugsy Siegel and a number of Hollywood stars, including Frank Sinatra. Such contributions, however generous, could not compensate for the Haganah's shortage of artillery and tanks and for its lack of even a single warplane.

That deficiency became acute as bands of Arab irregulars crossed into Palestine to join with local Arab militias in launching an all-out assault on the *Yishuv*. Fearing that the outbreak of civil war in Palestine would frighten the world into rethinking its earlier approval of partition, Ben-Gurion ordered his troops to exercise restraint (Hebrew: *Havlagah*) and stay on the defensive. But then the policy backfired. Arab forces effectively isolated and laid siege to Jewish settlements and transformed the meandering, mountainous road to Jerusalem into a deathtrap for Jewish vehicles. The Jewish community, it seemed, might not hold out until May 15, the date now stipulated for Britain's withdrawal from Palestine. Ben-Gurion faced an excruciating choice: either fight back and jeopardize international support for partition or remain passive and risk annihilation.

The increasingly desperate situation in Palestine deepened Truman's sense of dismay. "The situation has been a headache to me for two and a half years," he confided to Eddie Jacobson. "The Jews are so emotional, and the Arabs are so difficult to talk with that it is almost impossible to get anything done. The British, of course, have been exceedingly noncooperative." Desperate for a means of averting further bloodshed, the president consented to a General Assembly review of the Palestine issue and asked the State Department to suggest alternative directions for American policy free of "political factors."

The department proceeded to devise a new trusteeship arrangement for Palestine to be administered jointly by the United States, Britain, and France. The plan, wrote the mannerly, Midwestern Loy Henderson, would "decide once and for all" that the United States "will not permit itself" to be dominated by Zionism and "result in freeing American Jews from the domination of American extremists." Truman's position on trusteeship remained unclear, though he seemed to view it as a precursor to partition rather than a substitute for it, as the State Department preferred. He certainly did not intend to sign it into policy as he did, unwittingly, with the numerous documents that were placed before him on the deck of the presidential yacht, *Williamsburg*, while cruising to St. Croix in February.

Returning to Washington, Truman continued to blame "British bullheadedness and the fanaticism of our New York Jews" for his Palestine headaches and to decline all meetings with Zionist leaders. Yet he could not bring himself to rebuff Eddie Jacobson. The president's old friend asked only one thing of him, to speak with Chaim Weizmann. Truman had met Weizmann once before, the preceding

November, and had been persuaded by him to include the Negev desert within the borders of the proposed Jewish state. The issue now, however, was no longer the contours of that state but its very existence. Truman resisted the idea, but Jacobson then pointed at a statue of Andrew Jackson. "Harry, all of your life you have had a hero," Jacobson reminded him, "and I too have a hero." Truman laughed, "You win, you baldheaded son-of-a-bitch." Secreted into the White House on March 18, Weizmann told Truman that the Jewish people stood between statehood and annihilation, and had no choice but to fight for independence. Truman expressed his desire to avoid further bloodshed in Palestine, but purportedly assured Weizman that he could "bank" on the United States. "I am for partition."

The next day, referring to the document that Truman had blindly signed on his yacht, Ambassador Warren Austin informed the General Assembly that the United States no longer supported partition and now preferred a trusteeship for Palestine. The Zionists were thunderstruck. The speech, for Rabbi Silver, represented a "shocking reversal" and "fatal capitulation" and, for Ben-Gurion, a "surrender to Arab terror." Their bitterness, though, did not exceed that of Truman. The State Department, the president raged, had "pulled the rug out from under" him and made him into a "liar and double-crosser." Austin's announcement was merely further proof that the "striped-pants boys," as Truman labeled them, "had always wanted to cut [his] throat."[12]

The government of the United States was now irrevocably divided between those officials who, fearful for America's strength, favored the trusteeship plan and others who, guided both by principle and by political considerations, still supported partition. That chasm further widened over the course of April, as Palestine plunged deeper into chaos.

Abandoning its policy of restraint and brandishing newly acquired Czech weapons, the Haganah went on the offensive. Jewish troops relieved beleaguered settlements and broke through the Jerusalem blockade. Dozens of Arab villages were also assaulted and in some cases their inhabitants were expelled. The violence climaxed on April 9, when Revisionist militiamen massacred more than one hundred Arab civilians, women and children included, in Deir Yassin, near

Jerusalem. Entering the village, Jacques de Reynier, the Swiss representative of the International Red Cross, saw "there were bodies strewn about. They had done their 'cleaning up' with guns and grenades and finished the work with knives." Less than a week later, Arab gunmen ambushed a Hadassah Hospital convoy, killing seventy-seven doctors, nurses, and patients. "When the buses burst into flames their occupants were shot down as they sought to escape," reported the *New York Times*. "This afternoon the street was littered with dead bodies." At the same time, Transjordan's British-officered Arab Legion began to occupy the West Bank, an area designated by the UN for inclusion in the independent Arab state. Ben-Gurion, anxious to avoid a clash with Transjordan, sent Golda Meir on a secret peace mission to Abdullah, but the king still opted for war. The legion subsequently overran the Etzion bloc of Jewish communities situated between Jerusalem and Hebron, killing 157 of its defenders, many of them after they surrendered.

The absolute breakdown of order in Palestine produced markedly different reactions in Arabs and Jews. Terrorized by Deir Yassin and by rumors of additional atrocities and deserted by many of their own leaders, Palestinian Arabs in massive numbers began to flee the country. Thousands of families, their belongings lashed hastily to donkeys or piled in bundles on their heads, choked the roads leading north to Syria and Lebanon, forded the Jordan River eastward or crowded into fishing boats bound for Gaza. "They are destitute of any belongings [and] without adequate shelter, medical supplies, sanitation and food," the State Department informed Truman. "Their average daily ration, made up exclusively of bread, is only 600 calories." Arab leaders did little to reverse this flight. Indeed, they seemed less concerned with the loss of Palestine's Arab population than with the territorial gains made by Abdullah in the West Bank. Anxious to counter Transjordan's advantage, the rulers of Egypt, Syria, and Iraq began contemplating their own military incursions into Palestine.

The Jews had neither the option of retreat nor the military capability of preempting a general Arab attack. Their energies consequently were directed to reinforcing the settlements' defenses, stockpiling small arms, and smuggling consignments of ammunition, heavy weaponry, and medical supplies. The Zionist leadership, meanwhile, in a display of unsubstantiated optimism, readied the *Yishuv* for statehood. Government ministries, complete with phone lines, desks, and secretaries were established and quickly issued paper currency and stamps. Missing only was the name of the anticipated state— Zion, Herzliya, and Judah were some of the possibilities suggested. Israel was another.

In light of these events, the issue of whether the United States should continue to back partition or switch its support to trusteeship was suddenly rendered irrelevant. By the second week of May, only two uncertainties remained: whether the impending Jewish state could survive the Arab onslaught and, if so, whether America would recognize Jewish statehood. Desperate to skirt both of these questions, the State Department proposed that the announcement of Jewish independence be indefinitely delayed and a general truce declared. Ben-Gurion accepted the truce but would not postpone the declaration, while Arab rulers agreed to a cease-fire but only if the partition were annulled. With war now virtually inescapable, the administration considered the Jews' ability to withstand a multifront incursion. Though estimates differed, Marshall, the most militarily experienced of the officials, believed that the Arabs would eventually prevail. "What will happen if there is a prolonged invasion?" he asked a high-ranking Zionist official. "It will weaken you."

Marshall, along with his undersecretary Robert Lovett, was present on May 12 at the meeting Truman convened on recognition. Also in attendance were the advisers Clark Clifford and David Niles. The president sat between them, the diplomats to his right and the counselors on his left. Lovett opened by summarizing the State Department's traditional arguments against the Jewish national home—the hazards it posed to vital American interests in the Middle East and the burden it would place on U.S. defense forces. He warned that the president might be perceived as engaging in "a very transparent attempt to win the Jewish vote." He also stressed the peril presented by "Bolshevik" Zionism and by the Soviet agents who were planted, Lovett claimed, among the refugees. The United States should not rush to recognize what might be a communist state, thus buying "a pig in the poke." Marshall expressed no objection to Lovett's curious metaphor, but he did resent the presence of political advisers at this crucial foreign policy meeting. Then, in a shocking remark for an acting secretary of state, he said, "If the President were to follow Mr. Clifford's advice and if in the elections I were to vote, I would vote against the President."

The threat of alienating the supremely esteemed Marshall no doubt terrified Truman, who was already lagging in the 1948 election polls. He remained expressionless, though, and gave the floor to Clifford. The counsel proceeded to refute each of the State Department's arguments, asserting that the Arabs needed money more than the United States needed their oil and that a swift recognition of the Jewish state was the best means of bolstering America's prestige in the world while outshining the Soviet Union. Truman absorbed the analysis as well, but was still noncommittal. Asked by reporters later which way he had decided on recognition, Truman obliquely replied, "I will cross that bridge when I get to it."

The bridge loomed before him two days later, May 14, when, as the British prepared to evacuate the last of their troops from Palestine, thirty-eight members of the provisional Jewish government assembled in the Tel Aviv Museum. Rising as the Palestine Symphony Orchestra led them in singing "Hatikvah," the representatives, Ben-Gurion and Golda Meir among them, lined up to sign a declaration of independence. This described the Land of Israel as the birthplace of the Jewish people, the cradle of their religious and national culture, and the wellspring of their spiritual gifts to the world. It recalled the milestones of the Zionist movement, from the creation of the first Jewish settlements to the Balfour Declaration, the resistance to Nazism, and the UN partition resolution. It remembered the Holocaust and offered peace to the neighboring states and to those Palestinian Arabs who accepted Jewish sovereignty. Reflecting, perhaps, Ben-Gurion's sojourn in the United States and his extensive reading on American democracy, the document pledged to uphold "the precepts of liberty, justice and peace," to safeguard the "full freedom of conscience, worship, education and culture," and to guarantee "the social and political equality of all its citizens, without distinction of race, creed or sex." The name of the Jewish state, the signatories agreed, was Israel.

Word of Israel's birth reached Washington at six o'clock in the evening of May 14. At that moment, the armies of Egypt, Lebanon, Syria, and Iraq were mobilizing to "restore peace and security in Palestine" by invading the nascent state. Egyptian planes had already bombed and strafed Tel Aviv. Arab refugees, fleeing out of fear or evicted by Jewish forces, continued to stream out of Palestine. In New York, the American delegation to the United Nations was still pressing for trusteeship, while in cities throughout America, Jewish communities and non-Jewish supporters of Zionism rejoiced. The question remained, though, would United States recognize this new nation of Israel and its self-proclaimed government?

Alone in the White House, Truman pondered the many and profound ramifications of that decision. "My soul [sic] objective in Palestine has been to prevent bloodshed," he had revealed in a personal note to Dean Alfange, an Istanbul-born labor activist who had championed the Zionist cause. "The way things look today we apparently have not been successful. Nobody in the country has given the problem more time and thought than I have." Against the anticipated damage that recognition would inflict on the image of United States in the Arab world, the fillip it would grant the Soviets, and the immense burdens it might place on Western defenses, the president had to weigh the need to render justice for the survivors of the Holocaust and to respond to public sympathies for Zionism. He had to consider America's past involvement in the Middle East—a legacy of support for nationalist movements, Arab as well as Jewish, and for the victims of oppression and war—along with the America's vital interests in the region, present and future.

At eleven minutes past six, an administration spokesman appeared before reporters at the White House. "This Government has been informed that a Jewish state has been proclaimed in Palestine and that recognition has been requested by the provisional government thereof," he matter-of-factly told the correspondents. Then, reading from a printed text, understating the momentousness of his message, the spokesman said, "The United States recognizes the provisional government as the de facto authority of the State of Israel."

I Am Cyrus!

The vision of renewed Jewish statehood described by Levi Parsons and Pliny Fisk from the pulpit of Old South Church 130 years earlier, which had animated Americans as diverse as Emma Lazarus and William Blackstone, Louis Brandeis and Mark Twain, was realized. But so, too, were some of the apprehensions expressed by Selah Merrill as early as the 1880s, by Charles Crane and Howard Bliss after World War I, and later by Allen Dulles and numerous government officials. Israel would grow into a militarily strong and increasingly valued American ally, a vibrant, if often rambunctious, democracy. It never turned Bolshevik or required American troops for its defense. But the Jewish state would radiate animosity throughout much of the Middle East and serve as the focus of a centuries-long Muslim animus toward the West. The Arab refugees who bore the name "Palestinian" with them into exile would constitute a core issue in an ongoing Arab-Israeli dispute and would consider the United States complicitous in causing their plight. Great quantities of Arab oil continued to flow to the United States after it recognized Israel—contrary to the State Department's predictions—but so did a profusion of Arab anger.

The creation of the State of Israel elicited luminous expectations in many Americans, but tenebrous anxieties in others, jubilation as well as fears. Harry Truman wavered between the two responses. Once described as a person whose mind could move in two different directions, at least, simultaneously and ingenuously, Truman had cursed the Zionists and their American supporters, often mimicking the very anti-Semites he despised. Yet, rising above his own rage and prejudice, he supported the right of Jewish refugees to immigrate to Palestine, endorsed partition, and acknowledged Israel's independence. Though he would often criticize Israel's policies, in particular its refusal to permit the return of Palestinian refugees, Truman never regretted his decision of May 14. On the contrary, he seemed to revel in the Jews' restoration and the role that he, a plain-speaking Baptist from Missouri, had played in it. Introduced by Eddie Jacobson to an American Jewish delegation as the leader who helped create the State of Israel, Truman snapped, "What do you mean 'helped create'? I am Cyrus, I am Cyrus!"[13]

Truman's boast was not entirely bluster. Cyrus the Great (576–529 BCE) not only repatriated Jewish exiles and authorized the rebuilding of a Judean state, he also presided over an immense Middle Eastern empire. The United States had emerged from World War II as the nonpareil power in the Middle East—not an empire in the formal sense but a hegemon nonetheless, a military and economic colossus capable of safeguarding the region's borders and fostering inchoate states. The United States had attained this dominion in an astonishingly short time, during which Americans transformed themselves from largely passive observers of Middle Eastern affairs into the region's primary architects and arbiters.

This was the country whose representative to the San Remo Conference in 1920 spent the proceedings in a courtyard reading a newspaper, whose policymakers refused to recognize Saudi Arabia when the kingdom was initially proclaimed, and which regarded Palestine—indeed much of the Middle East—as an inviolate European preserve. Twenty-five years later, however, the United States had come to wield unparalleled economic and strategic influence throughout the area. Its inhabitants, most of whom had yet to achieve complete liberty, looked to the United States for inspiration and relief from foreign domination. Many Middle Eastern countries, including several that would someday rank among America's deadliest opponents, owed their independence to the United States, while others received infrastructure, economic aid, and political guidance—the building blocks of sovereignty—as gifts of the American people.

Nineteenth-century American educators had helped to define a new Arab identity for many of the peoples of the Middle East and, in the period between the Paris Peace Conference and the creation of Israel, American soldiers and statesmen had helped remold the region. While it was still far from resembling the federation of enlightened and democratic nations that generations of Americans had envisaged, the Middle East was equally distant from the depressed backwater it had been under the Ottomans or the pre–World War II patchwork of European colonies. By the end of the 1940s, a substantially changed Middle East—resurgent, irrepressible, thrashing between modernity and tradition—would interact with a much altered, vastly empowered United States. The meeting would not always be amiable.

In spite of the assistance it rendered to emergent Middle East nations, the United States would, in time, come to be seen by many of them as the successor to imperialist Europe, a colonialist power that spoke of development and democracy while exploiting the area's resources and propping up oppressive native regimes. Arab nationalists assailed the United States for supporting nationalism only as long as it accorded with America's agenda, and Islamic radicals denounced the United States as the embodiment of Western liberalism, secularism, and decay. For well over a century, Americans had provided the Middle East with philanthropic support and ideological guidance, but starting in the postwar period they also furnished the region with a target for deep-seated and intensifying resentment.

After 1948, Americans would spend the next six decades struggling to balance the benefits they brought to the Middle East with the resources and military advantages they derived from it—to reconcile their image of themselves as educators, philanthropists, and peacemakers with the reputation they acquired throughout much of the area as arrogant and self-interested interlopers. They had to accommodate their commitment to the principles of self-determination and respect for national sovereignty to the need to counter global challenges, first from Soviet communism and later from Islamic extremism. Americans had to see through their long-held illusions about the Middle East—the dreamlike deserts, the erotic odalisques—in order to address credible threats to their security. The story of America's involvement in the postwar Middle East is one of determined attempts by statesmen, soldiers, and private citizens to attain that harmony, to safeguard vital interests, sustain valued ideals, and distinguish myth from reality.

Part Seven

In Search of
Pax Americana

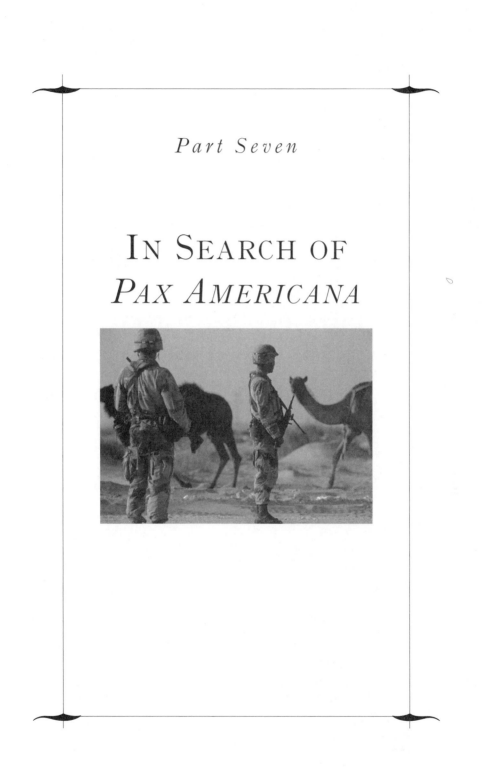

27

HARMONY AND HEGEMONY

THE PRECEDING CHAPTERS EXAMINED IN DETAIL THE diverse ways in which the United States has interacted with the Middle East since 1776. The purpose was to reveal the richness and substance of that history and to explore the foundations of America's involvement in the region today. Another goal was to fill a gap in the literature on the relationship between the United States and the Middle East in the 150 years separating the Revolutionary War from the end of World War II.

This final section deals with the past six decades, from the advent of the Cold War to the war in Iraq, a time of intense American engagement in the Middle East. In contrast to the 1776–1945 period, about which relatively few works exist, the contemporary phase has yielded vast quantities of articles and books. Many fine studies have been conducted on American efforts to mediate an Arab-Israeli peace prior to the 1973 war, for example, or on the evolution of the U.S.-Saudi alliance in the 1950s and 1960s, and little can be added to them in terms of original research. On the other hand, analysis of the major events of the last thirty years is hampered by lack of internal government documents—the bedrock of serious research—which are still classified and closed to the public. Any attempt to reconstruct American involvement in the Middle East from 1948 to the present risks either repeating what has already been written or speculating on what is not yet adequately known.

In view of these pitfalls, this concluding section attempts to provide not an exhaustive study of this period but rather an overview of its crucial turning points and trends. The emphasis is on the continuity between the post–World War II phase of this history and earlier stages and on the persistent themes of power, faith, and fantasy. American policymakers, it will be shown, wrestled with many of the same challenges faced by their prewar predecessors and similarly strove to reconcile their strategic and ideological interests in the area. Mythic images of the Middle East, meanwhile, remained a mainstay of American popular culture.

By focusing on the consistency of America's involvement with this crucial region and by placing its current involvement there within a historical context, the chapter aims to deepen the understanding of the nature of U.S.–Middle East relations. The objective is to enable Americans to read about the fighting in Iraq and hear the echoes of the Barbary Wars and Operation Torch or to follow presidential efforts to mediate between Palestinians and Israelis and see the shadows of Teddy Roosevelt and Woodrow Wilson. The same illusions that lured John Ledyard to explore the Middle East, they will learn, still entice Americans to attend movies with Middle Eastern motifs. After more than two hundred years, the interaction between the United States and the peoples and lands of the Middle East has remained remarkably vibrant, multifaceted, dynamic, and profound.

Cast between Communism and Nationalism

For a while, it seemed, Harry Truman managed to harmonize America's newfound status as the preeminent power in the Middle East with its traditional role of liberator and peacemaker. Hoping to heal the wounds opened by the creation of the Jewish state, the president supported United Nations efforts to establish peace between Israel and the Arabs. The task fell to the UN special mediator on Palestine, Ralph Bunche, a former UCLA basketball star, accomplished editor, and one of the first African Americans to receive a Harvard Ph.D. "Have a look at these lovely plates!" the dapper but straight-talking Bunche told the Arab and Israeli delegates who dined with him on the island of Rhodes. "If you reach an agreement, each one of you will get one to bring home—if you don't, I'll break them over your heads!" By July 1949, Bunche had ironed out armistice agreements between Israel and the neighboring Arab states of Egypt, Lebanon, Jordan, and Syria and established a precedent for more permanent treaties. His achievement earned him the Nobel Peace Prize and appeared to restore America's reputation as a principled mediator.[1]

Truman also sought to balance Cold War concerns with the ascending tide of Middle Eastern nationalism. The first test of the president's prowess came in Iran, where the prime minister, a seventy-year-old Swiss-educated lawyer named Mohammad Mossadegh, declared himself the champion of the people and the adversary of all forms of foreign domination. He worked to steer the country clear of Soviet influence but also maneuvered to ease the British out of Iran by nationalizing the Anglo-Iranian Oil Company (AIOC).

Mossadegh was a forerunner of the nonaligned movement, composed mostly of developing countries that declared their neutrality in the Cold War, affiliated with neither the Soviet Union nor the West. Such a position could well have antagonized the United States, but Mossadegh, to the contrary, became something of an American hero. Iran, in the eyes of many Americans, was still the enchanted land of *A Thousand and One Arabian Nights*. They continued to flock to Middle Eastern fantasy films such as *The Son of Ali Baba* (1952) and *The 7th Voyage of Sinbad* (1953) and to the 1953 Broadway sensation *Kismet*, in which a love-struck caliph croons to a lissome Iraqi slave, "Take my hand, I'm a stranger in paradise." They remained mesmerized by the myth of the liberty-loving Middle Easterner, which Mossadegh seemed to embody. The American press consequently compared him to Paine and Jefferson, and *Time* magazine named him its 1951 Man of the Year. Truman invited the prime minister to the White House and, much to Britain's annoyance, supported his claims to Iranian oil.

Another example of Truman's ability to juggle America's strategic and ideological interests occurred in Egypt. There, too, the nationalist movement mobilized to expel the British, disband parliament, and overthrow the monarchy of King Farouk. In scenes evocative of the 'Urabi revolt seventy years earlier, rioters rampaged through the streets of Cairo and Alexandria in January 1952, torching foreign-owned buildings. Among the classic structures destroyed was the Shepheard's Hotel, which had once hosted Mark Twain. Such chaos, Truman feared, was liable to be exploited by the Soviets in order to penetrate Egypt politically. He consequently assigned Kermit Roosevelt and other CIA agents to identify an Egyptian nationalist figure, "a Moslem Billy Graham," who could restore order in the country and enroll it in a NATO-like Middle East Defense Organization (MEDO). Their search took them to a cell of self-described Free Officers who were plotting to stage a coup and to their thirty-four-year-old leader, Lieutenant Colonel Gamal Abdul Nasser.[2]

Articulate and strikingly handsome, Nasser looked like a modern incarnation of 'Urabi, as well as a hero culled from the pages of *A Thousand and One Arabian Nights*. He was also the product of the nationalist ideas introduced to Egypt by American veterans of the Civil War and by Arab graduates of the Syrian Protestant College. Nasser indeed seemed to be the leader whom the CIA, for the first time in its Middle East operations, sought to install, and the agency assured him and his co-conspirators of America's sub rosa support. Emboldened by this backing, the officers seized government buildings on July 23, 1952, dissolved the parliament, and deposited Farouk on a yacht bound for Europe. The British responded with horror to these events, but the United States promptly recognized the new regime and initiated a dialogue with Nasser.

By the last year of his presidency, Truman had succeeded in mediating between Arabs and Israelis, in supporting nationalists, and in blocking Soviet aggression. A *pax Americana* in the Middle East suddenly appeared within grasp. But that proximity proved to be a mirage. The Arab states declared that the armistice was little more than a provisional truce and that a state of war continued to exist between them and Israel. Egypt blockaded Israel-bound cargoes from traversing the Suez Canal or from passing through the Straits of Tiran, at the entrance to the Red Sea, to Israel's southern port of

Eilat. In violation of the armistice, the Jordanians banned Israelis from entering the Old City in East Jerusalem, home to the holiest of Jewish shrines, the Western Wall. Israel, for its part, refused to repatriate the Palestinian refugees without a peace agreement and retaliated for Palestinian infiltration across its border with large-scale raids into Arab territory.

Burned-out vehicles and the bullet-ridden dead once again littered the landscape sacred to millions. Scenes elsewhere in the Middle East, though, were scarcely less appalling. Much of the region from Morocco to Iraq was agitated by nationalist demonstrations and sporadic guerrilla attacks against the French and British authorities. The tumult coincided with renewed Soviet provocations against Iraq and Iran and by the Kremlin's decision to embrace the Middle Eastern nationalists whom it had formerly shunned as "bourgeois lackeys" as its natural allies in the Cold War. A convergence of communism and radical nationalism imperiled the Middle Eastern oil on which the West depended for its well-being and even its survival.

The inability of the Western allies to stabilize, much less redress, the multiple conflicts rocking the Middle East was apparent as early as 1950, when Britain, France, and the United States issued the Tripartite Declaration. The document implicitly admitted the powers' growing frustration with Arab-Israeli peace efforts and called on both disputants to exercise restraint. Rather than shoot at one another, the powers urged all states in the Middle East to aim their guns at their common Soviet foe by cooperating on regional defense.

The Tripartite Declaration marked another attempt to reconcile the incompatible components in America's Middle East policy. The Truman administration naïvely believed that the United States could befriend both Israel and the Arab world, and that it could support demands for Middle Eastern independence while expecting Britain and France to defend the region from communism. Those assumptions were baseless, however, and by 1952, with the rise of Arab-Israeli tensions and the resurgence of nationalist revolts, the United States again faced agonizing choices. Either it could continue supporting Israel and further inflame Arab anger or back away from the Jewish state and garner Arab goodwill. America could either stand beside Britain and France in protecting the Middle East from Soviet aggression or abandon them in favor of native nationalists, some of whom were already in contact with the Kremlin.

Truman would not have to make those decisions. In January 1953, the Democratic White House passed into the hands of the Republicans under the square-jawed former general and World War II icon, Dwight David Eisenhower. "We who are free must proclaim anew our faith," Eisenhower, a Kansan, drawled in his first inaugural address. Appearing no fewer than fourteen times in the text, the word "faith," for the new president, meant confidence in America's ability to protect freedom worldwide while respecting "the special heritage of each nation." The United States had at last achieved the supremacy necessary to disseminate its values around the globe, but so, too, had the Soviet Union. And the "special heritage" of those nations still languishing under imperial rule contained at least as much hostility toward the West as it did fear of Soviet aggression. "Faith," Eisenhower proclaimed, "defines our full view of life," but that weltanschauung still overlooked the contradiction between nurturing nationalism and combating communism in an increasingly labyrinthine Middle East.

Dull, Duller, Dulles

Never adept at foreign policy, Eisenhower ceded responsibility for the Middle East—indeed for much of the world—to his secretary of state, John Foster Dulles. Prim and stodgy, his gaze frigid behind steel-rimmed glasses and his smile precluded by a pipe, Dulles was notorious for his lack of pathos. Winston Churchill, who again served as British prime minister in the early 1950s, epitomized him in three words: "Dull, Duller, Dulles." A Princeton graduate and a pious Presbyterian, the secretary was Wilsonian in his anticolonialism but Jacksonian in his determination to safeguard America's interests abroad. He regarded communism as a global evil and viewed nonaligned countries such as India and Indonesia as abettors of that evil. Radical nationalists were also considered dangerous by Dulles. "Whether it is in Indo-China or Siam or Morocco or Egypt or Arabia or Iran . . . the forces of unrest are captured by the Soviet

Communists," he told the Senate. Together with his brother, Allen, formerly of the State Department and now head of the CIA, Dulles vowed to rid the Middle East of those who furnished entrées for the Russians.

The first target of this campaign was Mohammad Mossadegh. Shedding his avuncular image, the prime minister emerged in 1953 as Iran's strongman. He severed relations with Britain, seized control of the army, and forged alliances with the communist Tudeh Party. The ineffectual but pro-Western shah, Mohammad Reza, was forced to flee the country. These events, in Dulles's mind, augured the imminent fall of the entire Persian Gulf to a nationalist-communist coalition and the loss of irreplaceable Middle Eastern oil. Determined to prevent this catastrophe, Dulles collaborated with the British in plotting Mossadegh's ouster. The operation, code-named Ajax, was carried out by the CIA's Kermit Roosevelt with the assistance of Loy Henderson, now serving as America's ambassador to Teheran, and General Norman H. Schwarzkopf, all of whom had supported Iranian nationalism in the past. The conspirators inserted virulent attacks on Mossadegh in the Iranian press and incited antigovernment riots in the streets. Civil war threatened to bifurcate Iran when, on August 19, 1953, Ajax finally succeeded. The shah regained his throne and eliminated hundreds of Mossadegh supporters. The deposed prime minister was placed under house arrest, where he remained until his death, in 1967.[3]

The Iranian coup served as a precedent for the CIA-orchestrated overthrow of the Guatemalan president Jacobo Arbenz Guzman in 1954. And yet, in countries in which the danger of communist takeover was not perceived as acute, the United States continued to foster nationalist movements, even at the expense of its European allies. Such was the case in North Africa. "We cannot give the French the support they desire for their North African policies without incurring the enmity of the native populations," the State Department averred in 1955. "The French are operating a police state in North Africa," raged the Republican senator from Nevada, George Malone, who assailed the United States for sinking "into the filthy business of bolstering colonial slavery" by aiding France. The United States in fact pressed for the repatriation of King Muhammad V of

Morocco and the Tunisian nationalist Habib Bourguiba, both of whom had been banished by the French, and helped their countries to achieve independence in 1956. The Eisenhower administration similarly urged France to show restraint in its suppression of Algerian nationalists. "Having gone so far to try to protect the independence of the Arab nations," the president said, the United States "did not want to back a French position which might destroy all the good we had done."

Resentment of America's role in the coup against Mossadegh would fester among many Iranians, but bitterness over America's support for the independence of other Middle Eastern states brewed in Britain and France. One senior British official regretted how "some Americans always saw a budding George Washington in every dissident or revolutionary movement," and another denigrated the "ideal dream" of creating "a chain of independent Muslim states from the Atlantic to the Indian Ocean working in grateful cooperation with the American Liberators." The French general Alphonse Juin railed against the "vast conspiracy" in which "the religious fanaticism and xenophobia of the Middle East joins with American anti-colonialism" to eject the French from North Africa.[4]

Frustration with America's vacillating policies in the Middle East increasingly roiled Europe and eventually boiled over in Egypt. The bonds between the United States and the Free Officers' junta thickened under the Eisenhower administration. Returning from a tour of Cairo and other Middle Eastern capitals in May 1953, Dulles publicly endorsed Nasser's demand for the complete withdrawal of British forces from Egypt. "From Foster's personal observation," Eisenhower wrote Churchill, "I have come to the conclusion that some step should be made soon to reconcile our minimum defense needs with the very strong nationalist sentiments of the Egyptian Government and people." Dulles was convinced that, once freed of Britain, Egypt would willingly join the Middle East Defense Organization. But the British believed that Nasser was inherently anti-Western and that by supporting him the United States would undermine, rather than fortify, MEDO. "The old colonial attitude toward the natives will drive them into the hands of the communists," Dulles complained. While British soldiers came under repeated attack from Egyptian guerrillas, Dulles intensified his pressure on London. Finally, in July 1954, Churchill capitulated and agreed to evacuate all British troops from Egypt. This ended a seventy-year occupation which had resulted in part from the rise and fall of Egyptian cotton prices during and after the Civil War.[5]

But Egypt did not enter MEDO. Nasser now explained that another obstacle to Egyptian membership in the organization remained: the conflict with Israel. Friction between Egyptian and Israeli forces had spiked in the wake of the British withdrawal and threatened to ignite the entire region. Restrain the Israelis, Nasser informed Dulles, and compel them to forfeit territory as a down payment on peace, and Egypt would surely join MEDO.

The offer deeply appealed to Dulles. Like many of the State Department officials who were descended from missionaries, he reviled the Jewish state—"the millstone around our necks," he called it—and generally empathized with the Arabs. He agreed with the department's assessment that Israel could achieve peace by ceding large portions of territory to the Arabs. But peace, for Dulles, was not only a means of assuring Middle East defense but also an exalted end in itself. Conditioned by his religious upbringing to feel a special attachment to Palestine, the secretary felt morally bound, if not celestially ordained, to restore tranquillity in the Holy Land.

The combined thrust of these strategic and theological impulses led Dulles to invite the British, only weeks after he had helped evict them from Egypt, to participate in an attempted mediation between Egypt and Israel. By the end of 1954, a team of Anglo-American planners had produced Alpha, a covert plan in which Israel relinquished swaths of territory to Egypt and Egypt promised to display nonbelligerency toward Israel. Predictably, Prime Minister Ben-Gurion of Israel rejected the proposal—Egypt should not be rewarded for its aggression in 1948, he explained—but Dulles was willing to pressure him to yield. All he needed was Nasser's approval.

The Egyptian leader had just then embarked on an ambitious project to establish his primacy in inter-Arab politics and his prominence, along with India's Jawaharlal Nehru, in the nonaligned movement. The first objective vitiated any chance that Nasser would make peace with the Arabs' ultimate enemy, while the second negated the possibility of Egyptian membership in MEDO. Rejecting Alpha's terms, Nasser proceeded to oppose Britain's military alliance with Turkey, Pakistan, Iran, and Iraq—the so-called Baghdad Pact—and to recognize Red China. In September 1955, he purchased massive quantities of Soviet arms via Czechoslovakia. Dulles nevertheless launched a second peace initiative, this one dubbed Gamma, in which a special presidential envoy shuttled between Nasser and Ben-Gurion in an attempt to arrange a meeting between the two. The emissary, the former defense secretary Robert B. Anderson, arrived in the region in the early spring of 1956 only to learn that Nasser had no intention of discussing peace and little interest in receiving him.

Dulles, enraged by this snub, authorized yet another operation, Omega, designed to effect regime change in Egypt by all means short of assassination. In addition to strengthening the friendly governments of Jordan and Lebanon and staging a pro-Western coup in Syria, Omega sought to promote King Saud as an "Islamic pope" who would supersede Nasser as the Arabs' leader. Most draconian, though, was Omega's stipulation for the withholding of U.S. aid for constructing the Aswan Dam. The project, first proposed by the American military explorer Erastus Sparrow Purdy in 1874, was the pride of Egypt's ruler.[6]

Nasser refused to bow to the sanctions, however, and on July 23, 1956, he stunned the world by announcing Egypt's nationalization of the Suez Canal. The move, Nasser, explained, was aimed at "the exploiters, the imperialists, and the stooges of imperialism" who had conspired to undermine Egypt by inhibiting the spread of its influence and cutting off funding for Aswan. In the eyes of the British, major shareholders in the Canal, Nasser had become a second Hitler and the seizure of Suez another *Anschluss.* "My object is to get rid of Colonel Nasser and his regime," swore Prime Minister Anthony Eden. Nasser was also bankrolling Algerian guerrillas, a gesture that scarcely endeared him to the French. If Egypt got away with the nationalization scheme, Foreign Minister Christian Pineau warned from Paris, France would be reduced to a third-rate power and Europe would be "totally dependent on the Arabs' goodwill."

French and British leaders immediately began drafting a military offensive against Egypt and seeking a green light for the attack, tacit or express, from the United States.[7]

The Suez crisis once again confronted the United States with difficult choices: either back a nonaligned nationalist with strong ties to Moscow or side with the two powers most capable of safeguarding the Middle East. The Americans had given priority to strategic over ethical concerns in Iran by colluding with Britain to oust Mossadegh, but in Egypt their ideology prevailed. The conflict, Dulles claimed, was not between Nasser and the West but rather between Middle Eastern nationalism and the imperialism of Europe. "The United States cannot be expected to identify herself one hundred per cent either with colonial powers or the power uniquely concerned with the problem of getting independence as rapidly and as fully as possible," he opined. Though he secretly assured the British and the French that he never ruled out the use of force against Egypt, Dulles publicly opposed any resort to arms.

"Such cynicism towards allies destroys true partnership," Eden protested. Pineau actually accused the United States of collaborating with the Kremlin to keep Nasser in power and prevent the emergence of a genuine Egyptian democracy. Exasperated by Dulles's double-talk, the French began clandestinely arming the Israelis and encouraging them to attack Egypt first. Ben-Gurion welcomed the proposal, convinced that Nasser's Soviet-equipped army mortally threatened the Jewish state. The British, who had never reconciled themselves to Israel's existence, initially hesitated, but by September they, too, were party to the plot. Israeli forces would strike within the vicinity of the Suez Canal and create a pretext for Anglo-French intervention to "protect" the vital waterway.

Just after daybreak on October 29, 1956, the sky over Sinai's Mitla Pass, twenty-five miles from the canal, was dotted with descending canopies. Landing, Israeli paratroopers fought a savage battle with Egyptian units in the pass while, farther to the north, Israeli armored formations smashed through Egyptian defenses en route to Suez and Gaza. France and Britain then threatened to intervene militarily unless all troops, Israeli and Egyptian, were withdrawn from the area of the canal. Egypt, as anticipated, rejected this ultimatum and an Anglo-French armada prepared to sail. Eden assured Dulles that the gathering invasion was not "a harkening back to the old colonial and occupational concepts" but rather an attempt to "strengthen the weakest point in the line against Communism." Dulles, however, fumed. He accused his former World War II allies of acting more barbarously than the Soviets whose tanks were just then crushing an anticommunist revolt in Hungary. "The United States would survive or go down on the basis of the fate of colonialism," the secretary bellowed. "Win or lose, we will share the fate of Britain and France."

While French and British planes bombed Egyptian airfields, the Americans and the Soviets together approved a General Assembly resolution condemning the aggression against Egypt and authorizing the deployment of UN peacekeeping forces along the canal. Ignoring the resolution, British and French forces landed in Egypt on November 5 with the intent of occupying the canal within a week. Two days later, however, amid fierce Egyptian resistance, the Soviets threatened to intervene militarily against the invaders and the United States levied massive economic pressure on Britain. Intimidated by these tactics, the Anglo-French expedition was compelled to withdraw, disgraced, leaving Suez under exclusive Egyptian control. Israel, too, buckled under the threat of American sanctions and withdrew its forces from Sinai and Gaza. Though UN forces continued to pacify these areas and Israeli ships now passed unhindered through the Straits of Tiran, the Arabs construed Israel's retreat as their triumph. As a result of the United States's actions, Nasser emerged from the Suez Crisis as the region's unrivaled master.[8]

Spurred by romantic notions of Middle Eastern nationalism and an anticolonialist creed, the United States had banded with its perennial Soviet enemy against its European friends and saved an Egyptian dictator whom Dulles had plotted to depose. In return for pursuing this meandering course, America earned contempt from the Soviet Union, acrimony from the British and the French, and antagonism from many Arabs. Rather than express gratitude to the nation that had saved him, Nasser denounced the United States as the new imperialist power in the Middle East. "The USA is being urged to take over the place of bankrupt and impotent Britain and France and to impose her influence over the Middle East," alleged Nasser's young spokesman, Anwar Sadat. Within a year of the Suez crisis, Nasserist agitation was undermining pro-Western governments throughout the area.

America, however, was virtually powerless to resist this onslaught. Having completed the work begun by Truman of ridding the Middle East of European imperialists, Eisenhower now found himself saddled with his allies' burdens but without the means of shouldering them. The United States did not maintain significant forces in the Middle East, nor did it have a legal basis for intervening forcibly in the region. "We have to act now or get out of the Middle East," he told Dulles. "To lose this area by inaction would be far worse than the loss in China, because of the [Middle East's] strategic position." Like Truman before him, Eisenhower needed a doctrine. Consequently, on January 5, 1957, the president asked Congress for $400 million to help steel Middle Eastern countries against any state "controlled by International Communism" and for permission to send American troops to defend them. "Seldom in history has a nation's dedication to principle been tested as severely as ours," he asserted, and Congress overwhelming concurred.

America's dedication would indeed be tested the summer of 1958, when mobs in Baghdad brutally overthrew the Iraqi government, publicly dismembering its prime minister and king. The conservative regimes of Jordan and Lebanon also faced anti-Western revolts. Panicked by the prospect of an Egyptian-executed, Soviet-backed takeover of the entire Middle East, Eisenhower invoked his doctrine. U.S. Air Force planes were dispatched to resupply the British paratroopers who were interceding in Jordan and U.S. forces were sent to bolster the beleaguered Lebanese government. On a scorching July morning, some 8,500 GIs splashed onto the beaches near Beirut. Unlike previous American amphibious landings in the region, this one encountered no opposition. Thousands of sightseers did turn out for the event, however, along with dozens of food and souvenir vendors who hawked their wares to the waterlogged soldiers.

The Lebanon operation marked an inauspicious end to a convoluted period in America's Middle East policies. The United States had first cooperated with Britain in overthrowing a popular Iranian

leader and then pressured the British to evacuate Egypt; it had supported North African nationalists against the French but plotted the
overthrow of the nationalists' sponsor, Nasser; it rescued Nasser
from the Anglo-French invasion in Suez but next intervened with
Britain to protect Arab governments from Nasser. Torn between the
antipodes of principles and realpolitik, the Eisenhower administration had effected a bewildering succession of reversals in the region,
embittering its allies and further provoking its foes. And yet, Americans in general believed that their government had acted both properly and prudently in Iran, North Africa, and Egypt, preserving their
crucial interests and promoting their democratic ideals. They remained,
as Mark Twain once portrayed them, innocents abroad in the Middle East, though they sometimes acted like "American vandals."

The guilelessness with which Americans continued to view the
increasingly complex and morally ambiguous Middle East was
reflected in *Ben-Hur*, a Hollywood extravaganza released in 1959.
Based on the novel written eighty years earlier by Lew Wallace, America's ambassador to the Porte, the movie was a remake of a silent film,
but this new version contained a wistful political message. The script
has Judah Ben-Hur, a nationalist Jewish prince, befriending an Arab
sheikh named Ilderim and together resisting their common enemy,
the Roman tribune Messala. Ilderim (played by the British actor
Hugh Griffith) delivers his lines in a generic Middle Eastern accent,
but Ben-Hur (Charlton Heston) speaks like a typical Midwesterner—
the conflation, once again, of the new American and the ancient Jew.
The Romans, however, sound like British lords. Judah and Ilderim
predictably emerge victorious, humbling the vengeful Messala.[9] In
the real Middle East, though, there was little affinity between Jewish
nationalist Israel and the government of the United States, and scant
Arab affection for either. To the ears of many of the region's inhabitants, moreover, the tribunes of imperial power no longer sounded
like Englishmen but rather, unmistakably, like Americans.

Yet the peoples of the Middle East soon heard a new inflection
emanating from the United States, one that combined Old World
refinement with a modern noblesse oblige. That voice described a
different vision of America's relations with the area, a partnership
based on equality rather than dominance, on the peaceful resolution

of conflict and mutual respect between leaders. Resonating to Egyptians and Jordanians and to Palestinians and Israelis alike were the Boston Brahmin tones of John Fitzgerald Kennedy.

Camelot Comes to the Middle East

Though raised a Roman Catholic, Kennedy embraced the Puritan concept of America as the "city on the hill" and the missionary commitment to disseminate American values throughout the world and promote native independence. "The single most important test of American foreign policy today is how we meet the challenge of imperialism," Kennedy, while still a senator, proclaimed. "On this test more than any other, this nation shall be critically judged by the uncommitted millions in Asia and Africa." In the Middle East, America could meet this test by supporting the few nationalist movements that had yet to succeed in casting off European rule and by reaching a modus vivendi with those newly independent regimes that remained nonaligned. Ascending to the presidency in January 1961, Kennedy endorsed Algeria's quest for independence from France and reconsidered America's antipathy toward Nasser.

Among Kennedy's first acts in office was to write the Egyptian leader and offer to resuscitate the friendship between the two countries forged after the Civil War. The United States, he reminded Nasser, had once been like the Arab world: an assortment of liberated colonies that longed to combine into a viable commonwealth. He congratulated Nasser on the anniversary of the creation of the United Arab Republic—the ultimately short-lived merger between Egypt and Syria—on February 22, "the birthday anniversary of our own first president, Washington." The gesture was promptly and warmly requited. Nasser expressed "immense satisfaction and appreciation" for Kennedy's letters and emphasized the "love and admiration" with which he and his countrymen had always regarded Americans.

Camelot, the Arthurian court to which the idealistic administration was often likened, appeared to have opened a new and gallant chapter in U.S.–Middle Eastern relations. A concrete sign of that chivalry came in the form of massive economic aid and wheat shipments; 60 percent of all Egyptians were soon receiving their daily bread courtesy of the United States. The revived amity between Nasser and the United States, and America's enduring romance with the unencumbered nomad, was intuited by the movie industry in *Lawrence of Arabia*, a 1962 classic. In one illuminating scene, a brassy American journalist named Bentley—clearly a stand-in for Lowell Thomas—declares his support for Prince Feisal and the struggle for Arab independence during World War I. "Your Highness," Bentley tells Feisal, "we Americans were once a colonial people and we naturally feel sympathetic to any people, anywhere, who are struggling for their freedom." The prince, played by the august Alec Guinness, laconically replies, "Very gratifying."

Hollywood myth and Middle Eastern realities once again parted, however, that same year, 1962, with the collapse of Kennedy's initiative in Egypt. The breakdown began with the overthrow of the pro-Western imam of Yemen by a group of Free Officers closely associated with Nasser. When Saudi Arabia stepped in to restore the royalists, Nasser responded by transferring tens of thousands of his troops to Yemen. Egyptian planes also started bombing Saudi targets, some with poison gas. The sight of a Soviet-armed and Soviet-advised army so close to the oil reserves on which America's economy depended keenly upset a Kennedy administration that had scarcely recovered from the Cuban missile crisis. Though never favorably disposed toward the Saudis, who, he felt, "somehow represented yesterday rather than tomorrow," Kennedy nevertheless had to decide between his reconciliation with Nasserism and the defense of the Persian Gulf. The choice, in the end, was virtually made for him when Nasser violated an American-brokered cease-fire. Two years after posting his first letter to Cairo, in November 1963, Kennedy sent warplanes to defend Riyadh.[10]

Stymied in his attempts at rapprochement with Nasser, Kennedy refocused his energies on Israel and its ongoing dispute with the Arabs. Since the failure of operations Alpha and Gamma in the 1950s, American policymakers had concluded that there was no chance for peace in the region. Instead, they resolved to keep the Arab-Israeli conflict "in the icebox" by preventing another outbreak of war. Enraptured by the image of Ari Ben Canaan, played by a strapping Paul Newman, leading gallant Israelis against Arab anti-heroes in the 1960 blockbuster *Exodus*, many Americans had romanticized the conflict. Kennedy, though, who had never forgotten the violence he witnessed in Jerusalem in 1939, had a more nuanced view. As a first step toward resolving the dispute, he proposed resettling thousands of Palestinian refugees in the arid Jordan Valley, which would be irrigated by Jordan River water. But Ben-Gurion, reluctant to share Israel's major water source with its enemies, balked at the idea, while Arab leaders rejected any degree of cooperation with Israel. Flustered by his failure to make peace, Kennedy turned to preventing a new outbreak of Arab-Israeli bloodshed. He was particularly concerned about the secret production of nuclear weapons by Israel, a project that, he feared, would precipitate an unbridled arms race in the Middle East.

"A woman should not only be virtuous, but also have the appearance of virtue," Kennedy told Ben-Gurion at New York's Waldorf-Astoria Hotel in May 1961. The president enjoyed excellent relations with the American Jewish community, whose support was widely credited with having helped to propel him to a narrow electoral victory in 1960, and was openly friendly toward Israel. Privately, though, Kennedy rejected the claim that Israel was developing nuclear power for peaceful purposes only and railed at Ben-Gurion's refusal to allow American inspectors to verify the "virtue" of the Israeli reactor at Dimona. "It is to our common interest that no country believe that Israel is contributing to the proliferation of atomic weapons," Kennedy advised the much older, far shorter, and less gainly Ben-Gurion. But the more seasoned Israeli statesman brushed aside the president's concerns. He reassured his host of Israel's peaceful intentions while apostrophizing how Nasser, if ever victorious, "would do to the Jews what Hitler did."

Unresolved, the issue of Israel's atomic capabilities remained a source of friction in Kennedy's relations with Israel. In an attempt to assuage Ben-Gurion's fears of Egypt, the president offered to supply him with Hawk ground-to-air missiles, setting a precedent for American arms sales to Israel. Ben-Gurion merely deployed the Hawks around Dimona and continued to block the American inspections. By the summer of 1963, an irate Kennedy was warning the Israelis

522   /   Power, Faith, and Fantasy

that their relations with the United States were liable to be "seriously jeopardized" by their intransigence on the nuclear issue.[11]

Jack Kennedy had set out to distinguish his policies toward the Middle East from those of the preceding president only to be repeatedly frustrated. He strove for reconciliation with Nasser and for a nonproliferation agreement with Ben-Gurion, but was brazenly rebuffed by both. Arab-Israeli reconciliation remained an elusive American dream. Such disappointments ultimately compelled Kennedy to abandon his righteous policies in favor of Eisenhower-era measures to shield the region from communism and to guarantee the outflow of oil. In the Middle East, perhaps more flagrantly than in any other realm, Camelot's magic had failed.

The president who descended onto Love Field in Dallas on the morning of November 22, 1963, had despaired of achieving a breakthrough in any area of American–Middle Eastern relations. Kennedy's assassination later that day would conventionally be remembered as a transformative juncture in U.S. history, inaugurating a spate of revolutionary changes within American society and a scourge of calamities in the nation's foreign affairs. Little of this upheaval exerted any impact, however, on America's interaction with the Middle East. The postcolonial regimes of Syria, Egypt, and Iraq had devolved into repressive military dictatorships, inimical to the West and hostile to one another. The lines between Soviet-backed rulers such as Nasser and the pro-Western monarchies of Jordan and the Persian Gulf were ineffaceably drawn. The public might still be charmed by the sight of a scantily clad Barbara Eden wafting from an Aladdin-esque lamp in the midsixties sitcom *I Dream of Jeannie*, but American policymakers had largely wearied of such myths. Before terminating at the Berlin Wall, the front in the Cold War ran through the hellish jungles of Vietnam to the oases and deceptively idyllic dunes of the Middle East.

From the Alamo to El Alamein

The thirty-sixth president was not a romantic. Fathomlessly ambitious, ruthlessly shrewd, as resolute in his fight for civil rights at home as in his ill-fated struggle against communism in Southeast Asia, Lyndon Baines Johnson exhibited none of Kennedy's penchant for Middle Eastern fantasies. Nor were events in the region conducive to reverie. Nasser was waging vicious propaganda wars against America's Jordanian and Saudi allies, blatantly collaborating with the Soviets, and pressing for the closure of the Wheelus air base, America's sole strategic asset in Libya. In November 1964, rioters in Cairo burned down the U.S. embassy's library. When the American ambassador protested the vandalism, Nasser told him to "go drink from the sea" and threatened to "cut out the tongue" of anybody who spoke ill of Egypt. "We are not going to accept gangsterism by cowboys," he pledged, alluding to the president from Texas. Johnson, in reply, suspended all further wheat shipments to Egypt.[12]

Johnson's hardheaded approach to the region did not prevent him from displaying an almost mawkish sentimentality toward Israel. "You have lost a very great friend," he told an Israeli diplomat shortly after Kennedy's murder. "But you have found a better one." Some of the new president's closest advisers, including Undersecretary of State Eugene Rostow and UN Ambassador Arthur Goldberg, were American Jews with pronounced pro-Israeli views. On a political level, Johnson's affection for Israel flowed from his gratitude for the overwhelming support that American Jews continued to show to the Democratic Party, and yet that affection continued in spite of mounting American Jewish opposition to the Vietnam War. A deeper reason for Johnson's pro-Israel policies lay, rather, in religion. "Take care of the Jews, God's chosen people," his strict Baptist grandfather had exhorted him, and his aunt warned, "If Israel is destroyed, the world will end." The State Department conversely continued to caution that America's ties to Israel would alienate the Arabs and jeopardize oil supplies, but the president remained unperturbed. Israel, for him, was a latter-day Alamo, surrounded on all sides by compassionless enemies, and Nasser was the reincarnated Santa Ana, the Mexican general who laid siege to that fort.[13]

The analogy became eerily apt on May 15, 1967, the day Nasser placed his nation on a war footing. Tensions in the region had been inexorably rising as a result of Palestinian guerrilla raids into Israel staged by the Syrian-backed al-Fatah organization, led by a rough-shaven and unflinching former engineer named Yasser Arafat. In response to this challenge to Egypt's leadership of the Arab world, Nasser established a rival movement, the Palestine Liberation Organization (PLO), and instructed to it to launch its own operations. Israeli reprisals for these attacks led to large-scale clashes with Syrian forces on the Golan Heights, overlooking northern Israel, and finally to Soviet claims of an imminent Israeli invasion of Syria. Though Nasser quickly ascertained that these predictions were false, he exploited them as an excuse for evicting the peacekeeping forces that the UN had maintained in Sinai and the Gaza Strip since the end of the Suez crisis. A week later, Nasser closed the Straits of Tiran to Israeli shipping and concluded military pacts with Jordan, Syria, and Iraq. Mass demonstrations erupted throughout the Arab world, clamoring for all-out war. "Our goal," declared President 'Aref of Iraq, "is clear—to wipe Israel off the face of the map."

But who would shoot first? With nearly half a million Arab soldiers converging on its borders and the Soviets encouraging them to strike, Israel faced a potentially existential situation. Israeli hospitals were frantically stockpiling bandages and units of blood, while rabbinical authorities dug thousands of graves for the war's anticipated casualties. The sudden decision of the French, Israel's erstwhile allies, to switch to the Arab side, only amplified Israel's need to neutralize Nasser immediately. But Levi Eshkol, Israel's bland but sagacious prime minister, and Abba Eban, the urbane foreign minister, fretted over the American reaction. Would the United States act as it did in 1956, they worried, rescuing Nasser and forcing an Israeli retreat?

Though he shared many of the Israelis' concerns, Johnson did, in fact, oppose a preemptive strike, which he feared might drag the entire Middle East and perhaps the world into war. "Israel will not be alone unless it decides to go it alone," the president repeatedly told Eban at the White House on May 26. More portentously, Secretary of State Dean Rusk warned, "If Israel fires first, it'll have to forget the U.S." In a desperate effort to avoid a perilous war, the president proposed to assemble a convoy of ships from two dozen nations and sail it through the blockaded Tiran Straits to Eilat. If the Egyptians opened fired on the convoy, Johnson explained, the ships and planes of the U.S. Sixth Fleet would bombard strategic targets in Egypt. The plan, clandestinely known as Regatta, impressed the Israelis, who agreed to delay their offensive in order to give Johnson time to implement it. Congress, though, already reeling from America's entanglement in Vietnam, recoiled from any operation that was liable to lead to another foreign imbroglio. The Europeans, in a fashion reminiscent of their forebears' refusal to join a U.S.-led coalition against the Barbary pirates, rejected the proposal outright. "I failed. They're going to go," Johnson, referring to the Israelis, admitted to his aides. "They're going to hit. And there's nothing we can do about it."

Johnson's only consolation came from U.S. intelligence agencies that predicted Israel would swiftly overpower Egypt or any combination of Arab armies. The Israelis more than confirmed that forecast. In a surprise attack that began at eight o'clock in the morning of June 5, Israeli warplanes strafed and bombed Egyptian jets, most of which never left the ground, destroying 286 of them. Israeli tanks and mechanized units then punched through the fortified Egyptian lines in Sinai and Gaza. Honoring their treaties with Nasser, Jordanian and Syrian forces entered the fighting, only to be crushed by Israeli counteroffensives. Tortuous columns of destroyed Egyptian vehicles stretched the length of Sinai, while retreating Syrian and Jordanian troops left a trail of smoldering tanks and fallen comrades on the Golan Heights, throughout the West Bank, and across East Jerusalem. Jewish soldiers, by contrast, were planting the Israeli flag on the peak of Mount Hermon, wading with raised rifles into the Suez Canal, and dancing, their shoulders draped with bullet belts instead of prayer shawls, before the Western Wall.

Privately, at least, Johnson applauded Israel's triumph. While assuring the Soviets that America was making every effort to stop the fighting, the president, in fact, maneuvered to delay approval of a UN cease-fire until the Arabs' defeat was assured. Even after Israeli jets and missile boats on June 8 mistakenly fired on an American spy ship, the USS *Liberty*, killing thirty-four sailors and wounding 171, the president's position remained staunchly pro-Israel. His devotion was further tested the following day when the Soviets, in a move reminiscent of the 1956 crisis, announced their intention to intervene militarily. But Johnson refused to flinch. "Find out exactly where the Sixth Fleet is," he instructed his advisers, "and tell it to turn around." The Soviets backed down and continued to watch as Israel concluded its rout.

The Six-Day War, as it would be remembered by Israel and the West, represented the greatest military triumph in the Middle East since the British defeat of the Germans at El Alamein twenty-five years earlier. Israel suddenly controlled territories more than three times its original size and placed at least two million Palestinian Arabs—residents of East Jerusalem, the West Bank, and Gaza—under occupation. The geographical, political, and human consequences of the war owed much to Johnson's decision making, but so did the peacemaking efforts that followed the fighting. No sooner was the cease-fire accepted than the president asked Undersecretary of State Rostow to draw up a comprehensive peace plan. "Let us not forget that a crisis is also an opportunity," Rostow told his staff. "Many patterns become loosened, and doors open. Let your minds rove over the horizon."[14]

The American formula called for Israeli withdrawals from occupied Arab territories in exchange for Arab recognition of the rights of all states in the region to exist in peace "within secure and recognized boundaries." The proposal also cited the need for a "just settlement" of the Palestinian refugee problem. These guidelines served as the basis of UN Resolution 242, enacted that November, and as the starting point for what soon became known as the peace process. The chances for the initiative's success did not, however, appear auspicious. Though Israel offered to relinquish all of Sinai and the Golan Heights in return for formal peace treaties with Egypt and Syria, it also unilaterally annexed East Jerusalem. The Arab states, meeting in Khartoum, enacted the notorious "three no's"—no negotiating with Israel and no granting it peace or recognition. The Palestinians were furious over the failure of 242 to address their right to self-determination and resolved to carry on the armed struggle to eliminate Israel. The effort would be spearheaded by the PLO, which, breaking free of Egyptian control, came under al-Fatah's sway and the chairmanship of Arafat.

The 1967 war, the reverberations of which continue to convulse the region, was a primary juncture in the making of the modern Middle East. Arab nationalism, a largely secular ideology, suffered a setback from which it would never recover and which accelerated the rise of its rival, Islamic extremism. Zionism was conversely reinforced by Israel's victory and, through the Jewish people's reunion with their spiritual homeland in Jerusalem and the West Bank, galvanized by a new religious zealotry. The war was also pivotal for America's relations with the region. For the millions of evangelical Americans who had always valued Israel as the fulfillment of biblical prophecies, the Six-Day War was an act of divine intervention designed to hasten the coming of the messianic age. But the victory also persuaded American policymakers, many of whom had previously advised against maintaining close relations with the Jewish state, to view Israel as America's small but muscular cohort in the Cold War.

Israel's transformation in American eyes from distant friend to de facto ally was scarcely lost on the Arabs. In spite of Johnson's efforts to achieve peace and to restore their captured lands, six Arab states followed Egypt's lead in severing relations with Washington. Nasser proceeded to launch a war of attrition in which Egyptian and Israeli forces facing each other across the Suez Canal exchanged daily salvos of high-explosive shells, sniper fire, and aerial strafing. From Jordan, PLO units regularly bombarded Israeli border towns and settlements. If intended to hamper the intensifying ties between Washington and Jerusalem, these assaults had precisely the opposite effect. Johnson sold 150 warplanes to the Israeli air force, completing the process through which the United States replaced France as Israel's principal arms supplier.

Though hardly conducive to mediation, these developments seemed only to stiffen Johnson's resolve to mount a major Middle East peace effort in 1968. The need for such an initiative appeared to be underscored by the assassination of Robert F. Kennedy, the late president's younger brother and a contender for the presidency, by a deranged Palestinian named Sirhan Sirhan. The murder took place on the first anniversary of the Six-Day War, but by that time Johnson had dropped out of the electoral race, a victim of domestic backwash from Vietnam. The Johnson period, a turbulent interlude in which Cold War considerations vied with religious stimuli in the making of America's Middle East policies, had ended. Faith, however, would play little or no role in shaping the next administration's attitudes toward the region, nor would fanciful illusions. Starting in 1969, piety and illusions gave way to a staid and almost purblind focus on power.

American Metternichs in the Middle East

The Middle East inherited by Richard Milhous Nixon was a doleful place, war-wracked and ideologically fractured, but the president had the bleak, disjointed personality to match it. Though he was raised in a God-fearing Quaker family, religion played an imperceptible role in Nixon's handling of Middle Eastern affairs. Rather, his policies were informed solely by his sense of the Soviet threats facing the region and of the potency America needed to meet that menace. All other objectives—the attainment of Arab-Israeli peace or the broadening of Arab-American understanding—became, in Nixon's mirthless mind, subordinate to Cold War exigencies.

Nixon's worldview was to a large extent shared by his brilliant but inscrutable adviser on national security, Dr. Henry A. Kissinger. As a teenage Jewish refugee from Nazi Germany, Kissinger had learned the perils of political chaos and, conversely, the paramount value of stability. The hero of his Harvard doctoral dissertation was Metternich, the artful Austrian prince who managed to preserve his empire's interests throughout the Sturm und Drang of post-Napoleonic Europe and to maintain a finely wrought balance between the powers. Kissinger sought to replicate Metternich's achievement on a global scale, fortifying America's role internationally and establishing a durable equilibrium with Moscow.

The challenge was far from trivial, especially in the Middle East. "The difference between our goal and the Soviet goal in the Middle East is very simple," Nixon explained. "We want peace. They want the Middle East." Accordingly, the administration sought to prevent the outbreak of another Arab-Israeli war, which would render the Arabs even more dependent on Soviet arms and advisers, and to protect the friendly regimes of Jordan, Iran, and Saudi Arabia. Israel's security also preoccupied the president. His attachment to the Jewish state owed little to his Quaker legacy or to his desire for electoral support—less than 8 percent of America's Jews had voted for him—but once again to his need to repel the Russians. "Israel is the current most effective stopper to the Mideast power of the Soviet Union," he told a delegation of senior legislators. "I am supporting Israel because it is in the interest of the United States to do so." But Nixon also believed that an Israel that felt secure in its alliance with America would take the risks necessary for attaining peace. Less than a year after assuming office, the president authorized his secretary of state, William P. Rogers, to mediate an end to fighting between Egypt and Israel and to press Israel to accept a territory-for-peace arrangement on the basis of Resolution 242. In keeping with the spirit of détente, Nixon invited the Soviets to co-sponsor the initiative.

Nixon had embarked on a proactive and calculating course in the Middle East, but events converged to derail its progress. In Libya, the dashing and often delusional Colonel Muammar Qadhafi (or Qaddafi) had ousted King Idris, closed the Wheelus air base, and warmly allied himself with the Kremlin. Soviet arms streamed into Algeria and Sudan, and thousands of Red Army advisers deployed in Egypt, South Yemen, Syria, and Iraq. Rogers secured a cease-fire between Egypt and Israel, but then Nasser violated it by moving his Soviet-made missiles into the truce zone. The Israeli prime minister, Golda Meir—the former Golda Meyerson of Milwaukee—was happy to receive Rogers's assistance in ending the attrition war and eager to accept Nixon's offer of additional arms sales. But she refused to give up the territories Israel captured in 1967 for anything less than full peace. Nasser still recoiled from the notion of talking with Israel, much less reconciling with it.[15]

The administration's inability to achieve even its minimum policy goals in the Middle East was exemplified by the escalating lawlessness in Jordan. The PLO had established a virtual state within a state in the country; it regularly sent guerrilla bands across the Jordan River into the occupied West Bank and fired rockets at Israeli border settlements. Israel retaliated massively for these raids, perpetuating yet another round of spiraling violence. But tensions took on a sharper, international edge on September 6, 1970, when Palestinian guerrillas waylaid three passenger planes belonging to TWA, Swissair, and Pan Am and forced them to land in the Jordanian desert. The hijackers took fifty-four hostages, thirty-four of them Americans, and sequestered them in an Amman hideout. They then set charges under the aircraft and, with cameras whirring, blew them apart.

The explosions ignited the long-simmering confrontation between the PLO and Jordan, the period preserved in Palestinian memory as Black September. Vicious fighting broke out between Palestinian militias and forces loyal to Hussein, Jordan's bantam king. The royalists quickly subdued the rebels, but then the Syrians threatened to intervene on the Palestinians' behalf. A panicked Hussein appealed to the United States to save him from the numerically superior Syrian army, but the administration demurred. Though Nixon admired Hussein and appreciated Jordan's value in the Cold War, he feared that any attempt to aid the kingdom militarily would provoke the Soviets to intercede in Syria and trigger a direct superpower clash. Only one alternative remained. Using a secret phone line that had been installed between the White House and the Israeli embassy, Kissinger asked Ambassador Yitzhak Rabin, the chief of staff during the Six-Day War and the son of a former New Yorker, whether Israel would move its army into northern Jordan to block the Syrians' advance. Jewish troops were being asked to sacrifice their lives for the sake of an Arab monarch and for the security of the United States. Rabin conveyed the request to Meir in Jerusalem, who promptly approved it.

Israeli assistance, as it turned out, proved unnecessary. Jordanian jets picked off Syrian tank formations as they rumbled across the border. Arafat and the PLO were banished to Lebanon and Hussein reigned on as the unvanquished Hashemite king. The White House, though, would long remember Israel's readiness to fight at America's behest. Over the next three years, American military aid to the Jewish state multiplied tenfold and pressure for Israeli territorial concessions ceased.

The emerging alliance between Israel and the world's paramount superpower made an immense impression on Arab rulers. While the Soviet Union might provide them with the wherewithal of war, only the United States could furnish the diplomatic leverage needed to pry captured Arab lands from Israel's grip. And few Arab leaders understood this subtle but momentous change better than Anwar Sadat. Having risen to power after Nasser's death—literally, from heartbreak, while trying to resolve the Black September crisis—the dark and gangly Sadat was widely viewed as an unsubstantial lackey. His anti-American utterances were legion. Yet Sadat would soon reveal himself to be an astute and farsighted statesman, a visionary who foresaw the importance of wooing the Americans away from Israel and back into the Arab fold. The road to Sinai ran not through Damascus or Moscow, Sadat realized, but through the capital of the United States.

Sadat lost little time in signaling his openness to Washington. "You would be mistaken to think that [Egypt] was in the sphere of Soviet influence," he informed Nixon, assuring him that if the United States "proves friendly to us, we shall be ten times as friendly." Sadat further indicated that, in return for an interim agreement that facilitated the reopening of the Suez Canal, closed since the Six-Day War, and the return of a symbolic number of Egyptian troops to Sinai, he would evict the Soviet advisers from Egypt. "There is no reason why the Arabs should be closely aligned to the Soviet Union," he said. "My people like the West better." Sadat branded 1971 as his year of decision and stressed that the direction in which Egypt turned, whether toward peace or war, hinged principally on America.

Nixon was eager to explore Sadat's intentions, but events—international, regional, and domestic—again conspired to obstruct him. Deeply engaged in secret negotiations to end the Vietnam War and in efforts to reach an agreement with the Soviets on limiting nuclear arms, the administration shied away from any policies that were liable to irritate Moscow. Instead, in May 1971, the superpowers pledged to work collectively toward an overall Arab-Israeli settlement. A year later, Sadat abruptly expelled as many as fifteen thousand Soviet advisers from Egypt, but his coup de main failed to effect a change in American policy. Détente with the Soviets still took precedence over Arab-Israeli peacemaking.

The chances for diplomatic breakthroughs further receded over the course of 1972. Among the worst hindrances to peace were actions by the PLO and other Palestinian organizations that, in the wake of the 1967 defeat, had attained a new heroic status in Arab eyes. Eager to build on this popularity and to focus international attention on their cause, the Palestinians launched a series of increasingly brazen and bloody attacks against Israeli targets. These reached a climax in September 1972, when masked members of Black September, a PLO offshoot named for the preceding year's war in Jordan, slaughtered eleven Israeli athletes at the Munich Olympic Games. The Munich massacre was the first major terrorist action to be captured live on television and watched by much of America. It was also the harbinger of far deadlier violence to come. Nixon nevertheless reacted perfunctorily to Munich, refusing to denounce the PLO's Soviet and Arab backers or even to lower the White House flag to half-staff. More pressing for the president was the need to counter accusations of deep-seated corruption in the White House and charges that his staffers had burglarized the offices of the Democratic National Committee in Washington's Watergate Hotel.

As long as the United States remained committed to joint diplomacy with the Soviets, and with much of the Middle East in flames and the president politically hamstrung, Sadat could not hope to achieve a negotiated accord. Kissinger, who replaced Rogers as secretary of state in September 1973, proposed a step-by-step process of Egyptian commitments to Israeli security and Israeli recognition of Egyptian sovereignty over Sinai, but his efforts proved tardy.[16] At two o'clock in the afternoon of October 6—a day after Kissinger discussed his plan with Sadat's foreign minister—Egypt went to war.

The attack, coordinated with a Syrian assault across the Israeloccupied Golan Heights, caught the United States completely off guard. The country's attention was riveted on Watergate and Nixon, retreating to his Florida home, left much of the decision making to Kissinger. The secretary had accepted intelligence assessments that war in the Middle East was highly improbable—"We were brainwashed by the Israelis who brainwashed themselves," one American official complained—and was successfully misled by Sadat. The Israelis were no less shocked. Most of them were at home that day or in synagogue observing the holiest Jewish holiday of Yom Kippur. Prime Minister Meir had earlier been warned about the offensive and considered striking Egypt preemptively as Israel had done in 1967, but Kissinger dissuaded her. The international community no longer viewed Israel as a David fighting the Arab Goliath, he explained, and would condemn the Israelis as aggressors. Meir concurred and the cost of her decision proved exorbitant. Under a nearly impenetrable umbrella of artillery shells and ground-to-air missiles, some eighty thousand Egyptian troops stormed over bridges and ferried across the Suez Canal. They overran the outnumbered and unprepared Israelis and established an inextricable foothold in Sinai. Hundreds of Syrian tanks meanwhile plowed through the minefields and redoubts on the Golan Heights. The scenes of desert roads lined with charred tanks and blackened bodies were revisited, only this time most of the wreckage was Israeli.

The Yom Kippur War or, as the Arabs called it, the October War, was the crucible of Kissinger's realist approach to Middle Eastern politics. His goals in the crisis were threefold: to stop the bloodshed as rapidly as possible, to prevent the Soviets from gaining any political advantages from the crisis, and to lay the groundwork for postwar American mediation. The United States would accordingly place its diplomatic weight behind UN efforts to achieve a cease-fire and flex its military muscle to discourage Soviet intervention in the war. Though Israel was expected to rally and quickly repulse the Arab invaders, the administration assumed it would make extensive territorial concessions once the fighting ended. "We could not make our policy hostage to the Israelis," Kissinger said, emphasizing that anti-Americanism in the Arab world suited Israel's interests but was, for the United States, "a disaster."

Events in the field, however, once again failed to conform to America's agenda. The anticipated Israeli counterattack did not materialize and the embattled Jewish state soon found itself desperately bereft of supplies. The Arabs, by contrast, were receiving continuous shipments of guns and ammunition from the Soviets. Kissinger deliberated whether or not to respond to the Soviets' move; the Defense Department claimed that restocking Israel would harm America's war effort in Vietnam. But the prospect of victory for communist arms was sufficiently horrific to rouse Richard Nixon from his seclusion. "Whatever it takes," the president commanded, "save

Israel." Galaxy and Starlifter aircraft subsequently flew the 6,000-mile journey to Tel Aviv some three hundred times—Operation Nickel Grass—and delivered more than 22,000 tons of matériel. The replenished Israeli forces doggedly turned the tide, driving the Syrians back to Damascus within a week and encircling the Egyptian army in Sinai.

Washington initially welcomed this battlefield turnaround, until it precipitated two unexpected and ominous results. First, the Arab oil producers whose families had been doctored by American missionaries, enriched by American oil companies, and protected by every president cut off oil supplies to the United States and other industrialized countries, ostensibly in retaliation for their support of Israel. Production lines and power stations all but shut down and long lines of vehicles waited with empty tanks at gas-depleted filling stations throughout America. Far more harrowing than the Arab use of the oil weapon, however, was the Soviets' decision to place their ground and naval forces on the highest alert, hazarding a nuclear exchange.

The United States suddenly confronted the specter of an American economy paralyzed by lack of fuel and, more nightmarishly, of a global war with Russia. "We may have to take [the Soviets] on," Kissinger conceded. "We have to be tough as nails now." Demonstrating that tenacity, war-ready state of DEFCON-III was declared for American troops in Europe and for the Sixth Fleet in the eastern Mediterranean. At the same time, the White House concentrated immense pressure on the Israelis to halt their drive on Damascus and to ease their stranglehold on the Egyptian army. Several cease-fire efforts foundered and American and Soviet battleships nearly scraped prows. Nevertheless, by October 28, Israeli soldiers were delivering jerry cans of water to their Egyptian counterparts and cooperating with them on tension-reducing measures. The UN Security Council passed Resolution 338, calling for a "just and durable peace" on the basis of 242 and providing for an international conference to achieve it. An exultant Kissinger reported to Nixon, "It was a tremendous victory."[17]

The secretary was perhaps overly generous in his self-praise. By concentrating almost exclusively on global strategic factors, the United

States had failed to prevent a regional conflict and, by dallying on diplomatic efforts, may even have hastened its eruption. As many as fifteen thousand Arabs lay dead and more than twenty-five hundred Israelis. The war had also exposed serious splits within the Western alliance, as many NATO countries closed their airspace to American planes flying to Israel. "The Europeans behaved like jackals," Kissinger later commented. "Their behavior was a total disgrace."

Could realism alone suffice to rectify this devastation and clear a pathway toward peace? The dispiriting answer was provided in Geneva, where, in December 1973, the international peace conference convened. The Arab delegates refused to discuss a political settlement in advance of a total Israeli withdrawal from the occupied territories; the Syrians boycotted the proceedings entirely. Propelled by the Arab embargo, meanwhile, the price of oil skyrocketed nearly 400 percent, and Palestinian organizations that had been excluded from Geneva carried out massacres in two northern Israeli towns. This was the seismic environment in which Kissinger undertook his most delicate diplomatic task.

Fifty years after the State Department abandoned the tradition of appointing Jewish immigrants from Germany like Simon Wolf, Oscar Straus, and Henry Morgenthau as intermediaries between America and the Muslim world, replacing them with the descendants of missionaries, another German-born American Jew was mediating in the Middle East. Employing the tactic pioneered by Robert B. Anderson in the 1950s, the secretary shuttled between Arab and Israeli capitals in a step-by-step effort to separate the warring armies. Unlike Anderson, though, who traveled incommunicado, Kissinger peregrinated in public. A typical day began with a visit to Cairo and kisses of greeting from Sadat followed by a stopover in Damascus, to be kissed by the Syrian dictator Hafez al-Assad, and concluded in Tel Aviv, where Kissinger finally embraced Golda Meir. "Oh, Mr. Secretary," the prime minister quipped, "I didn't know you kissed girls, too." But behind the bonhomie, the negotiations were strained, especially with the Israelis, whom Kissinger often had to browbeat into compliance. The result was separation-of-forces agreements on the Egyptian and Syrian fronts and the renewal of diplomatic ties between America and the Arab world.

Buoyed by these successes, Kissinger was poised to progress toward more far-reaching Arab-Israeli agreements, but obstacles sprouted in his path. Desperate for a respite from Watergate and to revel in his last diplomatic success, Nixon deplaned in the Middle East in June 1974. Exuberant crowds turned out to greet the president in Egypt, Syria, Jordan, and Saudi Arabia, and the Israelis treated him deferentially. The adulation did little to improve his status at home, however, and Nixon resigned shortly after returning. His replacement, the affable but lackluster Gerald Ford, had little experience in statecraft and was generally unversed in the Middle East. Golda Meir, who stepped down four months after Nixon, was succeeded by Yitzhak Rabin, a deceptively quiet politician who proved equally hawkish on territorial issues. The infelicitous combination of Ford and Rabin produced the direst crisis in U.S.-Israel relations since Suez, with Ford announcing a "reassessment" of American support for the Jewish state. Rabin responded by mobilizing the American Israel Public Affairs Committee—AIPAC, the pro-Israel lobby—against the president. Though founded in 1953, AIPAC had only now, in the mid-1970s, achieved the financial and political clout necessary to sway congressional opinion. Confronted with opposition from both houses of Congress, Ford rescinded his "reassessment."

Still, Kissinger, who remained as Ford's secretary of state, succeeded in mediating a second treaty between Israel and Egypt, in September 1975. Israel agreed to further pullbacks in Sinai in return for Egyptian pledges of nonbelligerency and American security guarantees. The accord perhaps owed less to Kissinger's Metternichian approach, though, than to the deepening desire of Egyptians and Israelis for peace. A more notorious example of Kissinger's dispassionate diplomacy in the Middle East occurred that same year when, during a border dispute between Iran and Iraq, the secretary clandestinely encouraged Iraqi Kurds to revolt against Iraqi rule. The Kurds rebelled, but the shah and Saddam Hussein soon resolved their differences, freeing the Iraqi army to crush the insurrection. The Kurds appealed to Kissinger for help, but the secretary was now impervious. "Covert action should not be confused with missionary work," he said.[18]

For seven years, throughout the terms of Nixon and Ford, the United States had weathered relentless upheavals in the Middle East. It had braved a whirlwind of battles, coups, and boycotts and had skirted Soviet squalls. Both presidents strove to restore America's status in the Arab world and restrict that of Russia, all the while nurturing a delicate strategic balance. Their achievements, in the final reckoning, were impressive. Egypt, the predominant Arab state, had been coaxed back into the American orbit and Soviet influence in the region, though still strong in Syria, Iraq, and Libya, was contained. Arabs and Israelis for the first time since the 1949 armistice had initialed diplomatic agreements and renounced further recourse to war. Peace, in the view of many of the conflict's parties, was attainable— not under the watch of the UN or the Soviet Union, however, but solely under the auspices of the United States.

Yet peace remained a remote destination toward which American leaders still had to trudge. Israel was already building settlements in the territories it had captured in 1967, signaling its resistance to the concessions intimated by Resolution 242. Hafez al-Assad sent forty thousand Syrian soldiers into civil war–torn Lebanon, beginning a brutal thirty-year occupation. The terror first unleashed against the Israelis soon lashed out at Americans. Cleo Allen Noel Jr., the U.S. ambassador to Sudan, and his chargé, George Curtis Moore, were abducted and shot by the PLO in March 1973—freeing Sirhan Sirhan was one of the organization's demands—and three years later, Palestinian gunmen killed Ambassador Francis Meloy and the economic counselor Robert Waring in Beirut. On September 8, 1974, a TWA jet en route from Tel Aviv to New York was destroyed in midair by a bomb planted in its cargo hold, killing all eighty-eight passengers. Islamic radicalism smoldered and fumed throughout the region, fanned by the Arabs' failure to vanquish Israel militarily and by the dominance of dictatorial regimes, some of them sustained by America. Attaining interim truces in such an environment, much less a *pax Americana*, would require not just realism but ethics and imagination as well. Those qualities, precisely, distinguished Ford's successor, the most faith-guided and fantasy-infused president to date.

Deacons, Doyens, and Shahs

Peanut farmer, Annapolis-trained submariner, governor of Georgia—Jimmy Carter had consummated several careers before becoming America's thirty-ninth president. Throughout, though, Carter remained a believing Christian, a Baptist deacon, and a daily reader of the Bible. "I want the fullness of Christ in my life more than I want anything—even politics," he confessed. That piety persisted after Carter entered the White House in January 1977. Like Woodrow Wilson, he dreamed of establishing a "fellowship of faith" in international relations and of pursuing a humanitarian policy overseas. His apostolic approach to foreign affairs often proved peculiar to world leaders, even those who shared his righteousness. "After a couple of hours with President Carter, I had the feeling that two religious leaders were conversing," recalled Pope John Paul II.

Carter's religious fervor was also evident in his almost obsessive focus on the Middle East. The area contained the Holy Land, which had always been a source of passion for the new president, and the State of Israel, support for which he regarded as a "significant moral principle." Such views remained exceedingly popular among the evangelical Christians whose congregations now surpassed those of mainline Protestant churches in size and political influence. Restorationism was resurgent and so was the notion, once pervasive in colonial America, of Islam as a tool of the anti-Christ. But Carter dissented from these tenets in his criticism of Israeli policies in the West Bank and Gaza and his sympathy for the Palestinians' plight. In contrast to Nixon and Kissinger, who addressed the conflict purely on the plane of power, Carter sought to reconcile the belligerents on the basis of their common devoutness. "The blood of Abraham . . . still flows in the veins of Arab, Jew, and Christian," Carter avowed. "The spilled blood in the Holy Land still cries out to God—an anguished cry for peace."[19]

In response to that lamentation, Carter relinquished the monopoly over Middle East peacemaking meticulously built by the preceding administration. He invited the Soviets to join him in hosting another international peace conference and declared his intention to seek Israel's withdrawal from all of the occupied territories. Most surprisingly Carter pledged to realize "legitimate Palestinian rights"—a euphemism for creating a Palestinian state—and to negotiate with the PLO once it accepted Resolution 242.

These measures hardly endeared Carter to evangelical leaders who, in widely circulated advertisements, stated, "The time has come for evangelical Christians to affirm their belief in biblical prophecy and Israel's divine right to the land." The president's positions also antagonized Menachem Begin, the commander of the Irgun militia in 1948, head of the right-wing Likud party, and now Israel's newly elected prime minister. But while alienating evangelicals and many Israelis, Carter failed to impress Sadat. The Egyptian ruler was appalled by Carter's willingness once again to subject the peace process to Soviet, Syrian, and PLO whims and by his apparent reluctance to arm-twist the Israelis. Instead of waiting for a change in Washington's policies, Sadat opened direct secret channels to Begin. The outcome of these talks was broadcast to the world on November 19, 1977, when Sadat, illuminated by hundreds of flashbulbs, stepped onto the tarmac at Tel Aviv's airport and became the first Arab leader to visit the Jewish state.

The United States had almost no part in that historic event, nor was it involved in the ensuing treaty discussions between Begin and Sadat. The talks quickly became deadlocked, however, and both sides concluded that progress toward peace was unattainable without American mediation at the highest level. Carter consequently became the first president since Teddy Roosevelt arbitrated the Algeciras conference in 1906 to engage personally in Middle East mediation and the first to style himself a "full partner" with Arabs and Israelis, seeking a common ground.

The task of locating that median, however, proved grueling. Sadat demanded that the Israelis vacate all of the occupied territories and provide for Palestinian self-determination. Begin would not hear of conceding the West Bank, Gaza, and the Golan and insisted on retaining Israeli positions in Sinai as well. Carter almost unreservedly accepted the Egyptian position and assiduously rejected Israel's. Especially galling for Carter were the Israeli settlements that had proliferated in the occupied territories. "We all felt that the Egyptian leader had gone out on a limb in order to promote peace in the region and that Begin was busily sawing the limb off," remembered Carter's national security adviser, Zbigniew Brzezinski. But beyond policy differences, the president evinced a personal aversion to Begin's abrasiveness and the rough-and-tumble of Israeli democracy. He preferred the courtly Sadat, who, regularly reelected by more than 95 percent of his citizens, was unrestrained in his decision making—another exemplar of the noble, unfettered nomad. "There was also a bit of hero worship," Brzezinski added, recalling how Carter told Sadat, "You are probably the most admired statesman in the United States."

Carter's devotion to peace for peace's sake, not as a vehicle for sidelining the Soviets, and his affection for Sadat converged at Camp David in September 1978. He had summoned Israeli and Egyptian leaders to the presidential retreat in a final, intensive effort to forge a compromise between them. Shuttling now between bungalows rather than capitals, Carter threatened Begin with a cutoff of American aid to Israel and cajoled Sadat with promises of augmented support. The combination of admonishments and largesse proved fruitful, producing two interlocking treaties collectively called the Camp David Accords. In the first of these, establishing peace between Israel and Egypt, Israel consented to withdraw completely from Sinai in exchange for normal ties with Egypt, including an end to anti-Israel incitement in the Egyptian press. The United States served as guarantor of the agreement by maintaining observers on the Egypt-Israeli border and by providing billions of dollars of aid annually to both countries. The second accord furnished a framework for peace between Israel and the other Arab countries and a solution for the Palestinian problem. A five-year period of Palestinian autonomy in the West Bank and Gaza would be followed by talks on the territories' final status, potentially leading to statehood.

The three-way handshake with which Begin, Sadat, and Carter sealed their agreement on the White House lawn in March 1979 became the emblem of America's preeminence in Middle East peacemaking and the high-water mark that later presidents would aspire to match. "The Camp David Accords had now become almost like the Bible," Carter commented, but he alone seemed to regard those texts as scripture. Israel agreed to grant autonomy to the Palestinian residents of the territories but not to the land, which it continued to stake out with settlements. The Egyptians never normalized relations with Israel or ended incitement against it—and Jews in general—in state-controlled media. Most of the Arab world, meanwhile, led by Syria, Iraq, and Libya, denounced the treaty as treasonous and declared a total boycott of Egypt. Arafat also rebuffed the autonomy scheme and called for Sadat's assassination. No less adamant in their damning of the accords were the Islamic radicals whose influence was burgeoning throughout the Middle East. While watching a military parade in Cairo on the eighth anniversary of the October War in 1981, Sadat was gunned down by Egyptian members of Islamic Jihad, who continued to shout "Death to the Pharoah!" as they raked his breathless body with bullets.[20]

CARTER HAD come to the Middle East committed to Christian and American ideals but, apart from one dazzling moment on the White House lawn, was unable to realize any of them. Rather, the region remained a maelstrom of inter-Arab tensions and Cold War stress, of friction between Arabs and Israelis and rising fundamentalist opposition to insecure despotic regimes. The turbulent state of the Middle East in the 1970s might have dispelled any enduring illusions about the area, certainly the sexual aura with which Westerners had long endowed it. But myth once again proved more durable than reality, especially among the Hollywood doyens of mythmaking.

One of the most persistent of those reveries, that of the free-ranging Arab who absconds with a fair-skinned Western maid, again captivated audiences in 1975. *The Wind and the Lion* boasted of being based on a true story: the kidnapping of Ion Perdicaris by the Berber chieftain Raisuli seventy years earlier. But dramatic tension could not be served by the sight of Raisuli, played by the perennially virile Sean Connery, decamping with a plump and balding businessman of sixty-four, and so the film transmuted Ion Perdicaris into Eden Perdicaris, fetchingly portrayed by Candice Bergen. The movie took further license with history when it depicted Teddy Roosevelt dispatching U.S. Marines to Morocco in order to rescue Perdicaris, but not before romance blooms between her and the red-blooded Raisuli.

The image of the Middle East as a realm of dark and limitless sexuality also inspired one of the most popular American songs of the 1970s—"Midnight at the Oasis," sung by a sultry Maria Muldaur. The theme was the same as that of *The Sheik of Araby* of fifty years earlier, only the seducer this time had become a seductress. "You won't need no harem, honey, when I'm by your side," she cooed, "And you won't need no camel, no, no, when I take you for a ride." Yet not even the entertainment industry could remain impervious to the upheaval convulsing the Middle East. Americans of the 1970s, much like their forebears two hundred years earlier, were not only titillated by phantasms about the region but also unnerved by its threats. In the suspense thriller *Black Sunday* (1977), Hollywood for the first time spotlighted the subject of Palestinian terrorism. A master bomber named Muhammad Fasil (played by Bekim Fehmiu, a Bosnian) sought revenge against the American-Israel alliance by blowing up the Goodyear blimp over the Superbowl. Though the plot was foiled in the last minute by Israeli agents, the idea of Middle Eastern extremists committing mass murder on American soil had been seeded in the public's imagination.

These countervailing images of the Middle East, one romantic and the other brutally real, once again coexisted in the American mind. But a fundamental schism in the interpretation of Middle Eastern cultures and politics was also surfacing in universities. Two eminent scholars were offering antithetical views of the region, one radical and unexceptionally sympathetic and the other traditional and fault-finding.

Edward Said, an Arab Christian raised in Cairo and Jerusalem, attended Princeton and Harvard before receiving a professorship in English at Columbia. Handsome, articulate, and musically gifted, he gained prominence as a literary critic and a spokesman for Palestinian rights. Then, in 1978, Said departed from literature and politics and published *Orientalism*, an assault on the traditional academic interpretations of the Middle East. Unable "to discover any period in European or American history . . . in which Islam was . . . thought about *outside* a framework created by passion, prejudice and political interests," he accused Western scholars of inventing a place they called the Middle East, a culturally inferior and politically hostile "other." By dissecting and analyzing this region, Said asserted, these experts rendered it more easily conquerable by the West.

As history, Said's thesis was difficult to sustain—Edward Salisbury, America's first professor of Arabic in 1841, was hardly an imperialist—yet *Orientalism* served to expose the biases that had long marred Western writing about the Middle East, as exemplified by the works of Melville, Mark Twain, and Edith Wharton. The manifesto also appealed to a generation of American academicians who, in reaction to the Vietnam fiasco and the West's exploitation of developing countries, had grown skeptical of their own civilization's virtue. They agreed with Said that the field of Middle Eastern studies was little more than an ancillary to colonialism and that the only authentic Middle East scholar was one who remained "engaged and sympathetic . . . to the Islamic world" and who "identified . . . wholeheartedly with the Arabs." Those failing to meet these criteria were dismissed as Orientalists, beginning with the Orientalist par excellence, Bernard Lewis.

A British-born Jew, Lewis immigrated to America and joined the faculty of Near Eastern studies at Princeton, where he occupied the chair named for the missionary-minded philanthropist Cleveland Dodge. He authored numerous works on Ottoman history and the emergence of the Arab world, becoming one of the nation's foremost authorities on Middle Eastern affairs. In contrast to Said, though, who imputed most Middle Eastern deficiencies to the West, the genteel and eloquent Lewis indicted the region for creating its own malaise and blaming it on Europe and America. "Compared with its millennial rival, Christendom, the world of Islam had become poor, weak, and ignorant," he wrote. The United States bore no responsibility for those failures, Lewis contended, though it could help rectify them by supplanting Middle Eastern tyrannies with American-style republics.

Such allegations were, for Said, the epitome of Orientalist disdain. He accused Lewis of positing "willful political assertions in the form of scholarly arguments" and of hiding "beneath the umbrella of academic respectability" his true identity as "lobbyist and a propagandist." The fact that Lewis was outspoken in his support of Israel—the apotheosis, according to Said, of Western imperialism—further discredited his views. Lewis countered by characterizing *Orientalism* as a tragedy that "takes a genuine problem . . . and reduces it to the level of political polemic and personal abuse."[21]

A debate on the disparate ways of perceiving the Middle East had unfolded on American campuses and from there radiated into society at large. One position held that the construction of clinics and universities and the construing of myths were merely precursors to conquest and that, to purge themselves of such evils, Americans had to distance themselves from the legacy of European and Israeli imperialism and abstain from demonstrations of power. But another school maintained that Americans had enriched the area with their visions and beliefs and could further enhance it with their might, by liberating the Middle East from despotism.

Jimmy Carter tried to take a middle road between these divergent paths. He expressed empathy for the Middle Eastern peoples and eschewed the use of force. Yet he insisted that American principles could rectify many of the region's shortcomings, while American strength—diplomatic and financial—would redress some of its most irresolvable conflicts. His approach, though, brought only momentary success in Arab-Israeli mediation and elsewhere failed entirely. And in no country was that failure more glaringly registered than in Iran.

IN SPITE of his avowals to promote freedom and democracy throughout the world, Carter overlooked the pervasive human rights abuses committed by friendly Middle Eastern states such as Egypt and Saudi Arabia. Few regimes were as systematically oppressive of their own populations, however, and more ardently allied with the United States, than Iran. Since his reinstatement by the CIA's anti-Mossadegh coup in 1953, the shah had proven to be fiercely anti-Soviet but also ruthless toward any Iranians he considered disloyal. His secret service, Savak, tortured and executed thousands. The Carter administration nevertheless continued its predecessors' policy of propping up the shah politically, indulging his sumptuous lifestyle, and equipping him with cutting-edge arms. Feted in Teheran on December 31, 1977, Carter toasted Iran as an "island of stability" in the Middle East and lauded its leader for his wisdom, sensitivity, and insight.

Carter's support for the shah remained undiluted throughout 1978, even as a popular revolt fermented against him. Finally, on January 16, 1979, the monarch was compelled to flee the country and two weeks later the exiled Ayatollah Ruhollah Khomeini, the grim-faced Shi'ite imam who had inspired the rebellion from abroad, returned triumphantly to Teheran. "Our relations with the United States are the relations of the oppressed with the oppressor, the relations of the plundered with the plunderer," Khomeini proclaimed. His words induced near ecstasy among his innumerable supporters, none of whom seemed to have remembered America's role in assuring Iran's independence after World War II. They surged through the streets chanting "Death to the Three Spreaders of Corruption, Sadat, Carter, and Begin!" and "Death to the Great Satan," meaning the United States.

Much like previous presidents, Carter was confounded by the appearance of a popular Middle Eastern leader who, though never enamored of the Soviets, showed scant affection for the West. He was further confused by the refusal of a religious man like Khomeini to respect even the most basic civic rights. "It's almost impossible to deal with a crazy man," Carter wrote. Despairing of chances of negotiating with the newly declared Islamic republic, the president permitted the shah, now sick with cancer, to receive medical treatment in United States. The gesture appeared noble to most Americans, the least Carter could do for an exiled and ailing ally, but Iranians were incensed by this display of hospitality to a tyrant, a fugitive they considered a war criminal.

On November 4, 1979, hundreds of Iranian students shouting "allahuakbar" and waving laminated photographs of Khomeini vaulted over the walls of the U.S. embassy compound in Teheran. They smashed into the chancery and residence buildings and captured sixty-six Americans—diplomats, administrative staff, Marine guards, and CIA officials. "We will teach you about God," one of the students ranted. "We will teach the CIA not to interfere with our country." In exchange for freeing the prisoners, the kidnappers demanded the shah's extradition and the transfer of his American holdings to Iran. They also insisted that the president apologize for a long list of American crimes against the Iranian people, beginning with the overthrow of Mossadegh.

The Iranian hostage crisis, as it came to be known, confronted Carter with a dilemma no less daunting than that which plagued Thomas Jefferson two hundred years earlier. The president could either try to reason with the piratical regime and purchase the hostages' release or forgo negotiations and fight. In a Jeffersonian manner, Carter first attempted to establish back channels to the inimical Middle Eastern government. "The people of the United States desire to have relations with Iran based on equality, mutual respect and friendship," he attested, and approved of the establishment of a UN commission to investigate America's iniquities against Iran. But Khomeini rejected these tokens, boasting how the Iranian revolution had "undermined the political, economic, and strategic hegemony of America in the region." Weary of this bad faith, the president finally resorted to power. He severed ties with Teheran, froze its American assets, and prohibited the import of Iranian oil into the United States. Proposals for imposing a broader boycott on Iran failed to gain international support, however, even from the Europeans.

The American hostages remained in Iranian custody, meanwhile, held in primitive conditions where they were frequently interrogated and occasionally threatened with execution. Force alone, it seemed, would restore their freedom. Carter considered many options, from destroying refineries and mining Iranian harbors to dropping an atomic bomb on Teheran. He ultimately decided on a rescue operation no less daring than William Eaton's trans-desert assault against Tripoli in 1805. Helicopter-borne commandos would fly into Teheran, retake the U.S. compound, and escape with the liberated captives.

Intensive training for the mission began immediately and lasted many months, during which time America's position in the Middle East continued to deteriorate. The closing weeks of 1979 saw a radical Wahhabi uprising in Saudi Arabia; hundreds were killed in an attempt to seize the Grand Mosque in Mecca. In Iraq, a bullish Soviet-backed dictator named Saddam Hussein grabbed power in a blood-soaked coup and proceeded to liquidate his rivals. Most stressful of all for the administration, however, was the Soviet invasion of Afghanistan. The presence of hordes of Soviet soldiers and multitudes of tanks along the Middle East's borders revived Truman's nightmare of a Red Army takeover of Dhahran and other petroleum lodes. "An attempt by any outside force to gain control of the Persian Gulf region will be regarded as an assault on the vital interests of the United States of America," Carter combatively informed Congress, warning that such attempts would be "repelled by any means necessary, including military force." An American president had once again declared a doctrine on the Middle East, but its impact on events now seemed negligible. A pincer of pro-Soviet and radical Islamic forces continued to close on America's interests in the area, while American hostages languished in captivity.

The sole hope for ameliorating this situation was Operation Eagle Claw, the raid to release the American prisoners, launched on the night of April 24, 1980. Landing in the Iranian desert, Delta Force and Ranger troops prepared to refuel their Sea Stallion helicopters for the flight to Teheran. But caught in a sudden sandstorm, two of the choppers broke down and a third crashed into a C-130 cargo plane, igniting a ball of flame that consumed both aircraft. Seven helicopters were left behind, some containing highly classified documents, along with the scorched corpses of eight American servicemen.[22] Iranian authorities exhibited some of the bodies at a press conference, evoking another image from the Barbary Wars—of the pasha of Tripoli displaying the remains of U.S. sailors killed by the *Intrepid*'s explosion. That atrocity spurred Jefferson to enter his second term determined to defeat the pirates with the help of Stephen Decatur and other stalwart warriors. But there would be no Decatur for Jimmy Carter, nor was there a second term.

The dust churned up by American helicopters fleeing Iran and by the Soviet tanks subduing Afghanistan obscured the glimmer of Carter's contributions to Arab-Israeli peace. Voters in the 1980 presidential elections were less impressed by his faith-inspired policies than by the perils of appearing to project weakness in the Middle East. Fittingly, Carter's last act in office was to negotiate an end to the hostage crisis. His method no longer recalled Jefferson's, though, but rather that of John Adams. Using Algeria, the former pirate state, as a go-between, he offered to pay the modern form of tribute by unfreezing Iranian bank accounts in the United States and indemnifying Iran from future lawsuits by the prisoners. Temporarily pacified, the Iranians ended their captives' 444-day incarceration—roughly one hundred days shorter than the imprisonment of Captain Bainbridge and the *Philadelphia*'s crew in Tripoli, but no less traumatic for Americans.

THE CONCLUSION of the hostage crisis represented the closing of a chapter in America's postwar relations with the Middle East. Throughout the preceding thirty years, the United States had tussled with the twin menaces of Soviet aggression and nationalist agitation in the area, navigating perilously between the two. Successive administrations sought to cast America as the champion of anticolonialism and at times even sided with native leaders in their struggles with Britain and France. But many people in the Middle East saw little difference between the Soviet Union and the United States, which, in their eyes, had superseded Europe as the ultimate imperialist power. America's support for the Jewish state further alienated the Arabs, especially after 1967, when the United States ceased viewing Israel as a liability in the Cold War and began embracing it as an asset. The attempts of every president, starting with Truman, to resolve the Arab-Israeli dispute tended to tarnish, rather than burnish, America's image in the area.

Decision makers in Washington nevertheless persisted in their peacemaking efforts throughout the period after 1980, all the while supporting an often recalcitrant Israel. The United States still sought a balance between maintaining its hegemony in the Middle East and preserving its essential values. Yet the nature of the threat to American interests was changing. Neither the Ba'athist-style dictators nor the customary kings had succeeded in raising the region's peoples from their political and economic malaise. On the contrary, the manifestations of backwardness, oppression, and military incompetence had only multiplied under both radical and conservative regimes. But now a resurgent movement rose to tap into the resentment generated by three hundred years of Muslim humiliation by the West, the suffering inflicted by autocratic Middle Eastern regimes, and the effrontery caused by a lax and impertinent modernity. Starting in 1979, Islamic extremism superseded socialist nationalism and conservative monarchism as the Middle East's most dynamic political force and the paramount challenger to American supremacy in the area. The Cold War coalition with Europe meanwhile continued to dissolve, leaving the United States increasingly unaided in confronting this new and implacable foe. Two hundred years after the Tripolitan envoy 'Abd al-Rahman lectured Jefferson and Adams on the Islamic injunction to fight "all Nations who should not have acknowledged [the Muslims'] authority," America would again fight holy warriors alone.

28

THE THIRTY
YEARS' WAR

THE DECADE THAT BEGAN IN 1981 WOULD BE REMEMBERED as a time of appalling disasters, from the explosion of the space shuttle *Challenger* to the spread of the AIDS epidemic. Less recollected, perhaps, was the era's distinction as a span of almost uninterrupted upheaval in America's relations with the Middle East. Preemptive attacks and regional conflicts, revolutions, international conspiracies, and terrorist strikes—punctuated the period and provoked a series of increasingly violent reactions from Washington. Over the course of those ten years, the image of the Middle East in the United States steadily hardened from that of a vaguely menacing conglomeration of states to a phalanx of bloodthirsty regimes that specifically targeted Americans.

Grappling with that transformation would prove to be a Sisyphean task for Carter's successor, a man of scarcely less rigorous convictions and an even greater fondness for Hollywood-spun myths. Inaugurated on the day of the hostages' release in Iran, Ronald Reagan, a former California governor and an actor in more than twenty-five movies and fifty television dramas, assumed responsibility for redressing America's Middle East failures. The new president indicated his intention of returning to the stern Cold War tactic of checking Soviet encroachments on the region and of restoring the Jeffersonian model of countering terrorists. "I don't think you pay ransom for people who have been kidnapped by barbarians," he said.

A Decade of Disorder

Reagan had barely settled into the White House when his first Middle East contest commenced. A radical socialist whose rhetoric had taken on a new religious bend, Muammar Qadhafi represented the shift from a pro-Soviet to an Islamic orientation that was subtly transforming Arab politics. The change was manifest in May 1981 when the Libyan leader proclaimed his support for Iran's struggle against "the Great Satan" and instructed a mob to burn down the U.S. embassy in Tripoli. "He's not only a barbarian, he's flaky," said Reagan, whose florid complexion and soft-spoken style contrasted starkly with the swarthy and blusterous Qadhafi. In retaliation for the embassy sacking, the president closed the Libyan People's Bureau in Washington and banned oil imports from the North African state. But then Qadhafi again taunted the United States by extending Libya's territorial waters twenty kilometers into the Mediterranean. Reagan retrieved this gauntlet and ordered a naval task force to demonstrate in the Gulf of Sidra, adjacent to Libya's coast. A squadron of Soviet-supplied SU-22 fighters flew out to challenge the flotilla, but Navy pilots speedily shot down two of them. For the first time since the Madison administration, American servicemen had engaged an Arab adversary in combat.

The dogfight over Sidra succeeded in quelling America's contretemps with Libya—for a while. Less than a month later, however, on June 7, a formation of F-16's was again soaring into action, this time against Iraq. But in place of five-pointed American stars, these aircraft were emblazoned with the sky-blue hexagrams of the Israeli air force. Their objective was the Osirak nuclear reactor, eighteen miles south of Baghdad. After flying 1,100 miles across enemy airspace, the Israeli pilots unleashed their payloads over the French-built facility and in eighty seconds reduced it to a smoking shell. Operation Opera, as it was code-named, was one of history's most daring aviation raids, but by destroying an Iraqi plant with fighters purchased from the United States, the Israelis placed the White House in a bind.

Reagan's relationship with Israel was, and would remain, complex. He still regarded oil as America's paramount interest in the Middle East and resisted any Israeli action that was liable to jeopardize it. In 1981, for example, he supplied AWACS surveillance aircraft to Saudi Arabia, defeating intense AIPAC efforts to block the sale, and when Arab oil producers protested Israeli steps to annex the occupied Golan Heights, the president suspended a strategic cooperation agreement with Israel. Prime Minister Begin complained that America treated Israel "like a banana republic," but Reagan in fact revered the Jewish state. Much of this admiration stemmed from his Manichean view of the Cold War, in which Israel had aligned itself with the West against the wicked Soviet empire. More fundamentally, Reagan, raised in the restorationist-minded Disciples of Christ church and closely associated with pro-Zionist American evangelicals, was religiously attached to Israel. He consistently endorsed measures to strengthen Israel militarily and economically and to assist Soviet (and later Ethiopian) Jews to immigrate to their ancestral homeland.

Israel's bombing of the Osirak reactor challenged that commitment. Fresh from his run-in with Qadhafi, Reagan could commiserate with Israeli fears of a Soviet-backed Arab dictator such as Saddam Hussein, but he also appreciated the fact that the Iraqis had recently launched a full-scale war against Iran. The enemy of America's enemy in the Middle East had automatically become its friend. Eager to dispel any semblance of collusion in an attack against America's new de facto ally, Reagan delayed the delivery of additional jet fighters to Israel. He also permitted America's pertinacious ambassador to the UN, Jeane Kirkpatrick, to confer with her Iraqi counterpart in drafting a Security Council condemnation of the raid. The Osirak raid did not, in the end, impair U.S.-Israel relations— later American presidents would thank Israel for denying nuclear capabilities to Iraq—but it did inaugurate ties between America and Saddam Hussein.[1]

The United States was once again placing its trust in a nationalist

Arab leader, though no longer as an anticommunist bastion but rather as a bulwark against Islamic radicals. Still, the policy of backing Arab secularists against Muslim extremists, on the one hand, and of supporting Israel against Soviet proxies, on the other, ultimately proved incompatible. The contradictions between the two were tragically unveiled a year after the raid on the Osirak reactor, with the Israeli invasion of Lebanon.

The Israelis had long prepared for this offensive. The PLO, which had transplanted its state within a state from Jordan to southern Lebanon, was regularly striking at Israeli settlements in the Galilee. But in addition to neutralizing this threat, Israel's portly, pugnacious defense minister, Ariel Sharon, sought to eliminate the PLO as a competitor for control over the West Bank and Gaza. An audacious commander who had led Israeli retaliation raids in the 1950s and had masterminded the encirclement of Egyptian forces in 1973, Sharon argued for a lightning strike to evict both Arafat and the Syrians from Lebanon and to install an amenable government in Beirut. The plan deeply cleaved Reagan's White House. The fiercely anticommunist Secretary of State Alexander Haig favored any move that was likely to harm the Soviets and their clients in the Arab world. Defense Secretary Caspar Weinberger, on the other hand, less bellicose and more pragmatic, worried about the damage the war would inflict on America's Middle East standing. The debate became academic, though, on June 3, 1982, when Palestinian gunmen shot and grievously wounded Israel's ambassador in London. Three days later, Israel invaded Lebanon.

Piercing the country in a two-pronged assault, some thirty thousand Israeli troops stormed up the coast and into the mountainous Lebanese interior, obliterating an estimated five hundred Syrian tanks and one hundred planes and driving six thousand Palestinian fighters northward to Beirut. Pursuing them, the Israeli army surrounded the city and proceeded to bombard PLO positions and headquarters. A dense murky pall hung over the city, backlit by flares and penetrated only by incendiary rounds. Operation Peace for Galilee, originally described as a limited incursion to secure Israel's northern border, had mushroomed into a massive siege of a major Arab capital containing tens of thousands of civilians.

"No matter how villainous the attack on Israel's diplomat in London had been, it has not given Israel cause to unleash its brutal attack on Beirut," the president scolded Begin. The images of bombed-out neighborhoods, limbless children, and roads teeming with refugees were effacing whatever reverence America still commanded in the Arab world. More perilously, the defeat of Moscow's Syrian and Palestinian proxies revived the danger of direct Soviet intervention in the conflict. "We're walking a tightrope," wrote Reagan. He insisted that the Israelis halt their shelling immediately and pull their forces back from Beirut. Apart from prompting Haig's resignation, though, these demands went largely ignored. The Israeli bombardment intensified. Desperate, finally, to defuse the crisis, Reagan offered to oversee the transfer of Arafat and his followers to Tunis. Eighty years after Teddy Roosevelt dispatched the Marines to Beirut to protect the Americans living there, Reagan was sending them back to the city to supervise a Palestinian retreat.

Undertaken in conjunction with French and Italian forces, the Marines' evacuation of PLO fighters and personnel was an unequivocal success. Reagan marked the event by revealing a new Middle East peace plan. Israel, he declared, would pull out of the West Bank and Gaza, which would then be federalized with Jordan. The president subsequently sent a personal emissary, the affable Arab-American diplomat Philip Habib, to try to implement the program. Habib embarked under what appeared to be propitious circumstances. A looming disaster in Lebanon had been averted and a fissure to peace exposed. Under banners proclaiming "Job Well Done," the Marines waded onto their landing craft offshore.

They were back less than three weeks later. In the midst of Habib's mediation, on September 14, 1982, the Syrians assassinated the Lebanese president Bashir Gemayel, the Maronite leader with whom the Israelis had hoped to sign an accord. The murder provoked the Israelis into occupying much of Muslim Beirut and allowing Maronite militiamen to enter the Palestinian refugee camps of Sabra and Shatilla, where they massacred at least eight hundred civilians. The atrocity sparked an international outcry—Ariel Sharon was compelled to resign—and demands for American intervention to protect the Palestinians from further assault. Reagan, unable to resist this pressure, ordered the Marines to turn around and head back to war-shattered Beirut.

Their objective now was no longer to extricate Palestinians but to bolster the beleaguered government of Bashir Gemayel's brother, Amin. The Marines were once again cast in the role of innocents abroad, perceiving themselves as the defenders of democracy but seen by the Syrians, the Shiites, and the Druze as the imposers of a militant Maronite minority. Like the Iranians, these factions forgot America's contributions to Syrian and Lebanese independence and instead declared the United States a belligerent in Lebanon's interminable civil war. Landing, the Marines came under a withering fire, compelling them to shoot back with artillery and tanks and to bombard many of the same neighborhoods recently shelled by Israel. Not since World War II had U.S. ground forces been so actively engaged in Middle East combat. But even their firepower proved insufficient. Army units had to be sent in to reinforce the embattled Marines and warships from the Sixth Fleet positioned to pound enemy strongholds in the Shouf Mountains above Beirut.

And the enemy fought back, harder now and unconventionally. At midday on April 13, 1983, a suicide bomber belonging to Hizbollah (Party of God), an Iranian-backed Shi'ite organization, drove an explosives-laden truck into the U.S. embassy in Beirut. Seventeen Americans, many of them CIA officials, were killed, along with more than forty Lebanese. Six months later, on October 23, another Hizbollah bomber killed 241 servicemen—the deadliest single attack against Americans in the postwar period—at the lightly guarded Marine headquarters. Horrified, Americans watched on their living room TVs as rescue crews exhumed mangled bodies from the wreckage and listened as Reagan vowed to "resist those who seek to drive us out of that area." At first he seemed determined to fulfill that pledge. Fighters from the carriers *Kennedy* and *Independence* struck at Syrian targets—two planes were shot down and one of the pilots humiliatingly captured—and the battleship *New Jersey* fired its thunderous sixteen-inch guns at the Shouf. But by February 1984, Reagan realized that Lebanon was becoming a Vietnam-like quagmire and recalled all American troops.[2]

Reagan rebuffed charges that America had "cut and run" from

Lebanon, but the irrefragable fact remained that the United States had failed in its task of restraining Syria and its allies and, following the Iranian debacle, appeared to be retreating from the Middle East. The erosion of America's power in the region was underscored by Lebanon's cancellation of the peace treaty with Israel brokered by the United States and, more spectacularly, by a scourge of terrorist attacks against American citizens and institutions. Bombers, most likely belonging to Hizbollah, struck the American embassy in Kuwait on December 12, 1983, and the following September blew up an embassy annex in Beirut, killing two American soldiers. Hizbollah bombs killed eighteen American servicemen in a restaurant in Torrejon, Spain, in April 1984, and murdered twenty-two people that September in yet another Beirut embassy blast.

Hijackings and assaults on air terminals suddenly came back into vogue. Hizbollah terrorists executed two Americans when they forced a Kuwaiti plane to land in Teheran in December 1984, and six months later hijacked a TWA jet to Beirut, where they tortured and shot the U.S. Navy diver Robert Dean Stethem and dumped his body onto the tarmac. Five Americans were killed in grenade and machine-gun attacks staged by Abu Nidal, a Palestinian group, at the Rome and Vienna airports in December 1985. That March, Palestinian terrorists placed a bomb aboard an Athens-bound jet, killing another four Americans.

It seemed that a month could scarcely pass without Americans learning that some of their countrymen had been killed by nameless Middle Eastern thugs. The ubiquity of Arab terror—and the vulnerability of Americans—was hideously illustrated by the takeover of the Italian cruise ship *Achille Lauro*. Mimicking the Moroccan pirates who boarded the brig *Betsey* 201 years earlier, members of the Palestine Liberation Front overran the *Achille Lauro* and held its twelve American passengers at gunpoint. But in contrast to the *Betsy*'s capturers, the PLF gunmen did not merely incarcerate the Americans but decided to make an example of one of them. Their choice was a handicapped sixty-nine-year-old New Yorker named Leon Klinghoffer, an American Jew. The terrorists pushed Klinghoffer's wheelchair to the edge of the deck, shot him in the back, and pitched his still-twitching body into the sea.

"Once again, we had a crisis in the Middle East in which American lives were hanging in the balance," Reagan informed his diary. America's ability to respond to that threat was circumscribed by the absence of a credible deterrent but also by the dearth of dependable allies. Rather than arrest the *Achille Lauro* hijackers, Egypt offered them safe conduct to PLO headquarters in Tunis. U.S. Navy fighters intercepted the Egyptian jet carrying the Palestinians' ringleader, Abu Abbas, and forced it to land in Sicily, but Italian authorities promptly released the prisoner. In countering Middle Eastern terror, it seemed, America would have to respond unilaterally.

The United States indeed acted alone when it again confronted Libya, the primary sponsor of Abu Nidal, in March 1986. Hoping to provoke Qadhafi into a military clash, Reagan ordered the Navy to renew its patrols near the Libyan coast. "Any nation victimized by terrorism has an inherent right to respond with force to deter new acts of terror," the president explained. "I felt we must show Qaddafi that . . . we wouldn't let him get away with it." Qadhafi lunged at the bait. When Libyan missile boats opened fire on the fleet, Navy fighters blasted the vessels with missiles and bombed land-based radar sites as well.

Reagan had exacted justice for Abu Nidal's atrocities, but Qadhafi was far from deterred. Two weeks after the clash in Sidra, Libyan agents killed two American servicemen and wounded fifty with a bomb placed in a Berlin discotheque. Reagan retaliated by ordering more than sixty tons of ordnance dropped on Tripoli and Benghazi. Some of the explosives missed their target and killed a number of civilians, including, according to some reports, Qadhafi's adopted daughter. Operation El Dorado Canyon, as it was called, once again angered America's allies; France and Spain refused to allow the American fighters to overfly their territory en route to Libya. European sympathy for Libya did not, however, inhibit Qadhafi from staging yet another terrorist attack in Europe, his deadliest ever. On December 21, 1988, a bomb purportedly planted by Libyan operatives aboard Pan Am flight 103 blew up over Lockerbie, Scotland, killing all 259 passengers, thirty-seven American college students among them, and eleven villagers on the ground.

The United States had again projected its power, without European assistance, against a warlike North African despot. Unlike Yusuf Qaramanli, however, Tripoli's ruler in the beginning of the nineteenth century, Qadhafi could strike back almost anywhere in the world and with virtual impunity. And nowhere could revenge against the United States be more readily exacted than in Lebanon. In a further act of retribution for the Libya bombings, Qadhafi asked for the execution of Peter Kilburn, a librarian at the American University of Beirut who had been held by Hizbollah for two years. Hizbollah honored the request.

Kilburn's abduction and murder was symptomatic of the plague of hostage taking and assassinations that afflicted Americans living in Lebanon in the 1980s. Caught between warring factions in the vicious civil war, U.S. citizens became easy prey for the thousands of masked and heavily armed militiamen prowling Beirut's ruins. The first to be seized was David Dodge, the president of the American University of Beirut and the great-grandson of the university's founder, Daniel Bliss. Captured by Hizbollah in 1981 and incarcerated for a year, Dodge was released unharmed, but his successor, Malcolm Kerr, was less fortunate. Another son of Middle East missionaries and a renowned scholar of inter-Arab affairs, Kerr was exiting his AUB office in 1984 when two Hizbollah gunmen approached him and shot him in the head. The following year, Hizbollah kidnapped, tortured, and executed the CIA's Beirut bureau chief, William Buckley, and in 1988 abducted and hanged William Higgins, an American colonel serving with UN peacekeeping forces in Lebanon.

Lebanese factions detained nine other Americans during the decade 1981–91, one of them, the Associated Press correspondent Terry Anderson, for nearly seven years. "No noise, no speaking," Anderson recalled of his ordeal. "Even rolling from side to side . . . to relieve the painful muscle cramps brought on by lying still for hours would earn a slap or a poke with a gun."[3] More incensing than the bombing of U.S. facilities or the assassination of its citizens, the hostage crisis exasperated American leaders. A nation armed with untold numbers of tanks, assault aircraft, warships, and battle-ready divisions seemed impotent in the face of a few lightly armed kidnappers in the Middle East.

Teddy Roosevelt had been able to cable the Moroccan government, "We want Perdicaris Alive or Raisuli Dead," but for Reagan, faced with the Hobbesian state of Lebanon, there was simply no government to address. The only alternative was to deter the state sponsors of the kidnappers, foremost Iran, by military and economic means, but none of these measures had succeeded. Reagan spent much of his second term in office befuddled by the Iranian conundrum, uncertain whether to intimidate or placate the mullahs. Then, in the summer of 1985, the Israelis offered him a solution. They claimed that moderate elements within the Iranian leadership would obtain the hostages' release in return for antitank missiles that were desperately needed in the war with Iraq. Enticed by this arrangement, Reagan warranted a scheme in which Israel would secretly convey the missiles to Teheran and the United States would then replenish Israel's stocks. "We wouldn't be shipping any weapons to the people in Iran," the president consoled himself. "I did not think of the operation . . . as an 'arms-for-hostage' deal, because it wasn't."

At night, in unmarked boxes on neutral flag ships, Israel began transferring the projectiles. By August, six hundred of them had reached Iran, and another fifteen hundred by December. Yet even as these consignments restored some degree of communication between Tel Aviv and Teheran, they divided policymakers in Washington. While the CIA and the National Security Agency favored the operation, the notion of buying Iranian compliance with weaponry revolted George Shultz, the ursine former treasury secretary and Bechtel Corporation director who had replaced Haig as Reagan's secretary of state. The president nevertheless continued to sanction the arms transfers, even after November 1986 when the press leaked word of the operation. Reagan at first denied that he had sold missiles to a terrorist-sponsoring regime, but then, a week later, he reversed himself and admitted that the United States had, in fact, supplied some "defensive weapons" to Iran, albeit for an honorable cause. "Our government has a firm policy not to capitulate to terrorist demands," he insisted. "We did not—repeat, did not—trade weapons or anything else for hostages, nor will we."

Reagan's prevarications cost him enormously in terms of his credibility among Americans, and they failed to secure him credit in

Teheran. The Iranians refused to rein in Hizbollah in Lebanon and, in the Gulf, proceeded to launch missile boat attacks against unarmed Kuwaiti oil tankers. Reagan had ignored the seminal lesson of the Barbary Wars: providing arms to pirate states in the Middle East only produces more piracy. To defend America's oil supply from Kuwait, the president was obliged to send the Navy back into action. Over the course of 1987 and 1988, U.S. warships sank a number of Iranian naval boats and provided armed escorts for endangered Kuwaiti vessels. In the course of these operations, the *USS Vincennes* accidently downed a civilian Iranian airliner, killing all 290 of its passengers.

While American servicemen fought the Iranians in the Gulf, American arms shipments to the Islamic regime sparked a full-blown scandal in Washington. Proceeds from the missile sales, it was revealed, had been funneled to anticommunist Contra guerrillas in Nicaragua in violation of congressional law. The administration was subjected to a sweeping, nationally televised investigation, but that did not dissuade Reagan from pursuing controversial—and contradictory—policies in the Middle East. At the same time that the United States was arming Iran with antitank missiles, it was also supplying helicopters, mortars, and satellite intelligence to Iran's mortal enemies in Baghdad.

Though Iraq, no less than Libya, was a patron of Abu Nidal and other terrorist groups, Reagan removed Iraq from the list of terrorism-backing states. Twice, in 1983 and 1984, he sent the presidential envoy Donald Rumsfeld to meet with Saddam Hussein, ignoring evidence that the Iraqi dictator had employed poison gas against thousands of his enemies. "No one had any doubts about [the Iraqis'] continued involvement in terrorism," a document from the Defense Department confirmed. "The real reason was to help them succeed in the war against Iran." While unambiguously condemning Iraq's use of chemical weapons, Rumsfeld also assured Saddam that the United States still stood behind him in his struggle with the ayatollahs and desired "to improve bilateral relations, at a pace of Iraq's choosing." Ties between Washington and Baghdad continued to solidify even after an Iraqi Mirage jet mistakenly fired missiles at the *Stark*, a U.S. frigate patrolling the Persian Gulf in March 1987, killing thirty-seven sailors.

The administration's efforts to contain Iranian influence in the

Gulf coincided with a clandestine campaign to provide arms, military advisers, and financial assistance to the Arab irregulars battling the Soviet occupation of Afghanistan. Administration officials tended to romanticize this resistance, refusing to recognize the contempt which these mujahideen, or holy warriors, held the United States. Americans were also reluctant to acknowledge the hatred of their culture seething in Saudi Arabia or the willingness of Saudi authorities to deflect radical Islamic criticism of their own profligacy onto the United States. America, claimed one widely circulated Saudi cassette, was the enemy of all Muslims, a "nation of beasts who fornicate and eat rotten food." Few officials in Washington seemed alarmed that their country was fueling the spread of such anti-American propaganda through its purchases of Arab oil and funding some of the most militant Islamists, among them the son of a wealthy Saudi businessman, Osama bin Laden.[4]

The same Reagan administration famous for steering a straightforward course in its policies toward the Soviet Union was now notorious for running circles in the Middle East. Security concerns had led it to attack Libya while coddling Iraq and to arm both Saddam and the leaders of the Iranian revolution. Steeped in Middle Eastern myths, it provisioned the Arab freedom fighters in Afghanistan and succored the Saudi theocracy while ignoring the threats posed by both. Wavering between considerations of security and faith, the White House at first backed then protested Israel's invasion of Lebanon, expedited then delayed weapons shipments to the Jewish state, collaborated with Israeli intelligence on a controversial arms-for-hostages scheme but in 1985 prosecuted a former U.S. Navy Intelligence analyst, Jonathan Pollard, as an Israeli spy. Reagan helped evacuate the PLO from Beirut, only to boycott the organization thereafter, and then, in a final volte-face, engaged in a diplomatic dialogue with Arafat.

Parleys with the Palestinian leader represented a sharp departure from previous American policy. Though every administration since Nixon's had secretly communicated with the PLO, usually in an effort to shield Americans from Palestinian violence, the United States officially refused to recognize the group as long as it perpetrated terror and rejected Israel's right to exist. Reagan rigorously

upheld that policy—"hell no, PLO!" Shultz had led an AIPAC audience in chanting—until December 1987, when a large-scale civic
revolt, or *intifada*, broke out in the West Bank and Gaza. The scenes
of Palestinian youths pelting Israeli tanks with stones caught both
the Americans and the Israelis off guard, but it also stunned Arafat.
The young local leaders of the rebellion did not automatically take
their instructions from the Old Man, as he was known, in Tunis.
Arafat regained the initiative the following December, though, by
suddenly renouncing terror and recognizing Resolution 242. Now
that it had met America's preconditions for acceptance, Reagan had
no choice but to acknowledge the PLO as the Palestinians' representative and to open contacts with Arafat. Discussions between State
Department and Palestinian officials covered a range of issues,
including the possibility of creating a Palestinian state in the territories. But hopes that the president's record of consecutive debacles in
the Middle East would be crowned by a peacemaking success were
squelched by a terrorist assault on an Israeli beach led by Abu
Abbas, commander of the *Achille Lauro* raid. Arafat refused to condemn the attack and Washington suspended the talks.[5]

America's inability to sustain a constructive dialogue on Middle
Eastern disputes, much less resolve them, was symptomatic of a
more chronic malady. Though widely credited with achieving victory
in the clear-cut Cold War, Reagan had proved incapable of coping
with the complexities of the Arab-Israeli conflict, the Iran-Iraq war,
and tensions between secular and Islamic regimes. The vision of
establishing a *pax Americana* in the region had rarely seemed more
ephemeral.

Americans, though, seemed largely unaware of this muddle. Their
attention was riveted to the dazzling scenes of millions demonstrating
for freedom in Eastern Europe and pulverizing the Berlin Wall. Movie
audiences cheered as Michael J. Fox in *Back to the Future* (1985) and
Tom Cruise in *Top Gun* (1986) handily dispatched Libyan assailants,
and as Indiana Jones (Harrison Ford) smirked and shot a scimitar-
wielding Arab in the 1981 blockbuster, *Raiders of the Lost Ark*. They
delighted as a winsome Brooke Shields, cast as the naïve American
ingénue in *Sahara* (1983), was swept away by an Arab horseman in
black. They laughed at the bumbling Muslim terrorists who, in the

1982 comedy *Wrong Is Right*, experimented with suicide bombers and plotted to blow up New York's Twin Towers.

Hollywood was once again indulging in Oriental fantasies and conflating them with Middle Eastern facts. Reagan himself seemed confused. Exhibiting the first signs of the Alzheimer's disease that would later claim his life, he occasionally mixed up scenes from his earlier movies with actual world events. Such bewilderment, however, was rapidly becoming prohibitive for Americans. A disorderly decade had ended in the Middle East, but another was dawning, with war.

Sabers and Shields in the Sand

The prospect of large-scale conflict in the Middle East in fact looked distant the day in 1989 that Vice President George H. W. Bush dropped the "vice" from this title and became the nation's forty-first president. A trim former war hero, Yale baseball captain, and director of the CIA, Bush personified the vigor and skill with which the United States would tackle the region's quandaries. And the field seemed to have been leveled for his success. The Communist Bloc had crumbled, depriving several Arab dictators of Soviet political patronage and a reliable source of munitions. In the Persian Gulf, the armies of Iran and Iraq, exhausted after ten years of war and more than a million casualties, succumbed to an uneasy stalemate. The Palestinian *intifada* also appeared to have depleted its steam and the PLO to have rendered itself irrelevant. Though peace was as yet unattainable, the Middle East had at least been defused to the point where American policymakers could think of disposing of some of its more volatile disputes and clearing a lane toward stability.

The veneer of Middle Eastern tranquillity, though, soon proved transparent. Crippled by a war debt approaching a trillion dollars, Saddam Hussein frantically searched for a source of accessible cash and found it in neighboring Kuwait. Alleging that the oil-rich sheikhdom had been artificially detached from Iraq by British imperialists, Saddam laid claim to "Iraq's 19th province." In keeping with the fundamentalist trend sweeping the Arab world, the secular

Ba'athist Saddam refashioned himself as a modern Saladin and declared holy war against the ungodly Saudis, to whom he also owed billions. Starting in July 1990, thousands of Iraqi tanks and myriad troops began massing on the Kuwaiti border. The world braced for Iraq's imminent conquest of Kuwait and perhaps of the entire Arabian Peninsula, and the Bush administration confronted its first Middle Eastern crisis.

The president also faced a dilemma. In contrast to John Quincy Adams, who had to choose between asserting American ideals by aiding Greece in its struggle for independence and safeguarding the nation's commercial investments in Turkey, Bush had to decide between two strategic assets. True, Kuwait supplied the United States with oil, but Iraq's contributions to the country's welfare were no less vital. "Normal relations between the United States and Iraq . . . promote stability in both the Gulf and the Middle East," a national security directive issued in 1990 declared. The White House continued to value Iraq for exercising a crucial constraint on Iran and even exerting a moderating influence on the Palestinians. Unable to determine which of its allies to support in the Iraqi-Kuwaiti standoff, Washington strove to remain neutral. "We had no opinion on the Arab-Arab conflicts," April Glaspie, America's representative in Iraq and its first woman ambassador in the Middle East, purportedly assured Saddam. "All we hope is that these issues are solved quickly."

Americans in the past had tried to stay out of Middle Eastern disputes—in Palestine before 1948, for example—only to be violently dragged into them, and the conflict in the Gulf was unexceptional. When, on August 2, Saddam's army invaded and proceeded to pillage Kuwait, Bush's hope for a peaceful solution to the crisis evaporated while the specter of Iraqi-dominated Gulf region condensed. Neutrality was no longer an option. Summoning the UN Security Council, Bush demanded action to free Kuwait of all foreign forces and ordered the Navy to send a flotilla to the Middle East—Operation Desert Shield. "We cannot permit a resource so vital to be dominated by one so ruthless," he affirmed, "and we won't."

Patiently, conscientiously, Bush proceeded to assemble an international consensus on military intervention in Kuwait. The responses were serendipitously positive. In contrast to their previous reluctance to cooperate with America's battle against terror, the Europeans were anxious to join any effort to protect their Middle Eastern oil. More surprising still was the readiness of many Arab rulers, fearful of Iraqi threats to their own regimes, to enlist in an anti-Saddam coalition. Their only conditions were that the United States promise them millions of dollars in postwar aid and exclude Israel from the alliance. Fortified by this display of international solidarity, Bush tabled a series of UN resolutions authorizing the use of "all necessary means" to evict the Iraqis from Kuwait.

In a military buildup nearly ten times larger than Operation Torch forty-eight years earlier, more than a half a million U.S. troops, together with multitudes of tanks, planes, guns, and support vehicles, were stationed around Kuwait. Joining them were contingents from thirty-four nations, together constituting the greatest display of military hardware ever arrayed in the Middle East. And yet Bush refrained from unleashing that juggernaut, giving Saddam a final chance to withdraw. In several highly publicized meetings, Secretary of State James Baker, a taciturn Texan, impressed upon his Iraqi counterpart, the garrulous Tariq Aziz, the necessity of evacuating Kuwait. Baker's efforts proved fruitless. Saddam still refused to recall his forces; on the contrary, he extended his holy war to include Israel and the United States and vowed to wage "the mother of all battles" to retain the "19th province." The UN subsequently set January 15, 1991, as the deadline by which Saddam could either comply with its decisions or incur the coalition's wrath.

Bush had performed exemplarily in his first Middle Eastern trial, but the most formidable obstacle still confronted him. More taxing than maintaining an international alliance and sustaining an entire army in the Arabian desert was the president's task of persuading his fellow Americans of the need to go to war. Many indeed remained to be convinced, suspecting that young Americans would not be fighting for Kuwaiti freedom but rather for secure and affordable oil. Bush, accordingly, expunged any mention of oil from in his speeches and instead stressed the danger that Iraq posed to independent peoples everywhere. "Every day that passes brings Saddam one step closer to realizing his goal of a nuclear arsenal," the president warned. "He has never possessed a weapon he didn't use." British leaders had once compared Nasser to Hitler, but Saddam, in Bush's description, had surpassed the Führer in his barbarism. Even then, Congress remained divided over whether to authorize the president to rid Kuwait of the Iraqis. On the strength of a mere five-vote majority in the Senate, America went to war.

Operation Desert Storm opened on the evening of January 17 with a withering aerial barrage on Baghdad and other Iraqi command centers. Airfields, radar installations, and communication networks dissolved into flame and flying debris under the impact of precision-guided missiles and pulverizing cluster bombs. The Iraqis appeared to be ready for the blitz. Viewers around the world watched as dense volleys of Iraqi antiaircraft fire, transformed into green globules by night-vision cameras, pulsed across their televisions. But the fusillade proved ineffective in downing coalition jets, and instead of engaging the enemy, Iraqi warplanes fled en masse to Teheran. More lethally, Saddam fired Scud missiles at coalition camps in Saudi Arabia, in one case killing twenty-eight GIs.

The primary target of the Scuds was not Americans, but rather the Israelis. Eager to draw the Jewish state into the war and so drive Egypt, Saudi Arabia, and Syria out of the coalition, Saddam launched thirty-nine of the Soviet-made missiles at Tel Aviv and Haifa, destroying homes and paralyzing the country economically. Israelis stoically donned gas masks and took shelter in rooms specially sealed against chemical and biological attack, but even their forbearance was limited. Though Bush pleaded with Israeli leaders not to respond to Saddam's provocation, the Israeli army prepared for a search-and-destroy mission against the rocket launchers in Western Iraq. Israeli paratroopers were literally on the runways ready to depart when the president at last devised an answer. Batteries of U.S. Patriot antiballistic missiles and their crews would be rushed to Israel and arrayed against the incoming Scuds. Though most of the Patriots missed their mark, this first-ever sight of American soldiers on their soil hoisted the Israelis' morale. "I've been in the army for sixteen years and, I tell you, I've never been to a country that welcomed me like this," said one of the crews' commanders, Michael Woods. "It's, you know, like almost overwhelming."

Far more destructive than the Scuds, however, was Saddam's use of the oil weapon. In contrast to the Arab rulers who in 1973 sought to humble the West politically by depriving it of vital petroleum, the Iraqi leader sought to hamper the coalition's advance by literally saturating it with oil. Iraqi troops dumped more than one million tons of crude into the Gulf and torched Kuwait rigs, creating history's largest oil spill and fields of inextinguishable flame. Blackened waters and blackened skies combined to cause the deaths of countless fish and waterfowl and contaminate allied troops. The ecological disaster in the Middle East that George Perkins Marsh, the founder of the conservationist movement 150 years earlier, had hoped to avert was raging.

At the height of these atrocities and in spite of delaying tactics by Saddam, the coalition opened its ground campaign, Operation Desert Saber, on February 24. The offensive proved to be more lightning paced and more devastating than any of its planners divined. Charging into Kuwait and southern Iraq, armored and infantry formations outflanked and slaughtered Saddam's supposedly elite Republican Guards and demolished his tank divisions. "Saddam was what military theorists call an enemy center of gravity," the Desert Storm commander General Norman Schwarzkopf, whose father had helped overthrow an earlier Middle Eastern leader in Iran, explained. "[If] destroyed, [it] will cause the enemy to lose its will to fight." Within one hundred hours, Kuwait City was secured and a large portion of the Iraqi army, trapped while retreating on the aptly named Highway of Death, was incinerated. Advancing Marines and soldiers purportedly sang a song made famous by the rock band the Clash that told of bombs bursting between minarets and of muezzins defiantly shouting ragas. "Rockin' the casbah," the GIs chanted as they snuffed out the last of the Iraqi resistance. "Rock the casbah."

American leaders now had to decide whether or not to press the attack deeper into Iraqi territory in order to topple Saddam's regime. General Colin Powell, the Joint Chiefs of Staff chairman who supervised the campaign, was against pursuing the war. A warm-mannered man who had worked his way up from modest Jamaican origins in the Bronx, New York, Powell acted primarily on humanitarian grounds. The battle had become a "turkey-shoot," he said, and the

United States would merely sully itself morally by continuing to massacre Iraqis. But Powell was also a cunning strategist who saw a chastened, but still militarily viable, Iraq as an American asset. "Our practical intention was to leave Baghdad enough power to survive as a threat to an Iran that remained relentlessly hostile to the United States," he explained, and the Bush administration concurred. The vestiges of Saddam's army were allowed to limp unmolested back to Iraq. Once there, however, they turned their remaining guns on the northern Kurds and the Shi'ites in the south who, with America's covert encouragement, had rebelled against Ba'athist rule. With a sangfroid similar to that displayed by Kissinger in his earlier abandonment of the Kurds, Bush watched impassively while both communities were decimated.

Operation Desert Farewell, which opened on March 10, effected the rapid withdrawal of American troops from the war zone. Behind them lay a plundered but liberated Kuwait, tens of thousands of Kurdish and Shi'ite victims of Ba'athist savagery, as many as 400,000 Palestinians whom Kuwait had expelled for allegedly supporting Saddam, and an Iraq bereft of a civilian infrastructure but with its army largely intact. Many Persian Gulf leaders now viewed America as their savior. Among Saddam's innumerable victims in Iraq, however, the United States was seen as a turncoat. More venomous still was resentment aroused in the Arab mujahideen, including a still obscure Osama bin Laden, who had finally driven the Soviet unbelievers from Afghanistan only to find American infidels bivouacked near Mecca and Medina. "It is not the world against Iraq. It is the West against Islam," they contended, equating the West with America.

The long-term consequences of the conflict later known as the first Gulf War seemed of little concern to most Americans. Spared by military censors from seeing the grislier aspects of the fighting, relieved by the relatively low casualty rate—147 U.S. battle deaths—and by the willingness of coalition members to help pay the war's $61 billion bill, they reveled in their national might. "What the President did in the Gulf was simply the right thing to do," Secretary Baker determined. "George Bush took the difficult choices the world expects of American leadership." Yet not only at home but also abroad America's prestige had reached a postwar pinnacle, thanks to

Bush's policies in the Middle East. Much of the world had acknowledged America's hegemony in the region and harmonized with its goals. In contrast to Woodrow Wilson, whose refusal to make war on the Ottoman Empire weakened America's position at the Paris Peace Conference, the president had committed much of his army to the Gulf and stood poised to dictate its future. "Americans are the most religious people on Earth," he proclaimed. "And we have always instinctively sensed that God's purpose was bound up with the cause of liberty." Having brandished American power, Bush now flourished American ideals.

"We can see a new world coming into view, a world in which freedom and respect for human rights find a home among all nations." With these words Bush unveiled his vision of the new world order, a millennial era of peace and international fraternity that would begin in the Middle East. The president proceeded to outline his plan for maintaining a permanent U.S. naval presence in the Gulf, for providing funds for Middle East development, and for instituting safeguards against the spread of unconventional weapons. The centerpiece of his program, however, was the achievement of an Arab-Israeli treaty based on the territory-for-peace principle and the fulfillment of Palestinian rights.[6]

As the first step toward this noble objective, Bush announced his intention to reconvene the international peace conference, this one to be held in Madrid. Secretary Baker traversed the Arab world to rally support for the summit and generate pressure on Israel to forfeit land and uproot settlements. His efforts raised the ire of Yitzhak Shamir, the diminutive yet indomitable former underground leader who had replaced Begin as prime minister. Shamir accelerated the construction of settlements in the West Bank and Gaza and resisted all suggestion of negotiating with Arafat. "It was difficult not to believe that the Shamir government was simply expressing its disdain for American interests," Baker bitterly wrote. Withholding loan guarantees for resettling Soviet Jewish immigrants to Israel, the secretary told Congress that Shamir could call him when he was interested in peace and even revealed his White House phone number (202-456-1414). Browbeaten, the Israelis finally agreed to attend the conference, but only on the condition that Arafat not be invited. Bush readily accepted this demand; alone among Arab leaders, the PLO chairman had sided with Saddam during the war.

To much pomp and publicity, the peace conference opened on October 30, 1991, in the Spanish capital. Millions around the world delighted to the sight of Israeli and Arab leaders gathered in the rococo Royal Palace (from which a portrait of Charles V massacring Moors had been hastily removed) and seated around the same ornate table. "Like the walls of Jericho, the psychological barriers of a half century came tumbling down with resounding finality," Baker exulted. The seeming breakthrough, however, led only to culs-de-sac. Syria's crusty foreign minister, Farouk al-Shara, devoted his entire remarks to vilifying Shamir and Shamir offered paltry incentives to Palestinian representatives from the territories. The American delegation nevertheless managed to hammer out a two-tiered framework of bilateral peace talks and multilateral discussions on issues such as water resources, arms control, and refugee resettlement. But the bilateral discussions broke down over Israel's refusal to consider territorial concessions in the West Bank and Gaza and the Palestinians' rejection of anything less than a PLO-run state in both. Shamir objected to returning the entire Golan Heights to Syria and the Syrians were unwilling to offer real peace. In the absence of progress on the bilateral plane, many Arab delegations balked at even considering multilateral subjects.

Madrid, Baker concluded, was "a rich tale of determination, false starts, personal and political courage, blind alleys, perseverance, misjudgments, lost tempers, endless negotiations, scores of creative compromises, and both good faith and bad." It was also a nonstarter. By the end of 1991, the peace process was once again deadlocked. Facing a tough presidential contest, Bush blamed much of the impasse on Israel. The United States, he declared, had provided "nearly $1,000 [in aid] for every Israeli man, woman, and child" but had received only intransigence in return. Such imputations could not, however, camouflage the fact that the administration had committed all of its prestige and influence toward bridging the gap between Arabs and Israelis and had scarcely succeeded in narrowing them.[7]

American arms had defeated a brutal aggressor in the Middle East and liberated a loyal ally. But the United States had restored tribal rule to Kuwait, rather than instituting representative government, and enabled Saddam to retain his homicidal regime. It had convened a high-profile peace conference, only to fail at attaining even the most preliminary agreements. Though Bush had eschewed the Wilsonian reluctance to commit troops to the Middle East, he nevertheless shared Wilson's frustration with trying to transform the region along American-style democratic lines. The *pax Americana* the president had promised seemed almost as unattainable as it had been before the war; the new world order appeared virtually indistinguishable from the old. Arguably the most significant change occurred not in the Middle East but in the White House, which the Bush family vacated in January 1993 to make way for Bill and Hillary Clinton.

A Clash of Visions and Reality

Oh I come from a land, from a faraway place
Where the caravan camels roam
Where they cut off your ear
If they don't like your face
It's barbaric, but hey, it's home

With these irreverent lyrics, Walt Disney Productions opened its animated comedy *Aladdin* (1992), yet another *Thousand and One Arabian Nights* derivation. Making light of the presumed cruelty of Middle Eastern cultures had once been acceptable and even laudable in the United States, but the publication of *Orientalism* and the advent of political correctness had rendered such aspersions improper. Incensed by what they regarded as the latest attempt by Hollywood to disparage their heritage, Arab American groups strenuously protested the song. This time Disney relented. Songwriters quickly replaced the offensive couplet "Where they cut off your ear if they don't like your face" with the whimsical "Where it's flat and immense and the heat is intense." The movie industry nevertheless continued to insult Americans of Arab, Iranian, and Turkish heritage by perpetuating negative stereotypes of Middle Eastern peoples. The enraged Arab terrorist who tries to blow up an American city in *True Lies*, a 1994 Arnold Schwarzenegger comedy, had already become a staple.

The deepening schism in the depiction of the Middle East in the movie theaters was also widening in libraries and lecture halls. The field of Middle Eastern studies flourished in the United States of the 1990s. Well over one hundred colleges and universities were now offering courses on related subjects and the Middle East Studies Association—MESA, founded in 1966—boasted over twenty-six hundred members. Reared on multiculturalism and postcolonialist theories, many of these scholars voiced harsh disapproval of America's policies in the Middle East, in particular its support for Israel and for autocratic Arab rulers. They pressed for an explicit endorsement of the PLO and of democratic opposition forces in the region and, in some cases, lionized the anti-American leaders in Damascus and Teheran. Such sentiments were no longer confined to Middle East departments, however, but proliferated throughout the humanities and even into branches of science. "There is the fact that the U.S. has supported oppressive, authoritarian, harsh regimes, and blocked democratic initiatives," said Noam Chomsky, an esteemed MIT linguist and world-renowned liberal socialist, born in 1928 to Zionist parents in Philadelphia. "The U.S. is making a very clear statement: the U.S. is going to run this area of the world by force, so get out of the way."

Less pervasive were the views of Bernard Lewis, who continued to advocate robust ties between United States and Israel and saw America as the Middle East's principal, if not only, hope for democratic change. Among the few scholars to endorse publicly Lewis's pessimistic appraisal of the Middle East was Samuel P. Huntington, a Harvard specialist on government. In his seminal 1993 work *Clash of Civilizations*, the seemingly meek and retiring Huntington described a world no longer split between the rival ideologies of communism and capitalism, but torn rather by a visceral conflict between the Western, mostly Christian, countries and Islam. "The underlying problem for the West is not Islamic fundamentalism," he wrote. "It is Islam, a different civilization whose people are convinced of the superiority of their culture and are obsessed with the inferiority of their power." Unlike Lewis, though, Huntington did not foresee a cardinal role for the United States in averting this collision. America would, however, be its primary victim.[8]

Huntington's thesis appeared to be confirmed on the morning of February 26, 1993, when a van packed with explosives drove into the underground parking lot of the World Trade Center in Manhattan. A Kuwaiti, Ramzi Yousef, was driving the van, but the bomb was made by Abdul Rahman Yasin from Iraq. Both were carrying out the instructions of a blind Egyptian cleric named Omar Abdul-Rahman, who, from his mosque in Brooklyn, headed an extremist Islamic group with links to al-Qaeda (the Base) of Osama bin Laden. By toppling the Trade Center's Twin Towers, the tallest buildings in New York and one of the outstanding symbols of American mastery, Abdul-Rahman hoped to inaugurate a general holy war against the West. Ramzi lit the fuse on the 1,310-pound bomb and fled the lot on foot. The blast, which erupted just after midday, blew a ninety-foot-wide gap through four floors of concrete, killed six people, and wounded more than one thousand. Six of the conspirators were eventually arrested and remanded to prison for a total of 240 years.

The Twin Tower bombing was the first major terrorist strike on the continental United States, but though it clearly faced an unprecedented Middle Eastern menace, the federal government refrained from mobilizing all of its military and intelligence services. The month-old administration of Bill Clinton determined to treat terrorism as a crime rather than as a threat to national security. The president's reluctance to engage Muslim terrorists militarily was reinforced in October 1993 by the killing of eighteen American servicemen in a failed effort to capture the Somali warlord Mohamed Farrah Aidid—the Black Hawk Down incident. The murder, eighteen months later, of 168 civilians by the white supremacist bombers of the federal building in Oklahoma City, further strengthened Clinton's preference for combating terror with police officers rather than soldiers. "I was pleased with the effectiveness of our law-enforcement work, but troubled by the evident vulnerability of our open society to terror," he wrote.

Though a former Rhodes Scholar, law professor, and Arkansas governor, Clinton had only minimal experience in foreign affairs and no more than a passing familiarity with the Middle East. But he understood that part of Bush's defeat in the 1992 elections was due to his preoccupation with Iraq and Arab-Israeli mediation and his failure to focus on domestic issues. And Americans, enjoying a period of seemingly limitless prosperity, generally welcomed the president's inward-looking gaze. They shared Clinton's conviction that terrorism could be defeated by relieving the poverty and the ignorance that bred it and by isolating its bankrolling states. Relieved of the burdens of combating al-Qaeda and other extremist groups militarily, the people of the United States could enjoy the fruits of the century's final and halcyon decade.

In the Middle East, Clinton's approach meant avoiding major initiatives, either military or diplomatic, while maintaining the status quo in the Persian Gulf. Through a policy of "dual-containment," the United States would apply economic sanctions against Iran and Iraq and keep up the pressure on Saddam. In addition to enforcing the "no-fly zones" that prohibited Iraqi aircraft from operating over Kurdish and Shi'ite areas, Clinton twice ordered missile strikes against Iraqi installations—the first, in retaliation for Saddam's attempted assassination of former President Bush in 1993 and the second, five years later, as punishment for interfering with UN arms inspectors. Clinton was especially supportive of the inspectors' efforts to uncover weapons of mass destruction in Iraq. The Ba'athist regime, he believed, was the apex of an "unholy axis of terrorists, drug traffickers and organized international criminals" that would become "all the more lethal if we allow them to build arsenals of nuclear, chemical, and biological weapons."[9]

In general, though, Clinton refrained from resorting to force as a means of securing America's interests in the Middle East. There seemed little need. The Soviet challenge had faded into memory and native nationalism was essentially defunct. Terrorist bombers had indeed claimed multiple victims in the United States, but the Islamic threat could be met with vigilance rather than puissance, Clinton felt. Nor did he feel any compulsion to mediate between the Israelis and the Arabs. Raised a Baptist and warned by his childhood pastor, "God will never forgive you if you don't stand by Israel," Clinton was nevertheless content to cultivate amiable relations with the Jewish state without wasting precious presidential time on a futile peace process. That complacency might have continued if not for a phone call from Prime Minister Yitzhak Rabin of Israel on September 9, 1993, informing him that Israel and the PLO, after decades of mutual bloodletting, had reached a secret accord.

While the United States had yet to renew its dialogue with the Palestinian organization, representatives of the recently elected Rabin government had been covertly negotiating with Arafat's associates in the Norwegian capital of Oslo. Now, with the outlines of a treaty worked out, Rabin and Arafat sought to seal it with a presidential stamp. If disquieted by the fact that neither side had seen fit to consult him about the talks, Clinton was nevertheless happy to godfather their pact. Frenzied preparations ensued for a public signing at the White House to be held a mere four days later. The president's role was reduced to ensuring that both leaders attended the event and that Arafat would not attempt to kiss the reticent prime minister's cheeks. Clinton spent the sleepless night before the ceremony reading the book of Joshua—incongruously, a chronicle of Jewish conquest—and in the morning wore a tie adored with golden horns to remind him of those Joshua blew to topple Jericho's walls. "Now the horns would herald the coming of a peace that would return Jericho to the Palestinians," he thought. The next day, in the presence of thousands of Arab, Israeli, and American well-wishers, a radiant Clinton reenacted Carter's historic three-way handshake. "Shalom, salaam, peace," he bade the signatories, "go as peacemakers."

Like Sadat and Begin, Arafat and Rabin would go on to receive the Nobel Peace Prize, but the Declaration of Principles they initialed that day on the White House lawn was far from a fleshed-out treaty. Beyond providing for mutual recognition between Israel and the PLO, for the renunciation of terror and incitement, and for the gradual realization of Palestinian national rights, the popularly named Oslo process did not specify when the Israelis would vacate the West Bank and Gaza or how those territories would revert to Arab rule. Decisions on the final status of Jerusalem, claimed as a capital by both parties, and of the millions of Palestinian refugees and their descendants scattered worldwide, were postponed to an indefinite future. The Israelis exploited this ambiguity to expand their settlements in the territories, while Arafat and the Palestinian Authority created by Oslo made only desultory efforts to clamp down on terror or to educate Palestinians for peace.

Confronted by the inability of Arab and Israeli negotiators to move from general principles to concrete peace arrangements, Clinton, much like Carter, was compelled to mediate between the sides. Huge swaths of the president's schedule were blocked out to enable him to forge interim agreements between the parties. The White House hosted the battle-dressed Arafat so often that Clinton's critics, recalling his radical student days, charged him with reliving some Sixties fantasy of Third World guerrilla leaders. But the president in fact never bonded with Arafat. A far closer rapport blossomed between him and Jordan's King Hussein and his statuesque American wife, the Princeton-educated Queen Noor. Clinton's deepest affection, though, was reserved for Rabin, the quiet warrior and intrepid statesman, whom he came to view as the father he never fully had. "We had become friends in that unique way people do when they are in a struggle that they believe is great and good," Clinton remembered. "With every encounter, I came to respect and care for him more." Together with the king and the prime minister, as thousands of guests and the international media gathered in the Judean desert in October 1994, Clinton presided over the signing of an Israel-Jordan peace treaty. The clusters of blue, white, and green balloons released over the ceremony signaled the start of another peacemaking effort, as Clinton began exploring the possibility of exchanging the Israeli-held Golan Heights for Syria's reconciliation with Israel.

But the prospect of sacrificing the Golan, Gaza, and the West Bank infuriated those Israelis who revered those territories as sacred and vital to their nation's defense. Mass rallies were held denouncing Rabin's policies and excoriating him as a traitor. Arafat's failure to rein in terror groups, evidenced by the first bus bombing in Jerusalem, in August 1995, further fueled the opposition. After attending a peace rally in Tel Aviv on November 4, Rabin was shot by a lone Jewish gunman and died shortly afterward. Ashen and distraught, Clinton appeared before reporters at the White House and became the first president to utter an epitaph in Hebrew—"shalom, chaver," good-bye friend.[10]

Shimon Peres, Israel's perennial foreign minister and primary architect of Oslo, succeeded Rabin and tried to restore the process's momentum. But persistent bombings undermined his effort and, in 1996, caused him to lose the elections to the Likud's truculent, MIT-educated leader, Benjamin Netanyahu. The combination of a right-wing government in Israel and a Palestinian Authority rife with corruption and factional splits necessitated an even greater invest-ment of Clinton's energies. These produced yet another interim accord, negotiated at Maryland's Wye Plantation in October 1998, in which Israel ceded more territory and received further Palestinian pledges for peace. By that time, however, efforts to achieve Palestinian-Israeli accords were already being sidetracked by the need to defend Americans from yet another onslaught of Middle Eastern terror.

The latest spate of attacks began at ten in the evening of June 25, 1996, when a fuel truck crammed with five thousand pounds of dynamite blew up the Khobar Towers, a building used to billet U.S. servicemen in Dhahran, Saudi Arabia. Nineteen Americans were killed by the blast, which was attributed to Hizbollah and al-Qaeda, and 372 wounded. Two years later, on August 7, 1998, al-Qaeda killed 244 people and wounded more than 4,000 with simultaneous bomb blasts at the U.S. embassies in Kenya and Tanzania. The scenes of dazed rescue workers ferreting for bodies in the rubble, first wit-nessed in Beirut in the 1980s, and of rows of flag-enshrouded coffins being conveyed into American cargo planes, once again became com-monplace. Exultant, bin Laden announced the birth of a new organ-ization, the International Islamic Front for Jihad against Jews and Crusaders, and declared open war on the United States. "Every Mus-lim . . . in any country," he ordained, is obliged to "kill and fight Americans and their allies, whether civilians or military."

American intelligence services were convinced that al-Qaeda would eventually mount a major attack within the United States, yet Clinton's response remained minimal. Bound by a ban on political assassination issued by the Ford administration, the president pre-ferred to capture, rather than to kill, bin Laden, or to encourage Egyptian or Afghan agents to liquidate him. American forces, mean-while, were already committed in Kosovo, protecting Albanians from the Serbs, and bombing Belgrade—the public, Clinton believed, would not support a major operation in the Middle East. The president was under fire from Congress for attempting to cover up his dalliance with a White House intern. Legally and politically constrained, Clinton ordered a limited retaliation for the embassy bombings, launching cruise missile strikes against al-Qaeda training camps in Afghanistan and a Sudanese pharmaceutical factory suspected of making chemical weapons. America's battle, he stressed, was aimed at "fanatics and killers," not at Islam, and would be "a long ongoing struggle." Yet even this low-key response was denounced by Clinton's critics as an attempt to deflect attention from his impeachment and interpreted by the terrorists as a sign of weakness. Bin Laden escaped unscathed from the attack and though the missiles devastated the Sudanese camp, no traces of toxic substances were detected in its ruins.

By the end of his eight years in office, Bill Clinton had become an exceptionally seasoned—and indelibly scarred—veteran of the Middle East. He had refrained whenever possible from projecting America's military strength against Islamic extremists but then discovered that the extremists were determined to bring their battle to the United States. Upholding the highest American virtues, he had striven to achieve peace between Israelis and Palestinians, only to be repeatedly dismayed. The alliance between the United States and repressive Arab regimes, especially in the Persian Gulf area, was tighter than ever, while the gap between rich and poor in the Middle East grew wider. Clinton's original vision of Americans joining with the peoples of the region in the search for nonviolent resolutions of their disputes and in the quest for equitable development had, by the end of 1999, been shattered, the victim of intractable conflicts and cold economic calculations. Fittingly, Clinton's experience in the Middle East concluded with further disappointment and pain, in failures of faith and power.

In a last-ditch attempt to save the Oslo process, Clinton acceded to a request by Israel's new prime minister, Ehud Barak, a left-leaning former commando, to hold talks on a final peace treaty with Arafat. Convening the two leaders at Camp David in July 2000, a mere six months before the end of his presidency, Clinton spent nearly two weeks struggling to narrow the gap between them. According to the American and the Israeli participants, the Palestinians were offered an independent state in 90 (later expanded to more than 95) percent of the West Bank, all of Gaza, and in the eastern half of Jerusalem. Israel would also cede a small part of its Negev desert to Gaza. Israeli settlements were to be consolidated into blocks adjacent to the 1967 border and Palestinian refugees would receive significant monetary compensation. Arafat, however, contended that Clinton and Barak proffered him no more than noncontiguous areas—"Bantustans"—in the West Bank and refused to grant him sovereignty over Jerusalem's Haram al-Sharif or, as Jews call it, the Temple Mount, including the Western Wall. The Clinton bridging proposals also failed to provide the refugees full repatriation to Israel. Arafat departed from Camp David, pausing only to compliment Clinton on his greatness. "I am not a great man," Clinton sighed. "I am a failure, and you have made me one."

That September, following a visit to the Temple Mount by Ariel Sharon, now head of the Israeli opposition, the Palestinians accused Israel of attempting to destroy the al-Aqsa mosque on the Haram al-Sharif and launched a second *intifada*. In contrast to the first uprising, though, which was largely nonviolent, this rebellion was replete with suicide bombers and ambushes that soon claimed hundreds of Israeli lives. The Israelis lashed back by destroying Palestinian Authority buildings, isolating West Bank cities, and assassinating militant leaders. The bloodshed blotted out the once effulgent vision of Israeli-Palestinian peace and portended the strife that would soon blanket much of the region. Clinton devoted the last weeks of his presidency to a breakneck effort to establish a cease-fire and restart the talks. Secretary of State Madeleine Albright, teetering on her high heels, ran after Arafat as he bolted the American embassy in Paris, where truce negotiations were being held. "Close the gate!" she shouted at the Marine guards, as if sealing the entrance would not only confine Arafat within the grounds but also hold back the swells of Middle East mayhem. "Close the gate!" she hollered, in vain.

Americans, caught up in a bitterly close presidential election, were scarcely of a mind to monitor these events. The limited attention they could spare for the Middle East was taken up by an al-Qaeda suicide bomber who, on October 12, rammed an engine-powered inflatable boat into the U.S. destroyer *Cole* while it was docked in a Yemeni port. The boat held enough explosives to kill seventeen sailors and wound thirty-four. "We are at war," exclaimed CIA Chief George Tenet. "I want no resources or people spared in this effort."[11] Yet few of his countrymen seemed discomfited by the fact that the government had refrained from declaring war on terrorism or from bolstering national defense. The forty-by-sixty-foot hole ripped in the *Cole*'s hull seemed to symbolize the gap in America's strategic thinking on the Middle East. In the tradition of Wilson, Kennedy, and Carter, Clinton had preferred ideals over steel in his approach to the region and showed a warm predilection for myths. But none of these policies had proven effective either in attaining peace or in preventing terror. The United States never retaliated for the *Cole* attack—a fact duly noted in Afghanistan, now under the control of the puritanical Taliban regime, and in the headquarters of al-Qaeda.

Conflagration

The twenty-first century dawned on an America generally galvanized in its hopes for the future but also deeply fractured on a range of contemporary debates: free-market capitalism versus the welfare state, the demand for energy versus the desire to preserve the environment, relations between government and church. Differences also arose over America's involvement in the Middle East, over the country's alliance with Israel, and over the ties between big business and Arab oil. By contrast, there was little discussion on the dangers posed by Islamic extremism and the ways that the United States might defend itself. Americans seemed more agitated by the millennium's potentially debilitating impact on computers—the Y2K bug—than by the prospect of a terrorist assault at home. Back in 1789, the fear of attacks by Middle Eastern pirates on the new nation's shores prodded Americans to ratify their Constitution and unite. In 2000, though, the threat of a major terrorist strike within the United States went largely unnoticed by the citizens of the United States, who were busy disputing foundational issues.

Terrorism against America was foremost, however, in the mind of Osama bin Laden. He had already authorized an operation in which sleeper cells of al-Qaeda agents would awaken, hijack U.S. airliners, and fly them into major commercial and government buildings. Amply funded by Islamic charities from Saudi Arabia and the Persian Gulf, at least nineteen terrorists succeeded in infiltrating American cities, establishing new identities, and, in several cases, enrolling in flight training programs.

Numerous warnings regarding al-Qaeda's activities were received by the CIA and other intelligence services. "The system was blinking red," recalled Tenet. But American officials appeared to be slumbering at the helm. George W. Bush came into office declaring his intention to combat terror rigorously, but the new president in fact took few steps to strengthen the nation's defenses. The White House was ineffective in persuading Yemen to cooperate in the hunt for the *Cole*'s attackers and reluctant to pressure the Saudis to crack down on terrorist-funding charities. Even after a French citizen of Moroccan descent, Zacarias Moussaoui, was arrested at a Minnesota pilots' school in August 2001 and found in possession of 747 flight manuals, the administration reacted sluggishly. Bush raised the alert levels at American embassies and approved a plan to fire a drone-borne missile at bin Laden in Afghanistan, but refrained from upgrading domestic security. "The most important failure was one of imagination," a government commission later determined. "We do not believe leaders understood the gravity of the threat."

The American people should also have grasped the danger. Terrorist assaults, ending with the *Cole* and going back to hijackings and assassinations of the early 1970s, had become a reality of American life. The fact was reflected in popular culture, in films like *The Siege* (1998), in which New York is razed by Islamist bombers and reels under martial law, and *Three Kings* (1999) featuring childlike GIs bedeviled by Iraqi sadism. Menacing images of the Middle East, such as those sketched by Lewis and Huntington, were pervasive. Yet, confident in their military, Americans still had difficulty conceiving how a group of untrained men from Egypt, Saudi Arabia, and Lebanon could penetrate their country and attack its most prominent city and capital. Some, influenced by the theories of Said and

Chomsky, believed that Arabs and Iranians had far more to fear from Americans than vice versa. Others were still mollified by myths. Millions of Americans in 2000 thrilled at the Emmy-winning made-for-television movie *The Arabian Nights*, complete with a tale-telling Scheherazade, a swashbuckling Ali Baba, and Sindbad the Sailor. Many viewers of that film might have wondered why the inhabitants of so mystical a land, flying airliners rather than carpets, would strike at the United States, a nation that had never harmed them.

Those lingering Middle Eastern fantasies died, however, abruptly, at 8:46 in the morning of September 11, 2001. At that moment, a Los Angeles–bound American Airlines jet that had been commandeered by Al-Qaeda terrorists crashed, together with ninety-two people and 10,000 gallons of fuel aboard, into the North Tower of the World Trade Center. The sight of vermilion flames pluming from both sides of the building, of tons of debris, inanimate and human, plummeting to the streets below, would be cauterized into American memory. So, too, would the horror of hijacked United Airlines flight 175 striking the South Tower seventeen minutes later. "Please have fun in life and live your life the best you can," one of the passengers aboard that flight, Brian Sweeney, said in a message to his wife left moments before impact. "Know that I love you and no matter what, I'll see you again." Within less than half an hour, a third civilian airliner slammed into the western flank of the Pentagon in Washington, while a fourth, apparently intended for the White House or the Capitol but forced down by fearless passengers, plowed into a Pennsylvania field. By 10:30, the Twin Towers had collapsed and surrounding structures were teetering. A cloud of viscous, death-white smoke enveloped the southern portion of Manhattan, the very place from where, two hundred years earlier, the USS *Essex* had departed for America's first war in the Middle East.

Nearly three thousand Americans had been killed, the largest single massacre of civilians in the nation's history. The first reaction was shock. Confusion shrouded the identity of the hijackers, their motivation, and their modus operandi. Did other terrorist cells exist, people frantically asked, and, if so, what were their next objectives? As if to imitate *The Siege*, security forces grounded all flights, cordoned off tunnels and bridges, and detained hundreds of Arab and Muslim

Americans. National monuments were placed under heavy guard, among them the USS *Constitution*, anchored in Boston Bay, which authorities feared might be targeted for its role in the triumph over Barbary.

Americans of an earlier epoch might have reacted to such an attack by holding all Muslims responsible and declaring war on Islam. The clash of civilizations foretold by Huntington could not have been more luridly illustrated than by the crash of hijacked planes. And yet Americans were generally loath to lump the peace-abiding Muslim majority together with the mass murderers of 9/11. "[If] these are Islamic terrorists . . . they have defiled their own religion," Tom Clancy, a novelist who had written presciently of a terrorist plot to crash a plane into the Capitol, told CNN later that morning. "Islam does not permit suicide. It says you go to hell if you do something like this."[12] The fact that Clancy, a fiction writer, had been consulted as an expert on terrorism indicated the degree to which fantasy and fact remained blurred in America's Middle East perceptions. But the White House also underscored that the nation's enemy was Islamic fanaticism and not Muslims or the Islamic faith.

The United States, nevertheless, was irrefutably at war. The urgent questions were: with whom, where, and how would Americans strike back? The answers could be furnished only by the president, a man intimately and multifariously connected to the Middle East, the focus of intense loyalties and vehement opposition. The victor in an acrimoniously contested election, revered by some Americans for his defense of family values and his conservative social and economic policies, he was reviled by others for his artlessness, his insensitivity to welfare and ecological issues, and his simplistic piety. Nevertheless, in the panicky aftermath of 9/11, Americans rallied around George W. Bush and looked to him for leadership. And the president promptly complied. More than any other postwar president, Bush mapped the course of America's meandering relations with the Middle East.

He was the sum of many of America's diverse experiences in the region, a warrior-diplomat like George Bethune English and a warrior-evangelist like William Francis Lynch, an amalgam. In the manner of Jefferson and Theodore Roosevelt, Bush expressed few qualms about projecting force against America's adversaries in the area or changing hostile regimes. "The United States will hunt down and punish those responsible for these cowardly acts," he vowed after 9/11, pledging to "make no distinction between the terrorists who committed these acts and those who harbor them." Yet in the fashion of Teddy Roosevelt's fifth cousin, Franklin, Bush was deeply appreciative of the value of oil and reluctant to alienate its suppliers, especially in Saudi Arabia. He shared Andrew Jackson's solicitude for American trade with the Middle East and maintained his father's relationships with American corporations doing business there. In contrast to George H. W. Bush, though, a straitlaced Episcopalian, the junior Bush gravitated toward the vastly more popular and politically influential evangelical churches. This made him the spiritual heir and not merely the genetic descendant of Professor George Bush who in the 1840s advocated the creation of a Jewish state, and of the colonial theologians who warned of the dangers of militant Islam. Not inadvertently did Bush describe the struggle against Islamic terror as a "crusade to rid the world of evildoers." Along with this religious zeal, however, the president also espoused the secular fervor of the neoconservatives—many of them former liberals disaffected by the Left's abandonment of Israel and its leniency toward communist crimes—who preached the Middle East's redemption through democracy. The merging of sacred and civic missions in Bush's mind placed him firmly in the Wilsonian tradition. But the same faith that deflected Wilson from entering hostilities in the Middle East spurred Bush to decide in favor of war.

The location of America's reprisal was selected at Camp David on September 15. Deputy Secretary of Defense Paul Wolfowitz, a noted neoconservative, lobbied for retaliating against Iraq, which, he believed, was almost certainly linked to al-Qaeda. But Colin Powell, who was now the secretary of state, joined with Vice President Dick Cheney and National Security Adviser Condoleezza Rice in recommending Afghanistan, where the Taliban continued to harbor bin Laden. Bush agreed with Powell and set out to replicate the multinational coalition assembled by his father ten years earlier. Ridding Afghanistan of tyranny and terror would be a global, rather than a parochially American, campaign.

Aerial attacks against Taliban positions in Afghanistan began less than a month after 9/11. American jet fighters provided ground support for local anti-Taliban forces—the Northern Alliance—as they moved on the major cities of Kabul, Jalalabad, and Kandahar. By the end of November, the Marines were in action in Afghanistan as well, reducing pockets of Taliban resistance and hunting for bin Laden along the mountainous Pakistani border. Bush managed to persuade eighteen nations, including Britain, Russia, Germany, and France, to contribute troops to the campaign and to participate in the country's postwar reconstruction. Though bin Laden eventually escaped capture and Taliban guerrillas continued to operate from inaccessible redoubts, Operation Enduring Freedom was deemed successful. Now, with the military phases of the war largely completed, the United States could once again focus on matters of faith. Americans assisted in promulgating an Afghani constitution and in holding elections in which Afghani women, for the first time in history, stood for parliament.

Afghanistan's liberation might have sufficed to avenge the atrocity of 9/11, but Bush was convinced that America was embroiled in a long-term war with terror in which United States had only tenuously regained, but had yet to maintain, the initiative. The old policies of deterrence and containment first employed against the Soviets in the Middle East and later against Iran and Iraq no longer sufficed, he believed, to counter terrorist cells operating within the United States and potentially wielding weapons of mass destruction. Following the examples of Truman, Eisenhower, and Carter, all of whom had adopted new approaches to security threats from the region, Bush devised a doctrine. The United States would not wait and react to terrorist attacks but would rather combat any organization or country that engaged in or promoted terror. The tactic of preemption that Johnson and Nixon had opposed when wielded by Israel was now American policy. The United States would also devote its energies to furthering democracy in the Middle East, both as a matter of principle and as the best means of eliminating the hatred and backwardness in which terrorism thrived. "America has no empire to extend or utopia to establish," Bush told graduating cadets at West Point in June 2002. "We wish for others only what we wish for ourselves—

safety from violence, the rewards of liberty, and the hope for a better life." Once again, Americans would be striving to refashion the Middle East in their own image, beginning with Ba'athist Iraq.

Though proof of the ties between Saddam and bin Laden was scanty, Bush had determined to make Iraq the test case of his new doctrine. He did not lack for a casus belli. Saddam had tried to assassinate his father in 1993 and had consistently violated the no-fly zones. Most damning, though, for Bush, were Iraq's persistent attempts to produce weapons of mass destruction—WMD, for short—and to hide them from United Nations inspectors. Such actions betrayed a contempt for American power similar to that displayed by al-Qaeda and placed Iraq on an "axis of evil" alongside Iran and North Korea. Describing Saddam as a "grave and gathering danger" to world peace, Bush again began preparing for war.

Over the course of 2002, U.S. forces stepped up air attacks against Iraqi radar and defense installations and vastly expanded their presence in the Gulf. Massive depots of fuel and ammunition arose in the Kuwaiti desert together with veritable cities of air-conditioned military tents. On the diplomatic plane, the administration encouraged expatriate Iraqis opposed to Saddam Hussein, among them the MIT alumnus Ahmed Chalabi, a Shi'ite, to form a pro-Western and democratic government in exile. Bush was also busy domestically, persuading Americans of the necessity of war. To this end, the White House leaked classified CIA reports on Iraq's existing WMD programs and intimated that Saddam was conspiring to achieve nuclear capabilities as well. Some Americans took issue with these claims, but the public, eager to back the president so soon after 9/11, in general needed little persuading. Neither did Congress. By overwhelming majorities, both the House and the Senate in October approved the massive use of military power against Iraq. "The days of Iraq flouting the will of the world, brutalizing its own people, and terrorizing its neighbors must—and will—end," Bush declared. "Iraq will either comply with all U.N. resolutions, rid itself of weapons of mass destruction, and end its support for terrorists, or it will be compelled to do so."[13]

Unlike the first Gulf War, which many Americans opposed and Congress only narrowly authorized, this second offensive against Iraq commanded widespread domestic support. But while the world community joined with the United States in defeating Saddam in 1991, numerous countries now balked at enlisting in Bush's latest "coalition of the willing." Though Kuwait and Saudi Arabia begrudgingly allowed their deserts to be used as staging grounds for the attack, no Arab state would contribute troops to the invading force or actively participate in the overthrow of Saddam. A more grievous blow to Bush's alliance-building efforts was the opposition of Russia and several Western European states, most prominently Germany and France. Though they had closed ranks with America in freeing Kuwait in 1991 and in Afghanistan ten years later, many Europeans now expressed strong reservations about the proposed Iraqi incursion. They rejected America's attempts, through its regimen of international sanctions, to restrict their business dealings with Iraq and expressed resentment over Bush's unilateralist economic and environmental policies. As the image of the collapsing Twin Towers faded, the French and German governments resumed their long-standing efforts to distance themselves from America's antiterrorism tactics in the Middle East and to engage the region on an independent, nonconfrontational basis.

Divisions between the United States and Europe over Middle Eastern issues were further deepened by Bush's support for Israel and Ariel Sharon, who gained the premiership in 2001. Though widely expected to retaliate immediately for Palestinian suicide bombers, Sharon waited for over a year, strengthening his relations with Bush, before launching a major counteroffensive in the West Bank. Israeli forces killed hundreds of members of Hamas, Islamic Jihad, and the Al-Aqsa Martyrs Brigade and arrested thousands more. Arafat was confined to his half-ruined headquarters in Ramallah, where he would remain until his death two years later. Bush responded to these actions by recognizing Israel's right to defend itself and blocking UN Security Council efforts to intervene. His pro-Israeli positions pleased the majority of Americans who continued to favor the Jewish state, including the evangelicals, but angered many Western Europeans. Committed to the survival of the Palestinian Authority and concerned about rising disaffection among their own Muslim populations, members of the European Union moved to distance themselves from the U.S.-Israeli front. Bush took steps to mitigate this ire by becoming the first president in history publicly to endorse the creation of a Palestinian state and by offering to work with the EU on a "road map" for resolving the conflict. But the Europeans would not be appeased. Protesters teemed through the streets of Brussels, Antwerp, and Paris with posters decrying the "evil axis" of Bush and Sharon and comparing them both to Hitler.

Approaching the crucial Security Council vote on Iraq in February 2003, Bush could count only on Great Britain to back his Iraqi invasion plan. In a final bid to rally international support for the resolution, Bush emphasized the threat of Iraq's biological and chemical arms. "Leaving Saddam Hussein in possession of weapons of mass destruction for a few more months or years is not an option, not in a post-September 11th world," said Secretary of State Powell in a multimedia presentation to the council. The secretary presented tapes of intercepted transmissions and satellite photographs that presumably documented the existence of Iraqi WMD. Saddam had also collaborated with al-Qaeda, Powell alleged, and had conspired to acquire nuclear bombs.

Yet the council remained incredulous. The question was not whether Saddam possessed WMD—even Hans Blix, the chief UN inspector, believed he did—but whether that threat was effectively circumscribed by international monitoring and sanctions. A majority of the council's members agreed with Blix that the current measures were succeeding and that war was neither necessary nor warranted. Flummoxed, Bush resolved to proceed irrespective of the UN position and, on March 18, issued an ultimatum giving Saddam forty-eight hours to leave his country or face all-out invasion.

Two days later, a quarter of a million troops—more than 90 percent of them Americans—thundered into Iraq. Banned from entering northern Iraq through neighboring Turkey, the troops had set out from Kuwait, in the extreme southeast. Breaking a record set by Eaton and his Marines in the Western Desert, the modern Marines marched more than five hundred miles through inhospitable and nearly impassable terrain in order to engage the enemy. And engage they did, ruthlessly, annihilating Saddam's armored corps and his ostensibly elite divisions. A special Marine detachment, nicknamed

Task Force Tripoli in honor of the Barbary Wars, took Saddam's hometown of Tikrit. Coalition warplanes and cruise missiles meanwhile repeated their 1991 barrage on Baghdad and on other strategic locations in an intensive assault code-named Shock and Awe. Television screens around the world once again glowed with the greenish baubles of Iraqi antiaircraft fire raking the night sky ineffectually. But the haunting images of blazing rigs and blackened waters would not be revisited, due to the rapid-moving British and American units that seized Iraqi oil fields and refineries. Other outfits secured strategic bridges and airfields, facilitating the ground forces' advance.

Victory would come swiftly but not as handily or as resistance-free as in the first Gulf War. Fierce sandstorms pelted the coalition columns and Iraqi snipers harassed them as they slogged through the towns of Najaf, Kufa, and Nasiriya. But neither the grit nor the sleet of bullets and rocket-propelled grenades (RPGs) could stall the inexorable offensive. While Iraq's buffoonish information minister, Muhammad Saeed al-Sahaf, known to the press as Baghdad Bob, continued to insist that the Americans were "snakes moving in the desert" and that there was "no presence of infidels in the city," the invaders converged on the capital. On April 9, Iraqis thronged around Marine Corporal Edward Chin as he looped a steel cable around a statue of Saddam Hussein that had been draped with the Stars and Stripes. Late nineteenth-century Americans had celebrated their primacy by erecting an ancient Egyptian obelisk in Central Park and proclaimed their principles by building a torch-bearing colossus, originally intended for Suez, on Bedloe's Island. But now, just after the twenty-first century's turn, Americans flaunted their strength and advertised their idealism by tearing down an effigy in Iraq. Hooking the cable to his M88 tank retriever, Chin wrenched Saddam from his pedestal, while the Iraqis ululated and danced.

For one incandescent moment, America appeared to have reconciled the countervailing themes of its Middle East involvement. Victorious soldiers now patrolled the fabled city of *A Thousand and One Arabian Nights* and prepared to bestow liberty on a people yearning for it. After the disappointments of the nonaligned Mossadegh and Nasser, the autocratic Sadat and the gun-toting Arafat, America stood ready to realize its dream of a secular Middle Eastern leadership committed to democracy, nonviolence, and the West. For the first time, the vision of a *pax Americana* radiating out of Iraq and enlightening the entire region seemed reachable. Piloting a Viking jet, Bush descended deus ex machina–like onto the deck of the *Abraham Lincoln* on May 1 and declared the end of Operation Iraqi Freedom.

The battle had in fact scarcely begun. No sooner was Baghdad liberated than looters ransacked its buildings and vital services—water, electricity, and health care—broke down. Though Saddam was captured and his notorious sons Uday and Qusay were killed, opposition to the occupiers escalated. Thousands of former Iraqi troops, demobilized under an ill-advised de-Ba'athification policy, swelled the insurgency's ranks, while the overstretched American forces struggled to police a country twice the size of Idaho with a population of twenty-six million. Daily and with increasing deadliness, U.S. troops were blasted by improvised explosive devices and riddled in roadside ambushes. Several American civilians, many of whom were engaged in efforts to reconstruct Iraq, were kidnapped and filmed while knife-wielding Islamists beheaded them. Relations between the administration and the Iraqi opposition soured; Ahmad Chalabi switched his allegiance to Sayyid Ali Husaini Sistani, Iraq's leading Shi'ite cleric. And in spite of intensive searches throughout the country, no compelling physical evidence was uncovered of the existence of WMD.

Still, America's intervention in Iraq produced several positive outcomes, some of them of monumental import. Defying death threats from the insurgents, the Iraqi people succeeded in forging a constitution and in holding free elections. Muammar Qadhafi, the bête noir of successive American presidents, voluntarily abjured his search for nuclear weapons and sued for renewed relations with the United States. Aroused by the Iraqi example, a wave of democratization seemed to sweep the Middle East—in Egypt and Saudi Arabia, where opposition groups began to sprout, and in Lebanon, which finally succeeded in freeing itself from direct Syrian occupation. "We believe that freedom can advance and change lives in the greater Middle East," Bush, extolling these accomplishments, proclaimed. "Whenever people are given a choice in the matter, they prefer lives of free-dom to lives of fear."

The Egyptian and Saudi regimes quickly quashed these democratic stirrings, however, and Lebanon remained implicitly under Syria's thumb. Islamic extremist parties such as Hamas, which dominated the democratic Palestinian elections of 2006, gained popularity throughout the region at the expense of modernizing secular move-ments. Libya gave up its nuclear program, but Iran initiated one that was far larger, better defended, and vastly more threatening to the region. The Iraqis had united under a national constitution and lead-ership, but the country soon succumbed to sectarian bloodshed between Shi'ites and Sunnis and among Shi'ites, Sunnis, and Kurds. Suddenly, in addition to democraticizing, the United States was engaged in the even more herculean task of state-making in the Mid-dle East. American troops who came to unseat a tyrant now toiled at holding a nation together, braving shrapnel while shifting through the detritus of bombed-out marketplaces and mosques.

"You aren't going to war to change the Iraqis," a War Department handbook issued during World War II had assured the GIs who were stationed in Iraq. "Just the opposite. We are fighting this war to pre-serve the principle of 'live and let live.'" The handbook contained the usual list of do's and don'ts—"keep away from mosques, avoid any religious or political discussions, do not drink liquor or eat pork, never strike an Iraqi, and never make advances to Moslem women or try to attract their attention." Sixty years later, the mission assigned to American servicemen and women in Iraq had changed immeasurably, yet the warnings provided to them remained aston-ishingly similar. The laminated Iraqi Culture Smart Card issued to U.S. forces in Iraq advised them, "Shake hands only with your right hand, never offer a Muslim alcohol or pork, and don't engage in reli-gious discussions." In contrast to the World War II pamphlet, how-ever, the Smart Card also detailed the country's many mutually hostile factions and contained lifesaving hints on how to distinguish among them. But even this information often proved inadequate in negotiating Iraq's ethnic minefields and preserving American lives. Brian Turner, a poet who served as an infantry officer in Iraq, offered a more practical guide:

If you hear gunfire on a Thursday afternoon,
it could be for a wedding or it could be for you.

Inshallah means Allah be willing.
Listen well when it is spoken.

You will hear the RPG coming for you.
Not so the roadside bomb.

There are bombs under the overpasses,
in trashpiles, in bricks, in cars. . . .

Men wearing vests rigged with explosives
Walk up, raise their arms and say Inshallah.

There are men who earn eighty dollars
to attack you, five thousand to kill.

Small children who will play with you,
old men with their talk, women who offer chai—

and any one of them
may dance over your body tomorrow.

American troops struggled to maintain unity within Iraq while, back home, the consensus on the war rapidly unraveled. Mounting casualties among U.S. soldiers stoked the growing opposition to the fighting, as did proof of the massacre of Iraqi civilians by American troops and the abuse of Iraqi prisoners at Abu Ghraib. Critics of the president accused him of having exaggerated or even falsified evidence of Saddam's WMD and of violating civil liberties under the banner of Homeland Security. In response, Bush's defenders rallied to assert that America was in fact winning the war, that the Iraqi army had been reconstructed, and that the insurgency was on the wane. The states that survived an agonizing split between blue and gray were once again divided, this time between blue and red. So complete was the break that commentators, when writing about

Iraq, seemed to be describing entirely different countries. "We have given liberty to the stepchildren of the Arab world," determined the Middle East scholar Fouad Ajami. "We have overturned an edifice of material and moral power that dates back centuries." But the ex-neoconservative philosopher Francis Fukuyama lamented the "self-fulfilling prophecy" that Bush had created in Iraq, a land where "Jihadist gunmen can train on real-live American targets." The public intellectual Christopher Hitchens extolled the "federal and democratic Iraq" that "could undercut the Saudi and Iranian duopoly" and bring dignity to "a people immiserated by three decades of war and fascism." But the *New York Times* columnist Thomas Friedman, an early proponent of the war and acerbic critic of its conduct, excoriated the "faith-based" Bush for launching "a faith-based war in Iraq, on the basis of faith-based intelligence, with a faith-based plan for Iraqi reconstruction."[14]

The schism in public opinion regarding Iraq paralleled the deepening rifts in popular perceptions of the Middle East. College faculties grew increasingly polarized between those professors who still faulted America for the region's ills and those who accosted universities for varnishing the Islamist threat. At the same time, the movie industry continued to wrestle with the question of how best to depict the Middle East and its inhabitants. Produced in 2006, the film *Munich* portrays some Palestinian terrorists as articulate and sympathetic, while the al-Qaeda hijackers in *United 93*, also released that year, are unexceptionally murderous. *Syriana* (2005) features good and bad Arabs, suicide bombers and Pollyannaish Americans, but ultimately blames the Middle East's morass on avaricious oil companies and CIA assassins. Old myths meanwhile persisted, even in the post-9/11 years. *Hidalgo* (2004) tells the story of Frank Hopkins (Viggo Mortensen), a Pony Express rider who, disconsolate over the disappearance of the Old West, finds a fresh and unsullied frontier in the oases, dunes, and dreamlike encampments of Arabia.

The debate over the essential nature of the Middle East and its relations with the United States shows no signs of waning. The American people, who traditionally sought to transform the region into a mirror of the United States, can today see their own splintered reflection in Iraq's fractured face. And those fissures are likely to spread. Ahead loom possible large-scale collisions with Iran and with a profusion of Islamic militant groups. Americans may once again be dragged into eruptions of Arab-Israeli violence. Oil, an energy source for which the world has yet to find a replacement and which grows scarcer and costlier each year, may continue to fuel conflagrations that will consume American wealth and manpower. Though the domestic debate over Iraq has shifted from one of victory versus defeat to immediate versus phased withdrawal, American troops are expected to remain in the country at least through 2008. If so, then the United States will have concluded three decades of virtually uninterrupted clashes in the Middle East. But the end of one thirty years' war may merely herald the outbreak of other, potentially more devastating, conflicts lasting long into the twenty-first century.

Yet, in spite of these cataclysms, the United States can be expected to pursue the traditional patterns of its Middle East involvement. Policymakers will press on with their civic mission as mediators and liberators in the area and strive for a *pax Americana*. American churches and evangelist groups will still seek to save the region spiritually. And the producers of films about the mysterious, menacing Orient will never lack for audiences. The themes that evolved over the course of more than two centuries of America's interaction with the Middle East will continue to distinguish those ties, binding and animating them for generations.

————❦————

A PROFOUND AND
VISCERAL GRATITUDE

FOLLOWING THE TRADITION ESTABLISHED BY JOHN LEDYARD at the time of America's indepedence, Nathaniel Fick left Dartmouth College for the Middle East. Tall, broad-shouldered, and blond, he resembled Ledyard physically and shared his air of manly confidence and his easygoing dash. In contrast to Ledyard, however, Fick was not fleeing Dartmouth, but had rather graduated with honors. He departed not in a canoe on the Connecticut River but in a bus bound for Quantico, Virginia. He was also joining the Marines—not the Royal Marines, like Ledyard, but the Corps of the United States. Some 225 years after Ledyard landed in Egypt, Nathaniel Fick journeyed to Iraq.

"I felt totally disoriented, utterly adrift," Fick recalled of his initial impressions of the region, which he likened to "a hall of mirrors." As commander of a Special Operations platoon, driving Humvees with mounted fifty-caliber machine guns, Captain Fick had crossed the Kuwaiti border on March 20, 2003, ahead of the First Marine Division, to scout out Iraqi defenses. "How can you understand where you are when you can't even read the street signs?" The twenty-six-year-old Baltimorean watched as village elders stomped their feet and spat, only to be told by a native translator that the people were grateful to America and happy to be liberated from Saddam Hussein.

Many Iraqis in 2003 were in fact thankful and feted the advancing Americans. "I guess this is what it felt like in France in 1944," one of Fick's leathernecks remarked. One hospitable herdsman even offered the Marines a goat. The greetings ceased, however, in Nasiriya, where the Americans encountered spirited resistance, and in the towns outside of Baghdad, each of which they took with fire. Later, after the capital's fall, Fick and his men became the targets of rocket attacks and improvised bombings—the hallmarks of the Iraqi insurgency. "Hajj, an honorific term to Arab men, became the negative term we used for all Iraqis," Fick sadly remembered. "The 'gook' of our generation." Increasingly confused about the military's role in the conflict, with the home front divided over the war's validity and Iraq tottering between democracy and anarchy, Nathaniel Fick and his 130,000 fellow troopers focused on staying alive and, wherever possible, providing better lives for Iraqis.

By protecting themselves from Middle Eastern threats while simultaneously trying to assist native peoples, U.S. forces in Iraq were, in effect, revisiting the earliest American involvement in the region. The United States had scarcely achieved independence when the Barbary States began preying on its trade and imperiling its very existence. To endure, the incipient nation had to unite under a strong central government, create a formidable naval force, and wage a desperate campaign thousands of miles from its shores. American warships continued to patrol Middle Eastern waters after the Barbary Wars, enabling mechants to exchange New England rum and manufactured goods for opium, carpets, and figs. Bibles also arrived, along with a procession of missionaries. Though their original goal was to convert the native population to Christianity and to restore Palestine to the Jews, these evangelists eventually built schools and printed textbooks imparting Western-style education to their pupils. The missionaries later established the area's first universities and introduced concepts of American-style democracy and nationalism.

In addition to seeking national security, economic opportunity, and spiritual rewards, Americans sailed to the Middle East in search of adventure. From the earliest days of the Republic, residents of the former colonies had set out to explore this fabled realm, seduced by rumors of its eroticism and drawn to its murky dangers. The initial trickle of trailblazers and swashbucklers soon gave way to a deluge of sightseers and relic snatchers. Others, spurred by a blend of temerity and religion, established colonies in the Holy Land, navigated the Jordan, and pioneered the field of biblical archaeology. Returning home, Americans wrote poems and travelogues about their experiences; they created a fez-sporting fraternal order, a conservationist movement, and a camel corps. Less than a century after the first citizen of the independent United States had probed the reaches of the Nile, Americans had penetrated virtually every precinct of the region and dotted it with diplomatic legations.

But then, just as the bonds between America and the Middle East solidified, the Union began to unwind. The Civil War that ultimately saved the Republic exerted a far-reaching influence on Middle Eastern politics. Former enemies from the North and the South reunited to make the Egyptian army a catalyst for modernization and the vanguard of a patriotic movement. War-wrought fluctuations in the cotton market meanwhile caused radical shifts in the Egyptian economy, helping to bring about Britain's occupation of the country and accelerating Europe's conquest of the region. The industrialization spurred by the war enabled the United States to attain the status of world-class power in the Middle East. Its citizens, though bereft of their innnocence by the horrors of combat, remained no less avid in their desire to scale the pyramids and wade into the Dead Sea. But while their homeland enjoyed a new birth of freedom, the landmass between the Atlantic and Suez languished under foreign rule. A Statue of Liberty that the insolvent Egyptians could not afford to build instead arose in New York harbor, the gateway to freedoms for which Middle Eastern peoples might only yearn.

Antebellum America had faced keen dilemmas in the Middle East—whether to support the Greeks' righteous struggle against Ottoman occupation, for example, or pursue tangible economic interests with the Porte—and those quandaries only sharpened in the imperialist age. Should the United States side with the victims of the same colonialism against which it, too, had fought, or should it close ranks with the bearers of enlightened civilization against an allegedly stagnant Islam? Most Americans sympathized with the colonizers of the area and applauded those presidents who conducted their diplomacy through gunboats. An eminent minority, though, denounced displays of American militarism in the Middle East and worked for the region's independence. Others still sought sovereignty for specific peoples in particular lands, whether for the Jews in Palestine or for the Arabs of Syria and Mesopotamia. Americans as a whole, however, were content to consign such issues to their church or their newspapers while they marveled at Persian pageants and "genuine" Egyptian exhibitions. But the wonder of these reveries was soon infringed by the bleakness of Middle Eastern reality. Hundreds of thousands of Armenian corpses lined the path to even ghastlier slaughters in the area and to thornier American dilemmas.

As they entered World War I, Americans had to decide whether to commence hostilities against the Turks or to remain neutral in the fateful struggle for the Middle East. No longer a matter of ethics versus interests, the question now centered on which was more moral: defeating a genocidal empire or protecting the institutions that American philanthropy had cultivated over the course of one hundred years. The influence accumulated during that century by American missionaries and their supporters eventually proved decisive. The United States never sent an army to the Middle East, ceding an immense advantage to France and Britain, which did. American leaders consequently failed in any attempt to guarantee self-determination for Middle Eastern peoples, if that was indeed possible, and instead endorsed a mandate system that in effect perpetuated European rule. Though great numbers of Americans realized their dream of laying foundations for a Jewish home in Palestine, the desire of many others for the fulfillment of Arab national rights remained ungratified.

Repulsed by the carnage of World War I and the sordidness of the postwar settlement, Americans recoiled from further intervention in world affairs and from the Middle East especially. For the majority of Americans, the region was increasingly reduced to the romantic Hollywood images or bawdy vaudeville songs that had replaced books as the main purveyors of Middle Eastern myths. Prominent sectors of American society nevertheless remained actively involved in the area. Some mobilized to strengthen the Zionist enterprise in Palestine and to dislodge the U.S. government from its position of neutrality in that region's simmering dispute. Smaller but more influential groups of missionaries, adventurers, and businessmen established a historic rapport with the Saudi tribe in Arabia and a monopoly over its sole subterranean asset.

By 1939, Arabian oil had become an important component of America's economy, yet the United States still refrained from diplomatic, much less military, intervention in the region. That policy continued even after the outbreak of World War II and the Japanese attack on Pearl Harbor. It took the German conquest of much of the Mediterranean basin and the Axis's advance on the Suez Canal to prod the Americans into invading. Landing once again on the "shores of Tripoli," U.S. servicemen defeated the enemy and deployed across the theater, as far east as Iran. In contrast to its retreat into isolationism after World War I, the United States emerged from World War II as the preponderant power in the Middle East, an advocate for its development and a defender of its freedom.

With power, however, came responsibilities. Having failed to rescue European Jewry from Nazism, the United States was saddled with the hundreds of thousands of Holocaust survivors who insisted on resettlement in Palestine. But satisfying those demands brought America into conflict with Palestine's British trustees, who opposed further immigration into the country and its reconstitution into a Jewish state. Though the U.S. government needed Britain's assistance in defending the Middle East from a burgeoning Soviet threat, the American people also had a long-standing commitment to Zionism. America ultimately sided with the Jews and, in May 1948, became the first nation to recognize the State of Israel. In doing so, it hastened the process of Britain's retreat from the region and aroused the anger of many Arabs who, though grateful for this setback to imperialism, hated Zionism far more than they feared Soviet communism. The advent of the Cold War, escalation of the Arab-Israeli conflict, and deepening of America's dependence on Arab oil gave rise to Gordian questions. Could the United States maintain its support for

Israel and its alliance with Britain and France while sustaining its friendship with the Arabs? How could it rally a fractious Middle East and steel it against Soviet inroads?

Skirting these conundrums, America temporarily steered a cogent course through the region. A presidential doctrine—the first of several such pronouncements relating to Middle Eastern security— extended vital military aid to Greece and Turkey, and decisive American action in the UN barred the Soviets from North Africa and the Northern Tier. While standing by its European allies against communism, Washington aligned with native nationalists against imperialism. Libya, Syria, and Iran were among the countries that owed their independence partly or principally to the United States. Yet the countervailing requisites of the Cold War and the anticolonialist movement quickly proved irreconcilable. The United States banded with Britain in ousting a popular Iranian leader in 1953, but three years later it joined with the Soviets in preventing Britain, France, and Israel from overthrowing an Egyptian ruler whom America had secretly sought to depose. American leaders pressured Israel to abandon its nuclear program, but later backed Israel as a bulwark against Soviet aggression. The decision made the United States a target of an Arab oil embargo and of Palestinians who, disappointed by the failure of conventional efforts to vanquish Israel, increasingly turned to terror. Eager to defuse these hostilities, America offered its services as a mediator, urging Israel to relinquish captured territories in exchange for Arab promises of peace.

After thirty years of ascendancy in the Middle East, Americans could point to some proud achievements but also to painful setbacks. They had formed a steadfast alliance with Israel and negotiated a peace agreement between Cairo and Jerusalem. They had reduced Soviet influence in the Arab world and championed human rights. And yet, in the eyes of many peoples throughout the region, the United States remained the paladin of oppressive autocrats, the patron of Israeli settlements in the West Bank and Gaza, and the promoter of oil-fueled profligacy in the Persian Gulf. American policies in the Middle East had garnered an array of Nobel Prizes as well as a lengthening roster of terrorist attacks. Indeed, assaults rather than accolades became the norm for Americans as the period of East-West tensions in the region yielded to an era of intensifying clashes between the West and radical Islam.

Starting in 1979 with the takeover of the U.S. embassy in Teheran, Americans were repeatedly under fire from the Middle East. They were hijacked and bombed on airliners, gunned down in airports and at sea, blown apart in European discotheques, and buried under the rubble in Beirut. America fired back, dispatching its forces to Libya and Lebanon, but with little effect other than the emboldening of terrorists. Bewildered by the transition from Cold War to holy war, the United States supported an Iraqi dictatorship against an Iranian theocracy and secretly armed Teheran against Baghdad. It backed anti-American Islamists in their fight against the Soviets in Afghanistan and collaborated with the Saudis who were promulgating Islamic extremism. America at first endorsed and then opposed Israel's invasion of Lebanon, initially condemned and later appreciated the Israeli bombing of an Iraqi reactor, and collaborated with Israel in a covert arms-for-hostages scheme, only to imprison an American for life on the charge of spying for Israel. And while the government pursued these protean policies, the public perception of the Middle East vacillated between that of an Oriental dreamland and a netherworld of kidnappers and thugs. Scholars grappled with the question of whether the Middle East again threatened Americans mortally or whether the United States was the root of Middle Eastern ills.

Those questions appeared to be answered, albeit briefly, by America's war against a ruthless tyrant in Iraq and its campaign to liberate Kuwait. Exulting in that triumph, the United States promised to enact a new world order bestowing security and peace on the Middle East. In reality, the region received neither. Though American policymakers toiled to forge agreements between Palestinians and Israelis and to counter the Islamists nonviolently, the agreements disintegrated into bloodshed, and terror again claimed hundreds of lives. Reluctant to confront the danger at its sources, overconfident in its military, and still deluded by Middle Eastern myths, Americans were ill prepared for the ultimate jihadist aggression. With the crumbling of the Twin Towers, however, came the breakdown of romantic illusions and the collapse of American restraint.

Kabul fell to U.S. forces, followed by Baghdad, Faluja, and Tikrit. But the heat of America's victory over the fundamentalist Taliban and the secular Ba'ath seemingly welded the religious and nationalist elements in Iraq into an implacably galvanized insurgency. The United States fulfilled its centuries-long urge to instill American-style democracy in the Middle East, but with it came rapid dissolution. Initially mauled by Sunni and Shi'ite militiamen determined to drive them from the country, U.S. troops were soon trapped in the cross fires between Sunni and Shi'ite partisans aiming to kill one another. Internationally, the United States found itself isolated from the Western European states that refrained from enlisting in the coalition in Iraq, much as they had refused, two hundred years earlier, to join in an alliance against Barbary. Americans as a nation were also divided, disagreeing over the justification, the conduct, and the sacrifices of the war, as the casualty rate—military and civilian—soared. The Middle East that had helped unite Americans at the end of the eighteenth century was, early in the twenty-first, rending them apart.

"TERRIBLE MISTAKES were made," said Nathaniel Fick. "We failed to stop the looting, failed to seal the borders, and we disbanded the Iraqi army." The veteran Marine captain had just published a widely acclaimed book, *One Bullet Away*, a memoir of his military experiences, and was studying for advanced degrees in business and government at Harvard. "We were blind," he added. "We were strong but we weren't smart." He shared his views about Iraq with me, about the Middle East and America's role in it, in a coffee shop near the Cambridge campus. Outside, nattily bundled students bustled to class, angling against the February wind and clutching their books for warmth. We were far, impossibly far, from the sun-raked Nasiriya bridge where Fick and his men came under furious sniper fire and had to run doubled over their guns. Yet the war was still nearby, not only in Fick's memory but in the daily fears and hopes of virtually all Americans.

"I have been in four Middle Eastern countries, and I've never used a passport in any of them," Fick quipped, but only half sarcastically.

Though he had long ago exchanged his fatigues for a gray business suit, he once again became a soldier as he described the pitched gunfights his unit waged, his disappointments over the execution of the war, and sadness over the deaths of several of his comrades. Yet he remained proud of his service in Iraq—"I believed in the war and still do," he insisted—and optimistic about the Middle East. The United States can indeed assist the region to democratize, Fick explained, but the decision ultimately rests with its inhabitants. "They can go the way of modernization or they can go the way of Sub-Saharan Africa," he posited. "The choice is theirs."

He spoke, and for a moment I actually imagined myself listening to John Ledyard. The voices of Pliny Fisk, Charles Pomeroy Stone, Clara Barton, and the countless Americans who had served in the Middle East seemed to echo in his words. The history of U.S.-Middle East relations, I reminded myself, was not one of unqualified kindness and altruism. American oil companies pumped billions of barrels of Arabian oil not for the betterment of the indigenous population but for their own enrichment. Successive administrations had backed the oppressive regimes that advanced America's interests and conspired to overthrow popular leaders. Yet for all its demerits, the record of American interaction with the Middle East is rife with acts of decency and graced with good intentions. The United States was unrivaled in introducing modern education and health care to the area, in extending emergency relief and building infrastructure, in obtaining the freedom of colonized nations, and in attempting to achieve security and peace. On balance, Americans historically brought far more beneficence than avarice to the Middle East and caused significantly less harm than good.

Living up to that legacy and enhancing it are now America's challenges. The country's involvement in the Middle East may not be limited to waging war in Iraq or mediating the Arab-Israeli conflict. In the near future, Americans will have to cope with the threat of an expansionist Iran and with the dangers of al-Qaeda splinter groups. They will have to achieve a new understanding with Islam and invest in viable alternatives to oil. Above all, they will have to engage in brave introspection, reexamining their relationship to the Middle East and, through it, their relationship with the world.

Nathaniel Fick had already embarked on that journey. Unlike John Ledyard, who romanticized his voyage to the Middle East as a "passage to glory," Fick regarded his experiences in the region as a venue for gaining a deeper appreciation of the United States, confronting its faults but also acknowledging its virtues. "I felt a profound and visceral gratitude for the country in which I'd grown up," he noted. Persuading the peoples of the Middle East to share in that esteem will require resolute but prudent demonstrations of America's power and firm but tolerant applications of its faith. By responsibly wielding its strength and consistently upholding its principles, the United States might yet transform its vision of peaceful, fruitful relations with the Middle East from fantasy into reality.

Afterword

IN THE LONG AND DAZZLINGLY RICH HISTORY OF AMERICA IN THE Middle East, one year might not seem such a singular time. Throughout much of that history, between the end of the Barbary Wars and that of World War II, Americans rarely faced substantial threats from the region. Rather, they blithely regarded it as a realm for disseminating their values, for living out their Oriental fantasies, and for purchasing capers and dates. That complacency rapidly vanished, however, beginning in the late 1940s. The advent of the oil factor, the emergence of the Arab-Israeli conflict, and the fall of France and Britain as the principal Western powers in the region all intensified the U.S.-Middle East relationship, endowing it with an urgent, if not existential, edge.

Americans could no longer treat the Middle East merely as a quaint if fractured glass for casting and catching their reflection, as a potential simulacrum of the United States. Instead, disaffected groups in the region began viewing the United States as a reverse mirror of what they were not—libertine, decadent, democratic—and pondering ways for making Americans resemble them, even by violence.

The stakes in America's involvement in the Middle East have mounted exponentially, and no year better illustrated that ascent than the one that began on July 1, 2006, the day this book was completed. The ensuing twelve months saw the Middle East seized by paroxysms of warfare, political crises, and civil bloodshed. These cataclysms repeatedly challenged the United States to reassess its relations with the Middle East and to reexamine many of the fundamental assumptions about its role in the region and the world. The mirror had indeed become two-sided, compelling Americans to engage in deep and wrenching introspection.

An adumbration of the year's calamities appeared on the morning of July 12, 2006, when gunmen belonging to Lebanon's Shiite Hizbollah organization ambushed an Israeli border patrol, killing eight soldiers and kidnapping two. Israel lashed back with a massive bombing campaign against Hizbollah and the routes it used to receive munitions from Syria and Iran. Hundreds of civilians died and hundreds of thousands were displaced. The fighting forced the United States to choose between two allies—Israel, the object of an unprovoked terrorist attack, and Lebanon, an Arab democracy destabilized by Islamic radicalism. Struggling to reconcile its war on terror with its support for Middle East democratization, the Bush administration allowed Israelis the leeway to crush Hizbollah while pressuring them to avoid inflicting disproportionate injury on Lebanon. But these goals ultimately proved incompatible. Israel failed to stop the rain of thousands of Hizbollah rockets on its own cities while its bombing of civilian areas, turning entire streets into rubble and their residents into refugees, generated international pressure for a ceasefire. Though its headquarters were destroyed and much its fighting force eliminated, Hizbollah emerged from the war as the unbowed hero of the Arab and Muslim worlds, and the United States was blamed for further weakening Lebanon's beleaguered government. Popular opinion throughout the region perceived the war as a victory for Hizbollah's primary backer—and America's nemesis—Iran.

Iran loomed ominously over all of the year's convulsions, alternatively threatening and cajoling the United States. Iran's shrewd but unprepossessing president, Mahmoud Ahmadinejad, pledged to work for "a world without America and Zionism" in which liberalism and democracy were supplanted by "the Divine Word of the Holy Quran." He arrested U.S. citizens who were visiting Iran on spying charges and materially escalated Iranian support for anti-

American insurgents in Iraq. Yet the same Ahmadinejad addressed an open letter to the American people, blessing them and inviting them to join him in fruitful dialogue. He praised the "human values and spirit" of the United States, and proclaimed his dedication to "peace and tranquility" worldwide. Iran continued to defy United Nations sanctions by enriching the uranium necessary for producing nuclear arms, all the while reiterating Iran's commitment to UN principles of nonproliferation.

These vacillations again impelled the United States to confront the contradictions in its Middle East policies. Could a country long committed to the nonviolent resolution of the region's conflicts peremptorily brush aside Iranian offers of reconciliation? On the other hand, could the preeminent superpower allow Iran to flaunt the international strictures championed by the United States, to endanger its regional allies, and to murder its troops? And finally, if faithful attempts at diplomacy failed, would the United States, desperately bogged down in Iraq, still have the power necessary to defeat a geographically vast, densely populated, and lavishly armed Iran?

The question of whether America could counterbalance its republican beliefs with Middle Eastern realpolitik was poignantly raised in Gaza. Having promulgated free and open elections in the Palestinian Authority, American leaders watched horrified as representatives of Hamas, an Iranian-backed organization that opposed Israel's existence and espoused terror, swept the balloting. The Hamas victory presented Washington with a bitter choice: accept the Palestinians' preference, no matter how abhorrent, or back the avowedly moderate but fiscally corrupt and discredited al-Fatah faction, headed by PA President Mahmoud Abbas. Pressed with deciding between democracy and the possibility of peace, the Bush administration opted for the latter, furnishing funds and military assistance for Abbas and his militia.

Hamas, however, would not be subverted, and in July 2007—a year after the Lebanon war—it struck back. Hamas gunmen overran al-Fatah positions in Gaza, shooting prisoners in the head and hurling them off high-rise buildings. Within a week, Hamas's silky green flags furled unchallenged over the Strip. Washington hastened to impose a total embargo of the new Hamas mini-state and to augment its financial support for Abbas's West Bank government. But little could mitigate the militant Islamists' historic triumph at the expense of America and its allies.

Lebanon, Iran, and Gaza all obliged Americans to reevaluate their policies toward the Middle East and to reflect fundamentally on themselves. The most monumental crisis, however, and the mightiest impulse for self-scrutiny, remained Iraq. Now entering its fifth year, the war had claimed the lives of well over 3,500 U.S. soldiers and as many as 74,000 Iraqis. An average of one hundred Iraqis died each day during the last year, and insurgent attacks rose an estimated 77 percent.

Grisly scenes of carnage in Iraqi streets, of women wailing over their children's remains, became commonplace, as did reports of civilian contractor corruption and abuses by individual troops. Even the hanging of Saddam Hussein on December 30, 2006, an event intended to conciliate the Iraqi people and console his myriad victims, devolved into fission. The executioners taunted the former dictator with the name of his chief Shiite rival, and told him to "go to hell," as the trapdoor fell open.

The lightless horizon over Iraq accentuated the rising opposition to the war throughout the United States. Though support for the Bush administration's Iraqi policies stayed constant in conservative circles, especially among the families of the troops, a swelling majority of Americans demanded a radically changed course in Iraq, if not a precipitate pullout. "The victory we seek is . . . the restoration of America's role as peacemaker, not warmonger," James Clyburn, a Democratic congressman, averred, while his colleague, Vietnam veteran John Murtha, called for the withdrawal of all U.S. forces from Iraq.

Most Republican representatives, by contrast, rallied to the president's defense, warning of the dangers to America's interests in the Middle East as well as to its home security should the United States be perceived as defeated. "The enemy wants our men and women in uniform to think their Congress doesn't care about them," explained Texas Representative Sam Johnson, who had also served in Vietnam and who urged Americans to "learn from our mistakes" and not "leave the job undone." But other Republicans dared to dissent from their party's platform and assailed the president's approach. "It's a ping-pong game with American lives," affirmed Nebraska Senator Chuck Hagel. "[It's] the most dangerous foreign policy blunder in this country since Vietnam."

The cavalcade of the year's Middle Eastern crises elicited a multiplicity of American responses, many of them at cross purposes. In a national address on January 10, 2007, President Bush announced a New Way Forward in Iraq, where an additional 20,000 U.S. troops would uproot the rebels from urban centers and train the Iraqi army. The United States also augmented its naval presence in the Gulf, opposite Iran, and pledged an unprecedented $63 billion in defense assistance to Iran's principal adversaries—Saudi Arabia, Egypt, and Israel. "The world's free nations will not allow tyrants to develop a nuclear weapon," the president vowed. "America will not bow down to ants." This military "surge" was accompanied by a torrent of diplomatic activity designed to tighten sanctions against Iran and to secure an Arab-Israeli peace. Endorsing former British Prime Minister Tony Blair as a special Middle East envoy, Bush reiterated his support for Palestinian independence, offering them the choice between "chaos" and the chance to "reclaim their dignity."

A great many Americans, however, remained dissatisfied with Bush's choices, convinced that they led less to honor than to deepening disorder. Democrats in Congress insisted that the Iraqi government meet a series of benchmarks, such as equitably distributing oil revenues and disarming illegal militias, or face renewed demands for American withdrawal. A bipartisan Iraq Study Group, headed by former Secretary of State James Baker and ex-Congressman Lee Hamilton, also took exception to the president's path, prophesying an apocalypse of unbridled civil war in Iraq and expanded al-Qaeda terror should the United States fail to force Iraqi leaders to live up to their defense and democratic duties. The Bush administration had to embark on a concerted initiative to attain an Arab-Israeli agreement, Baker and Hamilton added, and inaugurate discussions with Syria and Iran. Bush publicly endorsed these proposals, sent Secretary of State Condoleezza Rice on repeated peace shuttles through the region, and even agreed—begrudgingly—to talks with Damascus and Teheran. But approaching the end of his term in the office, the president seemed determined to leave a pugnacious rather than pacific legacy. "Some can argue our withdrawal from Vietnam carried no price to American credibility, but the terrorists see it differently," he said. "We must defeat them overseas so we do not face them in the United States of America."

And in a few areas, at least, Bush's combativeness seemed to work. Combining urban combat tactics with delicate inter-clan diplomacy, American troops ousted al-Qaeda from some of Baghdad's most insurgent-infested neighborhoods. Yet, in the manner of legendary Dutch dams, the successful stemming of one breach was nullified by the rupture of dozens more. If humbled in Iraq, al-Qaeda emerged reinvigorated in Lebanon, Gaza, and Afghanistan. Terrorists continued to target the United States with narrowly averted attacks against Fort Dix, New Jersey, and Kennedy Airport. And while America's enemies remained robust, some of its allies grew recalcitrant. King Abdullah of Saudi Arabia denounced the "illegal foreign occupation" of Iraq, and a senior aid to Iraqi Prime Minister Nouri al-Maliki castigated the United States for treating his country as "an experiment in an American laboratory." Turkey, traditionally one of the Middle East's most avidly pro-American states, registered the highest level of anti-American sentiment anywhere in the region. Joshua Walker, an expert on modern Turkey, noted that such animus "cannot simply be erased with a special envoy to the Muslim world or with a new president in January 2009."

Bewildered by these events, internally cleft, Americans anguished over their future relationship with the Middle East. Many fell back on familiar patterns. Even while pressing for additional displays of American power in Iraq, President Bush emphasized the need to see "our faith in freedom redeemed." Power and faith again blended in the effort to transform the graft-ridden Palestinian Authority into a paragon state through the provision of American arms and military training. Faith also informed the "realist" assumptions of the Iraq Study Group that Arab-Israel peace would help resolve Shiite-Sunni feuding and that Iran and Syria shared America's interests in a stable Iraq—faith and a modicum of fantasy. Hollywood, for its part, continued to mass produce movies on Middle Eastern motifs, most of them spotlighting the trauma of those Americans who fought in the region and returned—like generations of their forebears going back to 1776—disoriented and shorn of innocence.

But while some of their countrymen looked to the past for models of how to proceed in the Middle East, others wondered whether the time had arrived to separate from the region entirely. For them, political commentator David Brooks observed, "the issue is no longer the Clash of Civilizations but a Gap of Civilizations, which many Americans believe is unbridgeable." There is a burgeoning sense that the Middle East can never be a reflection of the United States and that America's image refracted in the Middle Eastern glass is increasingly repulsive. Consequently, increasing numbers of Americans were prone to recoil entirely from the Middle East, leaving it to seethe in its own toxic environment.

The year that began in July 2006 might prove to have been the most pivotal in America's Middle East experience—the year that Americans turned away. And yet the United States cannot disengage from the Middle East for the ineluctable reason that the Middle East will remain engaged with America. For all the comparisons between Iraq and Vietnam, U.S. troops could withdraw from Vietnam in the 1970s confident that the enemy would not follow them home, but they will still confront Middle Eastern adversaries long after the last American leaves Baghdad. Rather than a self-contained war, Iraq represents a first and painful battle in a far more protracted struggle, more akin to Bull Run and Bataan than to Gettysburg and Midway. The rest of the region, meanwhile, is unlikely to gravitate toward greater stability—as the upheavals of 2006–2007 indicate—but rather toward further terror, internecine violence, and war.

Americans must do their utmost to avoid these perils while vigorously preparing to meet them. Needed is no mere revision but a revolution in the country's relationship with the Middle East. While enhancing their military ability to defend themselves from Middle Eastern threats, Americans will have to accept the limits of their power in the area. The United States should continue encouraging democratic movements in the Middle East while understanding that not all American values are transplantable to the region. Nationwide efforts can be mounted to educate Americans about the politics and cultures of the Middle East and conversely to disabuse Middle Easterners of their misconceptions about the United States. Voices of Islamic moderation can be amplified and scientific research financed to find substitutes for fossil fuels.

The goal is to attain a situation in which American power, though still predominant in the Middle East, is prudently and effectively employed, and all faiths are mutually revered. Distinguishing Middle Eastern myths from realities, however, remains the most daunting challenge facing Americans. Questions must be brutally asked. Can the Palestinians who consistently failed to sustain sovereign structures, and who violently rejected repeated offers of independence (in 1937, 1947, 1979, and 2000), possibly create a durable West Bank state? If so, is there an Israeli leadership capable of relocating tens of thousands of West Bank settlers to make way for such a state? Is the United States, on the other hand, able to restrain Hamas and Hizbollah from launching further attacks against Israel, or Syria from waging war, while preventing Israel from mounting massive retaliatory or preemptive strikes? Will Iran, having succeeded in extending its influence from the Persian Gulf to the Mediterranean, and which has systematically lied about its nuclear program in the past, be peacefully dissuaded from its quest for regional dominance and strategic arms? And will Iraq, even after decades of American sacrifice, ever cohere as a peaceful, democratic nation?

Answering these questions will undoubtedly prove difficult if not traumatic for Americans. History, however, can serve as their guide. By surveying the turbulent events of the past year and examining them in the context of more than two hundred years of multifaceted involvement, Americans can gain an understanding of the part they have played in modern Middle Eastern history and a foreshadowing of the future roles they can fill. A single year may be an insignificant time in the centuries-long relationship between the United States and the Middle East, yet, with a deeper appreciation of America's past in this crucial region, it could well inaugurate a new era.

Michael Oren
New Haven and Jerusalem
September 2007

Notes

A note on the notes: Because of the immense number of quotations and sources in need of citation, I have inserted endnotes at thematic breaks and transitions in the text.

Prologue: A Passage to Glory

1. Jared Sparks, *The Life of John Ledyard, the American Traveller* (Cambridge: Hillard and Brown, 1828), pp. 1–70. Helen Augur, *Passage to Glory: John Ledyard's America* (Garden City, N.Y.: Doubleday, 1946), pp. 142, 157–58, 173. Henry Beston, *The Book of Gallant Vagabonds* (New York: George H. Doran, 1925), p. 23. Laurie Lawlor, *Magnificent Voyage: An American Adventurer on Captain James Cook's Final Expedition* (New York: Holiday House, 2002), p. 203 ("the greatest traveler"). See also Clanance Ashton Wood, "Southhold's John Ledyard" and "John Ledyard the Traveler," longislandgenealogy.com/Ledyard/one.htm.

2. John Ledyard, *A Journal of Captain Cook's Last Voyage to the Pacific Ocean* (Hartford: Nathaniel Patten, 1783), pp. 33 ("dancing through life"), 72, 85, 157. Kenneth Munford, *John Ledyard: An American Marco Polo* (Portland: Binfords and Mort, 1939), p. 300. Beston, *Book of Gallant Vagabonds*, p. 43. James Zug, *American Traveler* (New York: Basic, 2005), p. 152. Lawlor, *Magnificent Voyage*, pp. 5, 59, 143, 197–98. S. G. Mantel, *Explorer with a Dream, John Ledyard* (New York: Julian Messner, 1969), pp. 121–23. Thomas Jefferson, *Autobiography* (New York: Capricorn, 1959), p. 80. Lawlor, *Magnificent Voyage*, p. 199 ("my brother"). See also Stephen D. Watrous, ed., *John Ledyard's Journey through Russia and Siberia, 1787–1788: The Journal and Selected Letters* (Madison: Univ. of Wis-

consin Press, 1966), and the website *Mutual Perceptions—Travel Accounts*, memory .loc.gov/intldl/mtfhtml/mfpercep/perceptledyard.html.

3. Henry Beaufoy, "Some Accounts of Mr. Ledyard's Method of Traveling," *Ladies' Magazine*, July 1792 ("manliness of his person"). Zug, *American Traveler*, p. 216 ("An American face"). Larzer Ziff, *Return Passages: Great American Travel Writing, 1780–1910* (New Haven: Yale Univ. Press, 2000), p. 36. Sparks, *Life of John Ledyard*, pp. 290, 293 ("My path will be"), p. 303. Augur, *Passage to Glory*, p. 268 ("Behold, I afford a new character"). Zug, *American Traveler*, pp. 173 ("I . . . do not think"), 220.

1. A Mortal and Mortifying Threat

1. Evan Thomas, *John Paul Jones: Sailor, Hero, Father of the American Navy* (New York: Simon & Schuster, 2003), pp. 30–34. James A. Field Jr., *America and the Mediterranean World, 1776–1882* (Princeton: Princeton Univ. Press, 1969), pp. 30–31. A. L. Tibawi, *American Interests in Syria, 1800–1901* (Oxford: Clarendon Press, 1966), pp. 1–2. Michael L. S. Kitzen, *Tripoli and the United States at War: A History of America's Relations with the Barbary States, 1785–1805* (Jefferson: McFarland, 1962), p. 10. Thomas A. Bryson, *American Diplomatic Relations with the Middle East, 1784–1975* (Metuchen, N.J.: Scarecrow, 1977), pp. 1–2. David H. Finnie, *Pioneers East: The Early American Experience in the Middle East* (Cambridge: Harvard Univ. Press, 1967), pp. 244–45 ("Go where you will"). A. Uner Turgay, "Ottoman-American Trade during the Nineteenth Century," *Journal of Ottoman Studies* 3, no. 1 (1982): 193–94.

2. Richard B. Parker, *Uncle Sam in Barbary: A Diplomatic History* (Gainesville: Univ. Press of Florida, 2004), pp. 5–6, 17–20. Robert Davis, *Christian Slaves, Muslim Masters* (New York: Palgrave Macmillan, 2003), pp. 4–5, 23, 36, 41–42, 74. Sir Godfrey Fisher, *Barbary Legend: War, Trade and Policy in North Africa, 1415–1830* (Oxford: Oxford Univ. Press, 1957), pp. 290–91. Max Boot, *The Savage Wars of Peace: Small Wars and the Rise of American Power* (New York: Basic, 2002), pp. 6–8. Maria Martin, *History of the Captivity and Sufferings of Maria Martin* (Philadelphia: Jacob Meyer, 1811), p. 37. Questions have been raised about the veracity of Martin's account, though her descriptions of the ordeals of captivity in North Africa accord with those of many other former prisoners. See James R. Lewis, "Savages of the Seas: Barbary Captivity Tales and Images of Muslims in the Early Republic," *Journal of American Culture* 13, no. 2 (Summer 1990): 68.

3. Joseph Wheelan, *Jefferson's War: America's First War on Terror, 1801–1805* (New York: Carroll & Graf, 2003), p. 36. Parker, *Uncle Sam in Barbary*, pp. 33–34 ("We had already lost five"). Charles A. Goodwin, *Narrative of Joshua Gee of Boston, Mass., While He Was Captive in Algeria of the Barbary Pirates, 1680–1687* (Hartford: Wadsworth Atheneum, 1943), pp. 1–29. Simon Smith, "Piracy in Early British America," *History Today* 46 (May 1996).

4. *Letters of Delegates to Congress, 1774–1789*, ed. Paul Smith (Washington,

D.C.: Library of Congress, 1995): Pierse Long to John Langdon, Aug. 6, 1786, p. 433. Alexander DeConde, *A History of American Foreign Policy* (New York: Scribner, 1971), pp. 21, 41 ("The Americans cannot protect"). *The Revolutionary War Diplomatic Correspondences of the United States*. ed. Francis Wharton (Washington, D.C.: GPO, 1889): Salva to Franklin, April 1, 1783, p. 357. Bradford Perkins, *The Cambridge History of American Foreign Relations,* vol. 1, *The Creation of a Republican Empire, 1776–1865* (Cambridge: Cambridge Univ. Press, 1993), pp. 33 ("No nation can be trusted"), 46, 69. Robert J. Allison, *The Crescent Obscured: The United States and the Muslim World, 1776–1815* (New York: Oxford Univ. Press, 1995), p. 3.

5. E. Dupuy, *Américains et Barbaresques* (Paris: R. Roger et F. Chernoviz, 1910), p. 8 ("to use its best offices"). *The Writings of Benjamin Franklin*, vol. 10, ed. Albert Smyth (New York: Haskell House, 1970): Franklin to Robert Livingston, July 7, 1783, p. 71 ("If there were no Algiers"). See also *The Papers of George Mason, 1725–1792*, ed. Robert Rutland (Chapel Hill: Univ. of North Carolina Press, 1970): George Mason to Hunter, Allison and Company, Aug. 8, 1783, pp. 788–89. Louis B. Wright and Julia H. Macleod, *The First Americans in North Africa: William Eaton's Struggle for a Vigorous Policy against the Barbary Pirates, 1799–1805* (New York: Greenwood, 1945), p. 15. Seton Dearden, *A Nest of Corsairs* (London: Butler and Tanner, 1976), p. 151. Parker, *Uncle Sam in Barbary*, pp. 218–19 ("there is no advantage").

6. Paul Baepler, ed., *White Slaves, African Masters: An Anthology of American Barbary Captivity Narratives* (Chicago: Univ. of Chicago Press, 1999), pp. 77–80. Stephen Clissold, *The Barbary Slaves* (London: Paul Elek, 1977), p. 3 ("They made signs"). A. B. C. Whipple, *To the Shores of Tripoli: The Birth of the U.S. Navy and Marines* (New York: Morrow, 1991), p. 26. H. G. Barnby, *The Prisoners of Algiers: An Account of the Forgotten American-Algerian War, 1785–1797* (New York: Oxford Univ. Press, 1966), pp. 2–3. Gardner W. Allen, *Our Navy and the Barbary Corsairs* (Boston: Houghton Mifflin, 1905), pp. 8–9 ("sabers grasped"). Donald Barr Chidsey, *The Wars in Barbary: Arab Piracy and the Birth of the United States Navy* (New York: Crown, 1971), p. 7.

7. *The Letters of Richard Henry Lee*, ed. James Ballagh (New York: Macmillan, 1914), vol. 2: Lee to Thomas Shippen, Oct. 14, 1785, p. 392 ("Curse and doubly curse"); Lee to Samuel Adams, Oct. 17, 1785, p. 396. John Jay Papers: 1968, 13031, Jay to William Bingham, Feb. 12, 1785; Jay to Bowen, May 24, 1786. *Naval Documents Related to the United States Wars with the Barbary Powers*, ed. Dudley Knox, 6 vols. (Washington, D.C.: GPO, 1939), vol. 1: O'Brien, Coffin, and Stevens to Thomas Jefferson, June 8, 1786, p. 2. David McCullough, *John Adams* (New York: Simon & Schuster, 2001), p. 352. Barnby, *Prisoners of Algiers*, pp. 3–9, 25–26. Allison, *Crescent Obscured*, pp. xiv–xv. Allen, *Our Navy*, pp. 13, 25, 21–22 ("perfectly dark"). Whipple, *To the Shores of Tripoli*, pp. 25–26, 69. *A Journal of the Captivity and Sufferings of John Foss* (Newburyport: Angier March, 1798), pp. 17 ("Now I have got you"), 20, 24, 33. DeConde, *History of American Foreign Pol-*

icy, p. 41 ("It will not be"). Lawrence A. Peskin, "The Lessons of Independence: How the Algerian Crisis Shaped Early American Identity," *Diplomatic History* 28, no. 3 (June 2004): 299–300 ("The Algerians are cruising"). Walter A. McDougall, *Promised Land, Crusader State: The American Encounter with the World since 1776* (New York: Mariner Books, 1997), p. 37.

8. *The Writings of Thomas Jefferson,* ed. Paul Ford (New York: Putnam, 1970): Jefferson to James Monroe, Nov. 11, 1783, pp. 10–11 ("We ought to begin"). Allen, *Our Navy,* p. 37 ("It will procure us"). See also Thomas Jefferson Papers: Gerard W. Gawalt, "America and the Barbary Pirates: An International Battle Against an Unconventional Foe," on memory.loc.gov/ammem/mtjhtml/mtjprece.html ("temper of my countrymen"). DeConde, *History of American Foreign Policy,* p. 83 ("sink us under them" and "erect and independent attitude"). Joseph J. Ellis, *American Sphinx. The Character of Thomas Jefferson* (New York: Vintage, 1998), p. 26 ("combined great depth"), and *Founding Brothers: The Revolutionary Generation* (New York: Vintage, 2002), pp. 233–42. William M. Fowler, *Jack Tars and Commodores: The American Navy, 1783–1815* (Boston: Houghton Mifflin, 1984), p. 5. I am aware of the controversy surrounding Jefferson's relationship with Sally Hemmings; geneticists have determined that Thomas Jefferson was almost certainly the father of Hemming's son, Eston.

9. *The Emerging Nation: A Documentary History of the Foreign Relations of the United States under the Articles of Confederation, 1780–1789,* vol. 2, ed. Mary Giunta (Washington, D.C.: National Historical Publications and Records Commission, 1996): Thomas Jefferson to James Monroe, Feb. 6, 1785, p. 543. *The Papers of George Washington,* ed. W. W. Abbit (Charlottesville: Univ. Press of Virginia, 1995): Lafayette to Washington, Jan. 13, 1787, p. 514. *Lafayette in the Age of the American Revolution,* vol. 5, ed. Stanley Idzerda and Robert Crout (Ithaca: Cornell Univ. Press, 1983): Lafayette to Adams, Jefferson, and Franklin, April 8, 1785, p. 315.

10. *Writings of Thomas Jefferson,* ed. Ford: Jefferson to James Monroe, Nov. 11, 1783, pp. 10–11 ("The states must see"). *The Writings of Thomas Jefferson,* ed. Andrew A. Lipscomb (Washington, D.C.: Thomas Jefferson Memorial Association, 1905): Jefferson to John Page, Aug. 20, 1785, p. 91 ("Honour as well as"). John Jay Papers: Jay to Jefferson, Adams, and Franklin, March 11, 1785 ("the Influence of . . . Courts"). Whipple, *To the Shores of Tripoli,* p. 23.

11. *Writings of Thomas Jefferson,* ed. Lipscomb: Jefferson to William Carmichael, Nov. 4, 1785, p. 194 ("His manners and appearance"). Barnby, *Prisoners of Algiers,* p. 75 ("I hope never to see"). Parker, *Uncle Sam in Barbary,* pp. 37–38, 217–19. Ray Irwin, *The Diplomatic Relations of the United States with the Barbary Powers, 1776–1816* (New York: Russell & Russell, 1970), pp. 49–50.

12. *Emerging Nation,* vol. 1: John Adams to John Jay, Feb. 17, 1786, p. 96. The John Jay Papers: 4605, Jay to Congress, Aug. 2, 1787. Walter Livingston Wright, "American Relations with Turkey to 1831" (Ph.D. diss., Princeton Univ., 1928), pp. 1–2 ("pestilence and war"). Allison, *Crescent Obscured,* pp. 8, 14–16. McCullough, *John Adams,* pp. 352–53. Allen, *Our Navy,* pp. 36–37.

13. Wright, "American Relations with Turkey," pp. 4–5 ("the Dignity of Congress"). *The Adams-Jefferson Letters: The Complete Correspondence between Thomas Jefferson and Abigail and John Adams,* ed. Lester J. Cappon (Chapel Hill: Univ. of North Carolina Press, 1959): Adams to Jefferson, July 13, 1786, p. 139. *Emerging Nation,* vol. 1: Letter from John Adams to John Jay, June 27, 1786, p. 207; vol. 2: John Adams to John Jay, Dec. 15, 1784, p. 513 ("unfeeling tyrants"). McCullough, *John Adams,* p. 366 ("We ought not to fight").

14. *Emerging Nation,* vol. 3: Jefferson and Adams to John Jay, March 28, 1786, pp. 135–36 ("It was . . . written"). *Adams-Jefferson Letters*: Adams to Jefferson, June 6, 1786, p. 133. *Writings of Thomas Jefferson,* ed. Ford: Thomas Jefferson to James Monroe, Aug. 11, 1786, pp. 264–65 ("an angel sent on this business"). *Writings of Benjamin Franklin:* Franklin to William Carmichael, March 22, 1785, pp. 301–2. McCullough, *John Adams,* p. 354. Wright, "American Relations with Turkey," pp. 7–10. Allen, *Our Navy,* pp. 30–31. Allison, *Crescent Obscured,* p. 12 ("a universal and horrible War").

15. *Revolutionary War Diplomatic Correspondences of the United States*: Franklin to Congress, May 26, 1779, pp. 192–93. *Diary and Autobiography of John Adams,* vol. 3, *Diary 1782–1804* (Cambridge: Harvard Univ. Press, Belknap Press, 1961), entries for March 19 and March 20, 1785, pp. 174–75. John Jay Papers: 3891, Jay to Congress, March 22, 1786. *Emerging Nation,* vol. 1: John Adams to John Jay, Feb. 16, 1786 ("Innocence and the Olive Branch"), p. 95. Jerome B. Weiner, "Foundations of U.S. Relations with Morocco and the Barbary States," *Hespris-Tamuda* [Morocco] 20–21 (1982–83), pp. 165–82. Field, *America and the Mediterranean World,* pp. 32–33, 40. Allen, *Our Navy,* pp. 27–30. Wright, "American Relations with Turkey," pp. 8–9. The text of the treaty is reproduced in J. C. Hurewitz, ed., *The Middle East and North Africa in World Politics: A Documentary Record,* vol. 1, *European Expansion, 1535–1914,* 2d ed. (New Haven: Yale Univ. Press, 1975), pp. 103–5.

16. *The Writings of Thomas Jefferson*: Jefferson to Humphreys, Aug. 14, 1786, p. 400 ("public treasury"). *The Writings of George Washington from the Original Manuscript Sources, 1745–1799,* vol. 38, ed. John Fitzpatrick (Washington, D.C.: GPO, 1938): Washington to Lafayette, March 25, 1787, p. 185 ("the highest disgrace"); Washington to Lafayette, Aug. 15, 1786, p. 521 ("Would to Heaven"). Whipple, *To the Shores of Tripoli,* p. 21. Boot, *Savage Wars of Peace,* p. 10. U.S. Naval History: *The Reestablishment of the Navy, 1787–1801,* on http://www.history .navy.mil/biblio/bibli04/bibli04a.htm. *The Documentary History of the Ratification of the Constitution,* ed. John Kaminksi and Gaspare Saladino (Madison: State Historical Society of Wisconsin, 2001): Russell to Adams, p. 47 ("Without a national system"). Parker, *Uncle Sam in Barbary,* p. 44 ("Our sufferings"). Field, *America and the Mediterranean World,* p. 33 ("See what dark prospect").

17. *Documentary History of the Ratification of the Constitution*: Speech by James Madison before the Virginia Constitutional Convention, June 12, 1788, p. 1206. *Writings of George Washington*: Washington to Lafayette, Aug. 15, 1787, p.

260. *Letters of Delegates to Congress*: Virginia Delegates to Edmund Randolph, Nov. 3, 1787, p. 539. James Madison, *Notes of Debates in the Federal Convention of 1787* (Athens: Ohio Univ. Press, 1966), p. 549. Perkins, *Cambridge History of American Foreign Relations*, p. 69. See also Julia H. Macleod, "Jefferson and the Navy: A Defense," *Huntington Library Quarterly* 8 (Feb. 1945): 154.

18. *Documentary History of the Ratification of the Constitution*, pp. 47, 160, 567 ("preposterous"), 1126 ("May not the Algerines"), 1417 ("our sailors . . . in Algiers"). *The Debate on the Constitution*, ed. Bernard Bailyn (Washington, D.C.: Library of America, 1993): Hugh Williamson's Speech, Nov. 8, 1787, p. 233. *The Republic of Letters: The Correspondence between Thomas Jefferson and James Madison, 1776–1826*, ed. James Morton Smith (New York: Norton, 1995): Jefferson to Madison, May 8, 1784, p. 314; Madison to Jefferson, Oct. 8, 1788, p. 555; Jefferson to Madison, Jan. 12, 1789, p. 583.

19. Alexander Hamilton, John Jay, and James Madison, *The Federalist Papers* (Cutchogue, N.Y.: Buccaneer Books, 1992), pp. 49-50 ("federal navy . . . of respectable"), 207–8 ("maritime strength" and "the rapacious demands"). John Jay Papers: 4572, Jay to Congress, May 29, 1786; 10876, Jay to Lafayette, Oct. 28, 1786; 4605, Jay to Congress, Aug. 2, 1787. Thomas A. Bailey, *A Diplomatic History of the American People* (Englewood Cliffs, N.J.: Prentice-Hall, 1980), p. 65 ("The more we are ill-treated"). See also George Pellew, *American Statesmen: John Jay* (Cambridge, Mass.: Riverside Press, 1890), p. 239.

20. Mary Chrysostom Diebels, *Peter Markoe (1752–1792): A Philadelphia Writer* (Washington, D.C.: Catholic Univ. of America Press, 1944), pp. 1–3, 16, 50–61. Peter Markoe, *The Algerine Spy in Pennsylvania; or, Letters Written by a Native of Algiers on the Affairs of the United States in America, from the Close of the Year 1783 to the Meeting of the Convention* (Philadelphia: Prichard and Hall, 1787), pp. 25–30, 78–79, 104–5 ("totally ruined" and "plundered without"), 113–14. Bailey, *Diplomatic History of the American People*, p. 65. See also Lotfi Ben Rejeb, "Observing the Birth of a Nation: The Oriental Spy/Observer Genre and Nation Making in Early American Literature," in Abbas Amanat and Magnus T. Bernhardsson, eds., *The United States and the Middle East: Cultural Encounters* (New Haven: Yale Center for International and Area Studies, 2002), pp. 253–89.

21. *Naval Documents Related to the United States Wars*, vol. 1: Jefferson to the Senate and the House of Representatives, Dec. 30, 1790, p. 22; Edward Church to Thomas Jefferson, Oct. 12, 1793, p. 45. *Writings of Thomas Jefferson*, ed. Lipscomb: Jefferson to the Board of Treasury, May 16, 1788, p. 11 ("sea-dogs"); Jefferson to John Jay, Aug. 11, 1788, p. 121 ("that pettifogging nest"). Ellis, *American Sphinx*, p. 162 ("Algerine"). Allison, *Crescent Obscured*, pp. 9–10 ("suspended between indignation").

22. *Writings of Thomas Jefferson*, ed. Lipscomb: Jefferson to John Paul Jones, June 1, 1792, p. 355; Jefferson to Thomas Barclay, June 11, 1792, p. 367. Charles Stuart Kennedy, *The American Consul: A History of the United States Consular Ser-*

vice, 1776–1914 (New York: Greenwood, 1990), p. 29 ("as a great People"). *Writings of Thomas Jefferson*, ed. Paul Ford: Jefferson to James Monroe, Nov. 11, 1783, pp. 10–11 ("John Paul Jones").

23. *Writings of Thomas Jefferson*, ed. Lipscomb: Jefferson to Thomas Barclay, June 11, 1792, p. 367. John Jay Papers: 5052, Temple to Jay, June 7, 1786. *The Papers of Alexander Hamilton*, ed. Harold Syrett, 27 vols. (New York: Columbia Univ. Press, 1961–87): Hamilton to William Seton, April 22, 1794, vol. 16, p. 312. *The Life and Correspondence of Rufus King*, ed. Charles King (New York: Putnam, 1894): John Alsop to Rufus King, Dec. 15, 1793, p. 505. Irwin, *Diplomatic Relations of the United States*, p. 80.

24. *Writings of George Washington,* vol. 33: Washington to Jonathan Trumbull, Aug. 20, 1793, p. 125; President's Sixth Annual Address to Congress, Dec. 13, 1793, p. 166 ("If we desire").

25. *Annals of the Congress of the United States: Third Congress* (Washington, D.C.: Gales and Seaton, 1849), pp. 433, 434 ("Bribery alone," "a Secretary of [the] Navy," and "we are no match"), 436 ("Our commerce is"), 439 ("at war with"), 447–48 ("pusillanimous measures"). Craig L. Symonds, *Navalists and Antinavalists: The Naval Policy Debate in the United States, 1785–1827* (Newark: Univ. of Delaware Press, 1980), pp. 27–37. See also *The Papers of Josiah Bartlett*, ed. Frank Mevers (Hanover: Univ. Press of New England, 1979): Paine Wingate to Josiah Bartlett, Feb. 24, 1794, p. 403.

26. *Papers of Alexander Hamilton*: John Quincy Adams to Hamilton, Dec. 5, 1795, vol. 17, pp. 420–21; Edmund Randolph to Hamilton, William Bradford, and Henry Knox, vol. 16, pp. 498–99. *Naval Documents Related to the United States Wars*, vol. 1: Samuel Calder to David Pearce, Dec. 4, 1793, p. 57; George Washington to Congress, Feb. 8, 1795, p. 93; Joel Barlow to Jefferson, March 18, 1796, pp. 140–41. Allison, *Crescent Obscured*, pp. 31, 141 ("stigma on the American"). Frances Diane Robotti and James Vescovi, *The USS Essex and the Birth of the American Navy* (Holbrook, Mass.: Adams Media Corp., 1999), p. 12. Field, *America and the Mediterranean World*, p. 7. Allen, *Our Navy*, p. 51 ("If I were to make peace").

27. Among the gifts given Tunis by the United States were "1 Fusee, 6 feet long, mounted with gold set with diamonds; 4 set with gold mounting, ordinary length; 1 pr. of pistols mounted with gold, set with diamonds; 1 poniard, enameled, set with diamonds; 1diamond ring; 1 gold repeating watch, with diamonds, chain the same, 6 pieces of brocade of gold; 30 pieces superfine cloth of different colors; 6 pieces Satin, different colors." See Irwin, *Diplomatic Relations of the United States*, pp. 100–1. Republic of Letters: Madison to Jefferson, Feb. 21, 1796, pp. 921–22; Jefferson to Madison, April 17, 1796, pp. 931–32. *Naval Documents Related to the United States Wars*, vol. 1: Barlow to Jefferson, March 18, 1796, pp. 140–41; O'Brien to Jefferson, Jan. 12, 1797, pp. 192–93 ("25 chests of tea"); Barlow to Jefferson, Aug. 18, 1797, p. 208 ("To what height"); Barlow to Jefferson, Aug. 24, 1797, p. 209 ("You are a liar"). Kennedy, *American Consul*, pp. 30–32. Allen, *Our Navy*, pp. 23–24, 53–54 ("Our people have conducted"), 56–57. Barnby, *Prisoner*

of Algiers, pp. 304, 318. Foss, *Journal of the Captivity*, p. 123 ("No nation of Christendom"). Milton Cantor, "Joel Barlow's Mission to Algiers," *Historian* 25 (1963). See also Library of Congress Country Studies, "Algeria, Relations with the United States," memory.loc.gov/cgi-bin/query/r?frd/cstdy:@field(DOCID+dz0025).

28. Royall Tyler, *The Algerine Captive; or, The Life and Adventures of Doctor Updike Underhill, Six Years a Prisoner among the Algerines* (Hartford: Peter B. Gleason, 1816), pp. 196, 239. Anonymous, *The American in Algiers; or, The Patriot of Seventy-six in Captivity* (New York: J. Buel, 1797), p. 16 ("Does Columbia"). Susanna Rowson, *Slaves in Algiers; or, The Struggle for Freedom* (Philadelphia: Wrigley and Berriman, 1794), p. 48 ("What, give it up").

29. James Leander Cathcart, *Tripoli* (LaPorte, Ind.: Herald Print, 1901): Cathcart to Pickering, Aug. 16, 1799, p. 67. *Naval Documents Related to the United States Wars*, vol. 1: Barlow to Jefferson, Aug. 24, 1797, p. 209. Kennedy, *American Consul*, pp. 2–3.

2. The Hostile and Ethereal Orient

1. Abbas, Hamdani, "Columbus and the Recovery of Jerusalem," Journal of the American Oriental Society 99, no. 1 (1979) pp. 43 ("As . . . enemies), 44 ("all the gain"). Robert Irwin, For Lust of Knowing: The Orientalists and their Enemies (London: Penguin, 2007), pp. 60–62, 87–88, 100. George Sandys, *Description of the Ottoman Empire* (Amsterdam: Theatrum Orbis Terrarum, 1973), p. 36. Philip L. Barbour, *The Three Worlds of Captain John Smith* (Boston: Houghton Mifflin, 1964), pp. 45–49. Timothy Worthington Marr, "Imagining Ishmael: Studies of Islamic Orientalism from the Puritans to Melville" (Ph.D. diss., Yale Univ., 1997), pp. 1–2, 30–33, 70 ("an emissary of Satan"), 87–89. Douglas Little, *American Orientalism: The United States and the Middle East since 1945* (Chapel Hill: Univ. of North Carolina Press, 2002), pp. 12–13, 73–74. Allison, *Crescent Obscured*, pp. xiv–xviii, 45–46, 61–64. Josiah Strong, "Anglo-Saxon Predominance (1891)," http://xroads.virginia.edu/~DRBR/strong.html ("The Eastern nations sink"). *Translating the Untranslatable: A Survey of English Translations of the Quran*, http://www.quranicstudies.com/article32.html. A. J. Arberry, *The Koran Interpreted* (New York: Macmillan, 1955), pp. 7 ("so viewing thine enemies"), 8 ("contradictions, blasphemies"), 10 ("attack the Koran"). Humphrey Prideaux, *The True Nature of Imposture Fully Displayed in the Life of Mahomet* (Fairhaven, Vt.: James Lyon, 1798), p. 108.

2. Henry Hugh Brackenridge and Philip Freneau, *Father Bombo's Pilgrimage to Mecca, 1770*, ed. Michael Davitt Bell (Princeton: Princeton Univ. Library, 1975), pp. 7 ("to change thy religion"), 92 ("I prostrated myself"). Ros Ballaster, *Fabulous Orients: Fictions of the East in England, 1662–1785* (Oxford: Oxford Univ. Press, 2005), pp. 8, 33, 54–56, 72, 77. Alain Grosrichard, *The Sultan's Court: European Fantasies of the East* (London: Verso, 1998), p. 79. Mohammed Sharafuddin, *Islam and Romantic Orientalism: Literary Encounters with the Orient* (London: I. B. Tau-

ris, 1994), pp. xxv–xxvi, 64, 107. Ben Rejeb, "Observing the Birth of a Nation," pp. 256–57. Claude Étienne Savary, *Letters on Egypt, Containing a Parallel between the Manners of Its Ancient and Modern Inhabitants* (London: G. G. J. and J. Robinson, 1787). Irwin, *For Lust of Knowing*, p. 109 ("the present terror"). Constantin-François Volney, *Voyage en Syrie et en Egypte, pendant les années 1783, 1784, et 1785* (Paris: Desenne et Volland, 1787).

3. Daniel Beaumont, *Slave of Desire: Sex, Love, and Death in 1,001 Nights* (Madison, N.J.: Fairleigh Dickinson Univ. Press, 2002), p. 42. Husain Haddawy, trans., *The Arabian Nights* (New York: Norton, 1990), pp. xv–xvii. *Novelists Magazine* 18 (Containing *The Arabian Nights Entertainment*) (London: Harrison, 1785). Adele L. Younis, "The Arabs Who Followed Columbus," *Arab World* 12, no. 3 (March 1966). Excerpt from *The Arabian Night Entertainment: Consisting of One Thousand and One Stories, the First American Edition, Freely Transcribed from the Original Translation by Galland* (Baltimore: H. & P. Rice and J. Rice, 1794). Susan Nance, "Crossing Over: A Cultural History of American Engagement with the Muslim World, 1830–1940" (Ph.D. diss., Univ. of California, Berkeley, 2003), p. 25. See also the *Arabian Nights Resource Center*, http://www.crock11 .freeserve.co.uk/arabian.htm.

4. Alexis de Tocqueville, *Democracy in America*, ed. J. P. Mayer, trans. George Lawrence (New York: Harper & Row, 1969), p. 536. Edward McNall Burns, *The American Idea of Mission: Concepts of National Purpose and Destiny* (New Brunswick: Rutgers Univ. Press, 1957), p. 125. Daniel Boorstin, *The Americans: The National Experience* (New York: Random House, 1965), pp. 219, 264. William H. Goetzmann, *New Lands, New Men: America and the Second Great Age of Discovery* (New York: Viking, 1986), pp. 1, 5, 14. Frederick Jackson Turner, *The Frontier in American History* (1920; reprint, New York: Henry Holt, 1947), pp. 2, 30, 37, 38.

5. Sparks, *Life of John Ledyard*, p. 305 ("Alexandria at large"). P. J. Vatikiotis, *The History of Egypt: From Muhammad Ali to Sadat* (Baltimore: Johns Hopkins Univ. Press, 1980), pp. 30–38. Samir Khalaf, *Persistence and Change in 19th Century Lebanon* (Beirut: American Univ. of Beirut, 1979), pp. 16–31. Bernard Lewis, *The Emergence of Modern Turkey* (London: Oxford Univ. Press, 1968), pp. 21–39, and *The Crisis of Islam: Holy War and Unholy Terror* (New York: Modern Library, 2003), pp. 64–65.

6. Augur, *Passage to Glory*, pp. 265, 276 ("The Mahometans [are] a superstitious"), 277–80. Zug, *American Traveler*, p. 222 ("infinitely below"). Sparks, *Life of John Ledyard*, pp. 306, 307 ("This was about" and "nothing merits more"), 309, 310 ("very, very humiliating"), 314–15. Finnie, *Pioneers East*, pp. 139–40 ("dust, hot"). See also Robert D. Kaplan, *The Arabists: The Romance of an American Elite* (New York: Free Press, 1993), pp. 16–17.

7. Finnie, *Pioneers East*, p. 140 ("a bilious complaint"). Wood, "John Ledyard the Traveler," ("full and perfect health"). Significant disagreement surrounds the date of Ledyard's death. Augur places it on March 4, 1789, and Dr. Wood on Jan.

17. Sparks, the official biographer, speculates that the time was late Nov. 1788 On the basis of Ledyard's last letter to Jefferson, I have remained with Sparks's date, albeit without certainty.

8. "An Egyptian Anecdote," *Ladies' Magazine*, April 1793 ("although generally tender"); "An Account of Egypt and Alexandria," Feb. 1793 ("absorbed in surprise"). Augur, *Passage to Glory*, p. 282 ("That Man"). J. Fred Rippy, *Joel R. Poinsett: Versatile American* (Durham: Duke Univ. Press, 1935), pp. 27–29. Finnie, *Pioneers East,* p. 14 ("long red pantaloons"). George Barrell, *Letters from Asia: Written by a Gentleman of Boston, to His Friend in That Place* (New York: A. T. Goodrich, 1819), p. 35 ("having perused"). Bruce G. Tigger, "Egyptology, Ancient Egypt, and the American Imagination," in Nancy Thomas, ed., *The American Discovery of Ancient Egypt* (New York: Abrams, 1995), pp. 21–22. Thomas Jefferson, *The Writings of Thomas Jefferson*, vol. 7 (Washington, D.C.: Thomas Jefferson Memorial Association of the United States, 1903), p. 78. Ziff, *Return Passages*, p. 53 ("Ledyard was a great favourite").

3. A Crucible of American Identity

1. Thomas Harris, *The Life and Services of Commodore William Bainbridge, United States Navy* (Philadelphia: Carey Lea and Blanchard, 1837), pp. 37, 45 ("You pay me tribute"). Robotti and Vescovi, *USS Essex*, pp. 70–72. Finnie, *Pioneers East*, pp. 48–50. Whipple, *To the Shores of Tripoli*, p. 56. Allen, *Our Navy*, pp. 75, 80–81. Wright, "American Relations with Turkey," pp. 31 ("To save the peace), 32–33 ("mortifying degradations"), 35–36. Richard Zacks, *The Pirate Coast: Thomas Jefferson, the First Marines, and the Secret Mission of 1805* (New York: Hyperion, 2005), pp. 13–15, 24.

2. Lord Kinross, *The Ottoman Centuries: The Rise and Fall of the Turkish Empire* (New York: Morrow Quill, 1977), pp. 429–36. Stanford Shaw, *History of the Ottoman Empire and Modern Turkey*, vol. 1, *Empire of the Gazis: The Rise and Decline of the Ottoman Empire, 1280–1808* (Cambridge: Cambridge Univ. Press, 1976), pp. 260–74. Henry A. S. Dearborn, *The Life of William Bainbridge, Esq., of the United States Navy* (Princeton: Princeton Univ. Press, 1931), p. 20. Barnby, *Prisoner of Algiers*, pp. 37, 84. Henry S. Osborn, *Palestine, Past and Present* (Philadelphia: James Challen and Son, 1859), p. 505. Field, *America and the Mediterranean World*, pp. 114–15. Lewis, *Crisis of Islam*, p. 66 ("heavenly bodies"). Turgay, "Ottoman-American Trade," p. 205.

3. Glenn Tucker, *Dawn like Thunder: The Barbary Wars and the Birth of the U.S. Navy* (New York: Bobbs-Merrill, 1963), pp. 15–18. Wright, "American Relations with Turkey," pp. 31–32 ("Had we 10 or 12"), 34 ("Did the United States know"), 37–41, 42 ("Capitaines Vilon"). Allen, *Our Navy*, pp. 85–86. Field, *America and the Mediterranean World*, pp. 115–16. Bainbridge letter to Stodder, in Robotti and Vescovi, *USS Essex*, p. 76. Harris, *Life and Services of Commodore William Bainbridge*, p. 60.

4. *Republic of Letters:* Jefferson to Madison, Aug. 28, 1801, pp. 1193–94 ("enemy to all these" and "send the powder"). Thomas Jefferson Papers: Jefferson to Wilson Cary Nicholas, June 11, 1801 ("There is no end"). *The Writings of Albert Gallatin,* ed. Henry Adams, vol. 1 (New York: Antiquarian Press, 1960): Gallatin to Jefferson, Dec. 1802, pp. 104–5. Kenneth J. Hagan, *This People's Navy: The Making of American Sea Power* (New York: Free Press, 1991), p. 55 ("deeply affected"). *Naval Documents Related to the United States Wars,* vol. 1: Cathcart to Dale, Sept. 17, 1801, Cathcart to Madison, April 18, 1802, p. 127 ("to buy peace").

5. Field, *America and the Mediterranean World,* p. 49 ("sinking, burning"). Herbert E. Klingelhofer, "Abolish the Navy!" *Manuscripts* 33, no. 4 (Fall 1981): 279–83. Macleod, "Jefferson and the Navy," p. 170. Allen, *Our Navy,* pp. 89–90 ("a delay on your part"), 94, 112–13. Wright, "American Relations with Turkey," pp. 31–36. Dumas Malone, *Jefferson the President: First Term, 1801–1805* (Boston: Little, Brown, 1970), p. 98.

6. The *Enterprise* was commanded by Lt. Andrew Sterrett. See *Naval Documents Related to the United States Wars,* vol. 1: National Intelligencer, Nov. 18, 1801, p. 539. Allen, *Our Navy,* pp. 89–91 92–93, 97–101. Robotti and Vescovi, *USS Essex,* pp. 78–79, 91–93. *Naval Documents Related to the United States Wars,* vol. 1: Dale to Cathcart, Aug. 25, 1801, p. 560 ("amuse"). Whipple, *To the Shores of Tripoli,* p. 79. Field, *America and the Mediterranean World,* p. 49. Boot, *Savage Wars of Peace,* pp. 13–14.

7. *Naval Documents Related to the United States Wars,* vol. 1: Dale to the Acting Secretary of the Navy, July 30, 1801, p. 535 ("the whole tribe"). *Circular Letters of Congressmen to Their Constituents, 1789–1829,* ed. Noble Cunningham (Chapel Hill: Univ. of North Carolina Press, 1978), vol. 1: Letter from John Stratton, April 22, 1802, p. 281. Whipple, *To the Shores of Tripoli,* p. 96 ("Shall we buy"). For a fuller discussion of the constitutional aspects of Jefferson's policy toward North Africa, see Robert F. Turner, "The War on Terrorism and the Modern Relevance of the Congressional Power to 'Declare War,'" *Harvard Journal of Law & Public Policy* 25 (2002). See also Gordon Silverstein, *Imbalance of Powers: Constitutional Interpretation and the Making of American Foreign Policy* (Oxford: Oxford Univ. Press, 1997), and David N. Mayer, "By the Chains of the Constitution: Separation of Powers Theory and Jefferson's Conception of the Presidency," *Perspectives on Political Science* 26 (1997).

8. *Republic of Letters*: Madison to Jefferson, March 17, 1802, p. 1265; Jefferson to Madison, March 22, 1802, p. 1267; Madison to Jefferson, July 22, 1802, p. 1231. Allen, *Our Navy,* pp. 89–93, 109–10, 130–31. Thomas Jefferson Papers: Jefferson to Albert Gallatin, March 28, 1803. *Naval Documents Related to the United States Wars,* vol. 2: Murray to Captain Richard Morris, Aug. 20, 1802, p. 242; Excerpt from the Journal of Henry Wadsworth, Feb. 26, 1803, p. 437 ("Twas good sport"); vol. 3: Captain Murray to Congressman Joseph Nicholson, Nov. 5, 1803, p. 201. Cathcart, *Tripoli,* p. 111 ("venal wretch"). Whipple, *To the Shores of Tripoli,* pp. 88, 90, 99. Boot, *Savage Wars of Peace,* pp. 14–15 ("best exertions").

9. *The Republic of Letters*: Madison to Jefferson, July 22, 1802, p. 1231; Jefferson to Madison, Aug. 17, 1802, p. 1264; Jefferson to Madison, March 19, 1803, p. 1266. *Life and Correspondence of Rufus King*: King to Madison, July 19, 1802, p. 149 ("Our security"). Whipple, *To the Shores of Tripoli*, pp. 65 ("rest the safety"), 113. *Naval Documents Related to the United States Wars*, vol. 3: Preble to the Secretary of the Navy, Sept. 22, 1803, p. 70 ("The Moors"); Preble to Cathcart, March 18, 1804, p. 501. Robotti and Vescovi, *USS Essex*, pp. 112–13 ("his savage highness").

10. *Naval Documents Related to the United States Wars*, vol. 3: Bainbridge to James Simpson, Aug. 29, 1803 ("I sincerely hope"); John Ridgeley to Susan Decatur, Nov. 10, 1826, p. 425. Robotti and Vescovi, *USS Essex*, p. 100. Whipple, *To the Shores of Tripoli*, pp. 114, 121. Allen, *Our Navy*, pp. 147–48 ("It is with deep regret"), 152–53, 164–65. Zacks, *Pirate Coast*, p. 48 ("Gift of Allah"). Harris, *Life and Services of Commodore William Bainbridge*, pp. 81, 92. Mohamed El Mansour, "The Anachronism of Maritime Jihad: The U.S.–Moroccan Conflict of 1802–1803," in Jerome Bookin-Weiner and Mohamed El Mansour, eds., *The Atlantic Connection: 200 Years of Moroccan-American Relations, 1786–1986* (Rabat: Edino Press, 1990).

11. *Naval Documents Related to the United States Wars*, vol. 3: Preble to the Secretary of the Navy, Dec. 10, 1803, pp. 256–57 ("Would to God"). James Tertius De Kay, *A Rage for Glory: The Life of Commodore Stephen Decatur* (New York: Free Press, 2004), pp. 38 ("We are now about"), 56. Allen, *Our Navy*, pp. 157, 160–73 ("The flames . . . ascending"). Robotti and Vescovi, *USS Essex*, p. 102. Whipple, *To the Shores of Tripoli*, pp. 121, 123, 136. Field, *America and the Mediterranean World*, p. 60.

12. MML: William Eaton, *Interesting Detail of the Operations of the American Fleet in the Mediterranean, Communicated in a Letter from W. E. Esq. to His Friend in the County of Hampshire* (Springfield, Mass.: Bliss & Brewer, 1804), p. 7 ("bayonet, spear"). De Kay, *Rage for Glory*, p. 67 ("Some of the Turks"). Allen, *Our Navy*, pp. 181–85, 192–94, 214, 217. *Niles' Weekly Register*, March 7, 1812, p. 12 ("done more for the cause"). Robotti and Vescovi, *USS Essex*, pp. 78–79, 91–93. Whipple, *To the Shores of Tripoli*, pp. 142, 156. Harris, *Life and Services of Commodore William Bainbridge*, p. 116. Field, *America and the Mediterranean World*, p. 60 ("The most bold"). *Naval Documents Related to the United States Wars*, vol. 3: Preble to the Secretary of the Navy, Feb. 19, 1804, p. 439 ("spend [his] life"); John Hall to William Burrows, Dec. 7, 1803, p. 254 ("eight oz. of bread); vol. 4: Preble to the Secretary of the Navy, Sept. 18, 1804, p. 301 ("I cannot but regret"). Jonathan Cowdery, *American Captives in Tripoli* (Boston: Belcher & Armstrong, 1806), pp. 13, 17 ("Such attempts served").

13. *Naval Documents Related to the United States Wars*, vol. 4: Diary of Surgeon Jonathan Cowdery, entry for Aug. 10, 1804, pp. 64–65. Thomas A. Bryson, *Tars, Turks, and Tankers: The Role of the United States Navy in the Middle East, 1800–1979* (London: Scarecrow, 1980), p. 14. Allen, *Our Navy*, pp. 176–77, 203–9, 217–18. Boot, *Savage Wars of Peace*, p. 22 ("like so many planets").

Robotti and Vescovi, *USS Essex*, p. 123. Whipple, *To the Shores of Tripoli*, pp. 149, 172, 221 ("You have done well").

14. *Writings of Albert Gallatin*: Gallatin to Jefferson, Aug. 16, 1802, pp. 88–89; Gallatin to Jefferson Jan. 18, 1803, 116. *Republic of Letters*: Jefferson to Madison, April 27, 1804, pp. 1324–25 ("the most serious one," "begging alms," and "beat . . . [the Algerians'] town"). Thomas Jefferson Papers, Princeton Univ.: Jefferson to Robert Smith, April 27, 1804. Allen, *Our Navy*, p. 197. *Naval Documents Related to the United States Wars*, vol. 1: Cathcart to Dale, Sept. 17, 1801, p. 572; Cathcart to Madison, April 18, 1802, p. 127. Nathan Schachner, *Thomas Jefferson: A Biography* (New York: Thomas Yoseloff, 1951), pp. 685–86.

15. William Eaton Papers (WEP) (San Marino, Calif.: Huntington Library). Negociations of the United States with the Kingdom of Tunis: William Eaton [no recipient], Feb. 21, 1799, p. 37 ("No man will"); roll 1: Eaton to Pynchon, Oct. 12, 1799 ("a man not overly"). Whipple, *To the Shores of Tripoli*, pp. 177–78 ("a great bulldog"). Kitzen, *Tripoli and the United States at War*, pp. 25–26. Wright and Macleod, *First Americans in North Africa*, p. 19.

16. WEP, Negociations of the United States with the Kingdom of Tunis: Remarks &c made at Algiers: Feb. 13, 1799, p. 28 ("Universal God"); William Eaton to "Honorable Secretary of the United States," April, 1799, 117 ("land of rapine," "Genius of my country!" and "There is but one"); Eaton to General Smith, Aug. 19, 1802 ("Are we then"); Continued Communications from Tunis in Barbary: Eaton to Cathcart, Aug. 8, 1802, p. 237 ("[The] Government may as well"). Zacks, *Pirate Coast*, p. 31 ("a *fiddle* bow"). Wright and Macleod, *First Americans in North Africa*, pp. 20–21, 49–50. Field, *America and the Mediterranean World*, pp. 41–42. Allen, *Our Navy*, pp. 68–69. Allison, *Crescent Obscured*, pp. 168, 177.

17. WEP, Negociations of the United States with the Kingdom of Tunis: Eaton to William Smith, Nov. 13, 1800 ("a cowardly Jew"); Eaton to General Smith, Aug. 19, 1802; Madison to Eaton, Aug. 22, 1802 ("zeal . . . and calculations"); William Eaton Journal, Sept. 4, 1804, p. 59 ("A whipt Spaniel!"). Whipple, *To the Shores of Tripoli*, pp. 54, 94–95, 183. Eaton to William Smith, May 24, 1801 ("buy[ing] oil of rose").

18. Eaton, *Interesting Detail of the Operations*, p. 29 ("sun-brown children"). See also R. C. Anderson, *Naval Wars in the Levant, 1559–1853* (Princeton: Princeton Univ. Press, 1952), p. 405. WEP, Continued Communications from Tunis in Barbary: Eaton to the Department of State, Sept. 5, 1801; Eaton to Samuel Lyman, Oct. 12, 1801; Eaton to Mr. James Uphorn, Aug. 11, 1802; Eaton to Hamet Dec. 14, 1804 ("God ordained"). *Republic of Letters*: Jefferson to Madison, Aug. 28, 1801, p. 1193. Robotti and Vescovi, *USS Essex*, p. 88. Allen, *Our Navy*, pp. 57–66, 110–12, 187, 217.

19. Zacks, *Pirate Coast*, pp. 184 ("Cash . . . is the only"), 188. WEP, William Eaton Journal, March 20, 1805, p. 20 ("o'er burning sands"); William Eaton Journal, March 30, 1805, p. 25 ("They have no sense"); Negociations of the United States with the Kingdom of Tunis: Eaton to the Governor of Derne, April 26, 1805

("Let no difference"). Allen, *Our Navy*, pp. 229–32, 235–39, 243–44. Finnie, *Pioneers East*, p. 258. Field, *America and the Mediterranean World*, pp. 53–54.

20. *Republic of Letters*: Madison to Jefferson, July 25, 1806, p. 1427; Madison to Jefferson, July 28, 1806, p. 1429; Madison to Jefferson, Sept. 4, 1806, p. 1438; Jefferson to Madison, Sept. 16, 1806, p. 1439. Robotti and Vescovi, *USS Essex*, p. 116. Field, *America and the Mediterranean World*, p. 55 ("Georgia, a Greek"). Whipple, *To the Shores of Tripoli*, p. 253 ("so unusually honorable").

21. *Naval Documents Related to the United States Wars*, vol. 2: Madison to Lear, July 14, 1805, p. 485. WEP, Negociations of the United States with the Kingdom of Tunis: Eaton to the Secretary of State, May 7, 1800; Eaton to Mr. Appleton, Feb. 18, 1800 ("covered with blood"); William Eaton to Com. Rodgers, on board the U.S. frigate Constellation, off Derne: June 13, 1805 ("uttering shrieks"). Zacks, *Pirate Coast*, p. 175. Whipple, *To the Shores of Tripoli*, pp. 235–37, 239, 244, 253. Harris, *Life and Services of Commodore William Bainbridge*, p. 123.

22. WEP, Hamet Bashaw Caramali to Eaton, June 29, 1805; Eaton to the President of the United States, Feb. 12, 1808 ("Honor recoils"). *Republic of Letters*: Jefferson to Madison, Aug. 2, 1806, pp. 1431–32. Allen, *Our Navy*, pp. 252–53, 256 ("You have acquired").

23. Whipple, *To the Shores of Tripoli*, p. 221. Thomas Jefferson Papers: Jefferson's Report to Congress, Dec. 3, 1805.

24. *Republic of Letters*: Jefferson to Madison, Sept. 1, 1807, p. 1494 ("to secure peace"). Perkins, *Cambridge History of American Foreign Relations*, pp. 145–46. Robotti and Vescovi, *USS Essex*, pp. 145–46. Hurewitz, *Middle East and North Africa*, p. 202. Field, *America and the Mediterranean World*, p. 57. Allen, *Our Navy*, pp. 277 ("Should our differences"), 279 ("My policy"). *An Affecting Narrative of the Captivity and Suffering of Thomas Nicholson Who Has Been Six Years a Prisoner among the Algerines* (Boston: N. Coverly, 1818), pp. 5–6, 11.

25. Jonathan D. Sarna, *Jacksonian Jew: The Two Worlds of Mordecai Noah* (New York: Holmes & Meier, 1981), pp. 13–27, 28 ("It might be well"), 29–33. Isaac Goldberg, *Major Noah: American-Jewish Frontier* (Philadelphia: Jewish Publication Society of America, 1936), pp. 76–80, 117–26. See also Mordecai Manuel Noah, *Correspondence and Documents Relative to the Attempt to Negotiate for the Release of the American Captives at Algiers Including Remarks on Our Relations with that Regency* (Washington, D.C.: n.p., 1816). "Judaic Treasures of the Library of Congress: Mordecai Manuel Noah," http://www.us-israel.org/jsource/loc/noah .html. For David Franks, see Frederick C. Leiner, *The End of Barbary Terror: American's 1815 War against the Pirates of North Africa* (Oxford: Oxford Univ. Press, 2006), p. 30.

26. Allen, *Our Navy*, pp. 283–84, 286–87, 289 ("swept from the seas " and "dictated from the mouths"). Field, *America and the Mediterranean World*, p. 58 ("liberal and enlightened"). Boot, *Savage Wars of Peace*, pp. 27–28 ("powder as tribute"). Leiner, *End of Barbary Terror*, pp. 46–47, 68–69 ("serious disasters"). William Shaler, *Sketches of Algiers* (Boston: Cummings, Hillard, 1826), pp. 38

("worthless a power"), 101 ("Islamism"), 126–27, 167–68. For the Madison-dey correspondence see Hurewitz, *Middle East and North Africa*, pp. 206–7. On the personality and foreign policy views of James Madison, see J. C. A. Stagg, *Mr. Madison's War: Politics, Diplomacy, and Warfare in the Early American Republic, 1783–1830* (Princeton: Princeton Univ. Press, 1983), p. 506. Drew R. McCloy, *The Last of the Fathers: James Madison and the Republican Legacy* (Cambridge: Cambridge Univ. Press, 1989), pp. 18, 22, 26. Robert A. Rutland, *The Presidency of James Madison* (Lawrence: Univ. Press of Kansas, 1990), pp. 2, 18–20, 25–26.

27. *Niles' Weekly Register*, April 15, 1815 ("The name of an American"); Oct. 15, 1815 ("energy which liberty"). Marshall Smelser, *The Democratic Republic* (New York: Harper & Row, 1968), p. 60. Boot, *Savage Wars of Peace*, p. 28. Allison, *Crescent Obscured*, pp. 33, 201–6. Allen, *Our Navy*, p. 295 ("It was not to be"). Irving Brant, *James Madison*, vol. 6 (New York: Bobbs-Merrill, 1961), p. 398. Dennis Caplan, "John Adams, Thomas Jefferson, and the Barbary Pirates: An Illustration of Relevant Costs for Decision Making," *Issues in Accounting Education* 18, no. 3 (2003). James Ellison, *The American Captive; or, The Siege of Tripoli: A Drama in Five Acts* (Boston: Joshua Belcher, 1812). Joseph Hanson, *The Musselmen Humbled; or, A Heroic Poem in Celebration of the Bravery Displayed by the American Tars, in the Contest with Tripoli* (New York: Southwick and Hardcastle, 1806).

28. Jefferson to Adams, May 27, 1813, in *Adams-Jefferson Letters*, p. 325. See also *Adams-Jefferson Letters*: John Adams to Thomas Jefferson, June 11, 1813, pp. 328–29. WEP, Eaton to General Bradley, Jan. 15, 1810 ("I am closely besieged"). William Harlan Hale, "'General' Eaton and His Improbable Legion," *American Heritage* 11, no. 2 (Feb. 1960): 106. Whipple, *To the Shores of Tripoli*, p. 280. Allison, *Crescent Obscured*, pp. 205–6. Field, *America and the Mediterranean World*, p. 336. Allen, *Our Navy*, pp. 265–66.

29. *Naval Documents Related to the United States Wars*, vol. 3: Statement by Mordecai Noah, Nov. 8, 1826, p. 232. John Martin Baker, *A View of the Commerce of the Mediterranean* (Washington, D.C.: Davis and Force, 1819), p. 67. Tibawi, *American Interests in Syria*, p. 2. Finnie, *Pioneers East*, pp. 32–33 ("What a reproof"), 119, 258. Smelser, *Democratic Republic*, p. 313.

4. Illuminating and Emancipating the World

1. Levi Parsons, *The Dereliction and Restoration of the Jews: A Sermon, Preached in Park-Street Church Boston, Sabbath, Oct. 31, 1819, Just before the Departure of the Palestine Mission* (Boston: Samuel T. Armstrong, 1819). Levi Parson, *The Memoir of Rev. Levi Parsons*, comp. Daniel Oliver Morton (New York: Arno Press, 1977), p. 219 ("The spirit of the missions"). Alvan Bond, *Memoir of the Rev. Pliny Fisk* (New York: Arno Press, 1977), pp. 63, 96–97 ("And now, behold"). Marty E. Martin, *Pilgrims in Their Own Land: 500 Years of Religion in America* (Boston: Little, Brown, 1984), pp. 146–47. Clifton Jackson Phillips, *Protestant America and the Pagan World: The First Half Century of the American*

Board of Commissioners for Foreign Missions, 1810–1860 (Cambridge: Harvard Univ. Press, 1969), p. 135. Finnie, *Pioneers East*, pp. 150–51. Tibawi, *American Interests in Syria*, pp. 13–16. Kaplan, *Arabists*, p. 21. Instructions to Fisk and Pliny, in Field, *America and the Mediterranean World*, p. 93.

2. Barbara W. Tuchman, *Bible and Sword: England and Palestine from the Bronze Age to Balfour* (New York: Ballantine, 1956), pp. 80 ("the genius and history"), 81, 124–25. Edward Robinson, *Biblical Researches in Palestine, Mount Sinai and Arabia Petraea*, vol. 1 (Boston: Crocker and Brewster, 1841), p. 46. Yona Malachy, *American Fundamentalism and Israel: The Relation of Fundamentalist Churches to Zionism and the State of Israel* (Jerusalem: Graph Press, 1978). Everett Emerson, *Puritanism in America, 1620–1750* (Boston: Twayne, 1977), pp. 71–72, 90–92. Cecelia Tichi, "The Puritan Historians and Their New Jerusalem," *Early American Literature* 6 (1971). John Davis, *The Landscape of Belief: Encountering the Holy Land in Nineteenth-Century American Art and Culture* (Princeton: Princeton Univ. Press, 1996), p. 14 ("Jerusalem was"). Shalom Goldman, ed., *Hebrew and the Bible in America: The First Two Centuries.* (Hanover: Brandeis Univ. Press and Dartmouth College, 1993), pp. xv–xxii, 105, and *God's Sacred Tongue: Hebrew and the American Imagination* (Chapel Hill: Univ. of North Carolina Press, 2004), p. 29 ("[In] New England").

3. Burns, *The American Idea of Mission*, pp. 5, 11, 18, 31, 261. Obenzinger, *American Palestine*, pp. 12, 28–29. Willard Sterne Randall, *Alexander Hamilton: A Life* (New York: Perennial, 2003), p. 18. Ron Chernow, *Alexander Hamilton* (New York: Penguin, 2004), p. 18 ("entirely out of the ordinary"). Davis, *The Landscape of Belief*, p. 15 ("instead of the twelve"). Conrad Cherry, ed., *God's New Israel: Religious Interpretations of American Destiny* (Chapel Hill: Univ. of North Carolina Press, 1998), pp. 40 ("City on the Hill"), 62–71, 82–85. Jon Meacham, *American Gospel: God, the Founding Fathers, and the Making of a Nation* (New York: Random House, 2006), pp. 79–84.

4. Tibawi, *American Interests in Syria*, p. 10. Bond, *Memoir of the Rev. Pliny Fisk*, p. 111 ("The Christian . . . ought"). Tocqueville, *Democracy in America,* pp. 418–19. Phillips, *Protestant America*, p. 8 ("We have now entered"), 12 ("the tabernacle of God"). Perkins, *Cambridge History of American Foreign Relations*, p. 4 ("an object so valuable "). Cherry, *God's New Israel*, p. 65 ("a great . . . design"). See also Brooke Allen, "Our Godless Constitution," *Nation*, Feb. 3, 2005.

5. Kenneth Latourette, *Missions and the American Mind* (Indianapolis: National Foundation Press, 1949), pp. 28 ("Though you and I"), 31–34. Phillips, *Protestant America*, p. 20. Walter Russell Mead, *Special Providence: American Foreign Policy and How It Changed the World* (New York: Routledge, 2002), pp. 151–52. Kaplan, *Arabists*, p. 19 ("Only the extension"). Rao H. Lindsay, *Nineteenth Century American Schools in the Levant: A Study of Purposes* (Ann Arbor: Univ. of Michigan School of Education, 1965), pp. 61–63, 67. Finnie, *Pioneers East*, pp. 50 ("the groans" and "Zion will now"), 114–15.

6. Israel Finestein, "Early and Middle 19th-Century British Opinion on the

Restoration of the Jews: Contrasts with America," in Moshe Davis, ed., *With Eyes toward Zion*, vol. 2: *Themes and Sources in the Archives of the United States, Great Britain, Turkey and Israel* (New York: Praeger, 1986), pp. 74–77, 79–80. Obenzinger, *American Palestine*, pp. 34, 37. Martin, *Pilgrims in Their Own Land*, pp. 181–82. Tuchman, *Bible and Sword*, p. 121 ("transport Izraell's sons"). Lester I. Vogel, *To See a Promised Land: Americans and the Holy Land in the Nineteenth Century* (University Park: Pennsylvania State Univ. Press, 1993), pp. 125–26. Cherry, *God's New Israel*, p. 91 ("the return of the twelve"). Marr, "Imagining Ishmael," pp. 32–33, 35 ("When that empire falls"), 37–40, 61.

7. *Niles' Weekly Register* Nov. 9, 1816, p. 168. Naomi Shepherd, *The Zealous Intruders: The Western Rediscovery of Palestine* (London: Collins, 1987), p. 39. Tibawi, *American Interests in Syria*, pp. 5–8. Field, *America and the Mediterranean World*, 281. Elias Boudinot, *A Star in the West; or, A Humble Attempt to Discover the Long Lost Ten Tribes of Israel, Preparatory to Their Return to Their Beloved City, Jerusalem* (Trenton, N.J: Fenton, Hutchinson, and Dunham, 1816), p. 43. Michael Schuldiner and Daniel J. Kleinfeld, *The Selected Writings of Mordecai Noah* (London: Greenwood, 1999), p. 127 ("a hundred thousand").

8. Twenty cities in the United States are named for Smyrna, which is twice mentioned in the New Testament (see Revelations 1:10–11 and 2:8). Papers of the American Board of Commissioners for Foreign Missions (PABCFM), 5/515/0039, Mission to the Jews, vol. 3: Journal of Eli Smith, Jan. 23, 1827 ("There seems to be"). Tibawi, *American Interests in Syria*, pp. 13–14 ("Do nothing rashly"), 17, 23. Parsons, *Memoir*, pp. 222 ("With the spirit"), 240 ("The permission to"). Finnie, *Pioneers East*, p. 151 ("wear a turban").

9. PABCFM, 5/515/0039, Mission to the Jews, vol. 3: Journal of Eli Smith, Dec. 12, 1826 (estimation of Jerusalem's Jewish population). Rev. Harvey Newcomb, *Cyclopedia of Missions* (New York: Scribner, 1854), p. 734. Parsons, *Memoir*, pp. 263, 363 ("no place in the world"), 385 ("The door is already"), 390 ("the present commotions"). Moshe Davis and Yehoshua Ben-Arieh, *With Eyes toward Zion*, vol. 5, *Jerusalem in the Mind of the Western World, 1800–1848* (New York: Praeger, 1997), pp. 95–96, 144. Finnie, *Pioneers East*, pp. 24, 151–52. Joseph L. Grabill, *Protestant Diplomacy and the Near East: Missionary Influence on American Policy, 1810–1927* (Minneapolis: Univ. of Minnesota Press, 1969), p. 7 ("Thy spirit, Parsons").

10. Tibawi, *American Interests in Syria*, p. 22 ("Suffer not your minds"). *The Missionary Herald: Reports from Ottoman Syria, 1819–1870*, vol. 1, ed. Kamal Salibi and Yusuf Khoury (Amman: Royal Institute for Inter-Faith Studies, 1995): Journal of Jonas King, May 10, 1825, p. 405 ("the Arabs poured down"). Isaac Bird, *Bible Work in Bible Lands* (Philadelphia: Presbyterian Board of Publication, 1872), p. 15. Finnie, *Pioneers East*, pp. 154–55 ("He gave us").

11. PABCFM, 5/515/0039, Mission to the Jews, vol. 3: Journal of Eli Smith, March 1, 1827 ("She was brought"); May 13, 1824; April 18, 1825 ("It is by no means"), Gridley to Anderson, Nov. 16, 1826 ("Scarcely ten"). Newcomb, *Cyclopedia of Missions*, p. 735 ("Druses, Maronites"). Burns, *American Idea of Mission*, p. 261. Shep-

herd, *Zealous Intruders*, p. 40. Field, *America and the Mediterranean World*, pp. 94–95, 103, 129 ("missionaries loaded with books"). Julius Richter, *History of Protestant Missions in the Near East* (New York: AMS Press, 1970), p. 187. Tibawi, *American Interests in Syria*, pp. 28–29, 42. Grabill, *Protestant Diplomacy*, p. 8.

12. Tibawi, *American Interests in Syria*, pp. 25–26, 32–35, 37–39. Field, *America and the Mediterranean World*, pp. 98–99, 103. Finnie, *Pioneers East*, pp. 152, 171, 191–92.

13. George H. Scherer, *Mediterranean Missions, 1808–1870* (Beirut: Bible Lands Union for Christian Education, n.d.), p. 7. Adnan Abu-Ghazaleh, *American Missions in Syria: A Study in Missionary Contributions to Arab Nationalism in 19th Century Syria* (Brattleboro, Vt.: Amana Books, 1990), pp. 20–21. Kaplan, *Arabists*, p. 21 ("Christian workers"). Tibawi, *American Interests in Syria*, pp. 18 ("day of small things"), 35–37, 38 ("a wide and effectual"), 42.

5. Confluence and Conflict

1. Pierre Crabites, *Americans in the Egyptian Army* (London: Routledge, 1938), p. 25 ("pale, delicate-looking"). Finnie, *Pioneers East*, pp. 144–45, 146–47 ("to the prosperity"). Wright, "American Relations with Turkey," pp. 95–96. George Bethune English, *A Narrative of the Expedition to Dongola and Sennaar under the Command of His Excellence Ismael Pasha Undertaken by Order of His Highness Mehemmed Ali Pasha Viceroy of Egypt* (Boston: Wells and Lilly, 1823), p. 114 ("the land of the free"). George Bethune English, *The Grounds of Christianity Examined by Comparing the New Testament with the Old* (Boston: A.M., 1813), p. 113. George Bethune English, *A Letter to the Reverend Mr. Cary Containing Remarks upon His Review of the Grounds of Christianity Examined by Comparing the New Testament with the Old by the Author of That Work* (Boston: Printed for the Author, 1813), pp. 76 ("worship of angels"), 118 ("infernal wickedness"). George Bethune English, *Letter Respectfully Addressed to the Reverend Mr. Channing Relative to His Two Sermons on Infidelity* (Boston: Printed for the Author, 1813), pp. 9, 30.

2. English, *Narrative of the Expedition to Dongola and Sennaar*, pp. 18–20, 32 ("We are lost!"), 49, 59 ("luckless fornicators"), 61–62 ("monuments of his"). See also Finnie, *Pioneers East*, p. 147. Wright, "American Relations with Turkey," p. 96 ("Obstinate hostility to the truth"). *Adams-Jefferson Letters*: Adams to Jefferson, March 10, 1823, p. 591.

3. *Adams-Jefferson Letters*: Adams to Jefferson, June 6, 1785, p. 133. Republic of Letters: Jefferson to Madison, April 15, 1804, p. 1309. Kennedy, *American Consul*, pp. 94–95. Barrell, *Letters from Asia*, pp. 13–14. Field, *America and the Mediterranean World*, p. 118 ("bribery and brass"). Josiah Brewer, *A Residence at Constantinople in the Year 1827, with Notes to the Present Time* (New Haven: Durrie and Peck, 1830), p. 71. Bryson, *American Diplomatic Relations*, pp. 17–18. Wright, "American Relations with Turkey," pp. 58–63. Finnie, *Pioneers East*, pp.

26–29, 30 ("Imaginary Protection"). Ades Nimet Kurat, "Archival Documents concerning Relations between Turkey and the United States of America," *Journal of Historical Research* [Turkish] 5 (1964): 290 ("There is no benefit").

4. John Lewis Gaddis, *Surprise, Security, and the American Experience* (Cambridge: Harvard Univ. Press, 2004), p. 15. Mary W. M. Hargreaves, *The Presidency of John Quincy Adams* (Lawrence: Univ. Press of Kansas, 1985), pp. 29–30, 38. Field, *America and the Mediterranean World*, pp. 119–20 ("preserve him"). Finnie, *Pioneers East*, pp. 51–52. Wright, "American Relations with Turkey," pp. 28, 78–81, 89. Kurat, "Archival Documents," pp. 292 ("Though once only"), 308–9 ("Their cannon foundries").

5. Bryson, *American Diplomatic Relations*, p. 10 ("fellow-citizens of Penn"). Myrtle Cline, *American Attitude toward the Greek War of Independence, 1821–1828* (Atlanta: Higgins-McArthur, 1930), pp. 29 ("Sacred to the cause"), 63 ("My old imagination"), 98 ("Humanity, policy"). Edward Mead Earle, "Early American Policy Concerning Ottoman Minorities," *Political Science Quarterly* 42 (March 1927): 45 ("purge Greece"), 46 ("how spontaneously"), 47, 55–56. Field, *America and the Mediterranean World*, p. 121 ("see the language"). Little, *American Orientalism*, p. 12 ("Wherever the arms"). Thomas Robbins, *Diaries, 1796–1854* (Boston: Thomas Todd, 1886): vol. 2, entry for April 11, 1829, p. 90. Samuel Gridely Howe, *An Historical Sketch of the Greek Revolution* (New York: n.p., 1828), pp. 36–38.

6. Samuel Woodruff, *Journal of a Tour to Malta, Greece, Asia Minor, Carthage, Algiers, Port Mahon, and Spain* (Hartford: Cooke, 1831), p. 11. Bryson, *American Diplomatic Relations*, pp. 11–12 ("cherish[ed] sentiments"), 13–15. John Quincy Adams, *The American Annual Register, 1827–1829* (New York: Blunt, 1830), pp. 269 ("fanatic and fraudulent," "Ismael," and "doctrine [of] violence"), 274 ("the subjugation of others"), 299 ("the natural hatred"), 303. Samuel Flagg Bemis, *John Quincy Adams and the Foundations of American Foreign Policy* (New York: Knopf, 1956), p. 388. See also *American Philhellenes and the War for Independence,* http://www.ahepafamily.org/d5/Grk%20Inde-mar02.htm.

7. Hargreaves, *Presidency of John Quincy Adams*, 86. Wright, "American Relations with Turkey," pp. 96–97 ("You will inform me" and "American Mussulman"), 109–10 ("much engaged" and "his good offices").

8. Bemis, *John Quincy Adams*, p. 468. Hargreaves, *Presidency of John Quincy Adams*, pp. 85–86, 121. Finnie, *Pioneers East*, pp. 53–56. Wright, "American Relations with Turkey," pp. 109–10, 148 ("misconduct"). John Quincy Adams, *Chronology, Documents and Bibliographical Aids* (New York: Oceana Publications, 1970), p. 84 ("suffering Greeks"). Kurat, "Archival Documents," p. 293 ("See how these Franks").

9. For general histories of the reign and policies of Muhammad Ali, see Henry H. Dodwell, *The Founder of Modern Egypt: A Study of Muhammad ʿAli* (1931; reprint, New York: AMS Press, 1977), and Afaf Lutfi al-Sayyid Marsot, *Egypt in the Reign of Muhammad Ali* (Cambridge: Cambridge Univ. Press, 1984). See also Shimon Shamir,

"Egyptian Rule (1832–1840) and the Beginning of the Modern Period in the History of Palestine," in Gabriel Baer and Amnon Cohen, eds., *Egypt and Palestine: A Millennium of Association (868–1948)* (New York: St. Martin's, 1984), pp. 214–31.

10. The Senate approved the treaty, but objected to the provision of warships. Jackson chose to ignore the Senate's objections, and proceeded with arms sales to Turkey. Robert V. Remini, *Andrew Jackson and the Course of American Freedom, 1822–1832*, vol. 2 (New York: Harper & Row, 1981), p. 289 ("to leave no proper" and "the most friendly"). Kurat, "Archival Documents," pp. 293–94. John M. Belohlavek, *Let the Eagle Soar!: The Foreign Policy of Andrew Jackson* (Lincoln: Univ. of Nebraska Press, 1985), pp. 130–38. Donald B. Cole, *The Presidency of Andrew Jackson* (Lawrence: Univ. Press of Kansas, 1993), p. 128. Field, *America and the Mediterranean World*, pp. 145–46 ("Americans will be"). Lester D. Langley, "Jacksonian America and the Ottoman Empire," *The Muslim World* (Hartford: Duncan Black Macdonald Center, Hartford Seminary Foundation, 1978), pp. 46–49. Tungay, "Ottoman-American Trade," pp. 208–11. Text of the U.S.-Ottoman Treaty can be found in Hurewitz, *Middle East and North Africa*, pp. 246–47.

11. In appreciation of the sultan's purchases of his pistols. Samuel Colt presented him with a gold-plated revolver emblazoned with the images of George Washington and the Great Seal. The firearm, today valued at $5 million, is on display at New York's Metropolitan Museum of Art. Wright, "American Relations with Turkey," p. 138. Diplomatic Instructions of the Department of State, 1801–1906. Turkey. April 2, 1823–July 9, 1859. Microfilm 77, roll 162: John Forsyth to David Porter, May 16, 1837 ("improvement in seamanship"). Finnie, *Pioneers East*, pp. 16, 163–65, 175. Field, *America and the Mediterranean World*, pp. 168–69 ("balls without gunpowder"), 189 ("chairs and tables"), 191, 229. Sarah Rogers Haight, *Letters from the Old World by a Lady of New York* (New York: Harper, 1840), p. 193. Nathaniel Parker Willis, *Summer Cruise in the Mediterranean on an American Frigate* (New York: Scribner, 1853), p. 277. Brewer, *Residence at Constantinople*, p. 72. See also Thomas A. Bryson, *An American Consular Officer in the Middle East in the Jacksonian Era: A Biography of William Brown Hodgson, 1801–1871* (Atlanta: Resurgens, 1979), p. 42.

12. Edmund Roberts, *Embassy to the Eastern Courts of Cochin-China, Siam, and Muscat, in the U.S. Sloop-of-War Peacock, during the Years 1832–3–4* (New York: Harper, 1837) (courtesy of the New Hampshire Historical Society and the Tuck Library), pp. 343–45 ("the scene of"), 361 ("A strict lover"), 362–64. *New England Merchants in Africa: A History through Documents, 1802–1865*, ed. Norman Bennett and George Brooks (Boston: Boston Univ. Press, 1965): Edmund Roberts to Louis Mclane, May 14, 1834, pp. 156–57. Michael A. Palmer, *Guardians of the Gulf: A History of America's Expanding Role in the Persian Gulf, 1833–1992* (New York: Free Press, 1992), pp. 3–4. Among the coins presented to Sultan Sa'id was an extremely rare 1804 silver dollar now known as the Watters-Childs specimen, which last sold for $4.4 million. See http://www.geocities.com/

CollegePark/Union/8191/mcsh/Omanncss.html and http://www.coinfacts.com/ silver_dollars/1804_dollars/1804_Draped_Bust_Silver_Dollar.htm.

13. Finnie, *Pioneers East,* pp. 258 ("salutary effect"), 261 ("savage and uncivilized"). *Missionary Herald,* vol. 2: Letter from Eli Smith, Sept. 17, 1834, p. 431 ("multitude of Arab Christians"). John Israel and Henry Lundt, *Journal of a Cruize in the U.S. Ship Delaware 74 in the Mediterranean in the Years 1833 & 34* (1835; reprint, New York: Arno Press, 1977). George Jones, *Excursions to Cairo, Jerusalem, Damascus, and Balbec from the United States Ship Delaware, during Her Recent Cruise: With an Attempt to Discriminate between Truth and Error in Regard to the Sacred Places of the Holy City* (New York: Van Nostrand and Dwight, 1836). See also "An Audience with Sultan Abdul Mejud," by An American, *Knickerbocker* 19 (June 1842).

14. Frank E. Manuel, *The Realities of American-Palestine Relations* (1949; Westport, Conn.: Greenwood, 1975), pp. 9–10. Kennedy, *American Consul,* pp. 86–89, 97–98. Tibawi, *American Interests in Syria,* p. 88. Finnie, *Pioneers East,* pp. 250–53 ("Our whole consular"). Luella J. Hall, *The United States and Morocco, 1776–1956* (Metuchen, N.J.: Scarecrow, 1971), pp. 90–91. Ruth Kark, "Annual Reports of the United States Consuls in the Holy Land as a Source for the Study of 19th Century Eretz Israel," in Davis, *With Eyes toward Zion,* vol. 2, pp. 131–32.

15. USNA, Dispatches from U.S. Ministers to Turkey, 1818–1906 (Microfilm M46): David Porter to Nicholas Navoni, Sept. 23, 1831. W. M. Churchill to the Secretary of State, Aug. 10, 1833. *The Papers of Daniel Webster,* ser. 3, *Diplomatic Papers,* vol. 1 (Hanover: Univ. Press of New England, 1983), pp. 23–24. David Long, *Nothing Too Daring: A Biography of Commodore David Porter, 1780–1843* (Annapolis: U.S. Naval Institute, 1970), pp. 17–21. Tibawi, *American Interests in Syria,* pp. 3, 90. Archibald Douglas Turnbull, *Commodore David Porter, 1780–1843* (New York: Century, 1929), pp. 250–51. Field, *America and the Mediterranean World,* pp. 151, 168 ("There is no part"), 174. Finnie, *Pioneers East,* pp. 83–85 ("the head and neck"), 88 ("Salaams are"), 91, 94.

16. Field, *America and the Mediterranean World,* pp. 165–67, 170, 174. Finnie, *Pioneers East,* pp. 68, 71–73, 94–95 ("Had I the talent"), 259. Kennedy, *American Consul,* pp. 92–95. Tibawi, *American Interests in Syria,* p. 3. Cary Corwin Conn, "John Porter Brown, Father of Turkish-American Relations: An Ohioan at the Sublime Porte, 1832–1872" (Ph.D. diss., Ohio State Univ., 1973), pp. 48–49.

17. The pardon came too late, however, for two of the Syrians Jews, who were tortured to death. See Jonathan Frankel, *The Damascus Affair: "Ritual Murder," Politics, and the Jews in 1840* (Cambridge: Cambridge Univ. Press, 1997). Sarna, *Jacksonian Jew,* pp. 123–25. Tibawi, *American Interests in Syria,* pp. 3, 90. Malachy, *American Fundamentalism and Israel,* pp. 23–25. Diplomatic Instructions of the Department of State, 1801–1906. Turkey. April 2, 1823–July 9, 1859. Microfilm 77, roll 162: John Forsyth to David Porter, Aug. 17, 1840 ("atrocious cruelties").

18. *Papers of Daniel Webster,* pp. 273–74 ("Avoid doing anything"), 277–78 ("Frank residents of Beyrout"), 280. Stephen Vincent Benet, *The Devil and Daniel Webster and Other Writings* (New York: Penguin, 2000). Irving H. Bartlett, *Daniel*

Webster (New York: Norton, 1978), pp. 24, 44, 73, 85. Robert Seeger, *And Tyler Too: A Biography of John and Julia Gardiner Tyler* (New York: McGraw-Hill, 1963), pp. 104, 109. Field, *America and the Mediterranean World*, pp. 287–89, 350–51 ("A reading nation"). Finnie, *Pioneers East*, pp. 94–95, 126–27 ("at their own risk"). Franklin Steiner, *The Religious Beliefs of Our Presidents: From Washington to F.D.R.* (New York: Prometheus, 1995), pp. 95–97.

6. Manifest Middle Eastern Destiny

1. Brewer, *Residence at Constantinople*, pp. 25, 65, 361, 370. Finnie, *Pioneers East*, 36–37 ("Our *Pilgrim mothers*").

2. Newcomb, *Cyclopedia of Missions*, p. 737. Finnie, *Pioneers East*, pp. 50–51, 57, 171–72 ("I have not heard" and "roar of cannon"), 172–87. *Missionary Herald*, vol. 2: Journal of Mr. Thomson, April 16, 1834, p. 373 ("The Jordan"); Journal of Mr. Thomson [written in Nablus], April 23, 1834, p. 378 ("the wreck"); Whiting to Dodge, Nov. 17, 1834, p. 441. Davis, *Landscape of Belief*, p. 45. Newcomb, *Cyclopedia of Missions*, p. 737 ("not a single soul"). Yehoshua Ben-Arieh, *Painting the Holy Land in the 19th Century* (Jerusalem: Yad Izhak Ben-Zvi, 1997), p. 210. Tibawi, *American Interests in Syria*, pp. 100–1. Bird, *Bible Work in Bible Lands*, p. 87 ("a land of devils"). See also Shamir, "Egyptian Rule," pp. 214–31.

3. Tibawi, *American Interests in Syria*, pp. 40–43 ("The Turks . . . exhibit"). Board report in Newcomb, *Cyclopedia of Missions*, p. 737. Finnie, *Pioneers East*, pp. 35–38, 39 ("gloomy, austere"), 42 ("The thought of their"), 124, 193–94. Brewer, *Residence at Constantinople*, pp. 383–84.

4. Horatio Southgate, *Narrative of a Tour through Armenia, Kurdistan, Persia, and Mesopotamia* (London: Appleton, 1840), pp. 300–1 ("the first Americans"). Kaplan, *Arabists*, pp. 22–23 ("every species"), 24–25. Tibawi, *American Interests in Syria*, p. 79. Finnie, *Pioneers East*, pp. 208–9 ("I felt a stronger desire"), 216–17 ("The sick, the lame"), 196–97, 205-7, 214–15 ("his eye bright").

5. Finnie, *Pioneers East*, 118–19, 205–9 ("Enfeebled health"), 238–39 ("Let us have"). Louisa Hawes, *Memoir of Mrs. M. E. Van Lennep, by Her Mother* (Hartford: Belknap and Hamersley, 1849), p. 325 ("I sometimes fear"). Tibawi, *American Interests in Syria*, p. 73 ("The hour is near"). Hawes, *Memoir of Mrs. M. E. Van Lemep*, p. 325. *Missionary Herald*, vol. 2: Letter from Eli Smith, June 21, 1827, p. 247; Memoir of William Goodell, 1825, p. 431 ("a man's hat"). *The Reminiscences of Daniel Bliss* (New York: Revell, 1920), p. 106 ("You Americans think").

6. Robert T. Handy, *The Holy Land in American Protestant Life, 1800–1948* (New York: Arno Press, 1981), 85-86 ("Whereas, but"). Tibawi, *American Interests in Syria*, pp. 56, 82–83, 121–22, 170–76. Finnie, *Pioneers East*, pp. 109 ("liberty, property"), 200–1 ("Not only do"). Stephen Penrose, *That They May Have Life: The Story of the American University of Beirut, 1866–1941* (Princeton: Princeton Univ. Press, 1941), p. 6.

7. *Missionary Herald*, vol. 2: Letter from Mr. Marsh, Feb. 25, 1851, p. 299.

Field, *America and the Mediterranean World*, pp. 210 ("ought to know"), 250, 351 ("I do love"). Finnie, *Pioneers East*, p. 129 ("full extent" and "I am persuaded"). Phillips, *Protestant America*, p. 259. William Goodell, *Forty Years in the Turkish Empire* (New York: Robert Carter, 1883), p. 174 ("We have come") For insights into missionary views of Islam and Muhammad, see Thomas Laurie, *The Ely Volume; or, The Contributions of Our Foreign Missions to Science and Human Well-Being* (Boston: American Board of Commissioners for Foreign Missions, 1881), pp. 320–22, and the anonymous *Life of Mohammad* (Bombay: American Mission Press, 1851). The semidiplomatic role of European missionaries is discussed in Derek Hopwood, *The Russian Presence in Syria and Palestine, 1843–1914: Church and Politics in the Near East* (Oxford: Clarendon Press, 1969), p. 59.

8. Cyrus Hamlin, *My Life and Times* (Boston: Pilgrim Press, 1893), pp. 30, 62. Cyrus Hamlin, *Among the Turks* (New York: Robert Carter, 1878), pp. 57 ("a decided impression"), 62 ("rather leaky"). Finnie, *Pioneers East*, pp. 99–108, 109 ("indomitably self-willed"). Field, *America and the Mediterranean World*, p. 297 ("querulous" and "despotic"), 347–48.

9. Vogel, *To See a Promised Land*, pp. 118–19. Latourette, *Missions and the American Mind*, p. 33. Grabill, *Protestant Diplomacy*, p. 4. Lindsay, *Nineteenth Century American Schools*, p. 66. Phillips, *Protestant America*, p. 316. Tibawi, *American Interests in Syria*, pp. 97–98. Mead, *Special Providence*, pp. 143, 146–48, 150–51. Lewis, *Crisis of Islam*, p. 67 ("This country is"). PABCFM: Eddy to the American Board, Sept. 7, 1867 ("There are no rail"). Benjamin Foster, "Yale and the Study of Near Eastern Languages in America, 1770–1930," in Amanat and Bernhardsson, eds., *United States and the Middle East*, pp. 18 ("The countries of the West"), 19. Bruce Kuklick, *Puritans in Babylon: The Ancient Near East and American Intellectual Life, 1880–1930* (Princeton: Princeton Univ. Press, 1996), pp. 5, 20–22. John Thornton Kirkland, "Letter on the Holy Land," *Christian Examiner and General Review* 23, no. 2 (1842): 261. Elizabeth Cabot Kirkland, *Letters* (Cambridge: Massachusetts Historical Society, 1905), p. 503 ("These worthy people").

10. Robinson, *Biblical Researches in Palestine*, vol. 1, pp. 23–25, 75, 133 ("strangeness and overpowering" and "Although not given"). William Thomson, *The Land and the Book; or, Biblical Illustrations Drawn from the Manners and Customs, the Scenes and Scenery, of the Holy Land*, vol. 1 (New York: Harper, 1886), p. 6. Manuel, *Realities*, pp. 6–12. Ruth Kark, *American Consuls in the Holy Land, 1832–1914* (Jerusalem: Magnes Press, Hebrew Univ., 1994), pp. 84, 95, 127 ("There is no other"). Obenzinger, *American Palestine*, p. xvii. Vivian D. Lipman, "American-Holy Land Material in British Archives, 1820–1930," in Davis, *With Eyes toward Zion*, vol. 2, p. 28.

11. Robinson, *Biblical Researches in Palestine*, vol. 1, pp. 23–25, 75, 132, 162 ("stagnation and moral darkness"), 176, 262–63, 266–68, 350, 374 ("vast mass of tradition"). Edward Robinson, *Later Biblical Researches in Palestine and Adjacent Regions: A journal of travels in the year 1852* (London: John Murray, 1856), p. 73. Shepherd, *Zealous Intruders*, pp. 80–83. Handy, *Holy Land*, pp. 2–19. Neal Asher

Silberman, *Digging for God and Country: Archeology and the Secret Struggle for the Holy Land, 1799–1917* (New York: Knopf, 1982), pp. 40–47. Davis, *Landscape of Belief*, p. 36 ("American science").

12. William F. Lynch, *Narrative of the United States' Expedition to the River Jordan and the Dead Sea* (Philadelphia: Blanchard and Lea, 1853), pp. v ("teeming with sacred"), 18 ("hallowed by"), 76, 79 ("protection against"), 115 ("gun-shot wounds"), 119, 152 ("It must have been"), 230 ("wanderers in an unknown"), 259–60, 261, 284 ("The curse of God"), 293 ("in honour of), 287 ("the tents among"), 321 ("The thought of death"), 407. Edward P. Montague, *Narrative of the Late Expedition to the Dead Sea* (Philadelphia: Carey and Hart, 1849), pp. 116, 121–22 ("We Yankee boys"), 149, 218–19 ("float with perfect ease").

13. Lynch, *Narrative of the United States' Expedition,* pp. 360 ("Fifty well-armed"), 415 ("destined to be"). American Geographical and Statistical Society, *Report and Memorial on Syrian Exploration* (New York: New York Univ., 1857), p. 7. Andrew C. A. Jampoler, *Sailors in the Holy Land: The 1848 American Expedition to the Dead Sea and the Search for Sodom and Gomorrah* (Annapolis: Naval Institute Press, 2005), pp. 60, 142. See also Robert Edward Rook, "Blueprints and Prophets: Americans and Water Resource Planning for the Jordan River Valley, 1860–1970" (Ph.D. diss., Kansas State Univ., 1996), pp. 22–23.

14. Robbins, *Diaries, 1796–1854*, vol. 2, p. 573. Haight, *Letters from the Old World*, p. 110. George Bush, *The Life of Mohammed: Founder of the Religion of Islam, and of the Empire of the Saracens* (New York: Harper & Brothers, 1837), pp. 49 ("pseudo-prophet"), 160–61 ("man of superior"); *The Valley of Vision* (New York: Saxton and Miles, 1844), pp. 17 ("elevating"), 39 ("carnal inducements"), 41 ("It will blaze"), 56 ("link of communication"). Shalom Goldman, "Professor George Bush: American Hebraist and Proto-Zionist," *American Jewish Archives* 43, no. 1 (1991): 58–69. "Bush on Ezekiel's Vision," *Princeton Review* 16, no. 3 (1844): 384. Elaine B. Prince, "The Patrilineal Descent of Vice-President Bush," *NEXUS: The Bimonthly Newsletter of the New England Genealogical Society* 3 (1986): 124–25.

15. Truman G. Madsen, "The Holy Land and the Mormon Restoration," in Davis, *With Eyes toward Zion*, vol. 2, pp. 28–29. Obenzinger, *American Palestine*, pp. xvii, 116, 121, 126–27, 160 ("very weak minded"). Warder Cresson, *The Key of David* (Philadelphia: Self-published, 1852), p. 15 ("There is no salvation"). Frank Fox, "Quaker, Shaker, Rabbi: Warder Cresson: The Story of a Philadelphia Mystic," *Pennsylvania Magazine of History and Biography* 95 (1971): 147 ("I left the wife"), 157–63. Vogel, *To See a Promised Land*, p. 170 ("capacity & probity"). Sarna, *Jacksonian Jew*, pp. 153–55. *Selected Writings of Mordecai Noah*, pp. 125–26. William Makepeace Thackeray, *From Cornhill to Grand Cairo* (London: George Routledge, 1888), pp. 225–26, 242 ("has no knowledge").

16. Catherine A. Brekus, "Harriet Livermore, the Pilgrim Stranger: Female Preaching and Biblical Feminism in Early Nineteenth-Century America," *Journal of the Early Republic* 65 (Sept. 1996): 389–404. Elizabeth F. Hoxie, "Harriet Liver-

more: Vixen and Devotee," *New England Quarterly* 18 (March 1945): 41 ("Sick of the world"), 43 ("She is the most"). Diplomatic Instructions of the Department of State, 1801–1906. Turkey. April 2, 1823–July 9, 1859. Microfilm 77, roll 162: Louis Lane to David Porter, April 28, 1834 ("high character"). Finnie, *Pioneers East*, pp. 182–83 ("meet my lot"). Portraits of Lady Hester Stanhope can be found in Charles Lewis Meryon and Hester Lucy Stanhope, *The Travels of Lady Hester Stanhope* (London: H. Colburn, 1846). Michael Bruce, *The Nun of Lebanon* (London: Collins, 1951). "The Memoirs of Lady Stanhope," *Living Age* 6, no. 69 (Sept. 6, 1845).

17. John T. Brown, ed., *Churches of Christ* (Louisville: John P. Morton, 1904), pp. 440–41 ("criminally modest" and "they could all"). James Turner Barclay, *The City of the Great King; or, Jerusalem As It Was, As It Is, and As It Is to Be* (Philadelphia: James Challen, 1857), pp. 608–10. Handy, *Holy Land*, p. 84 ("God hath not"). Vogel, *To See a Promised Land*, p. 107.

18. Clorinda Minor, *Meshullam!; or, Tidings from Jerusalem: From the Journal of a Believer Recently Returned from the Holy Land* (Philadelphia: Self-published, 1851), pp. 52 ("His time to favor"), 91, 114 ("Many Christians profess"). Catherine A. Brekus, *Strangers and Pilgrims: Female Preaching in America, 1740–1845* (Chapel Hill: Univ. of North Carolina Press, 1998), p. 53 ("The conviction of my soul"). Henry L. Feingold, *Zion in America: The Jewish Experience from Colonial Times to the Present* (New York: Twayne, 1974), p. 199. Barbara Krieger, *Divine Expectations: An American Woman in 19th Century Palestine* (Athens: Ohio Univ. Press, 1999), pp. 38–39, 50, 113–16. Lipman, "American-Holy Land Material," pp. 29–32.

19. Field, *America and the Mediterranean World*, p. 280 ("the Modern Tabitha"). Tabitha—in Greek, Dorcas—was a righteous woman of Jaffa who, according to the New Testament (Acts 9:36–43), was resurrected after death by the apostle Peter. Yaron Perry, "John Steinbeck's Roots in Nineteenth-Century Palestine," *Steinbeck Studies* 15, no. 1 (Spring 2002): 51–52 ("our Hebrew friends"), 55. Abraham Karp, "The Zionism of Warder Cresson," in Isadore Meyer, ed., *Early Zionism in America* (Philadelphia: American Jewish Historical Society, 1958), pp. 9–14. Warder Cresson Biography, http://www.us-israel.org/jsource/biography/Cresson.html. Vogel, *To See a Promised Land*, p. 132. Field, *America and the Mediterranean World*, p. 281.

20. PABCFM, 5/546/16.8.1, Syrian Mission, vol. 7: Eddy to the American Board, Sept. 7, 1867 ("Europe is striving"). Tocqueville, *Democracy in America*, vol. 1, pp. 269 ("all-pervading"), 318 ("unquiet passions"); vol. 2, p. 622 ("strange unrest" and "in the midst").

7. Under American Eyes

1. Stanley T. Williams, ed., *Journal of Washington Irving, 1828 and Miscellaneous Notes on Moorish Legend and History* (New York: American Book Co., 1937), pp. 21–34. William H. Hedges, *The Old and New World Romanticism of*

Washington Irving (New York: Greenwood, 1986), pp. 20, 89–120. Philip Almond, "Western Images of Islam, 1700–1900," *Australian Journal of Politics and History* 49, no. 3 (2003). Fuad Shaban, *Islam and Arabs in Early American Thought: Roots of Orientalism in America* (Durham, N.C.: Acorn Press, 1991), p. 32. Malini Johar Schueller, *U.S. Orientalisms: Race, Nation, and Gender in Literature, 1790–1890* (Ann Arbor: Univ. of Michigan Press, 1998), pp. 68–70. Ahmed Mohamed Metwalli, "The Lure of the Levant: The American Literary Experience in Egypt and the Holy Land, 1800–1865," (Ph.D. diss., State Univ. of New York at Albany, 1971), p. 64 ("living in the *Arabian*"). Washington Irving and James Paulding, *Salmagundi* (Chicago: Belford, Clarke, 1807), pp. 34 ("positively assured"), 86 ("superlative ventosity"), 131 ("slangwhangging"). George S. Hellman, *Washington Irving, Esquire: Ambassador at Large from the New World to the Old* (New York: Knopf, 1925), pp. 155 ("A mighty potentate"), 207 ("a kind of Oriental"). Washington Irving, *The Conquest of Granada* (New York: Putnam, 1850), p. xx ("romantic adventures"). Washington Irving, *Alhambra* (Boston: Ginn, 1902), p. 90 ("naked realities").

2. Barrell, *Letters from Asia,* p. 10. Wright, "American Relations with Turkey," p. 155. Finnie, *Pioneers East,* pp. 4, 12–13, 160–65. Field, *America and the Mediterranean World,* p. 298. Joseph J. Malone, "America and the Arabian Peninsula: The First Two Hundred Years," *Middle East Journal* 30, no. 3 (Summer 1976): 407. Isaac M. Fein, *The Making of an American Jewish Community: The History of Baltimore Jewry from 1773 to 1920* (Philadelphia: Jewish Publication Society, 1971), pp. 24–25. Tigger, "Egyptology, Ancient Egypt," pp. 21–22.

3. Papers of William H. Seward: "Governor Seward's Journey from Egypt to Palestine," *New York Daily Tribune,* Dec. 24, 1859, p. 5 ("There are no berths"). Metwalli, "Lure of the Levant," p. 100. Prices to travel to the Middle East are listed in Warder Cresson, *King Solomon's Two Women and the Living and Dead Child or Messiah* (Philadelphia: Self-published, 1852), pp. 343–44. John Lloyd Stephens, *Incidents of Travel in Egypt, Arabia Petraea, and the Holy Land* (New York: Harper, 1855), pp. 4, 17–18. James Ewing Cooley, *The American in Egypt, with Rambles through Arabia Petra and the Holy Land during the Years 1839–1840* (New York: Appleton, 1842), pp. 16, 329. Wages in 1840 listed on "Senate Salaries since 1789," www.senate.gov/artandhistory/history/common/briefing/senate_salaries.htm and "Documenting the American South," http://docsouth.unc.edu/nc/helper/helper.html.

4. David F. Dorr, *A Colored Man round the World by a Quadroon* (N.p: Printed for the author, 1858), pp. 38 ("head-choppers"), 186. Cooley, *American in Egypt,* pp. 15 ("narrow, gloomy streets"), 16 ("Arabs, Armenians"), 262 ("ignorance and superstition"), 313 ("lunatics, idiots"). Stephens, *Incidents of Travel,* pp. 18 ("splendor and opulence" and "the dashing Turk"), 103 ("bigoted Musselmans"), 104, 120 ("false religion" and "haughty and deluded"). Haight, *Letters from the Old World,* pp. 30 ("I only saw"), 269 ("Mohammedanism").

5. Cooley, *American in Egypt,* pp. 259 ("civilized nations"). Stephens, *Incidents*

of Travel, pp. 174–75 ("When I heard"), 345 ("life hangs"). Haight, *Letters from the Old World*, pp. 45 ("penetrate the darkness"), 269 ("political crusade"), 270 ("kick the beam"). Walter Colton, *Visit to Constantinople and Athens*, vol. 2 (New York: Leavitt, Lord, 1836), pp. 105, 176–77 ("The same effort"), 181 ("Islamism"). Finnie, *Pioneers East*, pp. 155 ("There is a feeling"), 161. Valentine Mott, *Travels in Europe and the East* (New York: Harper, 1842), p. 269 ("His royal highness"). William H. Bartlett, *The Nile Boat; or, Glimpses of the Land of Egypt*. (London: Arthur Hall, Virtue, 1850), pp. 46 ("city of Saladin"), 135 ("Egypt, fallen"). Kirkland, *Letters*, pp. 480–81 ("a rich Jew"), 490 ("a man lying").

6. Stephens, *Incidents of Travel*, pp. 146 ("yellow slippers"), 84–85 ("that precious fragment"), 216. Mott, *Travels in Europe and the East*, p. 327. Dorr, *Colored Man round the World*, pp. 123 ("I would have given"), 177 ("jingling and a screwing"). Willis, *Summer Cruise*, pp. 254 ("the camel-driver's wife"), 268 ("a graceful creature"), 285. On nineteenth-century Western sexual fantasies of the Middle East, see Edward Said, *Orientalism* (New York: Vintage, 1979), pp. 119, 181–90.

7. Bayard Taylor, *The Lands of the Saracen; or, Pictures of Palestine, Asia Minor, Sicily, and Spain* (New York: Putnam, 1855), pp. 55 ("We kept our arms"), 56 ("heard the trumpets"). Finnie, *Pioneers East*, 181–83 ("plain man of steady habits"), 187. Field, *America and the Mediterranean World*, pp. 195–96. Stephens, *Incidents of Travel*, pp. 163 ("Can it be"), 188 ("witness of that great"), 318 ("I never saw"). Haight, *Letters from the Old World*, vol. 2, pp. 10 ("her friends have"), 130 ("How deplorable"). Cooley, *American in Egypt*, pp. 45 ("Surely the serpent"), 60 ("He that dippeth"). Dorr, *Colored Man round the World*, p. 187 ("not worth"). Mott, *Travels in Europe and the East*, p. 330 ("Nothing denotes"). Kirkland, *Letters*, p. 491 ("I wore my").

8. Davis, *Landscape of Belief*, pp. 33, 42. The review of Cooley's book can be found in *United States Democratic Review* 11, no. 50 (Aug. 1842): 219 ("a novelty quite unique"). Samuel Austin Allibone, *A Critical Dictionary of English Literature, and British and American Authors* (Philadelphia: Lippincott, 1871), pp. 415 ("replete with information"), 754 ("precious volumes"). *Cleveland Plain Dealer* archive, Sept. 20, 1858, p. 3 ("graphic and racy"). "A Kentuckian in the East," *Harper's New Monthly Magazine*, 6, no. 36, May 1853, p. 741. *The Works of the Late Edgar Allan Poe*, vol. 4 (New York: Arthur Gordon Pym, 1856), pp. 371–89. Washington Irving, *Mahomet and His Successors* (Chicago: Belford, Clarke, 1973), p. 200. J. Ross Browne, *Yusef; or, The Journey of the Frangi: A Crusade in the West* (New York: Harper, 1853), p. 177 ("Yes, sir").

9. John Freeman, *Herman Melville* (New York: Macmillan, 1926), pp. 32–34, 63–65. Robert L. Gale, *A Herman Melville Encyclopedia* (Westport, Conn.: Greenwood, 1995), pp. 106–7, 127, 143, 400. Herman Melville, *Redburn* (New York: Literary Classics of the United States, 1983), p. 10. Herman Melville, *Moby Dick* (New York: Hendrick's House, 1952), p. 30. Obenzinger, *American Palestine*, p. 63. Herman Melville, *Journals*, ed. Howard C. Horsford and Lynn Horth (Chicago: Northwestern Univ. Press, 1989), pp. 56 ("Imagine an immense"), 58, 61 ("horri-

ble grimy"), 62–63 ("Out of every"), 65 ("these millions"), 72–73 ("like a huge stick"), 75–76 ("Vapors below summits"). Herman Melville, *White-Jacket; or, The World in a Man-of-War* (Oxford: Oxford Univ. Press, 1990), p. 153. Metwalli, "Lure of the Levant," p. 353. Dorothee Metlitsky Finkelstein, *Melville's Orienda* (New Haven and London: Yale Univ. Press, 1961), pp. 3, 165–67, 189, 192.

10. Warder Cresson, *Jerusalem: The Center and Joy of the Universe* (Philadelphia: Self-published, 1844), p. 23 ("God hath chosen"). Frank Fox, "Quaker, Shaker, Rabbi," pp. 174, 182. Obenzinger, *American Palestine*, pp. 127, 133 ("sawdust of Christianity"), 134–35. Warder Cresson biography on http://www.us-israel.org/jsource/biography/Cresson.html ("settling forever"). Melville, *White-Jacket*, p. 153 ("peculiar chosen people"). Melville, *Journal*, pp. 83 ("It is against the will" and "Whitish mildew"), 85 ("An American turned Jew"), 87 ("confused and half-ruinous"), 90 ("No country" and "the color"), 91 ("Is the desolation" and "In the emptiness"), 94 ("preposterous Jew mania").

11. Melville, *Journal*, pp. 81 ("exponent of her aspirations"), 92 ("broken-down machinist"), 93 ("H.M.: Have you settled"). Herman Melville, *Clarel: A Poem and Pilgrimage to the Holy Land* (Chicago: Northwestern Univ. Press, 1991), p. 413 ("in the name of Christ"). Finkelstein, *Melville's Orienda*, pp. 60–61, 90. Obenzinger, *American Palestine*, pp. 68–89. Walter Herbert, "The Force of Prejudice: Melville's Attack on Missions in *Typee*," *Border States* 1 (1973). Perry, "John Steinbeck's Roots," pp. 52–55, 60–61 USNA, RG 59, Dispatches from the U.S. Consuls. Alexandria, Egypt, vol. 2: Gorham to Brown, Jan. 17, 1858: Testimony of Mary Steinbeck, Jan. 18, 1858 ("Oh! Father" and "We sat half"); Testimony of Caroline Dickson, Jan. 18, 1858. Vogel, *To See a Promised Land*, p. 133. Robert DeMott, "Steinbeck's Other Family: New Light on East of Eden?" *Steinbeck Newsletter* 7, no. 1 (Winter 1994).

12. USNA, RG 59, Dispatches from U.S. Consuls. Jerusalem, Palestine: De Leon to Bell, Jan. 27, 1858 ("prompt, stern"); De Leon to Cass, Feb. 22, 1858 ("unprotected heads"); De Leon to Cass, March 6, 1858 ("We regard the murder"); Gorham to Brown, Oct. 12, 1859; De Leon to Cass, July 28, 1860 ("It is the nature"). Edwin De Leon, *Thirty Years of My Life on Three Continents* (London: Ward and Downey, 1890), pp. 259 ("Are our countries"), 262 ("the Arab character"), 263 ("The audacity"). Feingold, *Zion in America*, p. 89. USNA, RG 84, *Records of Foreign Service Posts. Cairo, Egypt*: The State Department to Edwin de Leon, April 16, 1858. Papers of William H. Seward, Reel 58: Trabulsi to Seward, Sept. [n.d.], 1859.

13. Harold W. Felton, *Uriah Phillips Levy* (New York: Dodd, Mead, 1978), p. 34. Samuel Sobel, *Intrepid Soldier* (Philadelphia: Cresset, 1980), pp. 17, 15 ("I would rather serve"), 21. Sanford V. Sternlicht, *Uriah Phillips Levy: The Blue Star Commodore* (Norfolk: Norfolk Jewish Community Council, 1961), p. 41. Donovan Fitzpatrick and Saul Saphire, *Navy Maverick: Uriah Phillips Levy* (Garden City, N.Y.: Doubleday, 1963). Marc Leeson, *Saving Monticello: The Levy Family's Epic Quest to Rescue the House That Jefferson Built* (New York: Free Press, 2001). Field,

America and the Mediterranean World, pp. 292–93. Palmer, *Guardians of the Gulf*, pp. 6–8.

14. Douglas H. Strong, *Dreamers and Defenders: American Conservationists* (Lincoln: Univ. of Nebraska Press, 1988), pp. 29–30. *Life and Letters of George Perkins Marsh* (New York: Scribner, 1888), p. 7. Jane Curtis, Will Curtis, and Frank Lieberman, *The World of George Perkins Marsh* (Woodstock: Countryman Press, 1982), pp. 65, 90, 102. David Lowenthal, *George Perkins Marsh: Versatile Vermonter* (New York: Columbia Univ. Press, 1958), pp. 120 ("wretched place"), 121–22, 126, 134–36, 178 ("the Comanches" and "strike with a salutary"). Rook, "Blueprints and Prophets," pp. 34–35, 39–40. Melville, *Journals*, pp. 69–70. *Ninth Annual Report of the Smithsonian Institution* (Washington, D.C.: Beverley Tucker, 1855), pp. 100 ("Ship of the desert"), 120.

15. Younis, "Arabs Who Followed Columbus," p. 14. Felicity Allen, *Jefferson Davis: Unconquerable Heart* (Columbia: Univ. of Missouri Press, 1999), p. 210. Odie B. Faulk, *The U.S. Camel Corps* (New York: Oxford Univ. Press, 1976), pp. 30, 49, 102 ("What are these"), 185–86 ("Napoleon, when"). *The Papers of Jefferson Davis*, ed. Lynda Crist and Mary Dix, vol. 6 (Baton Rouge: Louisiana State Univ. Press, 1989), pp. 26–27, 87 ("These tests fully realize"), 385, 387. Ben Macintyre, *The Man Who Would Be King: The First American in Afghanistan* (New York: Farrar, Straus and Giroux, 2004), pp. 269–72. See also *U.S. Camel Corps Remembered in Quartzite Arizona*, http://www.outwestnewspaper.com/camels.html.

16. Khalaf, *Persistence and Change*, pp. 89–93. PABCFM: W. W. Eddy to Board, June 5, 1860. Henry Jessup, *Fifty-three Years in Syria*, vol. 1 (New York: Revell, 1910), pp. 175 ("terror-stricken, hungry"), 187–88 ("the blood at length"). *Reminiscences of Daniel Bliss*, pp. 142, 146, 152. Melvin Urofsky, *The Levy Family and Monticello* (Monticello: Thomas Jefferson Foundation, 2001), p. 83. Perry, "John Steinbeck's Roots," p. 70. Malini Johar Schueller, ed., *David F. Dorr: A Colored Man round the World* (Ann Arbor: Univ. of Michigan Press, 1999), p. xi.

8. Fission

1. *Writings of Benjamin Franklin*, vol. 10: Historicus to the Editor of the *Federal Gazette*, March 23, 1790, pp. 87–91. Ellis, *Founding Brothers*, pp. 81–119.

2. Lotfi Ben Rejeb, "America's Captive Freemen in North Africa: The Comparative Method in Abolitionist Persuasion" *Slavery and Abolition* 9 (1988): 60–61 ("If many thousands"). Arthur Zilversmit, *The First Emancipation: The Abolition of Slavery in the North* (Chicago: Univ. of Chicago Press, 1967), p. 171 ("doubtless shudder"). Marr, "Imagining Ishmael," p. 142 ("The American slaves") and ("the injustice and cruelty"). *The Family Letters of Thomas Jefferson*, ed. Edwin Bettis and James Bear Jr. (Columbia: Univ. of Missouri Press, 1966): Martha Jefferson to Thomas Jefferson, May 5, 1787, p. 39. *Documentary History of the Ratification of the Constitution*: Anonymous letter, Feb. 6, 1789, p. 872 ("six of one"). Tyler,

Algerine Captive, pp. 98 ("like so many head"), 111 ("fly to"). Anonymous, *American in Algiers,* p. 24.

3. James Stevens, *An Historical and Geographical Account of Algiers* (Philadelphia: Hogan and McElroy, 1797), p. 235 ("the execrable practice"). WEP, Negociations of the United States with the Kingdom of Tunis, roll 2: "Remarks &c Made at Algiers," Feb. 24, 1799, p. 38 ("Barbary is hell"). James Riley, *Sufferings in Africa: Captain Riley's Narrative* (New York: Potter, 1965), pp. 445 ("the cursed tree") 446–47 ("shiver in pieces"). Allison, *Crescent Obscured,* pp. 221–25. Gerald McMurty, "Influences of Riley's *Narrative* upon Abraham Lincoln," *Indiana Magazine of History* 30, no. 2 (June 1934): 136–38. Marr, "Imagining Ishmael," pp. 151–53. Charles Sumner, *White Slavery in the Barbary States* (Boston: J. P. Jewett, 1853), pp. 11, 12–13.

4. *Missionary Herald:* Journal of Pliny Fisk, Mary 8, 1823, p. 156. Shaban, *Islam and Arabs in Early American Thought.* Albert J. Raboteau, "Black Americans," in Davis, *With Eyes toward Zion,* vol. 2, pp. 312–14. Stephen Olin, *Travels in Egypt, Arabia Petra and the Holy Land* (New York: Harper, 1844), p. 318 ("great national calamities"). Handy, *Holy Land,* p. xiii ("A keen observer").

5. Ziff, *Return Passages,* p. 50. Mott, *Travels in Europe and the East,* pp. 390–91. Willis, *Summer Cruise,* pp. 282–83. Stephens, *Incidents of Travel,* p. 62. Cooley, *American in Egypt,* p. 349. Dorr, *Colored Man round the World,* p. 141.

6. *FRUS,* 1861: Brown to Aali Pacha, June 26, 1861, pp. 391–92 ("continue to cultivate"); Brown to Seward, July 17, 1861, p. 391 ("friendly sympathies"); Thayer to Seward, June 29, 1861; 1862: Message of the President to the Two Houses of Congress, Dec. 5, 1862, p. 5. Seward to Morris, April 1, 1862, p. 783 ("accustomed as they are"); 1863, vol. 2: Thayer to Seward, Nov. 5, 1862, p. 1101. Phillip Shaw Paludan, *The Presidency of Abraham Lincoln* (Lawrence: Univ. Press of Kansas, 1994), pp. 89–91, 218–19. Benjamin P. Thomas, *Abraham Lincoln: A Biography* (New York: Random House, 1968), pp. 281–83, 360. Wright, *United States Policy toward Egypt,* pp. 60–61. On the replacement of James Williams, see *Senate Executive Journal,* March 18, 1861, p. 310.

7. USNA, RG 59, Dispatches from U.S. Consuls. Tangier, Morocco, vol. 8: De Long to Seward; Feb. 15, 1862 ("so called Southern Confederacy"); De Long to Seward; Feb. 20, 1862 ("American Citizens"); De Long to Commander of the Sloop of War "Tuscarosa," Feb. 20, 1862 ("I want the presence"); De Long to Bargash, Feb. 26, 1862; De Long to Seward, Feb. 27, 1862 ("at least three thousand"); De Long to the French, Italian, Swedish, Spanish, and Portuguese Consuls in Tangier, March 1, 1862 ("If temporary civil war"); De Long to Seward, March 6, 1862 ("I have heard"); De Long to Seward, March 20, 1862 ("Moorish authorities"). *FRUS,* 1862: Bargash to De Long, Feb. 25, 1862, pp. 863–64. *Official Records of the Union and Confederate Navies in the War of the Rebellion,* ser. 1, vol. 1 (Washington, D.C.: GPO, 1894), pp. 310–20, 358–60, 392, 668, 676–79. Raphael Simmes, *Memoirs of a Service Afloat* (Baltimore: Baltimore Publishing Co., 1887), pp. 334–35, 336 ("political ignorance"), 337–40. Jay Monaghan, *Diplomat in Carpet*

Slippers: Abraham Lincoln Deals with Foreign Affairs (Indianapolis: Bobbs-Merrill, 1945), pp. 215–17. On the Tangier lighthouse convention, see Peter Larsen, *Theodore Roosevelt and the Moroccan Crisis, 1904–1906* (Princeton: Princeton Univ. Press, 1984), p. iv.

8. *FRUS*, 1861: Thayer to Seward, July 20, 1861, p. 424; 1863, vol. 2: Thayer to Seward, Nov. 5, 1862, p. 1101; 1864, vol. 4: Thayer to Seward, Jan. 23, 1864, p. 405; Hale to Seward, Oct. 22, 1864, p. 408 ("generous contribution"); 1864, vol. 1: Message of the President to the Two Houses of Congress, Washington, Dec. 6, 1864, p. 4.

9. *Studies in the National Military Victories of Egypt* [Arabic]. Cairo: Ministry of Information, 1984, pp. 153–63. *FRUS*, 1865, vol. 3: Hale to Seward, Aug. 26, 1865, p. 329 ("What the Pacha"). Wright, *United States Policy toward Egypt,* pp. 63–65. Bryson, *American Diplomatic Relations,* pp. 25–26. Field, *America and the Mediterranean World,* p. 385. Arnold Blumberg, "William Seward and Egyptian Intervention in Mexico," *Smithsonian Journal of History* 1 (Winter 1966–67): 31–34, 44–45. Howard Kerner, "Turko-American Diplomatic Relations, 1860–1880" (Ph.D. diss., Georgetown Univ., 1948), pp. 62–65.

10. Allen C. Guelzo, *Abraham Lincoln: Redeemer President* (Grand Rapids, Mich.: Eerdmans, 1999), p. 434 ("How I should like"). USNA, RG 84, *Records of Foreign Service Posts. Cairo, Egypt,* vol. 78: Seward to Hale, Dec. 4, 1866; Seward to Hale, Jan. 23, 1867 ("considerate and friendly"). Osborn Oldroyd, *The Assassination of Abraham Lincoln* (1901; reprint, Union, N.J.: Lawbook Exchange, 2001), pp. 65, 232–35, 239, 266. Edward Steers, *Blood on the Moon: The Assassination of Abraham Lincoln* (Lexington: Univ. Press of Kentucky, 2001), pp. 231–32.

9. Rebs and Yanks on the Nile

1. Zachary Karabell, *Parting the Desert: The Creation of the Suez Canal* (New York: Knopf, 2003), p. 184 ("Practically every"). David Christy, *King Cotton* (Cincinnati: Moore, Wilstach, Keys, 1855), pp. 68–79. Field, *America and the Mediterranean World,* pp. 193–94 ("a Southern plantation"), 248–49. The goats given to Davis became the progenitors of prize Angora herds in Texas and Oregon; see *Texas Department of Agriculture,* http://www.agr.state.tx.us/education/teach/mkt_fibernet.htm, and *The First Farmers of Oregon,* http://www.gesswhoto.com/centennial-farmers.html.

2. E. R. J. Owen, *Cotton and the Egyptian Economy, 1820–1914* (London: Oxford Univ. Press, 1969), pp. 89, 105. Edward M. Earle, "Egyptian Cotton and the American Civil War," *Political Science Quarterly* 41, no. 4 (Dec. 1926): 520–36. USNA, RG 84, *Records of Foreign Service Posts. Cairo, Egypt,* vol. 78: William Seward to William Thayer, Dec. 16, 1862 ("The . . . increase of cotton"). *FRUS*, 1861: Thayer to Seward, July 20, 1861, p. 423; 1863, vol. 2: Seward to Morris, Dec. 13, 1862, pp. 1090–91. Vatikiotis, *History of Egypt,* pp. 73–77, 125–28. Karabell, *Parting the Desert,* pp. 183–84. Wright, *United States Policy toward Egypt,* pp. 66–70.

3. Charles Dudley Warner, *Mummies and Moslems* (Toronto: Belford Brothers, 1876), p. 380. Wright, *United States Policy toward Egypt,* pp. 86–87 ("shorten by 2,000 leagues"), 219. USNA, RG 84, *Records of Foreign Service Posts. Cairo, Egypt*: W. L. Marcy to Edwin de Leon, June 17, 1854 ("cheerfully received"). *FRUS,* 1861: Thayer to Seward, July 20, 1861, p. 424; 1862, vol. 2: Thayer to Seward, Nov. 5, 1862, p. 1101; 1864, vol. 4: Thayer to Seward, Jan. 23, 1864, p. 405; 1864, vol. 1: Message of the President to the Two Houses of Congress, Washington, Dec. 6, 1864, p. 4 ("Our relations with Egypt"); 1865, vol. 3: Hale to Seward, Dec. 22, 1864, p. 315.

4. Pierre Crabitès, *Americans in the Egyptian Army* (London: Routledge, 1938), pp. 14, 39. Charles Chaillé-Long, *My Life in Four Continents,* vol. 1 (London: Hutchinson, 1912), pp. 17, 38, 231. William B. Hesseltine and Hazel C. Wolf, *The Blue and the Gray on the Nile* (Chicago: Univ. of Chicago Press, 1961), pp. 4 ("a soldier of misfortune"), 5–11, 18–19, 29–41, 43–44. Field, *America and the Mediterranean World,* pp. 395–96.

5. John Marlowe, *Spoiling the Egyptians* (New York: St. Martin's, 1975), pp. 104–17. Wright, *United States Policy toward Egypt,* p. 70.

6. James Morris Morgan, *Recollections of a Rebel Reefer* (Boston: Houghton Mifflin, 1917), pp. 268–69 ("That was about"), 270 ("An exact reproduction"). Chaillé-Long, *My Life,* pp. 20–22, 30–33. Crabitès, *Americans in the Egyptian Army,* pp. 41–42, 44. Hesseltine and Wolf, *Blue and the Gray,* pp. 65–66 ("discretion, devotion"), 72–73, 93–94 ("The East with its"), 98–100, 150–51.

7. William Wessels, *Born to Be a Soldier: The Military Career of William Wing Loring* (Fort Worth: Texas Christian Univ. Press, 1971), p. 78–79. Hesseltine and Wolf, *Blue and the Gray,* pp. 19–20, 51 ("The limits"), 66–72, 87 ("the express right" and "The army here"). Field, *America and the Mediterranean World,* pp. 392–93, 397. Wright, *United States Policy toward Egypt,* p. 81. Chaillé-Long, *My Life,* p. 35. Morgan, *Recollections of a Rebel Reefer,* pp. 271 ("I looked so much"), 287. See also Olive Risley Seward, ed., *William H. Seward's Travels around the World* (New York: Appleton, 1873), pp. 545–46, 620. Ralph Kirshner, *The Class of 1861: Custer, Ames, and Their Classmates after West Point* (Carbondale: Southern Illinois Univ. Press, 1999), pp. 6, 167. *Personal Memoirs of U.S. Grant,* vol. 1 (New York: C. L. Webster, 1885), p. 181.

8. Morgan, *Recollections of a Rebel Reefer,* pp. 277–81, 291 ("Christian prejudices"). William Loring, *A Confederate Soldier in Egypt* (New York: Dodd, Mead, 1884), p. 69 ("the same barbarous"), 135 ("born of the sword"). Hesseltine and Wolf, *Blue and the Gray,* pp. 60 ("they are better"), 61–62, 64–65 ("Christian intolerance"), 89 ("The army, both officers"), 106, 116–17, 125–26. William Dye, *Moslem Egypt and Christian Abyssinia* (New York: Negro Universities Press, 1969), pp. 38–39, 45–46 ("imaginative soul"), 102.

9. Frederick J. Cox, "The American Naval Mission in Egypt," *Journal of Modern History* 26, no. 2 (June 1954). Hesseltine and Wolf, *Blue and the Gray,* pp.

123–27, 130–34, 144–46, 147 ("In the philanthropist"), 220. Crabitès, *Americans in the Egyptian Army*, pp. 74 ("Although I am prostrate"), 77, 81.

10. Charles Chaillé-Long, *The Three Prophets: Chinese Gordon, Mohammed-Ahmed (El Maahdi), Arabi Pasha* (New York: Appleton, 1884), pp. 25–27, and *My Life*, pp. 68, 91 ("Prostrate upon their faces,"), 94 ("number of warriors"), 97 ("The entire Nile"), 102–6, 158, 195 ("This young officer"). H. E. Wortham, *Chinese Gordon* (Boston: Little, Brown, 1933), p. 181. Godfrey Elton, *Gordon of Khartoum* (New York: Knopf, 1955), pp. 127, 135 ("on what he *has* done"). Crabitès, *Americans in the Egyptian Army*, pp. 110–11 ("Give it to them"), 134–35, 151–62, 167–68 ("American pirate"), 167 ("My hair hung"), 185. See also David Icenogle, "The Expeditions of Chaille-Long," http://www.saudiaramcoworld .com/issue/197806/the.expeditions.of.chaille-long.htm, and "Americans in the Egyptian Army," http://www.home.earthlink.net/~atomic_rom/officers.htm.

11. William Loring, "The Egyptian Campaign in Abyssinia—From the Notes of a Staff Officer," in *Littell's Living Age* 34, no. 1729 (Aug. 4, 1877). Loring, *Confederate Soldier in Egypt*, p. 63 ("I need not repeat"). Hesseltine and Wolf, *Blue and the Gray*, pp. 176–82.

12. Loring, *Confederate Soldier in Egypt*, pp. 416 ("morally and physically"), 417 ("a splendid place"), 401 ("in any other army"), 419 ("The Egyptians not only"), 414 ("alive with the moving"), 420–21 ("hideous . . . howls"), 435 ("No sooner had he"). Chaillé-Long, *My Life*, p. 195. Hesseltine and Wolf, *Blue and the Gray*, pp. 184–86, 194–95 ("Loring has blockhouse"), 205, 211–13, 224–25. Morgan, *Recollections of a Rebel Reefer*, pp. 309–10. Dye, *Moslem Egypt*, pp. 167 ("as shriveled with lechery"), 139–40 ("They escaped"), 219–22, 235, 270–71, 369 ("surgeons and sheiks"), 371 ("one unsightly mass"), 483, 487–88.

13. *FRUS*, 1878: Farman to Evarts, July 3, 1878, pp. 922–23; Farman to Evarts, July 15, 1878, pp. 923–24. On the Ottomans' purchase of Civil War surplus, see *FRUS*, 1877: Mr. Maynard to Mr. Evarts Constantinople, May 25, 1877, p. 572. James Raab, *W. W. Loring* (Manhattan, Kan.: Sunflower Univ. Press, 1997), pp. 833, 890. Field, *America and the Mediterranean World*, pp. 312, 422 ("a crime against humanity"). Loring, *Confederate Soldier in Egypt*, p. 448 ("During the ten years"). Hesseltine and Wolf, *Blue and the Gray*, pp. 213–14, 223, 229–30 ("The whole confounded"), 243–24 ("Egypt has been kind"), 251. Bryson, *American Diplomatic Relations*, p. 27. Wessels, *Born to Be a Soldier*, p. 94. Wright, *United States Policy toward Egypt*, p. 83 ("No intelligent foreigner"). Dye, *Moslem Egypt*, p. 1 ("They were men").

10. The Trumpet That Never Calls Retreat

1. Edward Wilmot Blyden, *Christianity, Islam and the Negro Race* (Edinburgh: Edinburgh Univ. Press, 1967), pp. 6, 10 ("self-reliant, productive"), 13, 19–21, 186, 254. Edward Wilmot Blyden, *The Elements of Permanent Influence: A Discourse Delivered at the 15th Street Presbyterian Church* (Washington, D.C.: R. I. Pendle-

ton, 1890) ("the spirit" and "Not the author"). Obenzinger, *American Palestine*, pp. 230–31 ("with an awe"). Yvonne Chireau and Nathaniel Deutsch, *Black Zion: African American Religious Encounters with Judaism* (New York: Oxford Univ. Press, 2000), p. 15 ("I would earnestly"). Edith Holden, *Blyden of Liberia* (New York: Vantage Press, 1966), pp. 141–44. Hollis Lynch, "A Black Nineteenth Century Response to Jews and Zionism: The Case of Edward Wilmot Blyden, 1832–1912," in Joseph Washington, ed., *Jews in Black Perspective* (Rutherford, N.J.: Fairleigh Dickinson Univ. Press, 1984), pp. 43–45. See also "Edward Wilmot Blyden and Africanism in America," http://www.columbia.edu/~hcb8/EWB_Museum/EWB1.html, and George Bornstein, "A Forgotten Alliance: Africans, Americans, Zionists and Irish," *Times Literary Supplement*, March 4, 2005, p. 13.

2. *FRUS*, 1862: Morris to Seward, Oct. 25, 1861, p. 787; Morris to Seward, Oct. 16, 1862, p. 791; 1864, vol. 4: Morris to Seward, May 21, 1863, p. 368. Tibawi, *American Interests in Syria*, pp. 151 ("The providential history"), 170–76. Hanna F. Wissa, *Assiout: The Saga of an Egyptian Family* (Lewes, Sussex: Book Guild, 1994), pp. 93, 97, 105. Jessup, *Fifty-three Years in Syria*, p. 512 ("could place a Tammany"). Ellen Clare Miller, *Eastern Sketches* (New York: Arno Press, 1977), pp. 132–33. *Missionary Herald*, vol. 3: Letter from Mr. Perkins, Dec. 26, 1862, p. 341 ("This great struggle"). Harry N. Howard, "President Lincoln's Minister Resident to the Sublime Porte," *Balkan Studies* 5 (1964): 205–6.

3. John A. DeNovo, *American Interests and Policies in the Middle East, 1900–1939* (Minneapolis: Univ. of Minnesota Press, 1963), p. 15. Grabill, *Protestant Diplomacy*, p. 34 ("Mohammedans, Muscovites"). Tibawi, *American Interests in Syria*, pp. 220–21 ("enjoy[ed] a liberty"), 272. Wright, *United States Policy toward Egypt*, pp. 146–47 ("We had the Gospel"), 219. The murderers of the two missionaries, the Reverends Merriam and Coffing, were later apprehended and executed. As a sign of gratitude, Secretary of State Seward presented the Ottoman grand vizier with a brace of silver pistols. See *FRUS*, 1863, vol. 2: Morris to Seward, April 30, 1863, p. 1094; 1864, vol. 4: Morris to Seward, Dec. 4, 1863, p. 373; Seward to Morris, Jan. 11, 1864, p. 366; Morris to Seward, April 14, 1864, pp. 381–82.

4. Jessup, *Fifty-three Years in Syria*, p. 597 ("semi-secular" and "letting in the light"). Taylor, *Lands of the Saracen*, p. 78. Tibawi, *American Interests in Syria*, p. 145 ("From the same battlefields"). Finnie, *Pioneers East,* p. 134 ("more converts"). Henry M. Field, *From Egypt to Japan*, 19th ed. (New York: Scribner, 1905), p. 60 ("Christian Missions").

5. John Freely, *A History of Robert College* (Istanbul: Y.K.Y, 2000), pp. 11–12. "The History of Robert College," http://www.robcol.k12.tr/admin/headmaster/history.htm. Field, *America and the Mediterranean World*, pp. 355–56. Hamlin, *My Life and Times*, p. 286 ("The work has proved"), 446–49, 470–73. Marcia Stevens and Malcolm Stevens, *Against the Devil's Current: The Life and Times of Cyrus Hamlin* (Lanham, Md.: Univ. Press of America, 1988), pp. 246, 258 ("No one was about"), 269, 297–98, 330–31. Khalaf, *Persistence and Change*, p. 100.

6. Carleton Coon, ed., *Daniel Bliss and the Founding of the American University of Beirut* (Washington, D.C.: Middle East Institute, 1989), pp. 35 ("Their faces"), 62–63, 67–68, 75 ("a home for jackals"), 79. Tibawi, *American Interests in Syria*, pp. 161–62 ("necessary choice"). Jessup, *Fifty-three Years in Syria*, p. 595 ("the promised land"). Penrose, *That They May Have Life*, p. 23. Field, *America and the Mediterranean World*, p. 357 ("a man white").

7. Philip Hitti, *Lebanon in History from the Earliest Times to the Present* (London: Macmillan, 1962), pp. 450, 454, 462–67. Albert Hourani, *Arabic Thought in the Liberal Age, 1798–1939* (Cambridge: Cambridge Univ. Press, 1962), pp. 243, 246–49. Holden, *Blyden of Liberia*, pp. 143–44 ("to the day"). Elie Kedourie, "The American University of Beirut," *Middle Eastern Studies* 3 (1966): 75. Bernard Lewis, *The Arabs in History* (London: Hutchinson's Univ. Library, 1950), pp. 173–74. Abu Ghazaleh, *American Missions in Syria*, pp. 31, 41–42, 59, 67–68. George Antonius, *The Arab Awakening* (London: Hamish Hamilton, 1938), pp. 42–43. *Missionary Herald*: "Recent Intelligence" (Mr. Wolcott), Feb. 1841, p. 255. Daniel Bliss, *Letters from a New Campus: Written to His Wife Abby and Their Four Children during Their Visit to Amherst, Massachusetts, 1873–1874* (Beirut: American Univ. of Beirut, 1994), pp. 159 ("Oh that all"), 280–81.

8. USNA, RG 84, *Records of Foreign Service Posts. Cairo, Egypt:* William Seward to Charles Hale, Nov. 16, 1867. Glyndon Van Deusen, *William Henry Seward* (New York: Oxford Univ. Press, 1967), pp. 212–13. *FRUS*, 1864, vol. 4: Seward to McMath, Dec. 9, 1863, p. 410 ("exert all proper").

9. *A Maine Family's History*, http://www.calaisalumni.org/Maine/tales9.htm ("lips shut tight"). Reed M. Holmes, *The Forerunners* (Independence, Mo.: Herald, 1981), pp. 189 ("The great Restitution"). John Swift, *Going to Jericho* (New York: A. Roman, 1868), p. 201 ("Johnson's patent"). Vogel, *To See a Promised Land*, pp. 135. Obenzinger, *American Palestine*, pp. 181 ("The reign of Christ"), 182–83. Shlomo Eidelberg, "The Adams Colony in Jaffa (1866–1868)," *Midstream* 3 (Autumn 1957): 52–53. Peter Amann, "Prophet in Zion: The Saga of George J. Adams," *New England Quarterly* 37 (Dec. 1964): 481–86.

10. In his response to the Reverend Monk, Lincoln also mentioned that his chiropodist and close confidant, Isachar Zacharie, was a Jew who had "put me upon my feet" so often that he would gladly aid the doctor's countrymen to "get a leg up" in moving to Palestine. Peter Grose, *Israel in the Mind of America* (New York: Knopf, 1983), pp. 25–26 ("There can be no"). See also Naphtali J. Rubinger, *Abraham Lincoln and the Jews* (New York: Jonathon David, 1962), p. 42, Bertram Korn, *American Jewry and the Civil War* (New York: Jewish Publication Society of America, 1951), p. 202, and Steiner, *Religious Beliefs*, pp. 110–45. Vogel, *To See a Promised Land*, p. 203. Little, *American Orientalism*, p. 13 ("We know far more"). Henry White Warren, *Sights and Insights; or, Knowledge by Travel* (New York: Nelson and Phillips, 1874), p. 246 ("This is the first country"). John Russell Young, *Around the World with General Grant: A Narrative of the Visit of General U. S.*

Grant, Ex-President of the United States, to Various Countries in Europe, Asia and Africa, in 1877, 1878, 1879 (New York: American News Co., 1879), p. 335 ("Somehow you always").

11. Vogel, *To See a Promised Land*, p. 83 ("shall yet be brought home"), 220 ("So much has"). *Princeton Review* 38, no. 4 (1866): 670–74. Warren, *Sights and Insights*, pp. 283–84 ("the greatest temptation"). Philip Schaff, *Through the Bible Lands* (New York: American Tract Society, 1878), pp. 233, 237, 249 ("squalid and forbidding"). David S. Landes, "Passionate Pilgrims and Others: Visitors to the Holy Land in the 19th Century," in Davis, *With Eyes toward Zion*, vol. 2, pp. 10–11. Henry A. Riley, *The Restoration at the Second Coming of Christ: A Summary of Millenarian Doctrines* (Philadelphia: Lippincott, 1868), pp. 41–42 ("be gathered from"). Sarah Barclay Johnson, *Hadji in Syria* (New York: Arno Press, 1977), pp. 16 ("rightful owner"), 119 ("the Hebrew race"). William C. Prime, *Tent Life in the Holy Land* (New York: Harper, 1857), pp. 2 ("cast in holy radiance"), 99–100 ("imported by Jaffa"). Henry W. Bellows, *Restatement of Christian Doctrines in 25 Sermons* (Boston: American Unitarian Association, 1869). Holmes, *Forerunners*, p. 19 ("The sons of Ephraim").

12. Amann, "Prophet in Zion," p. 486 ("he would rather"). Eidelberg, "Adams Colony in Jaffa," pp. 55–60. Obenzinger, *American Palestine*, p. 183 ("The exhalations"). Field, *America and the Mediterranean World*, pp. 281, 325 ("churches, hotels"). Holmes, *Forerunners*, pp. 119–21, 187 ("Put your faith"). Vogel, *To See a Promised Land*, pp. 138 ("adventurer, a charlatan"), 139 ("our warmest friends"), 140–41, 144 ("a monster in human"), 145–46, 147 ("We the colony"). Henry W. Bellows, *The Old World in Its New Face* (New York: Harper, 1869), pp. 262–62 ("religious fanatic"). Charles Elliot, *Remarkable Characters and Places in the Holy Land* (Hartford: J. B. Burr, 1867), p. 586 ("unprotected as they would be"). Swift, *Going to Jericho*, pp. 197–98 ("modern Mayflower"), 199–200 ("American eagle"), 201. On the death of Walter Cresson, see USNA, RG 59, Dispatches from U.S. Consuls. Jerusalem, Palestine: Page to Cass, Nov. 8, 1860.

13. National Library of Israel, Jerusalem, Manuscript Archive, Miscellaneous File 519: Petition of Colonists to Governor Chamberlain, Aug. 31, 1867. USNA, RG 84, *Records of Foreign Service Posts. Cairo, Egypt*, vol. 4: William Seward to Charles Hale, Oct. 7, 1867; RG 59, Dispatches from U.S. Consuls. Beirut, Lebanon, vol. 5: Letter for Jaffa Colonists to Beauboucher, March 20, 1867 ("How can we confide"); *Records of Foreign Service Posts: Jerusalem, Palestine*. March 8, 1857–Dec. 21, 1869, vol. 24: Johnson to Beauboucher, Dec. 3, 1867. Lipman, "American-Holy Land Material," pp. 32–33 ("The failure of the"). Vogel, *To See a Promised Land*, pp. 140 ("pale faced"), 147 ("recede and become"), 149. Obenzinger, *American Palestine*, pp. 184–85 ("American citizens"). Field, *America and the Mediterranean World*, p. 326 ("An Appeal!"). Eidelberg, "Adams Colony in Jaffa," p. 61. Holmes, *Forerunners*, p. 226.

11. American Onslaught

1. USNA, RG 59, Dispatches from the U.S. Consuls. Alexandria, Egypt, vol. 2: De Leon to Appleton, July 5, 1859. Vogel, *To See a Promised Land*, pp. 56, 59 ("The number of American"). Charles Dudley Warner, *Mummies and Moslems* (Toronto: Belford, 1876), p. 382 ("the perfumes of Arabia"). Jeffrey Alan Melton, *Mark Twain, Travel Books, and Tourism: The Tide of a Great Popular Movement* (Tuscaloosa: Univ. of Alabama Press, 2002), pp. 17, 18 ("nomadic era"). Kark, "Annual Reports," p. 164 ("unfavorable for the foreigner"). *The Memoirs of Rose Eytinge* (New York: Frederick A. Stoker, 1905), p. 151 ("most irksome"). Schaff, *Through the Bible Lands*, p. 26. Goldman, *God's Sacred Tongue*, pp. 160–61 ("The few Englishmen"). Field, *From Egypt to Japan*, pp. 7–8 ("Ah, you Americans").

2. Warner, *Mummies and Moslems*, pp. 357 ("Antiquity" Smith), 411 ("the conclusive verdict"). Vogel, *To See a Promised Land*, pp. 88 ("with few ideas" and "These cousins"), 91–92 ("miserable fellaheen"), 177. Crabitès, *Americans in the Egyptian Army*, p. 65 ("They usually come" and "They often think"). Morgan, *Recollections of a Rebel Reefer*, p. 267. Young, *Around the World*, pp. 301–2 ("Powell Tucker,"). *Journals of Ralph Waldo Emerson,* ed. Edward Emerson, vol. 10 (Boston: Houghton Mifflin, 1914), pp. 406, 407–8 ("The people . . . are"), 409 ("The lateen sail"). Frederick Douglass, *Autobiographies* (New York: Library of America, 1994), pp. 1006 ("combat American prejudice"), 1007 ("half brothers").

3. Papers of William H. Seward, reel 58: Seward to Johnson, Sept. 28, 1859; "Governor Seward's Journey from Egypt to Palestine," *New York Daily Tribune*, Dec. 24, 1859, p. 5. Thornton Kirkland Lothrop, *William Henry Seward* (Boston: Houghton Mifflin, 1896), pp. 396–97. George E. Baker, ed., *The Life of William H. Seward with Selections from His Works* (New York: J. S. Redfield, 1855), p. 224 ("To the oppressed masses"). Frederic Bancroft, *The Life of William H. Seward*, vol. 2 (New York: Harpers, 1899), pp. 521–23. Walter LaFeber, *The Cambridge History of American Foreign Relations*, vol. 2, *The American Search for Opportunity, 1865–1913* (Cambridge: Cambridge Univ. Press, 1993), p. 10. *William H. Seward's Travels around the World*, pp. 525–32, 616 ("double thralldom"), 634–35 ("former chief minister"), 654–55 ("a remarkable rabbi"). USNA, RG 84, *Records of Foreign Service Posts. Cairo, Egypt*, vol. 78: Seward to Hale, Jan. 5, 1867. Olive Risley Seward, *Around the World Stories* (Boston: D. Lothrop, 1889), pp. 265–80, 281 ("It used to be"), 282 ("It is not enough), 283–86.

4. George B. McClellan, "A Winter on the Nile," *Scribner's Monthly* 13, no. 3 (Jan. 1877): 368–83; 13, no. 4 (March 1877): 670–77; "The Bombardment of Alexandria," *North American Review* 142, no. 355 (June 1886): 593 ("so long as we"), 594 ("little but life").

5. USNA, RG 59, Dispatches from U.S. Consuls, Cairo, Egypt, vol. 2: Beardsley to Fish, Jan. 22, 1872. William T. Sherman Family Papers, CSHR9/59: Sherman to Thomas Sherman, March 29, 1872 ("Their Faith in Mohamet" and "the most

repulsive"). Michael Fellman, *Citizen Sherman: A Life of William Tecumseh Sherman* (New York: Random House, 1995), p. 307 ("a hard-looking" and "undertake to move"). Morgan, *Recollections of a Rebel Reefer*, p. 266. Chaillé-Long, *My Life*, p. 231. *Memoirs of Rose Eytinge*, p. 201. J. C. Audenreid, "General Sherman in Europe and the East," *Harper's New Monthly Magazine* 47, no. 280 (Sept. 1873): 232, 234–35, 236, 240, 486–95.

6. USNA, RG 59, Dispatches from U.S. Consuls, Cairo, Egypt, vol. 5: Farman to Evarts, Feb. 12, 1878. *The Papers of Julia Dent Grant*, ed. John Simon (New York: Putnam, 1975), pp. 220 ("One might easily think"), 221 ("We had only to clap"), 222–23, 224 ("One could not but"). Vogel, *To See a Promised Land*, pp. 54–55 ("the most remarkable journey"). Young, *Around the World*, pp. 257 ("Welcome General Grant"), 299. Elbert Farman, *Along the Nile with General Grant* (New York: Grafton Press, 1904), pp. 26, 32–33, 92, 99. William McFeely, *Grant* (New York: Norton, 1981), pp. 466–67. Geoffrey Perret, *Ulysses S. Grant* (New York: Random House, 1997), p. 454 ("It looks as if" and "I have seen"). Dye, *Moslem Egypt*, p. 491. Wessels, *Born to Be a Soldier*, pp. 80–81 ("Why there's Loring"). Hesseltine and Wolf, *Blue and the Gray*, pp. 232–33 ("I wouldn't sit down").

7. *Papers of Julia Dent Grant*, p. 233 ("a gorgeous gleaming" and "a poor place"). Vogel, *To See a Promised Land*, p. 149. Young, *Around the World*, pp. 234–35, 329, 351. McFeely, *Grant*, p. 467. Perret, *Ulysses S. Grant*, p. 454. Steiner, *Religious Beliefs*, pp. 71–76. See also William N. Still, *American Sea Power in the Old World: The United States Navy in European and Near Eastern Waters, 1865–1917* (Westport, Conn.: Greenwood, 1980), p. 76.

8. References to "Cairo," "Turk," "Arab," and "Arabian Nights" in Twain's writing, can be located on *Mark Twain and His Times*, http://etext.lib.virginia.edu/railton/about/srchmtf.html. Mark Twain website, http://www.boondocksnet.com/twaintexts/letters/letter670607.html: Letter to Jane Clemens and Family, June 7, 1867 ("tired of staying"). "Mark Twain's Correspondence with the San Franciso *Alta California*," http://www.twainquotes.com/altaindex.html: April 9, 1867 ("Isn't it a most attractive"). Dayton Duncan and Geoffrey C. Ward, *Mark Twain: An Illustrated Biography* (New York: Knopf, 2001), pp. 10, 48 ("the necessary stock "), 54 ("permanently miserable"), 60–61. Mark Twain, *The Innocents Abroad; or, The New Pilgrims' Progress: Being Some Account of the Steamship Quaker City's Pleasure Excursion to Europe and the Holy Land* (Pleasantville, N.Y.: Reader's Digest Association, 1990), pp. 11 ("picnic on a gigantic," "scamper about the decks," and "green spectacles"), 17 ("The Synagogue"), 418 ("a funeral without"). Albert Bigelow Paine, *Mark Twain: A Biography: The Personal and Literary Life of Samuel Langhorne Clemens* (New York: Harper, 1912), pp. 324–31.

9. Twain, *Innocents Abroad*, pp. 51 ("Tangier is a foreign"), 52 ("The emperor of Morocco"), 53 ("Christian dogs"), 54 ("thinks he has five" and "They slice around"), 56, 419 ("strange horde"), 424 ("Travel is fatal").

10. Twain, *Innocents Abroad*, pp. 80–81 ("a short, stout"), 228 ("in all the outrageous"), 229 ("the three-legged woman"), 233, 239 ("nothing of romance"), 262

("The picture lacks"), 290–91 ("an island of pearls"), 284, 289–90 ("wretched nest"), 303 ("couldn't smile"), 351 ("To glance at").

11. Twain, *Innocents Abroad*, pp. 302 ("The gods of my"), 306, 311, 317 ("If all the poetry"), 319–20, 324, 332 ("frescoed . . . with disks"), 342, 358, 361, 385, 391. Paine, *Mark Twain*, pp. 333-36, 337 ("Is it any wonder"), 338, 394 ("hopeless, dreary"). Justin Kaplan, *Mr. Clemens and Mr. Twain* (New York: Simon & Schuster, 1966), p. 52.

12. USNA, RG 84, *Records of Foreign Service Posts. Cairo, Egypt*, vol. 78: William Seward to Charles Hale, Oct. 30, 1867. Twain, *Innocents Abroad*, pp. 397–98 ("shamefully humbugged"), 401 ("Palestine is no more"), 406 ("American vandals"). Mark Twain website, http://www.boondocksnet.com/twaintexts/letters/letter670607.html: Twain to the San Francisco *Alta California*, Jan. 8, 1868 ("Moorish haiks"). Paine, *Mark Twain*, p. 341 ("gospel of sincerity"). Kaplan, *Mr. Clemens and Mr. Twain*, p. 233. Obenzinger, *American Palestine*, pp. x ("right along with"), 188, 256.

13. "A Short History of the Shrine," http://www.shrinershq.org/shrine/short history.html. Eric Davis, "Representations of the Middle East at American World Fairs, 1876–1904," in Amanat and Bernhardsson, eds., *United States and the Middle East*, pp. 352–53, 354 ("the oldest people"), 355–58, 359 ("from Tangiers").

12. Resurgence

1. USNA, RG 59, Dispatches from U.S. Consuls, Damascus: Johnson to Seward, April 3, 1867 ("that Americans sympathize"); Governor General of Syria to Johnson, Oct. 3, 1868; Johnson to Seward, Oct. 10, 1868; Johnson to Seward, July 22, 1868; Johnson [L.] to Johnson [A], Oct. 31, 1868; Johnson to Seward, Nov. 12, 1868; Dillon to Johnson, Dec.19, 1868; Johnson to Seward, Dec. 31, 1868. *New York Times*, Dec. 7, 1880.

2. *FRUS*, 1880: Evarts to Fairchild, March 12, 1880, pp. 893–94. USNA, Dispatches from U.S. Consuls, Tangiers: Cohen to Mathews, May 5, 1880 ("It is to America"); Dispatches from U.S. Consuls, Jerusalem: Meizel, Alexander and Lipkin to deHass, May 3, 1877. Bryson, *American Diplomatic Relations*, pp. 29, 47. Brainerd Dyer, *The Public Career of William M. Evarts* (Berkeley: Univ. of California Press, 1933), pp. 217–18. Cyrus Adler, *Jews in the Diplomatic Correspondence of the United States* (Baltimore: Friedenwald, 1906), pp. 39–45. Ron Bartur, "American Consular Assistance to the Jewish Community of the Land of Israel at the End of the Ottoman Period to the Outbreak of World War I, 1856–1914 [Hebrew]" (Hebrew Univ., 1984), p. 364 ("The stars and stripes").

3. David Harris, *Britain and the Bulgarian Horrors of 1876* (Chicago: Univ. of Chicago Press, 1939), p. 410 ("In Paniguischte"). *New York Times*, Sept. 9, 1876 ("the remains of babes"). Field, *America and the Mediterranean World*, pp. 365–72. Bryson, *American Diplomatic Relations*, pp. 29–30. Sir Edwin Pears, *Forty Years in Constantinople*, 1873–1915 (New York: Appleton, 1916), pp. 16–18.

4. Palmer, *Guardians of the Gulf*, p. 311 ("There is no place"). Field, *America and the Mediterranean World*, p. 312 ("now gets its"). Jonathan Grant, "The Sword of the Sultan: Ottoman Arms Imports, 1854–1914," *Journal of Military History* 66 (Jan. 2002), pp. 9–36. John Dunn, "Egypt's Nineteenth-Century Armaments Industry," *Journal of Military History* 61 (April 1997), pp. 231–54. Jeffrey D. Wert, *General James Longstreet* (New York: Simon and Schuster, 1993), p. 419. Marty H. Krout, ed., *Lew Wallace: An Autobiography* (New York: Harper, 1906), pp. 962–63. See also "Meet Lew Wallace: American Minister to Turkey, 1881–1885," on http://www.ben-hur.com/meet_ambassador.html.

5. *FRUS*, 1877: Mr. Maynard to Mr. Evarts, Nov. 26, 1877, p. 141; 1878, Mr. Heap to Mr. Hunter, Jan. 25, 1878, pp. 929–31; 1879: Farman to Evarts, May 22, 1879, p. 1003 ("long remain"); Message of the President, Dec. 1, 1879, p. xiv ("a generous mark"); 1880, Farman to Evarts, May 5, 1880, pp. 1108–12. Elbert Eli Farman, "Negotiating for the Obelisk," *Century Illustrated Monthly Magazine* 24 (Oct. 1882): 882–83 ("The population," "another souvenir," and "It is not for"). Elbert Farman, *Egypt and Its Betrayal* (New York: Grafton Press, 1908), pp. 148–49, 166. Seaton Schroeder, *Fifty Years of Naval Service* (New York: Appleton, 1922), pp. 133–36, 140–43. Labib Habachi, *The Obelisks of Egypt* (Cairo: American Univ. in Cairo Press, 1984), pp. 176–78, 181–82. Bob Brier, "Saga of Cleopatra's Needles," *Archaeology* 55, no. 6 (Nov.–Dec. 2002): 48–51. Martina D'Alton, *The New York Obelisk* (New York: Metropolitan Museum of Art, 1993), pp. 2, 11 ("point the finger" and "It would be absurd"), 16–21, 63. James Field, "Near East Notes and Far East Queries," in John Fairbank, ed., *The Missionary Enterprise in China and America* (Cambridge: Harvard Univ. Press, 1974).

13. Empires at Dawn

1. Conn, "John Porter Brown," pp. 10–11. USNA, RG 59, Dispatches from U.S. Consuls, Algiers, Algeria: Lee to French Consul, Feb. 20, 1830 ("the Frenchman"); Lee to Van Buren, July 15, 1830; Porter to Van Buren, Sept. 22, 1830. Haight, *Letters from the Old World*, pp. 260, 262. *FRUS*, 1882: Wallace to Frelinghuysen, Feb. 1, 1882, p. 501. Akira Iriye, *From Nationalism to Internationalism: U.S. Foreign Policy to 1914* (London: Routledge and Kegan Paul, 1977), p. 65 ("we cannot follow"). Potts, "National Boasting," *New York Times*, Nov. 26, 1852. E. J. Hobsbawm, *The Age of Empire, 1875–1914* (New York: Pantheon, 1987), p. 59.

2. USNA, RG 59; Dispatches from U.S. Consuls, Tunis: Fish to Hunter, April 22, 1881 ("It looks as though"); Fish to Hunter, May 5, 1881 ("In plain Anglo-Saxon"). David M. Pletcher, *The Awkward Years: American Foreign Relations under Garfield and Arthur* (Columbia: Univ. of Missouri Press, 1962), pp. 224–25 ("Civilization gains"). General Lewal, "The French Army," *Harper's New Monthly Magazine* 82, no. 491 (April 1891): 657.

3. USNA, RG 59, Dispatches from U.S. Consuls, Cairo, Egypt: Beardsley to Page, April 24, 1874; Beardsley to Fish, Dec. 11, 1875. Wright, *United States Policy toward Egypt*, pp. 92, 108–9 ("What folly"), 120, 123. Adam Badeau, "The Bom-

bardment of Alexandria," *North American Review* 142, no. 355 (June 1886): 592.
"American Trade Opportunities in Egypt Destroyed," *Los Angeles Times,* July 26,
1882, p. 2 ("shameful act"). "A Mohammedan Revival," *New York Times,* Sept.
22, 1881, p. 4 ("fanatic . . . Arabs "); "The Conquest of Egypt," Sept. 15, 1882, p.
4 ("everlasting shame"); "The Bondage of Egypt," Feb. 6, 1882, p. 4 ("taxation
without representation").

4. Chaillé-Long, *My Life,* pp. 245–48, 251, 259 ("In the sea"), 271 ("Men,
women"), 302–3 ("We dominate"), 307 ("the Americans . . . who"). Still, *American Sea Power,* pp. 83–84, 85 ("I corralled"), 86–87. Frederick J. Cox, "Arabi and
Stone: Egypt's Military Rebellion, 1882," *Cahiers d'Histoire Egyptienne* 8 (April
1956): 173–74. *Messages and Papers of the Presidents, 1789–1897,* vol. 8, ed.
James D. Richardson (New York: Bureau of National Literature, 1917): Second
Annual Address of Chester Arthur to Congress, Dec. 4, 1882, p. 126. *FRUS,* 1882:
Sackville West to Frederick T. Frelinghuysen, Sept. 17, 1882, p. 325 ("sailors and
marines").

5. Farman, *Egypt and Its Betrayal,* pp. 286 ("evil genius"), 289 ("Shylock"), 290
("aggressive European Powers"), 302 ("He was the idol"), 303 ("instigated by").
Egyptian State Information Service, "Orabi Pasha," http://216.239.41
.104/search?q=cache:O8sDNNWobzsJ:www.sis.gov.eg/calendar/html/c1310397.htm
+orabi&hl=en&start=2. For a reference to the Arabic roots of the name "'Urabi,"
see Hans Wehr, *A Dictionary of Modern Written Arabic* (Beirut: Librairie du Liban,
1980), p. 601.

6. USNA, RG 59, Dispatches from U.S. Consuls, Cairo: Wolf to Blaine, Sept. 12,
1881 ("act cautiously"); Wolf to Blaine, Sept. 15, 1881 ("Here on this"); Wolf to
Blaine, Oct. 29, 1881 ("the natives and owners"); Wolf to Blaine, Nov. 11, 1881
("in no way"); Urabi to Wolf (n.d.) ("management and wisdom"); Wolf to Frelinghuysen, March 21, 1882 ("There is scarcely"). Esther L. Panitz, *Simon Wolf: Private Conscience and Public Image* (Rutherford: Fairleigh Dickinson Univ. Press,
1987), pp. 71–78. *Selected Addresses and Papers of Simon Wolf* (New York: Bloch,
1926), pp. 15–16. Simon Wolf, *The Presidents I Have Known from 1860–1918*
(Washington, D.C.: Byron S. Adams, 1918), pp. 124–30.

7. Cox, "Arabi and Stone," pp. 155–58. Charles P. Stone, "Stone Pacha and the
Secret Dispatch," *Journal of the Military Service Institution of the United States* 8,
no. 29 (March 1887): 95. Fanny Stone, "The Diary of an American Girl in Cairo
during the War of 1882," *Century Illustrated Monthly Magazine* 28, no. 2 (June
1883): 29 ("quietly eating"), 43 ("death to the Christians"), 38 ("There never
lived"), 34 ("be brave"), 45 ("For once"). Crabitès, *Americans in the Egyptian
Army,* p. 263. USNA, RG 59, Dispatches from U.S. Consuls, Cairo: Gomanos to
Frelinghuysen, July 23, 1882.

8. Chaillé-Long, *My Life,* pp. 139 ("Egypt for the Egyptians"), 201 ("a very bad
soldier"). Farman, *Egypt and Its Betrayal,* p. 333 ("Tel el-Kebir"). USNA, RG 59,
Dispatches from U.S. Consuls, Cairo: Wolf to Blaine, Oct. 29, 1881 ("The cup is
full"). Later in life, Wolf seems to have altered his opinion of the British administra-

tion in Egypt, crediting it with bringing it into "new light." See Wolf, *Presidents I Have Known*, p. 134.

9. Cox, "Arabi and Stone," p. 158 ("Egypt had become"). Bernard A. Weisberger, *Statue of Liberty: The First Hundred Years* (Boston: Houghton Mifflin, 1985), pp. 22–23 ("Granite beings"), 24–25, 33. Willadene Price, *Bartholdi and the Statue of Liberty* (Chicago: Rand McNally, 1959), pp. 27–29, 42–45, 63–65, 119–20. Marvin Trachtenberg, *The Statue of Liberty* (New York: Penguin, 1986), pp. 46, 53–54, 57. Grabill, *Protestant Diplomacy*, p. 56 ("When will you turn").

10. On the use of the Middle East model by American imperialists in the Far East, see Field, "Near East Notes," pp. 24 ("The Muslim societies"), 25–27. Field also makes the remarkable observation (p. 41) that "all the countries in which women have recently exercised significant political power—Israel, India, Ceylon, and China—were nineteenth-century targets of American missionary endeavor." Mark Twain, "An Anti-Imperialist," *New York Herald,* Oct. 15, 1900.

14. Imperial Piety

1. Eve Merriam, *The Voice of Liberty: The Story of Emma Lazarus* (New York: Farrar, Straus and Cudahy, 1959), pp. 140–41. Mark A. Raider, *The Emergence of American Zionism* (New York: New York Univ. Press, 1998), pp. 12 ("We consider ourselves"), 70–71 ("Wake, Israel"). Bette Roth Young, "Emma Lazarus and Her Jewish Problem," *American Jewish History* 84 (Dec. 1996): 299 ("opens up such"), 309 ("a home for" and "artisans, warriors"). Martin Feinstein, *American Zionism, 1884–1904* (New York: Herzl Press, 1965), pp. 18, 58–59. Emma Lazarus, "Epistle to the Hebrews," *American Hebrew* 13 (Feb. 2, 1883): 137; "The Jewish Problem," *Century Illustrated Monthly Magazine* 36, no. 6 (Feb. 1883). Daniel Marom, "Who Is the 'Mother of Exiles'?: Jewish Aspects of Emma Lazarus's *The New Colossus,*" *Prooftexts* 20, no. 3 (2000): 250 ("renew their youth"). Abram S. Isaacs, "Will the Jews Return to Palestine," *Century* 26, no. 1 (May 1883). See also Ranen Omer-Sherman, "Emma Lazarus, Jewish American Poetics, and the Challenge of Modernity," *Journal of American Women Writers* 19 (2003). Gregory Eiselein, "Emotion and the Jewish Historical Poems of Emma Lazarus," *Mosaic* 37 (2004). Arthur Zeiger, "Emma Lazarus and Pre-Herzlian Zionism," in Shulamit Reinharz and Mark A. Raider, eds., *American Jewish Women and the Zionist Enterprise* (Waltham, Mass.: Brandeis Univ. Press, 2004), pp. 13–17.

2. T. De Witt Talmage, *Talmage on Palestine* (New York: W. D. Rowland, 1890), pp. 7, 10 ("that curse of nations"), 24 ("All the fingers" and "They would be foolish"). John Rusk, *The Authentic Life of T. DeWitt Talmage* (New York: L. G. Stahl, 1902), pp. 79–82, 104, 125–26. Handy, *Holy Land*, pp. 125–28. See also T. De Witt Talmage, *New Tabernacle Sermons* (New York: George Munro, 1886).

3. William E. Blackstone, *Jesus Is Coming* (Chicago: Revell, 1908), pp. 240–41. Paul Charles Merkley, *The Politics of Christian Zionism, 1891–1948* (London: Frank Cass, 1998), pp. 60–63, 69–71. Obenzinger, *American Palestine*, pp. 268–69.

Vogel, *To See a Promised Land*, pp. 228–29. The full text of the Blackstone Memorial can be found in Joseph Celleni, ed., *Christian Protagonists for Jewish Restoration* (New York: Arno Press, 1977), pp. 13–14.

4. In his first State of the Union Address, in 1885, Grover Cleveland assailed the Porte for its attempts to impose "religious tests as a condition of residence [in Palestine]," but otherwise refrained from endorsing the Jewish state idea. See *Messages and Papers of the Presidents: 1789–1897*, vol. 8 (Washington, D.C.: GPO, 1898), p. 335. *FRUS*, 1882: Wallace to Said Pasha, June 3, 1882, p. 508; Ascher and Weinberg to Wallace, June 13, 1882, pp. 517–18; 1885: Bayard to Cox, Oct. 15, 1885, p. 871; 1888: Straus to Said Pasha, May 17, 1888, p. 1589 ("inquisitorial"); Rives to Gilman, Oct. 12, 1888, p. 1618; 1898: Straus to Hay, Nov. 22, 1898, p. 1092. Merle Curti, *American Philanthropy Abroad* (New Brunswick: Rutgers Univ. Press, 1963), p. 108. Jacob M. Landau and Kemal Mim Oke, "Ottoman Perspectives on American Interests in the Holy Land," in Davis, *With Eyes toward Zion*, vol. 2, pp. 269–72. Cyrus Adler, *Jacob H. Schiff: His Life and Letters*, vol. 2 (London: William Heinemann, 1929), pp. 162–63. Naomi Wiener Cohen, *A Dual Heritage: The Public Career of Oscar S. Straus* (Philadelphia: Jewish Publication Society of America, 1969), pp. 88–89, 171, 283. Regina S. Sharif, *Non-Jewish Zionism: Its Roots in Western History* (London: Zed Press, 1983), pp. 92–93.

5. Bertha Spafford Vester, *Our Jerusalem: An American Family in the Holy City* (1950; reprint, New York: Arno Press, 1977), pp. 56–57, 63 ("American-made"), 98 ("He taught me"), 134, 158. Vogel, *To See a Promised Land,* pp. 114 ("post-Protestant period"), 152–53 ("When sorrows"), 155 ("hoping to be").

6. Supporters of the American Colony were also instrumental in securing the recall of Merrill's successor, Edwin S. Wallace. Wallace accused Mrs. Spafford of holding "such power over her victims as to make them swear to be true what they know to be false," and of "doing much harm to injure the good name of America in this part of the world." See USNA, RG 59, Dispatches from U.S. Consuls. Jerusalem: Wallace to Cridler, Dec. 7, 1897; Merrill to Wharton; Oct. 3, 1891 ("one of the wildest"); Merrill to Quincy, Aug. 17, 1893; Merrill to Cridler, Jan. 30, 1899; Merrill to Cridler, July 8, 1901 ("They hate the United"). Shalom Goldman, "The Holy Land Appropriated: The Careers of Selah Merrill, Nineteenth Century Christian Hebraist, Palestine Explorer, and U.S. Consul in Jerusalem," *American Jewish History* 85, no. 2 (June 1997): 152–67. Ruth Kark, "Annual Reports," pp. 173–74. Alexander Fume Ford, "Our American Colony at Jerusalem," *Appleton's Magazine* 8 (1906): 643–55.

7. Carl Dolmetsch, *"Our Famous Guest"—Mark Twain in Vienna* (Athens: Univ. of Georgia Press, 1992), pp. 45, 128–31, 25, 270. Cynthia Ozick, "Mark Twain and the Jews," *Commentary* 99, no. 5 (May 1995): 56–62. Theodore Herzl, "Mark Twain and the British Ladies: A Feuilleton," *Commentary* 28, no. 3 (Sept. 1959): 243–44 ("a short, spare"). Twain, *Innocents Abroad*, p. 324. Amos Elon, *Herzl* (New York: Holt, Rinehart and Winston, 1975), pp. 66, 245. Obenzinger, *American Palestine*, pp. 266 ("The difference between the brain"), 267–68 ("If that con-

centration"). "Concerning the Jews" first appeared in *Harper's New Monthly Mazagine* in Sept. 1899; see also Charles Neider, ed., *The Complete Essays of Mark Twain* (Garden City, N.Y.: Doubleday, 1963), pp. 235–50, and Dan Vogel, *Mark Twain's Jews* (Jersey City, N.J.: KTAV Publishing House, 2006), pp. 61–88.

8. USNA, RG 59, Dispatches from U.S. Consuls, Cairo: Wolf to Frelinghuysen, March 25, 1882. Field, *America and the Mediterranean World*, p. 350. Tibawi, *American Interests in Syria*, pp. 249–50, 275. DeNovo, *American Interests*, pp. 9, 13–14, 18, 31. Kaplan, *Arabists*, pp. 39–40. Grabill, *Protestant Diplomacy*, p. 21. Wright, *United States Policy toward Egypt*, p. 229 ("Americans occupy Egypt").

9. American diplomatic records are rife with correspondence describing assaults on, and even the murder of, missionaries. See, e.g., *FRUS*, 1901: Negotiations for the Settlement of Indemnity Claims of United States Citizens, Hay to Straus, Jan. 11, 1900, p. 906. Laurie, *Ely Volume*, pp. 84, 457. Cagri Erhan, "Ottoman Official Attitudes towards American Missionaries" in Amanat and Bernhardsson, eds., *United States and the Middle East*, pp. 317–19. Vogel, *To See a Promised Land*, pp. 116–17. Tibawi, *American Interests in Syria*, pp. 237, 269 ("In the war"), 275, 280. DeNovo, *American Interests*, pp. 12, 35 ("No man ever came"), 42. Wright, *United States Policy toward Egypt*, p. 331. Field, *America and the Mediterranean World*, p. 437. Grabill, *Protestant Diplomacy*, pp. 30–31 ("modern missionaries").

10. J. Christy Wilson, *Apostle to Islam: A Biography of Samuel M. Zwemer* (Grand Rapids, Mich.: Baker Book House, 1952), pp. 40–44, 72–73. Henry Harris Jessup, *The Setting of the Crescent and the Rising of the Cross; or, Kamil Abdul Messiah, a Syrian Convert from Islam to Christianity* (Philadelphia: Westminster Press, 1898), pp. 51–53, 65, 72, 127, 137–39, 143. Alfred DeWitt Mason and Frederick J. Barny, *History of the Arabian Mission* (New York: Board of Foreign Missions Reformed Church in America, 1926), pp. 76–77, 86 ("very heart of Islam"), 90–91. Samuel Zwemer and James Cantine, *The Golden Milestone: Reminiscences of Pioneer Days Fifty Years Ago in Arabia* (New York: Revell, 1938), pp. 18–19, 30, 43, 92, 135. A. E. Zwemer and S. M. Zwemer, *Zigzag Journeys in the Camel Country: Arabia in Picture and Story* (New York: Revell, 1911), pp. 27, 31 ("Pioneer journeys"), 50, 92, 103 ("A country [without]"). Paul W. Harrison, *Doctor in Arabia* (London: Robert Hale, 1943), p. 264. Stuart Knee, "Anglo-American Relations in Palestine, 1919–1925: An Experiment in Realpolitik," *Journal of American Studies of Turkey* 5 (1997): 5 ("American religious-philanthropic").

11. Josiah Strong, *Our Country: Its Possible Future and Its Present Crisis* (New York: American Home Mission Society, 1885), pp. 218–19. USNA, RG 59, Diplomatic Instructions of the Department of State, Persia: Bayard to Pratt, Aug. 23, 1887; Bayard to Pratt, July 7, 1886. *FRUS*, 1881: Foster to Blaine, May 21, 1881, pp. 1016–17; Vol. XLII, 1883: Benjamin to Felinghuysen, June 13, 1883, pp. 703–6 ("the most brilliant"); 1886, Pratt to Bayard, Nov. 29, 1886, p. 913 ("iron, coal, copper"); 1887: Pratt to Bayard, May 4, 1887, pp. 916–17. Bryson, *American Diplomatic Relations*, pp. 39–40. Abraham Yeselson, *United States–Persia Diplomatic Relations, 1883–1921* (New Brunswick: Rutgers Univ. Press, 1956), pp.

23–25. Palmer, *Guardians of the Gulf*, pp. 6–9. DeNovo, *American Interests*, pp. 296–97. Michael Zirinsky, "American Presbyterian Missionaries at Urmia during the Great War," *Journal of Assyrian Academic Studies* 12, no. 1 (April 1998): 8–11.

12. Field, "Near East Notes," pp. 51, 54. Still, *American Sea Power*, pp. 79 ("The wayward Turks"), 103–4 ("Even the head").

13. USNA, RG 59, Dispatches from the U.S. Consuls, Erzerum: Chilton to Use, Oct. 9, 1895. *New York Times*, Dec. 28, 1894 ("if not by"). Peter Balakian, *The Burning Tigris: The Armenian Genocide and America's Response* (New York: HarperCollins, 2003), pp. 11 ("Armenian Holocaust"), 23, 64, 73, 93. Arman Kirakossian, ed., *The Armenian Massacres, 1894–1896: U.S. Media Testimony* (Detroit: Wayne State Univ. Press, 2004), pp. 37 ("blot upon civilization"), 47 ("Not all the perfume"). Grabill, *Protestant Diplomacy*, p. 43 ("the demon of damnable"). Clyde E. Buckingham, *Clara Barton: A Broad Humanity* (Alexandria, Va.: Mount Vernon Publishing, 1977), p. 262 ("the warships").

14. Angell later served as president of the University of Michigan, where an impressive hall still bears his name. *FRUS*, 1900: Griscom to Hay, Dec. 12, 1900, p. 515. USNA, RG 59, Dispatches from U.S. Consuls, Constantinople: Judson Smith to Olney, Nov. 19, 1895; Olney to Terrill; Jan. 16, 1896. Frederick Davis Greene, *Armenian Massacres; or, The Sword of Mohammed* (Philadelphia: National Publishers Co., 1896), p. xvii ("The policy of the United"). Grabill, *Protestant Diplomacy*, pp. 41–44, 45 ("rattle the Sultan's"). Kirakossian, *Armenian Massacres*, p. 71 ("Yankees of the Orient"). Erhan, "Ottoman Official Attitudes," p. 332. Still, *American Sea Power*, pp. 99–100, 105–6, 107. George Washburn, *Fifty Years in Constantinople* (Boston: Houghton Mifflin, 1909), pp. 246–49. Washburn relates how one American sailor, an African American whom the Turks mistook for a Muslim, succeeded in saving large numbers of Armenians.

15. Buckingham, *Clara Barton*, pp. 260–62. David H. Burton, *Clara Barton: In the Service of Humanity* (Westport, Conn.: Greenwood, 1995), pp. 128–30. Curti, *American Philanthropy Abroad*, pp. 124, 127 ("I shall never counsel"). Balakian, *Burning Tigris*, pp. 10, 62–65, 69–70. Kirakossian, *Armenian Massacres*, pp. 42–43. "Profiles in Caring: Clara Barton," http://www.nahc.org/NAHC/Val/Columns/SC10-1.html ("perhaps the most perfect"). McDougall, *Promised Land*, pp. 104–5.

15. Imperial Myths

1. Clarence Clough Buel, "Preliminary Glimpses of the Fair," *Century Illustrated Monthly Magazine* 45, no. 4 (Feb. 1893): 615. Davis, "Representations of the Middle East, 1876–1904," pp. 344–48, 370. Erik Larson, *The Devil in the White City: Murder, Magic, and Madness at the Fair That Changed America* (New York: Vintage, 2003), pp. 247–48, 250–51, 265–67.

2. *The Autobiography of Sol Bloom* (New York: Putnam, 1948), pp. 106 ("I came to realize"), 107–8 (I knew that"), 119 ("To have made"). Donna Carlton,

Looking for Little Egypt (Bloomington, Ind.: IDD Books, 1994), p. 27. A superb description of the Middle Eastern exhibitions at the Paris fair can be found in Timothy Mitchell's *Colonising Egypt* (Berkeley: Univ. of California Press, 1988), p. 1.

3. "The World's Columbian Exposition: Idea, Experience, Aftermath," http://xroads.virginia.edu/~MA96/WCE/title.html ("the strange music"). Mark Stevens, *Six Months at the World's Fair* (Detroit: Detroit Free Press, 1895), pp. 101, 103 ("Cairo was strikingly"). Larkin, *Devil in the White City*, p. 236. Gustav Kobbe, "Sights at the Fair," *Century Illustrated Monthly Magazine* 46, no. 6 (Sept. 1893): 653 ("The Midway Plaisance"). Carlton, *Looking for Little Egypt*, pp. 27, 35, 39 ("Such a jaunt"). Norman Bolotin and Christine Laing, *The World's Columbian Exposition* (Urbana: Univ. of Illinois Press, 2002), p. 139. Robert Muccigrosso, *Celebrating the New World: Chicago's Columbian Exposition of 1893* (Chicago: Ivan R. Dee, 1993), p. 164. David Burg, *Chicago's White City of 1893* (Lexington: Univ. Press of Kentucky, 1976), pp. 105, 221.

4. The cost of riding camels was twice that of riding donkeys—twenty-five cents. A quarter also gained admission to the Moorish Palace, the Persian Tent, the Turkish Pavilion, and the Bedouin encampment. See Bolotin and Laing, *World's Columbian Exposition*, p. 107. Stevens, *Six Months*, p. 102 ("This high art dancing"). Burg, *Chicago's White City*, pp. 221 ("splendid specimens"), 222 ("It is the coarse" and "Every motion"), 223 ("Now she revolves"). Carlton, *Looking for Little Egypt*, p. 23. Muccigrosso, *Celebrating the New World*, pp. 165, 166 ("genuine native muscle" and "a peaceful night's rest"), 167 ("simply horrid"). Larkin, *Devil in the White City*, pp. 311–12 ("whether the apprehensions").

5. Daniel Burnham, ed., *Final Official Report of the Director of Works of the World's Columbian Exposition* (New York: Garland, 1989), p. 40. "None Can Compare with It," *New York Times*, June 19, 1893, p. 5 ("The denizens"). Mrs. Mark Stevens, *A Lecture on What You Missed in Not Visiting the World's Fair* (Flint: n.p., 1895), p. 6 ("New Jerusalem"). Buel, "Preliminary Glimpses," p. 626 ("Haroun al-Raschid"). Muccigrosso, *Celebrating the New World*, pp. 167–68 ("We were all knocked"). *Autobiography of Sol Bloom*, pp. 122–23, 135 ("The crowds poured in" and "a masterpiece of rhythm"), 136. Burg, *Chicago's White City*, p. 223.

6. Blackstone's proposal for an international arbitrating organization, circulated at the 1893 fair, can be found in the William Blackstone Papers, collection 540, box 7, folder 1. Turner, *Frontier in American History*, p. 37.

16. A Region Renamed and Reordered

1. A. T. Mahan, *Retrospect and Prospect* (Boston: Little, Brown, 1902), pp. 233, 237, 243. A. T. Mahan, *The Problem of Asia* (Boston: Little, Brown, 1900), pp. 80–81, 83 ("the neck of land"). Numerous studies exist on the Mahan's naval theories in general and on his concept of the Middle East in particular. See, e.g., Roderic H. Davison, "Where Is the Middle East?" in Richard H. Nolte, ed., *The Modern Middle East* (New York: Atherton Press, 1963), pp. 15–17. Marwan R.

Buheiry, "Alfred T. Mahan: Reflections on Sea Power and on the Middle East as a Strategic Concept," in Lawrence I. Conrad, ed., *The Formation and Perception of the Modern Arab World* (Princeton: Darwin Press, 1990), pp. 157–62. W. D. Pulson, *The Life and Work of Captain Alfred Thayer Mahan* (New Haven: Yale Univ. Press, 1939), pp. 41–42.

2. Fareed Zakaria, *From Wealth to Power: The Unusual Origins of America's World Role* (Princeton: Princeton Univ. Press, 1996), pp. 46, 127. Walter Zimmerman, *First Great Triumph: How Five Americans Made Their Country a World Power* (New York: Farrar, Straus and Giroux, 2002), pp. 24–25, 30–31, 34–37. Walter LaFeber, *The New Empire: An Interpretation of American Expansion, 1860–1898* (Ithaca: Cornell Univ. Press, 1998), pp. 99, 105. Ernest May, *Imperial Democracy: The Emergence of America as a Great Power* (Chicago: Imprint Publications, 1961), p. 6.

3. Camel cigarettes first appeared in 1913, with a logo inspired by "Old Joe," a camel in the Barnum and Bailey Circus. Other "Middle Eastern" brands soon appeared, with names like Aga, Kismet, and Osman. See Nance, "Crossing Over," pp. 98–102. DeNovo, *American Interests*, pp. 16–22, 39–40. Wright, *United States Policy toward Egypt*, pp. 206–7. Turgay, "Ottoman-American Trade," p. 234 ("The newspapers"). Field, *America and the Mediterranean World*, pp. 327, 338. *The Complete Plays of Bernard Shaw* (London: Constable Press, 1931), pp. 320 ("As the search"), 323 ("The world").

4. *Theodore Roosevelt's Diaries of Boyhood and Youth* (New York: Scribner, 1928), pp. 227 ("I *felt* a great deal"), ("what we should call"), 276 ("How I gazed"), 278-79 ("the Arabs always talk"), 290, 304 ("a glimpse of"), 314-319. Theodore Roosevelt, *An Autobiography* (New York: Da Capo Press, 1985), pp. 20, 398–99, 548 ("so utterly incompetent"), 550, 561 ("dreadful scourge"). Nathan Miller, *Theodore Roosevelt: A Life* (New York: Quill Books, 1992), p. 54. Edmund Morris, *The Rise of Theodore Roosevelt* (New York: Modern Library, 2001), pp. 37, 40–41. Grabill, *Protestant Diplomacy*, p. 45 ("Spain and Turkey"). Steiner, *Religious Beliefs*, pp. 152–56. John Milton Cooper, *The Warrior and the Priest: Woodrow Wilson and Theodore Roosevelt* (Cambridge: Harvard Univ. Press, 1983), pp. 71–72 ("barbarous and semi-barbarous").

5. *FRUS*, 1901, vol. 4: Leishman to Hay, Sept. 5, 1901, p. 997; Lazzaro to Dickinson, Sept. 5, 1901, p. 998 ("dressed like Turks"); Stone to Peet, Sept. 20, 1901, p. 1006; Eddy to Hay, Dec. 13 1901; Leishman to Hay, March 1, 1902. Teresa Carpenter, *The Miss Stone Affair: America's First Modern Hostage Crisis* (New York: Simon & Schuster, 2003), pp. 30–31 ("Women have no earthly"), 32–35, 56–57, 94–96, 140–42.

6. USNA, RG 59, Dispatches from U.S. Consuls, Constantinople: Leishman to Hay, Sept. 10, 1903. "Unspeakable Turk to Be Called Upon to Settle for the Murder of American Vice-Consul," *Los Angeles Times*, Aug. 28, 1903. "Turkish Minister to Confer with Hay," *New York Times*, Aug. 30, 1903 ("We have allowed"). Still, *American Sea Power*, p. 159. Erhan, "Ottoman Official Attitudes," p. 332.

7. USNA, RG 59, Dispatches from U.S. Consuls. Tangier: Gummere to Hay, May 19, 1904 ("most prominent American"); Gummere to Hay, May 20, 1904; Gummere to Hay, June 15, 1904. *FRUS*, 1904: Hay to Gummere, June 9, 1904, pp. 498–99 ("Anything which may be regarded"). Edmund Morris, *Theodore Rex* (New York: HarperCollins, 2003), pp. 323, 324 ("all we hold sacred"), 329 ("PRESIDENT WISHES"), 325–26, 327 ("I had much rather"), 335 ("WE WANT PEDICARIS"), 337–38 ("that flag"). Baepler, *White Slaves*, pp. 291–97, 301 ("one of the most"). Peter Larsen, "Theodore Roosevelt and the Moroccan Crisis, 1904–1906" (Ph.D. diss., Princeton Univ., 1984), pp. 1, 21–22 ("surrender to the demands"), 40–41, 64, 66.

8. *FRUS*, 1906: International Diplomatic Conference at Algeciras: White to the Secretary of State, Jan. 30, 1906, pp. 1471–72. *The Letters of Theodore Roosevelt*, ed. Elting Morison (Cambridge: Harvard Univ. Press, 1954): Roosevelt to Whitelaw Reid, June 27, 1906, pp. 318–19; Roosevelt to Joseph Cannon, Sept. 12, 1904, pp. 923–24 ("Do they object"). *Selections from the Correspondence of Theodore Roosevelt and Henry Cabot Lodge, 1884–1918* (New York: Scribner, 1925): Roosevelt to Lodge, July 11, 1905, p. 166. USNA, RG 59, Special Missions: Root to White, March 2, 1906 ("side with either"). Frederick W. Marks, *Velvet on Iron: The Diplomacy of Theodore Roosevelt* (Lincoln: Univ. of Nebraska Press, 1979), p. 69. Howard K. Beale, *Theodore Roosevelt and the Rise of America to World Power* (Baltimore: Johns Hopkins Univ. Press, 1986), pp. 356–62, 366, 370–74, 377–78, 381–88. Raymond A. Esthus, *Theodore Roosevelt and the International Rivalries* (Claremont: Regina Books, 1970), pp. 70–79, 83–89, 104–9, 111 ("It would be enormously").

9. Franklin Matthews, *Back to Hampton Roads* (New York: B. W. Huebsch, 1909), pp. 282–83, 287–89, 290 ("We gave Cairo"). Roman J. Miller, *Around the World with the Battleships* (Chicago: A. C. McClurg, 1909), pp. 301–6, 308 ("About us swarmed"), 309, 315, 324–25. James A. Reckner, *Teddy Roosevelt's Great White Fleet* (Annapolis: Naval Institute Press, 1988), pp. 146–47. Robert A. Hart, *The Great White Fleet* (Boston: Little, Brown, 1965), pp. 272–74.

10. *Letters of Theodore Roosevelt*: Roosevelt to George Otto Trevelyan, Oct. 11, 1910, pp. 349–51. Wright, *United States Policy toward Egypt*, pp. 168–69. Vatikiotis, *History of Egypt*, pp. 203–4. David H. Burton, *Theodore Roosevelt: Confident Imperialist* (Philadelphia: Univ. of Pennsylvania Press, 1968), pp. 180–85, 191 ("I should have things"). Sheikh Ali Yousuff, "Egypt's Reply to Colonel Roosevelt," *North American Review* 191 (June 1910): 732–33, 755 ("Down with Roosevelt"), 737 ("when Egypt is").

11. Walter Scholes and Marie Scholes, *The Foreign Policies of the Taft Administration* (Columbia: Univ. of Missouri Press, 1970), pp. 30–31. Thomas Bentley Mott, *Twenty Years as Military Attaché* (1937, reprint, New York: Arno Press, 1979), pp. 171–74. DeNovo, *American Interests*, pp. 46–49, 52 ("an attitude"), 53 ("the veriest folly"), 76. Grose, *Israel in the Mind*, pp. 59–60. Robert A. McDaniel, *The Shuster Mission and the Persian Constitutional Revolution* (Minneapolis: Bibliotheca Islamica, 1974), pp. 115, 124–26, 134, 160–61, 170, 198 ("a monumental error").

17. Spectators of Catastrophe

1. Philip Roth, *The Plot against America* (Boston: Houghton Mifflin, 2004), p. 114. David Fromkin, *A Peace to End All Peace: The Fall of the Ottoman Empire and the Creation of the Modern Middle East* (New York: Avon, 1989), p. 534. Kinross, *Ottoman Centuries*, pp. 566–609. Stephen Hemsley Longrigg, *Oil in the Middle East: Its Discovery and Development* (London: Oxford Univ. Press, 1954), p. 25. Helen Davenport Gibbons, *The Red Rugs of Tarsus: A Woman's Record of the Armenian Massacre of 1909* (New York: Century, 1917), pp. 170 ("The only difference"), 179.

2. Grabill, *Protestant Diplomacy*, p. 38. DeNovo, *American Interests*, pp. 38, 96. *FRUS*, 1914, Supplement: Bryan to Morgenthau, Oct. 5, 1914, p. 9 ("I am much gratified").

3. *FRUS*, 1914, Supplement: Morgenthau to Bryan, Aug. 19, 1914, p. 758; Morgenthau to Bryan, Aug. 25, 1914, p. 75; Bryan to Morgenthau, Aug. 26, 1914, p. 77 ("in the interest").

4. *FRUS*, 1914, Supplement: Morgenthau to Bryan, Aug. 15, 1914, p. 66 ("grave immediate necessity"); Morgenthau to Bryan, Aug. 19, 1914, p. 758 ("reign of military terrorism"); Morgenthau to Bryan, Nov. 7, 1914, p. 139 ("never doubted"); Morgenthau to Bryan, Nov. 8, 1914, p. 781 ("For each Mussulman"); Lansing to Morgenthau, Nov. 18, 1914, p. 771 ("Should organized massacres"); Lansing to Morgenthau, Nov. 20, 1914, p. 771 ("any loss of life"); Bryan to Morgenthau, Dec. 20, 1914, pp. 777–78 ("it would be unsafe"); Morgenthau to Bryan, Dec. 22, 1914, p. 778; 1914–20, Lansing Papers, vol. 1: Rusem to Bryan, Sept. 12, 1914, pp. 70–71 ("who gave the world"); Wilson to Lansing, Sept. 17, 1914, pp. 72–73. See also Robert Trask, *The United States Response to Turkish Nationalism and Reform, 1914–1939* (Minneapolis: Univ. of Minnesota Press, 1971), p. 13. Arthur S. Link, *Wilson: The Struggle for Neutrality* (Princeton: Princeton Univ. Press, 1960), pp. 68–69. Robert L. Daniel, "The Armenian Question and American-Turkish Relations, 1914–1927," *Mississippi Valley Historical Review* 46 (Sept. 1959): 256.

5. "Missionaries Tell of Terrible Conditions—Raids by Turks," *New York Times*, Dec. 5, 1914; "20,000 Christians in Peril," Dec. 15, 1914; "Fear of General Massacre in Constantinople" ("There was no room"). Balakian, *Burning Tigris*, pp. 177–80.

6. Leslie A. Davis, *The Slaughterhouse Province: An American Diplomat's Report on the Armenian Genocide, 1915–1917* (New Rochelle: Aristide D. Caratzas, 1989), pp. 46–54, 67–69, 79 ("The Mohammedans"). *Statement by the Rev. William A. Shedd, of the American (Presbyterian) Mission Station at Urmia*, "Beth Aram—The Aramean homepage in Germany," http://www.beth-aram.de/dokumente3.html. "Agonies of Armenians Described by Dr. Richard Hill in Letter from Caucuses," *New York Times*, Feb. 7, 1916. Henry H. Riggs, *Days of Tragedy in Armenia* (Ann Arbor: Gomidas Institute, 1917), p. 48. Balakian, *Burning Tigris*, pp. 193–94 ("old men and old"), 346 ("The Government"), 180, 196, 200–201.

7. Jay Winter, ed., *America and the Armenian Genocide of 1915* (Cambridge: Cambridge Univ. Press, 2003), p. 192. Clarence Ussher and Grace Knapp, *An American Physician in Turkey* (Boston: Houghton Mifflin, 1917), pp. 236–44, 277. John D. Barrows, *In the Land of Ararat* (New York: Revell, 1916), pp. 128–34. *FRUS, 1915*, Supplement: Bryan to Gerard, March 12, 1915, p. 964 ("non-combatants"). "Turks Lock 1,000 in Wooden Building and Then Apply the Torch," *New York Times,* Sept. 3, 1915; "Spare Armenians Pope Asks Sultan," Oct. 13, 1915; "State Department Shows Quarter of a Million Women Violated," Oct. 22, 1915. Samantha Power, *A Problem from Hell: America and the Age of Genocide* (New York: Basic, 2002), pp. 4–6.

8. Barbara Tuchman, "The Assimilationist Dilemma: Ambassador Morgenthau's Story," *Commentary* 63, no. 5 (May 1977): 60. Henry Morgenthau III, *Mostly Morgenthau: A Family History* (New York: Ticknor & Fields, 1991), pp. 102–3, 127. *The Papers of Woodrow Wilson*, ed. Arthur Link (Princeton: Princeton Univ. Press, 1966–94), vol. 35: From the Diary of Colonel House, May 2, 1913, pp. 384–85; Henry Morgenthau to Woodrow Wilson, June 12, 1913 ("Would prominent Methodists"), p. 513. Central Zionist Archives (henceforth, CZA), A 243/150: Morgenthau to Wise, June 10, 1913; Wise to Morgenthau, Aug. 7, 1913.

9. Balakian, *Burning Tigris,* pp. 222–23 ("dazzling" and "intrigue, intimidation"). CZA, A 243/150: Morgenthau to Wise, Nov. 28, 1913 ("This is undoubtedly"). Henry Morgenthau Papers, reel 22; undated speech ("few rug merchants"). Henry Morgenthau, *All in a Life-Time* (Garden City, N.Y.: Doubleday, Page, 1922), pp. 175–76 ("I had hitherto"), 196, 203 ("the American spirit"), 204 ("gospel of Americanism"), 209 ("Here was I"). Henry Morgenthau, *The Murder of a Nation* (New York: Armenian General Benevolent Union of America, 1974), p. 18.

10. Lansing replaced Bryan, an adamant pacifist, who resigned in protest of Wilson's policies, which, he felt, were drawing America into the war. Balakian, *Burning Tigris,* pp. 227, 266–70. Merrill D. Peterson, *"Starving Armenians": America and the Armenian Genocide, 1915–1930 and After* (Charlottesville: Univ. of Virginia Press, 2004), p. 37 ("gigantic plundering"). "Armenians' Own Fault, Benstrof Now Says," *New York Times*, Sept. 29, 1915. Power, *Problem from Hell,* p. 6. Israel Charny, ed., *Encyclopedia of Genocide* (Santa Barbara: ABC-CLIO, 1999), p. 96. Lewis Einstein, *Inside Constantinople* (London: John Murray, 1917), p. 231. *FRUS, 1915*, Supplement: Morgenthau to the Secretary of State, July 10, 1915, p. 983 ("race extermination"); 1914–20, Lansing Papers, vol. 1: Lansing to Wilson, Nov. 15, 1916, p. 41.

11. *Papers of Woodrow Wilson*, vol. 35, p. 349 ("You may be sure"). *FRUS, 1914–20*, Lansing Papers, vol. 1: Lansing to Wilson, Nov. 21, 1916, p. 42 ("well-known disloyalty"). Winter, *America and the Armenian Genocide*, p. 104. "Government Sends Plea for Armenia," *New York Times*, Oct. 4, 1915 ("aroused strong sentiment"). Henry Morgenthau Papers, reel 7: Morgenthau to the Secretary of

State, July 16, 1915 ("Nothing short of"). Henry Morgenthau, *Ambassador Morgenthau's Story* (Garden City, N.Y.: Doubleday, 1918), pp. 333–34 ("not . . . as a Jew"). Morgenthau, *Murder of a Nation*, pp. 64 ("Our people will"), 68 ("They are all dead").

12. Henry Morgenthau Papers, reel 7: Morgenthau to Secretary of State, Aug. 11, 1915 ("It is difficult"). *FRUS*, 1915, Supplement, Morgenthau to Secretary of State, Sept. 3, 1915, p. 988. USNA, RG 59, Morgenthau to the Secretary of State, Nov. 25, 1915; Morgenthau to the American Consuls at Beiruth and Aleppo, Nov. 29, 1915. James Barton, *Story of Near East Relief (1915–1930)* (New York: Macmillan, 1930), p. 4. Ralph Elliot Cook, "The United States and the Armenian Question, 1894–1924" (Ph.D. diss., Tufts Univ., 1957), pp. 131–32. Balakian, *Burning Tigris,* pp. 279–80, 282. Power, *Problem from Hell,* pp. 9, 11–12. CZA, CM 241/2—roll 44: Clipping from the St. Louis Dispatch, Sept. 15, 1915 ("The United States might be"). Some Americans also opposed Morgenthau's plan for resettling Armenians in the United States. "Nothing is more stupid . . . than advocating that the solution of the Armenian question . . . is in emigration *en masse* to America," wrote the *New York Herald* correspondent Herbert Gibbons. "Their wholesale emigration . . . would mark the disappearance of the Armenians as a race and a nation." See Herbert A. Gibbons, *The Blackest Page of Modern History* (New York: Putnam, 1916), p. 50.

13. Richard Kloian, *The Armenian Genocide: News Accounts from the American Press* (Berkeley: Anto Press, 1985), p. 219 ("One group"). Balakian, *Burning Tigris,* pp. 242–43 ("arms or legs" and "hundreds of bodies"), 246–47. James Barton, ed., *"Turkish Atrocities": Statements of American Missionaries on the Destruction of Christian Communities in Ottoman Turkey, 1915–1917* (Ann Arbor: Gomidas Institute, 1998), p. 9 ("Women [who] escaped").

14. George Horton, *The Blight of Asia* (1926; reprint, Indianapolis: Bobbs-Merrill, 1953), pp. 54–57. Balakian, *Burning Tigris,* pp. 254–55. DeNovo, *American Interests,* p. 39. Morgenthau, *Ambassador Morgenthau's Story,* pp. 307, 321–22 ("The whole history"), 350. Morgenthau, *Murder of a Nation,* p. 114 ("I had reached"). See also *Marsovan 1915: The Diaries of Bertha B. Morley* (Ann Arbor: Gomidas Institute, 2000), p. 15.

15. *FRUS*, 1916, Supplement: Philip to Lansing, May 21, 1916, p. 851 ("Turkish authorities appear"); Philip to Lansing, July 15, 1916, pp. 932–33 ("In spite of"); Philip to Lansing, July 26, 1916, p. 934; Philip to Lansing, July 26, 1916, p. 935; 1914–20, Lansing Papers, vol. 2: Lansing to Wilson, May 17, 1917, pp. 17–19. Dennis R. Papazian, "Misplaced Credulity: Contemporary Turkish Attempts to Refute the Armenian Genocide," http://www.umd.umich.edu/dept/armenian/papazian/misplace.html ("unchecked policy of extermination"). Kaplan, *Arabists,* p. 65 ("The air was filled"). See also Grace D. Guthrie, Legacy to Lebanon (Richmond, Va.: Self-published, 1984), p. 17. Margaret McGilvary, *The Dawn of a New Era in Syria* (New York: Revell, 1920), pp. 94 ("The whole country"), 110 ("In Syria we were").

18. Action or Nonaction?

1. *Papers of Woodrow Wilson*, vol. 35: House to Wilson, Nov. 11, 1915, p. 191 ("Anything coming"); House to Wilson, Feb. 3, 1916, p. 124 ("The Central Empire runs"); Woodrow Wilson's State of the Union Address, Dec. 4, 1917, p. 200 ("do not yet stand"). *FRUS*, 1916, Supplement: Philip to Lansing, March 28, 1916, p. 849; 1914–20, Lansing Papers, vol. 1: Elkus to Lansing, Sept. 26, 1916, p. 782; Elkus to Lansing, March 2, 1917, pp. 787–88 ("What can we expect"); Elkus to Lansing, Feb. 11, 1917, p. 134 ("Our relations with Turkey"); Supplement 2: Secretary of State to Elkus, April 6, 1917, p. 11. See also Isaiah Friedman, *The Question of Palestine: British-Jewish-Arab Relations: 1914–1918* (New Brunswick: Transaction, 1992), p. 211.

2. Wilson's request for a congressional declaration of war appears on http://www.classbrain.com/artteenst/publish/article_86.shtml. Cornelius Engert Papers, box 1, folder 11.5: Engert to American Minister at The Hague, Nov. 11, 1917. *Papers of Woodrow Wilson*, vol. 35: Chambers to Wilson, Dec. 10, 1915, p. 337; vol. 45: Abram Elkus to Wilson, Nov. 14, 1917 ("Turkey is the weakest"). John H. Finley, *A Pilgrim in Palestine* (New York: Scribner, 1919), p. 55. "Senators Want War on Austria," *New York Times*, Nov. 27, 1917 ("Turkey's course"); Dec. 7, 1917 ("I should be sorry"). *Selections from the Correspondence of Theodore Roosevelt and Henry Cabot Lodge*: Lodge to Roosevelt, Oct. 2, 1918. *Letters of Theodore Roosevelt*: Roosevelt to Lodge, Oct. 23, 1918 ("We ought to declare"); Roosevelt to Paul Shimmon, July 10, 1918 ("surpassed the iniquity").

3. *Papers of Woodrow Wilson*, vol. 45: Dodge to Wilson, Dec. 2, 1917, pp. 185–86; Wilson to Dodge, Dec. 5, 1917 ("every word"); vol. 47: Lansing to Wilson, May 8, 1918, pp. 569–70; vol. 48: From the Diary of Colonel House, May 19, 1918, p. 70; Wilson to Lansing, May 24, 1918, p. 136; vol. 49: Sir William Wiseman to Sir Eric Drummond, Aug. 27, 1918, p. 365. DeNovo, *American Interests*, p. 106 ("I have thought"). *Letters of Theodore Roosevelt*, vol. 8: Roosevelt to Cleveland, May 11, 1918, pp. 1316–18 ("We are guilty"); Theodore Roosevelt to Andrew Fleming West, Dec. 28, 1918, p. 1418 ("It is rather bitter"). Joseph Grabill, "Cleveland H. Dodge, Woodrow Wilson, and the Near East," *Journal of Presbyterian History* 48 (Winter 1970): 249–54. Fromkin, *Peace to End All Peace*, p. 260 ("following its inclination"). See also David E. Cronon, ed., *The Cabinet Diaries of Josephus Daniels, 1913–1921* (Lincoln: Univ. of Nebraska Press, 1963), p. 246.

4. *FRUS*, 1914–20, Lansing Papers, vol. 2: Lansing to Wilson, May 17, 1917, pp. 17–19; 1917, Supplement 2: Morgenthau and Frankfurter to Secretary of State, July 8, 1917, pp. 120–22. *Papers of Woodrow Wilson*, vol. 43: Memorandum from an interview with Wilson written by Sir William Wiseman, July 13, 1917, p. 172; vol. 45: Morgenthau to Wilson, Nov. 26, 1917, p. 123 ("was the cancer"); Wilson to Lansing, Nov. 28, 1917, p. 147; vol. 49: Dodge to Wilson, Sept. 28, 1918, pp. 151–52 ("in the seventh heaven"). Jehuda Reinharz, *Chaim Weizman: The Making*

of a Statesman (New York: Oxford Univ. Press, 1993), pp. 153–54, 155 ("there was one chance"), 163 ("on no account"), 164–68. Richard Lebow, "The Morgenthau Peace Mission of 1917," *Jewish Social Studies* 32, no. 4 (Oct. 1970): 271 ("If it succeeds"), 272–80, 281 ("hot air impressions"), 284 ("wild goose chase"). William Yale, "Ambassador Henry Morgenthau's Special Mission of 1917," *World Politics* 1, no. 3 (April 1949): 311–15, 320 ("Morgenthau's trip"). Manuel, *Realities*, pp. 155–58. Chaim Weizmann, *Trial and Error: The Autobiography of Chaim Weizmann* (Philadelphia: Jewish Publication Society of America, 1949), pp. 196 ("Talk to Morgenthau"), 197–98.

19. An American Movement Is Born

1. Raider, *Emergence of American Zionism*, p. 12. Feinstein, *American Zionism*, pp. 99 ("a fatal blow"), 125. Rafael Medoff, *Zionism and the Arabs: An American Jewish Dilemma, 1898–1948* (Westport, Conn.: Praeger, 1997), p. 12 ("of merely being"). Gideon Shimoni, *The Zionist Ideology* (Hanover: Univ. Press of New England, Brandeis Univ. Press, 1995), p. 137 ("Their entire desire"). Grose, *Israel in the Mind*, p. 72 ("the most formidable"). Arthur Hertzberg, ed., *The Zionist Idea: An Historical Analysis and Reader* (New York: Atheneum, 1972), p. 500 ("We believe that"). Melvin I. Urofsky, *American Zionism from Herzl to the Holocaust* (Garden City, N.Y.: Anchor Press, 1975), p. 98. Oscar Straus Papers, box 4: Straus to Wolf, April 24, 1906.

2. Samuel Halperin, *The Political World of American Zionism* (Detroit: Wayne State Univ. Press, 1961), pp. 11–12 ("Will the Jews"). Hertzberg, *Zionist Idea*, p. 499 ("Is the German-American"). H. N. Hirsch, *The Enigma of Felix Frankfurter* (New York: Basic Books, 1981), p. 44. Michael E. Parrish, *Felix Frankfurter and His Times: The Reform Years* (New York: Free Press, 1982), pp. 129–30. Ben Halpern, "The Americanization of Zionism," *American Jewish History* 69, no. 1 (1979): 15–33. Melvin I. Urofsky, *A Voice That Spoke for Justice: The Life and Times of Stephen S. Wise* (Albany: State Univ. of New York Press, 1982).

3. Raider, *Emergence of American Zionism*, pp. 21, 25, 27. Grose, *Israel in the Mind*, pp. 48 ("these so-called dreamers"), 52 ("deep moral feeling"). CZA, A 243/13, Stephen S. Wise Papers: Wise to Frankfurter, Oct. 10, 1936 ("Sanity, soundness"). Ezekiel Rabinowitz, *Justice Louis D. Brandeis: The Zionist Chapter of His Life* (New York: Philosophical Library, 1968), pp. 14, 31. Evyatar Freisel, "Brandeis' Role in American Zionism Reconsidered," in Jeffrey Gurock, ed., *American Jewish History: The Colonial and Early National Periods, 1654–1840* (New York: Routledge, 1998), pp. 42–43, 105. Allon Gal, "In Search of a New Zion: New Light on Brandeis' Road to Zionism," in Gurrock, *American Jewish History*, pp. 79, 88, 90–91 ("the descendants"). Ben Halpern, *A Clash of Heroes: Brandeis, Weizmann, and American Zionism* (New York: Oxford Univ. Press, 1987), pp. 94–95, 100–5. Louis D. Brandeis, *The Jewish Problem: How to Solve It* (New York: Zionist Organization of America, 1919), pp. 19–20 ("There is no inconsistency").

4. USNA, Ducker to the Secretary of the Navy—Report on the Conditions in Palestine with Reference to Zionism, Feb. 10, 1915. Lansing to Brandeis, Feb. 16, 1915 ("general massacre"); Alexandria Palestine Committee to the Secretary of State, Jan. 25, 1915 ("In name of"); *FRUS*, 1914, Supplement: Morgenthau to Bryan, Aug. 13, 1914, p. 757; 1914–20, Lansing Papers, vol. 1: Elkus to Lansing, Nov. 17, 1916, p. 784. Manuel, *Realities*, pp. 128–31, 136–40. Ruth L. Deech, "Jacob de Haas: A Biography," in Raphael Patai, ed., *Herzl Year Book* 7 (New York: Herzl Press, 1971), pp. 340–41 ("If ever I have").

5. Morgenthau, *All in a Life-Time*, p. 175 ("Anything you can do"). Manuel, *Realities*, pp. 120–25, 126 ("unqualified loyalty"), 141–46. *FRUS*, 1916, Supplement: Morgenthau to Lansing, Dec. 1915, p. 830; Lansing to Glazebrook, Jan. 14, 1916, p. 925; Lansing to Philip, Sept. 13, 1916, p. 937. USNA, Ducker to the Secretary of the Navy—Report on the Conditions in Palestine with Reference to Zionism, Feb. 10, 1915 ("would long remain" and "undoubtedly one"). CZA, A 243/159, Correspondence on Matters of the Yishuv: Perlstein to Wise, Jan. 16, 1915; A 264/25, Papers of Felix Frankfurter: Primrose to Gaster, March 18, 1915. Alexander Aaronsohn, *With the Turks Palestine* (Boston: Houghton Mifflin, 1916), p. 85. Leonard Stein, *The Balfour Declaration* (London: Vallentine, Mitchell, 1961), p. 191 ("America was"). Scuttled by a tsunami in Aug. 1916, with the loss of thirty-eight hands, the *Tennessee* was mourned by the Jews of Palestine as "an eternal blessing." See Davis, *With Eyes toward Zion*, vol. 2, pp. 238–39.

6. Grose, *Israel in the Mind*, p. 68 ("The Jews from every"). Manuel, *Realities*, p. 83. *Letters of Theodore Roosevelt*: Roosevelt to Julian H. Miller; Sept. 16, 1918, p. 1372 ("It seems to me"); Roosevelt to Lioubomir Michailovitch, July 11, 1918, p. 1350 ("there can be"). *The Intimate Papers of Colonel House*, ed. Charles Seymour (Boston: Houghton Mifflin, 1928), vol. 1, pp. 43–44 ("It is all bad"). Ray Stannard Baker, *Woodrow Wilson and World Settlement* (Garden City. N.Y.: Doubleday, Page, 1923), p. 74 ("fine example"). Fromkin, *Peace to End All Peace,* pp. 257, 295 ("the English naturally want"). Stein, *Balfour Declaration*, p. 156. Elizabeth Monroe, *Britain's Moment in the Middle East, 1914–1956* (Baltimore: Johns Hopkins Univ. Press, 1963), p. 40 ("man to man"). Yaakov Ariel, *On Behalf of Israel: American Fundamentalist Attitudes toward Jews, Judaism, and Zionism, 1865–1945* (Brooklyn: Carlson, 1991), p. 45 ("the Zionist movement").

7. Grose, *Israel in the Mind*, pp. 63–66, 67 ("To think that"). *Cabinet Diaries of Josephus Daniels*, p. 267. Stein, *Balfour Declaration*, pp. 427–28, 505, 530. *The Letters of Louis D. Brandeis*, ed. Melvin I. Urofsky and David M. Levy (Albany: State Univ. of New York, 1973): Brandeis to de Hass, April 24, 1917, p. 283 ("I have heard much"), de Hass Memorandum, May 4, 1917, p. 286 ("a publicly assured"); Brandeis to de Hass, May 8, 1917, p. 288 ("I am a Zionist"); Brandeis to Weizmann, Sept. 24, 1917, p. 310 ("entire sympathy"). Richard Lebow, "Woodrow Wilson and the Balfour Declaration," *Journal of Modern History* 40, no. 4 (Dec. 1968): 501–13. Weizmann, *Trial and Error*, pp. 193–94, 208 ("one of

the most important"). Manuel, *Realities*, p. 168 ("the many dangers"). Merkley, *Politics of Christian Zionism*, p. 91 ("The vast mass").

8. Ben Halpern and Jehuda Reinharz, *Zionism and the Creation of a New Society* (New York: Oxford Univ. Press, 1998), pp. 175–77, 180–82. Robert Silverberg, *If I Forget Thee, O Jerusalem: American Jews and the State of Israel* (New York: Morrow, 1970), pp. 104, 105–6 ("The Americans brought"), 176. Martin Watts, *The Jewish Legion and the First World War* (London: Palgrave Macmillan, 2004), pp. 147–48. Elias Gilner, *War and Hope: A History of the Jewish Legion* (New York: Herzl Press, 1969), pp. 165–67, 170–71, 177.

9. Lansing's remark about Jewish guilt for the death of Christ was later leaked to the press, but the secretary denied having made it. *FRUS*, 1914–20, Lansing Papers, vol. 2: Lansing to Wilson, Dec. 13, 1917, p. 71 ("many Christian sects"); Lansing Note, Dec. 14, 1917, p. 71 ("very unwillingly"). Selig Adler, "The Palestine Question in the Wilson Era," *Jewish Social Studies* 10, no. 4 (Oct. 1948): 313 ("polluting and intolerable"). Medoff, *Zionism and the Arabs*, pp. 21–25. Grose, *Israel in the Mind*, pp. 70, 83 ("sentimental, religious"). William Yale Oral History, Columbia Univ., pp. 10 ("playboy"), 14 ("brass knucks"). Manuel, *Realities*, pp. 171, 172 ("400 million Christians"), 176 ("satisfaction" and "in the progress"), 184 ("younger and more hot-headed"), 185 ("young, hot-headed Jews"), 186 ("Religious fanaticism" and "If a Jewish State"), 189 ("disagreeable . . . type"), 190. Monroe, *Britain's Moment in the Middle East*, pp. 44–45.

10. Medoff, *Zionism and the Arabs*, pp. 21–25. Grose, *Israel in the Mind*, p. 81 ("The Arabs in Palestine").

20. Arise, O Arabs, and Awake!

1. John M. Munro, *A Mutual Concern: The Story of the American University of Beirut* (Delmar, N.Y.: Caravan Books, 1977), p. 65 ("I know why the Turks"). The study of the origins of Arab nationalism has generated a great many books and articles. See, e.g., Ernest C. Dawn, "The Origins of Arab Nationalism," in Rashid Khalidi, ed., *The Origins of Arab Nationalism* (New York: Columbia Univ. Press, 1991), p. 3. Ernest C. Dawn, *From Ottomanism to Arabism: Essays on the Origins of Arab Nationalism* (Urbana: Univ. of Illinois Press, 1973), pp. 132, 140. Adeed Dawisha, *Arab Nationalism in the Twentieth Century: From Triumph to Despair* (Princeton: Princeton Univ. Press, 2003), pp. 25–27, 32–34. Bassam Tibi, *Arab Nationalism: Between Islam and the Nation-State* (New York: St. Martin's, 1997), pp. 102–4. Eliezer Tauber, *The Emergence of the Arab Movements* (London: Frank Cass, 1993), pp. 15–18. Zeine N. Zeine, *The Emergence of Arab Nationalism*, 3d ed. (Delmar, N.Y.: Caravan Books, 1973), pp. 45, 79, 106. See also George Antakly, "American Protestant Educational Missions: Their Influence on Syria and Arab Nationalism, 1820–1923" (Ph.D. diss., American Univ., 1976), pp. 111–12, 115, 120.

2. Neville Mandel, *The Arabs and Zionism before World War I* (Berkeley: Univ. of California Press, 1976), pp. 42–55, 85–86, 211–12 ("The Jews' . . . right"). Mary

C. Wilson, "The Hashemites, the Arab Revolt, and Arab Nationalism," in Khalidi, *Origins of Arab Nationalism*, pp. 205, 219. Dawisha, *Arab Nationalism*, p. 34. Muhammad Y. Muslih, *The Origins of Palestinian Nationalism* (New York: Columbia Univ. Press, 1988), pp. 54–60, 67, 79, 87.

3. Alixa Naff, *The Arab Americans* (Philadelphia: Chelsea House, 1999), pp. 14, 33. Alixa Naff, "Arabs in America: A Historical Overview," in Sameer Abraham, ed., *Arabs in the New World: Studies in Arab-American Communities* (Detroit: Wayne State Univ., 1983), pp. 9–10, 13–19. Philip Keyal and Joseph Keyal, *The Syrian-Lebanese in America* (Boston: Twayne, 1975), pp. 34, 41, 63, 66, 82. Salom Rizk, *Syrian Yankee* (Garden City, N.Y.: Doubleday, Doran, 1943), p. 71 ("I could see America"). Because of a misspelling of his name in a Boston grammar school, Khalil Gibran's name is sometimes rendered Kahlil Gibran. See "Khalil the Heretic" in Gregory Orfalea, ed., *Grape Leaves: A Century of Arab American Poetry* (Salt Lake City: Univ. of Utah Press, 1988), pp. 24–25. Gibran Khalil Gibran, *The Prophet* (New York: Knopf, 1952), pp. 48–49. For further reference, see the Gibran Khalil Gibran website, http://leb.net/gibran/.

4. The Ameen Rihani Papers: From an unpublished manuscript, pp. 76 ("other educational institutions"), 111 ("proof of the aptitude"), 115 ("American spirit"), Bliss to Rihani, March 12, 1913 ("It was unfortunate"). Nada Najjar, "The Space In-between: The Ambivalence of Early Arab-American Writers" (Ph.D. diss., Univ. of Toledo, 1999), pp. 77, 96, 123, 126 ("Carry to the East"). *Theodore Roosevelt Papers*: Rihani to Roosevelt, April 20, 1917. Ameen Rihani, *The Path of Vision* (Beirut: Rihani House, 1970), pp. 97 ("in a land where"), 124 ("The voice of America"). Ameen Rihani, "Palestine and the Proposed Arab Federation," *Annals of the American Academy of Political and Social Science* 164 (Nov. 1932): 66 ("The Land of Promise"). Ameen Rihani, *The Fate of Palestine* (Beirut: Rihani House, 1967), pp. 25, 37, 80, 85 ("without prejudicing"). See also Suheil B. Bushrui, *The Thoughts and Works of Ameen Rihani*, http://www.alhewar.com/Bushrui_Rihani.html.

5. Laurence Evans, *United States Policy and the Partition of Turkey, 1914–1924* (Baltimore: Johns Hopkins Press, 1965), pp. 122 ("I have a kindly"). Stuart Knee, "The King-Crane Commission of 1919: The Articulation of Political Anti-Zionism," in Gurrock, *American Jewish History*, pp. 182–88, 188 ("Unitarians of the desert"). Grabill, "Cleveland H. Dodge," p. 254. Kaplan, *Arabists*, p. 70 ("the menace"). Frank W. Brecher, *Reluctant Ally: United States Foreign Policy toward the Jews from Wilson to Roosevelt* (New York: Greenwood, 1991), p. 19. David Philipson, *My Life as an American Jew* (Cincinnati: John G. Kidd, 1941), pp. 173–74.

21. The First Middle East Peace Process

1. Studies on the origins of Wilsonian diplomacy abound. See, e.g., Thomas J. Knock, *To End All Wars: Woodrow Wilson and the Quest for a New World Order* (Princeton: Princeton Univ. Press, 1992), pp. 3 ("A boy never gets"), 14, 33, 77.

August Heckscher, *Woodrow Wilson* (New York: Scribner, 1991), pp. 294, 434. Louis Auchincloss, *Woodrow Wilson* (New York: Penguin, 2000), pp. 74, 92. Arthur Walworth, *Woodrow Wilson* (New York: Norton, 1978), pp. 343, 344 ("go to the ends"), 345 ("do the thinking"). Ray Stannard Baker, *Woodrow Wilson: Life and Letters, 1856–1890* (Garden City, N.Y.: Doubleday, 1927), pp. 49, 211, 312. Lloyd E. Ambrosius, *Woodrow Wilson and the American Diplomatic Tradition* (Cambridge: Cambridge Univ. Press, 1987), pp. 1–2, 9. Cooper, *Warrior and the Priest*, pp. 15, 273, 323. David M. Kennedy, "What 'W' Owes to 'WW,'" *Atlantic Monthly*, March 2005, p. 36.

2. *FRUS*, 1919, Paris Peace Conference Papers, vol. 5: Proceedings, April 21, 1919, p. 107; May 13, 1919, p. 584 ("docile people"); vol. 6: June 25, 1919, p. 676 ("cleared out"). *Intimate Papers of Colonel House*, vol. 1: Diary entry for Dec. 18, 1912, p. 96 ("There ain't going"). Harley Notter, *The Origins of the Foreign Policy of Woodrow Wilson* (Baltimore: Johns Hopkins Press, 1937), p. 46 ("abnormal"). Walworth, *Woodrow Wilson*, p. 497 ("America believes in helping").

3. *FRUS*, 1919, Paris Peace Conference, vol. 1: Excerpt from "The Inquiry," Dec. 22, 1917, p. 52; Lippmann to the Secretary of War, May 16, 1918, pp. 97–98. Manuel, *Realities*, pp. 212, 213–14. William L. Westermann Paris Peace Conference Diaries, entry for Dec. 29, 1918, p. 14 ("thrown in the waste"). Lawrence E. Gelfand, *The Inquiry: American Preparations for Peace, 1917–1919* (New Haven: Yale Univ. Press, 1963), pp. 227, 231–32, 244, 248–49, 255 ("fanaticism and bitter"), 256 ("It was the cradle"). Taner Akçam, *A Shameful Act: The Armenian Genocide and the Question of Turkish Responsibility* (New York: Metropolitan Books, 2006), pp. 227–30.

4. Manuel, *Realities*, p. 217 ("Will not the Mohammedans"). George Noble, "The Voice of Egypt," *Nation* 110, no. 2844 (Jan. 3, 1920): 862 ("No people").

5. *FRUS*, 1919, Paris Peace Conference, vol. 1: Jusserand to Lansing, Nov. 29, 1918, p. 367. *Papers of Woodrow Wilson*, vol. 47: Memorandum by William Westermann, April 17, 1919, p. 443 ("the great loot"). Link, *Wilson*, p. 414 ("call through a crack"). Margaret MacMillan, *Paris 1919: Six Months That Changed the World* (New York: Random House, 2002), pp. 30–32, 386 ("the complete and definite"). Edward House, ed., *What Really Happened at Paris* (New York: Scribner, 1921), pp. 178–79 ("Not having declared"). Fromkin, *Peace to End All Peace*, pp. 373 ("The other governments").

6. Grose, *Israel in the Mind*, p. 84 ("In spite of"). MacMillan, *Paris 1919*, p. 386 ("knowing in the bottom" and "The obstacle is"). Frederick Palmer, *Bliss, Peacemaker* (New York: Dodd, Mead, 1934), p. 418 ("Wherever a mandate"). *FRUS*, 1919, Paris Peace Conference, vol. 3: Proceedings, Jan. 30, 1919, p. 807 ("I can think of"). Smuts envisaged three types of mandates—A, B, and C, where A mandates were intended for those territories most ready for independence. All of the Middle East mandates were type A. See F. S. Crafford, *Jan Smuts: A Biography* (Garden City. N.Y.: Doubleday, Doran, 1943), p. 148. H. C. Armstrong, *Grey Steel* (London: Arthur Barker, 1937), p. 316.

7. *Felix Frankfurter Reminisces: Recorded in Talks with Harlan B. Phillips* (New York: Reynal, 1960), p. 156 ("Here was little me"). Joseph P. Lash, *From the Diaries of Felix Frankfurter* (New York: Norton, 1975), p. 26 ("cousins in race"). *FRUS*, 1919, Paris Peace Conference, vol. 3: Proceedings, Feb. 6, 1919, p. 891; Bliss Address to the Council of Ten on Feb. 13, 1919, pp. 1016–17; vol. 4: Proceedings, Feb. 27, 1919, p. 169 ("They are intelligent"). Walworth, *Woodrow Wilson*, p. 500 ("startling resemblance"). John Allen, "Inventing the Middle East," *On Wisconsin* (Winter 2004): 36–39. Paul C. Helmreich, *From Paris to Sèvres: The Partition of the Ottoman Empire at the Peace Conference of 1919–1920* (Columbus: Ohio State Univ. Press, 1974), p. 67. Robert Lansing, *The Big Four and Others of the Peace Conference* (Boston: Houghton Mifflin, 1921), pp. 163–64 ("ancient seer"), 169 ("His voice seemed"). Manuel, *Realities*, pp. 221–22, 229 ("prominent American Jews"), 234–35, 238 ("The opposition of the Moslems"), 257 ("Jerusalem will be").

8. Helmreich, *From Paris to Sèvres*, pp. 22 ("So long as"), 67. Edith Wharton, *In Morocco* (New York: Scribner, 1920), pp. 79 ("Nothing endures in Islam"), 266 ("from Persia to Morocco"). Evans, *United States Policy*, p. 29. James Shotwell, *At the Paris Peace Conference* (New York: Macmillan, 1937), pp. 130–31, 176–78. Harry N. Howard, *The King-Crane Commission* (Beirut: Khayats, 1963), pp. 50–51 ("widespread trouble"). MacMillan, *Paris 1919*, pp. 152–53, 154 ("I cannot imagine"). Walworth, *Woodrow Wilson*, p. 492 ("America is the only").

9. *FRUS*, 1919, Paris Peace Conference, vol. 5: Proceedings, March 20, 1919, pp. 10 ("scrap"), 12; vol. 11: Minutes of Meeting, March 27, 1919, p. 133 ("knew nothing about"). Brecher, *Reluctant Ally*, pp. 19–20. Manuel, *Realities*, p. 245 ("a very experienced"). *Papers of Woodrow Wilson*: Feisal to Wilson, vol. 47: April 20, 1919, p. 525 ("I am confident"); vol. 48: Wilson Remark in Paris, May 3, 1919, p. 401 ("Our [Allied] governments"). *Felix Frankfurter Reminisces*, p. 151 ("A crazy idea"). Howard, *King-Crane Commission*, pp. 35, 37 ("is about to cheat"), 38–39, 44–45 ("too honest"). William L. Westermann Paris Peace Conference Diaries, entry for Jan. 12, 1919, pp. 19 ("the root of all good"), 24.

10. Thomas Bailey, *Woodrow Wilson and the Great Betrayal* (New York: Macmillan, 1947), pp. 264–66. Justin McCarthy, *Death and Exile: The Ethnic Cleansing of Ottoman Muslims, 1821–1922* (Princeton: Darwin Press, 1995), p. 263 ("Old men, unarmed"). MacMillan, *Paris 1919*, pp. 349, 353–54. Fromkin, *Peace to End All Peace*, pp. 393–95. Howard M. Sachar, *The Emergence of the Middle East, 1914–1924* (New York: Knopf, 1969), p. 349. *FRUS*, 1919, Paris Peace Conference, vol. 5: Proceedings, May 14, 1919, p. 618; May 19, 1919, p. 708; May 22, 1919, p. 812. Grabill, *Protestant Diplomacy*, p. 260 ("with all my heart"). William L. Westermann Peace Conference Diaries, entry for May 22, 1919, p. 81. *Documents on British Foreign Policy, 1919–1939*, ed. Rohan Butler and J. P. T. Bury (London: Her Majesty's Stationery Office, 1963), vol. 13: Geddes to Curzon, May 11, 1919, pp. 70–71; Geddes to Curzon, May 19, 1919, p. 76. *Intimate Papers of Colonel House*, vol. 3: entry for May 20, 1919, p. 468 ("something of a scandal").

11. Donald M. Love, *Henry Churchill King of Oberlin* (New Haven: Yale Univ. Press, 1956), pp. 215–16. Howard, *King-Crane Commission*, pp. 56, 221 ("Every part of the Turkish"). Manuel, *Realities*, pp. 249–51 ("Whereas injustice"). *FRUS*, 1919, Paris Peace Conference, vol. 12; Crane and King to the Commission to Negotiate Peace, July 10, 1919, pp. 749–50 ("A real great lover"); King-Crane Commission, pp. 792, 794 ("be seriously considered" and "It is simply impossible"), 797 ("On account of her" and "no other Power"), 799 ("The people of the area"), 801, 833 ("Constantinopolitan State"). William Yale Oral History, pp. 64, 70. For an overview of the commission, see James Gelvin, "The Ironic Legacy of the King-Crane Commission," in David Lesch, ed., *The Middle East and the United States* (Boulder: Westview Press, 1999), pp. 13–26.

12. Erik Goldstein, "The Eastern Question: The Last Phase," in Michael Dockrill, ed., *The Paris Peace Conference, 1919: Peace without Victory* (New York: Palgrave, 2001), p. 145 ("Lloyd George is a cheat!"). MacMillan, *Paris 1919*, pp. 33 ("God himself was content"), 145.

13. *FRUS*, 1919, Paris Peace Conference, vol. 11: Proceedings, July 1, 1919, p. 184; July 8, 1919, p. 284 ("perfectly useless proposition"). Lansing, *Peace Negotiations*, p. 149. Manuel, *Realities*, p. 255 ("whole disgusting scramble"). Herbert Hoover, *The Memoirs of Herbert Hoover* (New York: Macmillan, 1957), p. 385. William L. Westermann Paris Peace Conference Diaries, p. 69. Feroz Ahmad, *The Making of Modern Turkey* (New York: Routledge, 1993), p. 55 ("America, which knows"). James B. Gidney, *A Mandate for Armenia* (Kent, Ohio: Kent State Univ. Press, 1967), pp. 17, 184–87, 188 ("Here is a man's job"). General James G. Harbord, *Conditions in the Near East: American Military Mission to Armenia* (Washington, D.C.: GPO, 1920).

14. *Papers of Woodrow Wilson*, vol. 64: "The President's State of Health," Lansing Memorandum, Nov. 5, 1919, pp. 56–57. Henry Cabot Lodge, *The Senate and the League of Nations* (New York: Scribner, 1925), p. 184 ("obligation to preserve"). Sachar, *Emergence of the Middle East*, pp. 349, 361. Heckscher, *Woodrow Wilson*, p. 609 ("the American people").

15. Marjorie Housepian Dobkin, *Smyrna 1922: The Destruction of a City* (Kent, Ohio: Kent State Univ. Press, 1988), pp. 101, 103, 112, 166 ("I'll never forget"). Horton, *Blight of Asia*, p. 113 ("a fittingly lurid"). *FRUS*, 1923, vol. 2: Child and Grew to Hughes, Dec. 13, 1922, p. 921 ("find [the] means"); Child and Grew to Hughes, Jan. 3, 1923, p. 946; Harding to Hughes, Jan. 15, 1923, p. 950 ("The most ardent"). *Documents on British Foreign Policy, 1919–1939*: British Secretary's Notes, April 10, 1920, pp. 20–21; April 20, 1920, pp. 60–61. Daniel, "Armenian Question," p. 262.

16. William L. Westermann Paris Peace Conference Diaries, pp. 179–80 ("When boldness"). Lansing, *Peace Negotiations*, p. 175 ("The seeds of discontent"). Palmer, *Bliss, Peacemaker*, p. 370 ("there never had been"). DeNovo, *American Interests*, pp. 299–301. Gelvin, "Ironic Legacy of the King-Crane Commission," p. 13 ("It is not possible"). Sachar, *Emergence of the Middle East*, p. 365.

22. Fantasies Revived

1. One could easily dedicate a book to the innumerable books written about Lawrence of Arabia. See, e.g., David Fromkin, "The Importance of T. E. Lawrence," *New Criterion* 10, no. 1 (Sept. 1995). John E. Mack, *A Prince of Our Disorder: The Life of T. E. Lawrence* (Oxford: Oxford Univ. Press, 1990), pp. 221 ("limelight of history"), 265 ("On the whole"), 275. Phillip Knightley and Colin Simpson, *The Secret Lives of Lawrence of Arabia* (London: Thomas Nelson, 1969), pp. 52–53. Lawrence James, *The Golden Warrior* (New York: Paragon House, 1993), pp. 272, 276–77. See also Shotwell, *At the Paris Peace Conference*, p. 131 ("younger successor of Mohammed").

2. Norman Bowen, *Lowell Thomas: The Stranger Everyone Knows* (Garden City, N.Y.: Doubleday, 1968), pp. 39–40. Lowell Thomas, *Good Evening Everybody* (New York: Morrow, 1976), pp. 131–39. Lowell Thomas, *With Lawrence in Arabia*, pp. 12 (the Uncrowned King" and "one of most picturesque"), 20 ("He walked rapidly"), 22 ("restored the sacred places"), 75 ("united the wandering tribes"), 76 ("reincarnation of a prophet"), 114 ("400 Turks"), 264 ("a great scoop"). Joel Hodson, *Lawrence of Arabia and American Culture* (Westport, Conn.: Greenwood, 1995), pp. 43, 61, 62 ("quite without intention" and "the George Washington"). Knightley, *Secret Lives*, p. 53 ("break up the Islamic"). Knock, *To End All Wars*, p. 213 ("chuckled in the desert"). Mack, *Prince of Our Disorder*, pp. 276 ("I saw your show"), 277 ("I don't bear him"). Hodson, *Lawrence of Arabia*, pp. 30, 43, 66 ("Come with me").

3. Michael North, *Reading 1922: A Return to the Scene of the Modern* (New York: Oxford Univ. Press, 1999), pp. 21–24. Willa Sibert Cather, *My Ántonia* (Boston: Houghton Mifflin, 1977), pp. 6 ("more inscribed"), 10 ("the beard of an Arabian"). Little, *American Orientalism*, pp. 17–18.

23. From Bibles to Drill Bits

1. Harrison, *Doctor in Arabia*, pp. 24 ("not even their religion"), 30. DeNovo, *American Interests*, p. 361 ("of little commercial importance"). USNA, Records of the Department of State Relating to Internal Affairs of Saudi Arabia: Brandt to the Secretary of State, May 5, 1930 ("demonstrated that the Arabs"). Eleanor Calverley, *My Arabian Days and Nights* (New York: Crowell, 1958), p. 7 ("until that moment"). Mary B. Allison, *Doctor Mary in Arabia: Memoirs* (Austin: Univ. of Texas Press, 1994), p. 25 ("like being born"). Thomas W. Lippman, *Inside the Mirage: America's Fragile Partnership with Saudi Arabia* (Boulder: Westview Press, 2004,) pp. 10–11 ("I know you are"). Paul L. Armerding, Doctors for the Kingdom: The Work of the American Mission Hospitals in the Kingdom of Saudi Arabia, 1913–1955 (Grand Rapids, Mich.: Eerdmans, 2003), p. 115. See also Miriam Joyce, *Kuwait, 1945–1956: An Anglo-American Perspective* (London: Frank Cass, 1998), p. xviii, and Thomas Lippman, "The Pioneers," *Saudi Aramco World* 55, no. 3

(May–June 2004), and Eleanor A. Doumato, *Getting God's Ear: Women, Islam, and Healing in Saudi Arabia and the Gulf* (New York: Columbia Univ. Press, 2000), pp. 43–48. According to Doumato, the most common ailment Harrison treated was "inability," i.e., male sexual dysfunction.

2. Anthony Sampson, *The Seven Sisters: The Great Oil Companies and the World They Shaped* (New York: Bantam, 1991), p. 83. Longrigg, *Oil in the Middle East*, pp. 38–39. Bryson, *American Diplomatic Relations*, pp. 103–5. Anthony C. Brown, *Oil, God, and Gold: The Story of Aramco and the Saudi Kings* (Boston: Houghton Mifflin, 1999), pp. 24–28. Benjamin Shwadran, *The Middle East, Oil, and the Great Powers* (Jerusalem: Israel Universities Press, 1973), pp. 237–38, 288. H. St. John Philby, *Saudi Arabia* (London: Ernest Benn, 1955), p. 330.

3. In spite of his seminal role in the establishment of U.S.-Saudi relations, Twitchell has yet to be the subject of a serious study, and the descriptions of him remain fragmentary. See, e.g., William Yale, *The Near East: A Modern History* (Ann Arbor: Univ. of Michigan Press, 1958), p. 362. D. Van der Meulen, *The Wells of Ibn Saud* (New York: Praeger, 1957), p. 136. George Kheirallah, *Arabia Reborn* (Albuquerque: Univ. of New Mexico Press, 1952), pp. 239–40. Moukhtar Ani, *Saudi Arabia: Its People, Its Society, Its Culture* (New Haven: HRAF Press, 1959), p. 234.

4 Daniel Yergin, *The Prize: The Epic Quest for Oil, Money and Power* (New York: Touchstone, 1992), pp. 289–91. George Stocking, *Middle East Oil: A Study in Political and Economic Controversy* (Kingsport, Tenn.: Vanderbilt Univ. Press, 1970), p. 76. Sampson, *Seven Sisters*, pp. 109–11. Joseph W. Walt, "Saudi Arabia and the Americans, 1928–1951" (Ph.D. diss., Northwestern Univ., 1960), p. 87 ("Some of these firms"). H. J. B. Philby, *Arabian Oil Ventures* (Washington, D.C.: Middle East Institute, 1964), p. 124. Philby relates that the king in fact slept through much of the discussions on the agreement and that his—Philby's—advice weighed decisively in favor of the Americans.

5. Sampson, *Seven Sisters*, p. 111 ("descending from the skies"). Wallace Stegner, *Discovery: The Search for Arabian Oil* (Beirut: Export Press, 1971), pp. 3–54.

6. Aaron Miller, *Search for Security: Saudi Arabian Oil and American Foreign Policy, 1939–1949* (Chapel Hill: Univ. of North Carolina Press, 1980), p. 25 ("We should let matters"), 26–27. Irvine H. Anderson, *ARAMCO, the United States, and Saudi Arabia: A Study of the Dynamics of Foreign Oil Policy, 1933–1950* (Princeton: Princeton Univ. Press, 1981), p. 25. Kaplan, *Arabists*, p. 71 ("the real bulwark"). DeNovo, *American Interests*, p. 337. Lippman, *Inside the Mirage*, p. 117 ("Saudi Arabia is presumably"). William Eddy Papers, box 17: Excerpt from Eddy's unpublished memoirs ("We Muslims"). Karl Twitchell Papers, box 5: Twitchell to Cleveland Dodge, March 3, 1932. Stegner, *Discovery*, p. 65 ("If utter faith").

7. USNA, Records of the Department of State relating to the Internal Affairs of Saudi Arabia, 1930–1944: 890f.00/53, Fish to the State Department, April 12, 1940 ("German ruthlessness"); 890f.00/60, Twitchell to Murray, May 14, 1941; 890f.00/73, Memorandum on conditions in Saudi Arabia based on an interview with a reliable informant (American) returned recently from there Oct. 29, 1941. Parker

T. Hart, *Saudi Arabia and the United States: Birth of a Security Partnership* (Bloomington: Indiana Univ. Press, 1998), p. 37. Rex J. Casillas, *Oil and Diplomacy: The Evolution of American Foreign Policy in Saudi Arabia, 1933–1945* (New York: Garland, 1987), pp. 33, 37, 40. Miller, *Search for Security*, pp. 33–34 ("It can easily").

8. Shwadran, *Middle East*, p. 317. Brown, *Oil, God and Gold*, pp. 106–7 ("extending financial assistance"). USNA, Records of the Department of State relating to the Internal Affairs of Saudi Arabia, 1930–1944: 890f.00/73 Memorandum on Conditions in Saudi Arabia, Oct. 29, 1941; 890f.00/81, Strictly confidential for Secretary and Under Secretary, April 17, 1943 ("Jews had been hostile").

24. An Insoluble Conflict Evolves

1. The study of the origins of the Arab-Israeli conflict has generated innumerable books. Few of these, however, are free of an expressed bias toward one side or the other in the conflict. For a sample of some of the more highly regarded scholarly works on the subject, see Philip Mattar, *The Mufti of Jerusalem: Al-Hajj Amin al-Husayni and the Palestinian National Movement* (New York: Columbia Univ. Press, 1988), pp. 12–49. Christopher Sykes, *Crossroads to Israel, 1917–1948* (Bloomington: Indiana Univ. Press, 1973), pp. 41–232. J. C. Hurewtiz, *The Struggle for Palestine* (New York: Greenwood, 1968), pp. 3–94.

2. Irwin Oder, "The United States and the Palestine Mandate, 1920–1948: A Study of the Impact of Interest Groups on Foreign Policy" (Ph.D. diss., Columbia Univ., 1956), pp. 75 ("an influential and noisy"), 320. Gideon Biger, "The American View of the Tel Hai Affair," *Journal of Israeli History* 19, no. 1 (1998): 91–94. Manuel, *Realities*, pp. 272, 277 ("[We] should avoid"), 280–84, 291–92 ("They would turn Trotsky"), 293–99. Barry Rubin, *The Great Powers in the Middle East, 1941–1947* (London: Cass, 1980), p. 22 ("decidedly anti-Jewish"). See also Knee, "Anglo-American Relations," pp. 13–17.

3. Naomi Cohen, *The Year after the Riots: American Responses to the Palestine Crisis of 1929–30* (Detroit: Wayne State Univ. Press, 1988), pp. 22, 23 ("A crowd of savage Arabs"), 27–28, 29 ("ordinary law-abiding"), 33 ("The Jews are always"). USNA, RG 59: Palestine Internal Affairs: Knabenshue to Stimson (n.d.) ("Jewish financial influence"); Knabenshue to Stimson, Aug. 24, 1929 ("provocative acts"); Knabenshue to Stimson, Aug. 26, 1929; Hamilton Fish Jr. to Stimson, Aug. 28, 1929; Knabenshue to Stimson Oct. 19, 1929. CZA, A243/104, Stephen S. Wise Papers: Memorandum of Meeting of SSW with Secretary of State Stimson on the S.S. *Leviathan*, Sept. 1, 1931. Manuel, *Realities*, pp. 302–3. "Says Syria Admires Us," *New York Times,* Jan. 11, 1929; "4th in Jerusalem Brings Out Throngs," *New York Times*, July 5, 1929. "U.S. Investigates Palestine Consul," *Washington Post*, Sept. 7, 1929. Oder, "United States and the Palestine Mandate," p. 156.

4. CZA, A 243/178, Stephen S. Wise Papers: Wise to Frankfurter, July 29, 1937; O'Toole to Wise, July 30, 1937; Wise to Felix Frankfurter, Oct. 16, 1938. *FRUS*, 1937, vol. 4: Memorandum by Wallace Murray, July 12, 1937, p. 893 ("Any dispo-

sition"); 1938, vol. 2: Memorandum submitted to the Secretary of State by American Jewish Delegation, Oct. 14, 1938, p. 956 ("radical departure"). USNA, Palestine Internal Affairs: Wadsworth to Secretary of State, July 7, 1938 ("Palestinian Jews"); Murray to Secretary of State, Feb. 1, 1939 ("In America there is"); Wadsworth to Secretary of State, June 27, 1939. John Fitzgerald Kennedy Presidential Library, President's Office Files, box 135, Series: Special Events, Folder: 1939 ("It seems to me"): Letter Written to His Father following Trip to Palestine. Halperin, *Political World of American Zionism*, pp. 21–26. Louis Rapoport, *Shake Heaven and Earth: Peter Bergson and the Struggle to Rescue the Jews of Europe* (Jerusalem: Gefen, 1999), p. 43 ("Americans don't like Jews"). Phillip J. Baram, *The Department of State in the Middle East, 1919–1945* (Philadelphia: Univ. of Pennsylvania Press, 1978), pp. 263, 268.

5. The proposal for transferring 300,000 Palestinian Arabs was first tabled by Edward Norman, a non-Zionist Jew and heir to a family fortune made from food concessions from the 1893 world's fair. The cost of the project was estimated at $300 million, to be contributed by the Western powers and wealthy American Jews. Neither Britain nor France, however, showed enthusiasm for the idea and Roosevelt made no real effort to implement it. See Rafael Medoff, *Baksheesh Diplomacy: Secret Negotiations between American Jewish Leaders and Arab Officials on the Eve of World War II* (Lanham, Md.: Lexington Books, 2001), pp. 3, 140 ("less right there"), 141–43. On Roosevelt's foreign policy in general, and toward Palestine in particular, see Robert Dallek, *Franklin D. Roosevelt and American Foreign Policy, 1932–1945* (New York: Oxford Univ. Press, 1979), p. 20 ("a chameleon on plaid"). Willard Range, *Franklin D. Roosevelt's World Order* (Athens: Univ. of Georgia Press, 1959), p. 8. James MacGregor Burns, *Roosevelt: The Soldier of Freedom* (New York: Harcourt Brace Jovanovich, 1970), pp. 108, 397 ("I would put barbed"). Conrad Black, *Franklin Delano Roosevelt: Champion of Freedom* (London: Weidenfeld & Nicolson, 2003), p. 928. Frederick W. Marks III, *Wind over Sand: The Diplomacy of Franklin Roosevelt* (Athens, Georgia: Univ. of Georgia Press, 1988), p. 253. William Roger Louis, *The British Empire in the Middle East, 1945–1951* (New York: Oxford Univ. Press, 1984), p. 243 ("Holy Gehad"). *Memoirs of Cordell Hull*, vol. 2 (New York: Macmillan, 1948), p. 1530 ("It is something"). Steiner, *Religious Beliefs*, pp. 66–67. Grose, *Israel in the Mind*, pp. 113, 138–39 ("little baksheesh").

6. *FRUS*, 1936, vol. 3: Secretary of State to Ambassador in the United Kingdom, July 27, 1936, p. 444 ("influential Jewish circles" and "of course presume"); 1937, vol. 2: Memorandum from Secretary of State to the American Ambassador in the United Kingdom to be delivered to the British, p. 890 ("Large sections"). Manuel, *Realities*, pp. 306–8. PRO, FO 371: Mr. Mallet to British Embassy. Sept. 21, 1936 ("[It] is hardly worth"); Sir R. Lindsay to Viscount Halifax. Nov. 25, 1938. Grose, *Israel in the Mind*, p. 100. USNA, Palestine Internal Affairs: Knabenshue to Murray, May 25, 1935 ("The White Paper"). Henry L. Feingold, *The Politics of Rescue: The Roosevelt Administration and the Holocaust, 1938–1945* (New Brunswick:

Rutgers Univ. Press, 1970), pp. 126–31, 135 ("exponents of Communism"), 146 ("was 100%").

7. CZA, L66/22: Letter to Zionist Delegates (n.d.) ("At this time"); Letter to Heads of Organizations (n.d.) ("specializing in delicious"); L66/24: Brainin to Weisgal, Sept. 20, 1938 ("the most beautiful girl"); L66/59: Memorandum on the Opening of the Palestine Pavilion, May 13, 1939; Brainin to Bloom, June 30, 1939; L66/77: Press Release for Tuesday, Feb. 27, 1940; L66/69: Letter for Palestine Book by F. H. La Guardia (n.d.). See also James L. Gelvin, "Zionism and the Representation of Jewish Palestine at the New York World's Fair, 1939–40," *International History Review* 22, no. 1 (2000): 37–64. USNA, Palestine Internal Affairs: Wadsworth to Secretary of State, Sept. 11, 1938.

8. Golda Meir, *My Life* (New York: Putnam, 1975), pp. 30 ("New food"), 74 ("Crowds of beggars"), 81 ("I was profoundly happy"), 140 ("Look, Golda"). Ralph G. Martin, *Golda: Golda Meir, the Romantic Years* (New York: Scribner, 1988), p. 98 ("I owed America").

9. Edward Wagenknecht, *Daughters of the Covenant: Portraits of Six Jewish Women* (Amherst: Univ. of Massachusetts Press, 1983), pp. 153–56. Michael Brown, *The Israeli-American Connection: Its Roots in the Yishuv, 1914–1945* (Detroit: Wayne State Univ. Press, 1996), pp. 135–36, 141–45. Marvin Lowenthal, *Henrietta Szold: Life and Letters* (New York: Viking, 1942), pp. 244, 264. Simon Noveck, *Great Jewish Personalities in Modern Times* (Washington, D.C.: B'nai B'rith Department of Adult Jewish Education, 1960), pp. 324 ("first lady of Palestine"), 331. Michael Shire, *The Jewish Prophet: Visionary Words from Moses to Heschel* (London: Frances Lincoln, 2002), p. 93 ("Political scores"). CZA, Szold Papers, Speech before the Zionists of America Administration Committee, Jan. 9, 1936 ("I became a Zionist"). Jewish Women's Archive, "JWA—Henrietta Szold—Building the Yishuv," http://www.jwa.org/exhibits/wov/szold/yishuv.html (Oct. 6, 2005). See also Baila Round Shargel, "American Jewish Women in Palestine: Bessie Gotsfeld, Henrietta Szold, and the Zionist Enterprise," *American Jewish History* 90, no. 2 (June 2002).

10. Arthur Goren, *Dissenter in Zion: From the Writings of Judah L. Magnes* (Cambridge: Harvard Univ. Press, 1982), pp. 4–16, 23–24, 32–40, 276 ("a country of two nations"), 277–78, 279 ("I have learned"). Daniel P. Kotzin, "An Attempt to Americanize the Yishuv: Judah L. Magnes in Mandatory Palestine," *Israel Studies* 5, no. 1 (2000): 3–18. Neil Caplan, *Futile Diplomacy*, vol. 2 (London: Frank Cass, 1983), pp. 36–37, 87–90. Susan L. Hattis, *The Bi-national Idea in Palestine during the Mandatory Times* ([Haifa]: Shikmona, 1970), pp. 65–66, 100, 144–48, 171, 184. Shalom Ratzabi, *Between Zionism and Judaism: The Radical Circle in Brith Shalom, 1925–1933* (Leiden: Brill, 2002), pp. 252–53. Hagit Lavsky, *Before Catastrophe: The Distinctive Path of German Zionism* (Detroit: Wayne State Univ. Press, 1996), pp. 211, 212, 213–17. Michael J. Cohen, "Secret Diplomacy and Rebellion in Palestine, 1936–1939," *International Journal of Middle East Studies* 8, no. 3

(July 1977): 380, 383, 400–1. Menahem Kaufman, *The Magnes-Philby Negotiations, 1929: The Historical Record* (Jerusalem: Magnes Press, 1998), pp. 18, 100–1, 113. "Judah Magnes," http://www.wzo.org.il/en/resources/view.asp?id=1349& subject=70, Oct. 11, 2005 ("may have to live" and "We can establish").

11. James R. Kruger, *Turning On Water with a Shovel: The Career of Elwood Mead* (Albuquerque: Univ. of New Mexico Press, 1992), pp. 103, 107–8, 109 ("wards of the organization"). Robert E. Rook, "An American in Palestine: Elwood Mead and Zionist Water Resource Planning, 1923–1936," *Arab Studies Quarterly* 22, no. 1 (Winter 2000): 71–79. Elwood Mead, "The New Palestine," *American Review of Reviews* 70, no. 6 (Dec. 1924): 624 ("promise to be a replica"), 626 ("is as attractive"), 628 ("The Zionist movement").

12. Rook, "Blueprints and Prophets," pp. 91–92, 99 ("morgue of civilizations"), 101–10, 139–40. Walter C. Lowdermilk, *Palestine: Land of Promise* (New York: Harper, 1944), pp. 6–7 ("most remarkable devotion"), 8–24, 229 ("the lever that will lift"). Nathan Godfried, *Bridging the Gap between Rich and Poor: American Economic Development Policy toward the Arab East, 1942–1949* (New York: Greenwood, 1987), p. 168. Rory Miller, "Bible and Soil: Walter Clay Lowdermilk, the Jordan Valley Project and the Palestine Debate," *Middle Eastern Studies* 39, no. 2 (April 2003): 56–63. See also Walter C. Lowdermilk, *Conquest of the Land through Seven Thousand Years* (1948; reprint, Washington, D.C.: U.S. Department of Agriculture, Soil Conservation Service, 1953).

13. Shabtai Teveth, *Ben Gurion: The Burning Ground, 1886–1948* (Boston: Houghton Mifflin, 1987), pp. 97–98 ("absurd, resembling cages"), 109–20. Allon Gal, *David Ben-Gurion and the American Alignment for a Jewish State* (Bloomington: Indiana Univ. Press, 1991), pp. 15 ("bustling, industrious" and "We, who seek"), 16, 21, 103, 149, 196 ("London has not ceased"), 203, 216. See also Michael Bar-Zohar, *Ben-Gurion: A Biography,* translated by Peretz Kidron (New York: Adama Books, 1977). Dan Kurzman, *Ben-Gurion: Prophet of Fire* (New York: Simon & Schuster, 1983), pp. 115–19.

14. David S. Wyman and Rafael Medoff, *A Race against Death: Peter Bergson, America, and the Holocaust* (New York: New Press, 2004), pp. 19–29, 107 ("Mi samcha"). Rapoport, *Shake Heaven and Earth*, pp. 35–43, 56–57 ("An army with such").

15. David Shapiro, *From Philanthropy to Activism: The Political Transformation of American Zionism in the Holocaust Years, 1933–1945* (Oxford: Pergamon Press, 1994), pp. 71, 84. Silverberg, *If I Forget Thee, O Jerusalem*, pp. 188–90, 206 ("The more I think"). Raider, *Emergence of American Zionism*, pp. 205–6 ("battleground"). Halperin, *Political World of American Zionism*, p. 121. Gal, *David Ben-Gurion*, p. 69 ("Right now"). Walter Laqueur, *A History of Zionism* (New York: Simon & Schuster, 1989), pp. 546–47. For a detailed discussion of the *New York Times* treatment of the Holocaust, see Laurel Leff, *Buried by the Times: The Holocaust and America's Most Important Newspaper* (New York: Cambridge Univ. Press, 2005), pp. 2–3, 13, 42.

25. A Torch for the Middle East

1. *A Pocket Guide to North Africa* (Washington, D.C.: War and Navy Department, 1942), pp. 14, 19, 23, 28, 34, 39–41. William L. Langer and S. Everett Gleason, *The Undeclared War, 1940–1941* (Gloucester: P. Smith, 1968), pp. 380–81, 590, 592 ("We in the United"), 778 ("We should not get"). Michael J. Cohen, "American Influence on British Policy in the Middle East during World War Two: First Attempts at Coordinating Allied Policy on Palestine," *American Jewish Historical Quarterly* 67, no. 1 (Sept. 1977): 51–52 ("Our reputation"). Robert Murphy, *Diplomat among Warriors* (Garden City, N.Y.: Doubleday, 1964), p. 66–68, 91 ("The vice consuls"). George F. Howe, *Northwest Africa: Seizing the Initiative in the West* (Washington, D.C.: Center of Military History, 1991), pp. 57–58. *FRUS*, 1941, vol. 3: British and Free French Invasion and Occupation of Syria and Lebanon; Good Offices of the United States in Arranging Armistice: Personal to the President, June 7, 1941, pp. 725–26.

2. Dallek, *Franklin D. Roosevelt*, pp. 346–49, 262. Mark W. Clark, *Calculated Risk* (New York: Harper, 1950), pp. 50 ("Why stick your head"), 107. Rick Atkinson, *An Army at Dawn: The War in North Africa, 1942–1943* (New York: Henry Holt, 2002), pp. 12–13, 14 ("indirect contribution"), 16 ("was now our principal objective"), 17–18, 46–47. Hale, "'General' Eaton," p. 28. George S. Patton, *War as I Knew It* (Boston: Houghton Mifflin, 1995), p. 16. *Pocket Guide to North Africa*, pp. 4–5.

3. Arthur L. Funk, "Negotiating the 'Deal with Darlan,'" *Journal of Contemporary History* 8, no. 2 (April 1973): 81–117. Atkinson, *Army at Dawn*, pp. 3 ("North Africa was"), 287–88. Brown, *Oil, God, and Gold*, pp. 104–5 ("sons of the Mughreb"). Carleton S. Coon, *A North Africa Story: The Anthropologist as OSS Agent* (Ipswich, Mass.: Gambit Press, 1980), p. 14. Howe, *Northwest Africa*, pp. 108–9. Clark, *Calculated Risk*, pp. 155 ("I had constantly"), 269.

4. A. J. Liebling, *The Road Back to Paris* (Garden City, N.Y.: Doubleday, Doran, 1944), pp. 225 ("as examples"), 290 ("a wild competition"). Kenneth G. Crawford, *Report on North Africa* (New York: Farrar and Rinehart, 1943), pp. 45–46 ("warriors fighting"). Richard Breitman, "The Allied War Effort and the Jews, 1942–1943," *Journal of Contemporary History* 20, no. 1 (Jan. 1985): 140–41, 142 ("Arabs don't mind Christians"). *The Conferences at Washington, 1941–1942, and Casablanca, 1943* (Washington, D.C.: GPO, 1968): Conversation between President Roosevelt and General Noguès, Jan. 17, 1943, p. 608 ("eliminate . . . the understandable"). Carlo D'Este, *Eisenhower: A Soldier's Life* (New York: Henry Holt, 2002), p. 356 ("Many things done here"). There were few exceptions to the general Arab opposition to removing the wartime restrictions on Jews; see Robert Satloff, "In Search of 'Righteous Arabs,'" *Commentary* 118, no. 1 (July 2004).

5. Gaddis Smith, *American Diplomacy during the Second World War, 1941–1945* (New York: Knopf, 1985), pp. 96 ("A century"), 100–10. Stephane Bernard, *The Franco-Moroccan Conflict, 1943–1953* (New Haven: Yale Univ. Press,

1968), p. 3. Annie Lacroix-Riz, *Les Protectorats d'Afrique du Nord entre la France et Washington: Du débarquement à l'indépendance, Maroc et Tunisie, 1942–1956* (Paris: L'Harmattan, 1988), pp. 11–21. Benjamin Rivlin, "The United States and Moroccan International Status, 1943–1956: A Contributory Factor in Morocco's Reassertion of Independence from France," *International Journal of African Historical Studies* 15, no. 1 (1982): 64–65, 74. Egya N. Sangmuah, "Sultan Mohammed ben Youssef's American Strategy and the Diplomacy of North African Liberation, 1943–61," *Journal of Contemporary History* 27, no. 1 (Jan. 1992): 130. Kenneth Pendar, *Adventure in Diplomacy: The Emergence of General de Gaulle in North Africa* (London: Cassell, 1966), pp. 142, 146–47. Elliott Roosevelt, *As He Saw It* (New York: Duell, Sloan and Pierce, 1946), pp. 110 ("differ sharply), 111 ("French and British financiers"), 112 ("A new future" and "Glowering"). Ernie Pyle, *Here Is Your War* (New York: Henry Holt, 1943), p. 44 ("Arab farmers"). *FRUS, 1944,* vol. 5: Mayer to the Secretary of State, Jan. 5, 1944, pp. 527–29.

6. *FRUS,* 1945, vol. 8: Henderson to Truman, Nov. 10, 1945, p. 10 ("friendly disinterest"). Russell Buhite, *Patrick J. Hurley and American Foreign Policy* (Ithaca: Cornell Univ. Press, 1973), pp. 6–15, 27, 113 ("certain very rich"), 313. Don Lohbeck, *Patrick J. Hurley* (Chicago: H. Regnery, 1956), pp. 188–89, 190 ("Our President"), 191 ("My job"), 193 ("America could not"), 195 ("starvation was the easiest"), 210–11 ("the economy of colonial"). Franklin Delano Roosevelt Papers, Office Files, 1933–1945, pt. 4: Subject Files, reel 19; Hurley to Roosevelt, May 5, 1943 ("exploitation and imperialism"); Hurley to Roosevelt, June 9, 1943 ("similar to those embodied"). Abbas Milani, "Hurley's Dream," *Hoover Digest,* no. 3 (2003): 149 ("It is the purpose" and "free governments"), 150 ("unselfish American policy"). T. H. Vail Motter, *The Persian Corridor and Aid to Russia* (Washington, D.C.: Office of the Chief of Military History, 1952), pp. 6–7. See also Mark Hamilton Lytle, *The Origins of the Iranian-American Alliance, 1941–1953* (New York: Holmes & Meier, 1987), pp. 48–59, 60 ("messianic globaloney"). William R. Louis, *Imperialism at Bay, 1941–1945: The United States and the Decolonization of the British Empire* (Oxford: Clarendon Press, 1977), p. 226 ("the colonial system").

7. *FRUS,* 1943, vol. 4: Secretary of State to Wiley, Nov. 12, 1943, p. 1045; 1944, vol. 5: Morris to the Secretary of State, Oct. 9, 1944, p. 455. Phillip Baram, "Undermining the British: Department of State Policies in Egypt and the Suez Canal before and during World War II," *Historian* 40, no. 4 (Aug. 1978): 633–37, 641–45. Thomas A. Bryson, *Seeds of the Mideast Crisis: The United States Diplomatic Role in the Middle East during World War II* (Jefferson, N.C.: McFarland, 1981), pp. 85–89, 98–99. Rubin, *Great Powers,* pp. 141–42. Walter L. Browne, *The Political History of Lebanon, 1920–1950,* vol. 2 (Salisbury, N.C.: Documentary Publications, 1977), pp. 271, 386–87. Louis, *Imperialism at Bay,* p. 169. Steven L. Spiegel, *The Other Arab-Israeli Conflict: Making America's Middle East Policy, from Truman to Reagan* (Chicago: Univ. of Chicago Press, 1985), p. 13 ("New Deal" and "you will be"). On America's prewar refusal to encourage Egyptian nationalists, see Erez Manela, "Friction from the Sidelines: Diplomacy, Religion and Culture in

American-Egyptian Relations, 1919–1939," *The United States and the Middle East: Diplomatic and Economic Relations in Historical Perspective* (New Haven: Yale Center for International and Area Studies, 2000), pp. 28–35. On Hooker Doolittle's contribution to Tunisian independence, see David D. Newsom, "The Unsung Diplomat," *Christian Science Monitor*, April 12, 2000.

8. *FRUS*, 1944, vol. 5: Roosevelt to Landis, March 6, 1944, p. 2. James M. Landis Papers, box 164: Excerpt from a "Round Table" at the Univ. of Chicago entitled "The Middle East: Zone of Conflict?" July 22, 1945 ("The trouble is"). Donald A. Ritchie, *James M. Landis: Dean of the Regulators* (Cambridge: Harvard Univ. Press, 1980), pp. 3 ("I've been called"), 121–23, 124 ("A diffusion of power"), 126, 130. Robert Vitalis, "The New Deal in Egypt: The Rise of Anglo-American Commercial Competition in World War II and the Fall of Neocolonialism," *Diplomatic History* 20, no. 2 (Spring 1996): 213, 220–24. Martin W. Wilmington, *The Middle East Supply Centre* (Albany: State Univ. of New York Press, 1971), pp. 4–7, 62–72, 167. Peter L. Hahn, *The United States, Great Britain, and Egypt, 1945–1956: Strategy and Diplomacy in the Early Cold War* (Chapel Hill: Univ. of North Carolina Press, 1991), pp. 14–17. Godfried, *Bridging the Gap*, pp. 483–90. Arthur C. Millspaugh, *Americans in Persia* (Washington. D.C.: Brookings Institution, 1946), pp. 55, 64, 84–85 ("The Persian government").

9. Oder, "United States and the Palestine Mandate," pp. 326–27. On the Millspaugh and Schwarzkopf Missions, see *FRUS*, 1944, vol. 4: Ford to Secretary of State, Feb. 2, 1944, p. 391; Ford to Secretary of State, April 11, 1944, p. 395; Morris to Secretary of State Oct. 11, 1944, p. 430. James Bill, *The Eagle and the Lion: The Tragedy of American-Iranian Relations* (New Haven: Yale Univ. Press, 1988), pp. 24–25, 27. Michael K. Sheehan, *Iran: The Impact of United States Interests and Policies, 1941–1943* (Brooklyn: Theo Gaus' Sons, 1968), pp. 16–17. Lytle, *Origins of the Iranian-American Alliance*, pp. 112–16.

10. Wilmington, *Middle East Supply Centre*, p. 167 ("the time has come"). *FRUS*, 1942, vol. 4: Welles to Kirk, Feb. 26, 1942, p. 564; 1943, vol. 4: Secretary of State to the Secretary of the Interior, Nov. 13, 1943, p. 942 ("the oil of Saudi Arabia"); 1944, vol. 5: Hull to Winnant, Oct. 17, 1944, p. 666 ("a covert contest"); Davies to Murray, Dec. 27, 1944, p. 9; 1944, vol. 5: Murray to the Under Secretary of State, Nov. 23, 1944, pp. 35–36. David Long, *The United States and Saudi Arabia* (Boulder: Westview Press, 1985), pp. 14–15, 76. Bryson, *Seeds of Mideast Crisis*, p. 39. Miller, *Search for Security*, pp. 30–31, 43 ("Just how we could"), 51–55, 60–63, 71, 121, 237. Hart, *Saudi Arabia*, p. 29. Lytle, *Origins of the Iranian-American Alliance*, pp. 64, 71. Longrigg, *Oil in the Middle East*, pp. 133–34. Shwadran, *Middle East*, pp. 330–33.

11. Cecil Brown, *Suez to Singapore* (New York: Random House, 1942), p. 12 ("This is Baghdad"). Erasmus Kloman, *Assignment Algiers: With the OSS in the Mediterranean Theater* (Annapolis: Naval Institute Press, 2005), p. 17 ("never-never land"). Patton, *War as I Knew It*, p. 10 ("a city which combines"). Norman Schwarzkopf, *It Doesn't Take a Hero* (New York: Bantam, 1992), p. 11 ("magical,

faraway"). Roger Cohen and Claudio Gatti, *In the Eye of the Storm: The Life of General H. Norman Schwarzkopf* (New York: Farrar, Straus and Giroux, 1991), pp. 48–49. Humphrey Wynn, *Desert Eagles* (Osceola, Wis.: Motorbooks International, 1993), pp. 9 ("certainly a dirty place"), 10 ("the last place"), 13 ("Even the beer"). Ernest D. Whitehead, *World War II: An Ex-Sergeant Remembers* (Kearney: Morris Publishing, 1996), 36 ("What are we doing"). *The Papers of Dwight David Eisenhower*, ed. Alfred Chandler (Baltimore: Johns Hopkins Univ. Press, 1970), vol. 2: Dwight Eisenhower to John Eisenhower, Nov. 20, 1942, p. 746 ("beautiful and picturesque"). Clark, *Calculated Risk,* p. 157 ("like illustrations"). Liebling, *Road Back to Paris*, p. 243 ("This is exactly"). "Hey, Jack, which way to Mecca?" appears in Peter Arno, *Peter Arno* (New York: Perennial Library, 1990). *A Short Guide to Iraq* (Washington, D.C.: War and Navy Departments, 1944), pp. 3–4 ("you have seen").

12. Atkinson, *Army at Dawn*, pp. 124 ("Scrofulous, unpicturesque"), 169 ("useless, worthless" and "If they could have"), 255, 462 ("they were open"). D'Este, *Eisenhower*, p. 400 ("I would rather"). Patton, *War as I Knew It*, pp. 5, 47 ("the morning edition"), 49 ("the utter degradation"). Whitehead, *World War II*, pp. 41, 44 ("The Arab men"). *World War II Diary of Jean Gordon Peltier* (Groveland, Calif.: Perfect Art, 2000), pp. 37 ("The men spend"), 38 ("the animals lived"). Howard Wriggins, *Picking Up the Pieces from Portugal to Palestine: Quaker Refugee Relief in World War II* (Lanham, Md.: Univ. Press of America, 2004), p. 79 ("That may be so"). K. Ray Marrs, *I Was There When the World Stood Still* (Bloomington: 1st Books, 2003), p. 301 ("Their long flowing" and "kill the Arab"). David Rame, *Road to Tunis* (New York: Macmillan, 1944), pp. 14–15, 36. Liebling, *Road Back to Paris*, pp. 279, 291. *Stars and Stripes* (Cairo edition), July 2, 1942 ("Nobody ever taught"); July 30, 1943 ("buxom"), Oct. 8, 1943 ("sayeeda").

13. *The White House Papers of Harry Hopkins*, ed. Robert Sherwood, vol. 2 (London: Eyre and Spottiswoode, 1949), p. 860 ("horseplay"). Burns, *Roosevelt*, pp. 395–96 ("The mills of the gods"). *FRUS*, 1943, vol. 4: Ibn Saud to Roosevelt, May 11, 1943, pp. 773–74 ("Jews have no right"); 1944, vol. 5: Stettenius to Roosevelt, p. 649 ("It would seriously prejudice"), Berle to the Secretary of State, Jan. 28, 1944, pp. 561–62 ("opened for the free entry"); Satterthwaite to Secretary of State, Aug. 3, 1944, p. 607 ("moral as well as material"); Secretary of State to Roosevelt, Dec. 13, 1944, p. 649 ("economic concessions") Secretary of State to Roosevelt, p. 655 (n.d.); Tuck to Secretary of State, Nov. 21, 1944, p. 640 ("Democratic America"). Manuel, *Realities*, pp. 310–12.

14. Jim Bishop, *FDR's Last Year* (New York: Morrow, 1974), pp. 441, 443 ("the Moslem will not permit"), 435, 445 ("this prosperity" and "short of war"). John S. Keating, "Cruise of the USS *Flying Carpet*," *True* 33, no. 199 (Dec. 1953): 108–9, 110 ("lean and dark"), 111 ("serious damage"). William Eddy, *F.D.R. Meets Ibn Saud* (New York: American Friends of the Middle East, 1954), pp. 21, 30, 31 ("my most precious"), 34–35 ("Make the enemy"), 44–45 ("most precious pearl"). Black, *Franklin Delano Roosevelt*, p. 1068 ("whole party"). W. Barry McCarthy, "Ibn

Saud's Voyage," *Life*, March 19, 1945, pp. 62–64. *FRUS*, 1944, vol. 5: Secretary of State to Jidda, April 18, 1944, p. 687 ("thoughts, wants, needs"). Range, *Franklin D. Roosevelt's World Order*, p. 149. Burns, *Roosevelt*, pp. 378–79, 578. *White House Papers of Harry Hopkins*, pp. 860–61 ("horseplay" and "overly impressed"). Manuel, *Realities*, pp. 314 ("I will never rest"), 316–17 ("malicious misrepresentation").

26. The Middle East and the Man from Missouri

1. Walter Isaacson and Evan Thomas, *The Wise Men: Six Friends and the World They Made* (New York: Touchstone, 1986), pp. 255–56. Deborah Welch Larson, *Origins of Containment: A Psychological Explanation* (Princeton: Princeton Univ. Press, 1985), pp. 126–29, 134–35. Alonzo L. Hamby, *Man of the People: A Life of Harry S. Truman* (New York: Oxford Univ. Press, 1995), pp. 404–6. David McCullough, *Truman* (New York: Simon & Schuster, 1992), pp. 349 ("great, great tragedy"), 350, 353 ("I felt like the moon"), 597. Merle Miller, *Plain Speaking: An Oral Biography of Harry S. Truman* (New York: Putnam, 1974), p. 215 ("It wasn't just"). Michael T. Benson, *Harry S. Truman and the Founding of Israel* (Westport, Conn.: Praeger, 1997), pp. 29–33, 34 ("God has created us"), 35–38, 39 ("a matter of faith"), 53–54.

2. *FRUS*, 1945, vol. 8: Henderson to Matthews, Nov. 13, 1945, p. 1208; Acting Secretary of State to the Ambassador in France, May 23, 1945, p. 1092; 1946, vol. 7: Stettinius to Secretary of State, Feb. 7, 1946, p. 763; Secretary of State to Stettinius, Feb. 9, 1946, p. 766; Henderson to Truman, Nov. 10, 1945, pp. 10–11. Hahn, *United States, Great Britain, and Egypt*, pp. 20–21 ("the most deserving"), 26–29. David Lesch, *Syria and the United States: Eisenhower's Cold War in the Middle East* (Boulder: Westview Press, 1992), p. 17. G. W. Sand, ed., *Defending the West: The Truman-Churchill Correspondence, 1945–1960* (Westport, Conn.: Praeger, 2004), pp. 92–93, 94. H. W. Brands, *Inside the Cold War: Loy Henderson and the Rise of the American Empire, 1918–1961* (New York: Oxford Univ. Press, 1991), pp. 132 ("Your country has"), 134 ("Our refusal"). Robert Laffey, "United States Policy toward and Relations with Syria, 1941–1947" (Ph.D. diss., Univ. of Notre Dame, 1981), pp. 85–86. Irene L. Gendzier, *Notes from the Minefield: United States Intervention in Lebanon and the Middle East, 1945–1958* (Boulder: Westview Press, 1999), p. 51.

3. Geoff Simons, *Libya and the West: From Independence to Lockerbie* (Oxford: Centre for Libyan Studies, 2003), p. 18. William Roger Louis, "American Anticolonialism and the Dissolution of the British Empire," *International Affairs* 61, no. 3 (Summer 1985): 403–9. Scott L. Bills, *The Libyan Arena: The United States, Britain, and the Council of Foreign Ministers, 1945–1948* (Kent, Ohio: Kent State Univ. Press, 1995), pp. 8, 12, 24, 32. Ronald Bruce St. John, *Libya and the United States: Two Centuries of Strife* (Philadelphia: Univ. of Pennsylvania Press, 2002), pp. 40, 42–43.

4. *FRUS*, 1945, vol. 8: Morris to the Secretary of State, Jan. 4, 1945, p. 359; Minor to Acheson, June 2, 1945, p. 376; Henderson to the Secretary of State, Aug. 23, 1945, pp. 27–28. Bruce R. *Kuniholm, The Origins of the Cold War in the Near East: Great Power Conflict and Diplomacy in Iran, Turkey, and Greece* (Princeton: Princeton Univ. Press, 1980), pp. 157–65. Lytle, *Origins of the Iranian-American Alliance,* pp. 120–68. John Gaddis, *The United States and the Origins of the Cold War* (New York: Columbia Univ. Press, 1992), pp. 200, 310–11 ("Now we'll give"). Barry Rubin, *Paved with Good Intentions: The American Experience and Iran* (New York: Penguin, 1981), pp. 33–36. Louise L. Fawcett, *Iran and the Cold War: The Azerbaijan Crisis of 1946* (Cambridge: Cambridge Univ. Press, 1992), pp. 122–29, 139. Robert J. Donovan, *Conflict and Crisis: The Presidency of Harry S. Truman, 1945–1948* (New York: Norton, 1977), pp. 194–95. Willian Hillman and Harry Truman, *Mr. President: The First Publication from the Personal Diaries, Private Letters, Papers, and Revealing Interviews of Harry S. Truman, Thirty-second President of the United States of America* (New York: Farrar, Straus and Young, 1952), pp. 22–23: Truman to Byrnes, Jan. 5, 1946 ("We ought to protest").

5. *FRUS*, 1945, vol. 8: Harriman to the Secretary of State Moscow, March 21, 1945, p. 1220; Wilson to the Secretary of State, Sept. 25, 1945, pp. 1249; 1947, vol. 5: Smith to the Secretary of State, Jan. 8, 1947, pp. 2–3; MacVeagh to the Secretary of State, Feb. 11, 1947, p. 17; Report of the State-War-Navy Coordinating Committee (n.d.), pp. 76–77 ("There is, at the present"). Joseph C. Satterthwaite, "The Truman Doctrine: Turkey," *Annals of the American Academy of Political and Social and Science* 401 (May 1972): 74–84. Robert Frazier, "Acheson and Formulation of the Truman Doctrine," *Journal of Modern Greek Studies* 17, no. 2 (1999): 229–51. John Gaddis, *The Cold War: A New History* (New York: Penguin, 2005), p. 28. Kuniholm, *Origins of the Cold War,* p. 425. Fawcett, *Iran and the Cold War,* p. 128. Donovan, *Conflict and Crisis,* p. 251 ("Greece and Turkey"). Lawrence S. Kaplan, "The Monroe Doctrine and the Truman Doctrine: The Case of Greece," *Journal of the Early Republic* 13, no. 1 (Spring 1993): 2 ("Our foreign policy"). Laffey, "United States Policy," p. 71 ("star rising"). The text of Truman's speech to Congress is available online, through Yale Law School's Avalon Project.

6. James M. Burns and Susan Dunn, *The Three Roosevelts: Patrician Leaders Who Transformed America* (New York: Grove Press, 2001), p. 516 ("I cannot bear"). McCullough, *Truman,* p. 597 ("Everyone else"). Grose, *Israel in the Mind,* pp. 189 ("My sympathy"), 200 ("One is led"). Arnold Offner, *Another Such Victory: President Truman and the Cold War, 1945–1953* (Palo Alto: Stanford Univ. Press, 2002), p. 275 ("to make the whole world"). Louis, *British Empire in the Middle East,* p. 240 ("I have to answer").

7. Truman's policymaking on Palestine is one of the most lavishly researched subjects in modern Middle Eastern history. Notes relating to the episode contain a representative, but scarcely exhaustive, selection of these sources. Benson, *Harry S. Truman,* pp. 64–65 ("grievous harm"). Grose, *Israel in the Mind,* pp. 203 ("to the head"), 204 ("because they did not"). Zvi Ganin, *Truman, American Jewry, and*

Israel, 1945–1948 (New York: Holmes & Meier, 1979), p. 39 ("firmly believe"). David Schoenbaum, *The United States and the State of Israel* (New York: Oxford Univ. Press, 1993), p. 44.

8. Peter L. Hahn, *Caught in the Middle East: U.S. Policy toward the Arab-Israeli Conflict, 1945–1961* (Chapel Hill: Univ. of North Carolina Press, 2004), pp. 33–36. Michael J. Cohen, *Palestine and the Great Powers, 1945–1948* (Princeton: Princeton Univ. Press, 1982), pp. 96–112, 113 ("the further development"). Ganin, *Truman, American Jewry, and Israel*, p. 80 ("For the Jews"). Harry S. Truman, *Memoirs*, vol. 2: *Years of Trial and Hope* (Garden City, N.Y.: Doubleday, 1956), p. 57 ("the promised Jewish homeland"). Grose, *Israel in the Mind*, p. 206 ("Jesus Christ"). Truman Presidential Library: President's Secretary File: Jacobson to Truman, Oct. 7, 1947 ("Harry, my people"). Benson, *Harry S. Truman*, p. 96 ("Terror and Silver"). The Anglo-American Committee of Inquiry report is available on the Avalon Project website. See also Michael J. Cohen, ed., *The Anglo-American Committee on Palestine, 1945–46*, vol. 35 of *The Rise of Israel: A Documentary Record from the Nineteenth Century to 1948* (New York: Garland, 1987).

9. *FRUS*, 1947, vol. 7: Memorandum of Fraser Wilkins, Jan. 14, 1947, pp. 1003–4; Marshall to the Embassy in the U.K., Jan. 14, 1947, pp. 1005–6; Memorandum of Dean Acheson, Jan. 21, 1947, pp. 1008–11. Grose, *Israel in the Mind*, pp. 202 ("more concerned"), 214 ("sacrificial labors" and "the title deeds"). Dean Acheson, *Present at the Creation: My Years in the State Department* (Toronto: George-McLeod, 1969), p. 175 ("the most disliked power"). Benson, *Harry S. Truman and the Founding of Israel*, pp. 81 ("not in the light"), 93 ("crackpots"). Hahn, *Caught in the Middle East*, pp. 29, 34, 36 ("underground guerrilla warfare"), 40. *The Forrestal Diaries* (New York: Viking, 1951), pp. 180, 245, 303–4, 342, 345. Offner, *Another Such Victory*, p. 274 ("sixty-four dollar question").

10. Martin Gilbert, *Israel: A History* (London: Black Swan, 1998), p. 147 ("the thousands of years"). Cohen, *Palestine and the Great Powers*, p. 266 ("Zionist beachhead"). Manuel, *Realities*, p. 324 ("stuck his neck out"). Sykes, *Crossroads to Israel*, p. 325 ("relentless war"). *Forrestal Diaries*, p. 376. Mattar, *Mufti of Jerusalem*, p. 110. The minority UNSCOP plan was submitted by Iran, India, and Yugoslavia; the majority plan by Australia, Canada, Czechoslovakia, Guatemala, the Netherlands, Peru, Sweden, and Uruguay.

11. Truman Presidential Library: President's Diaries File, July 21, 1947 ("The Jews, I find"). *FRUS*, 1947, vol. 5: Marshall to Truman, April 29, 1947, p. 1080; Marshall to Certain Diplomatic Officers, June 13, 1947, p. 1103; Henderson to Marshall, Sept. 22, 1947, p. 1153; Memorandum of Paul Alling, Sept. 26, 1947, p. 1159; Wadsworth to Mattison, Nov. 13, 1947, p. 1257. Cohen, *Palestine and the Great Powers*, pp. 293–94, 295 ("get busy"). Hahn, *Caught in the Middle East*, pp. 39–41, 48.

12. FRUS, Vol. V, 1948: Kennan to Lovett, Feb. 12, 1948, pp. 589–92; Austin to Marshall, March 17, 1948, p. 736; Henderson to Lovett, April 22, 1948, pp. 841–42 ("decide once and for all"). Truman, *Years of Trial and Hope*, pp. 161, 164,

171, 173. Hahn, *Caught in the Middle East*, p. 46 ("British bullheadedness"). Truman Presidential Library: President's Secretary's File: Truman to Jacobson, Feb. 27, 1948 ("The situation has been"). Benson, *Harry S. Truman*, pp. 127 ("Harry"), 128 ("You win" and "bank"). McCullough, *Truman*, pp. 610–11 ("liar and a double-crosser"). Cohen, *Palestine and the Great Powers*, p. 358 ("shocking reversal" and "surrender to Arab terror"). Dan Kurzman, *Genesis 1948: The First Arab-Israeli War* (New York: Da Capo Press, 1992), pp. 83, 97. On Zionist fundraising efforts in the United States, see Yossi Melman and Dan Raviv, *Friends in Deed: Inside the U.S.-Israel Alliance* (New York: Hyperion, 1994), pp. 40–45.

13. *FRUS, 1948*, vol. 5: Rusk to Marshall, March 22, 1948, p. 751; Gross to Lovett, May 11, 1948, p. 959. Elsey Papers, May 12, 1948, p. 977 ("a very transparent attempt" and "pig in the poke"), State Department to Truman, Aug. 19, 1948, p. 1324 ("are destitute"). Howard M. Sachar, *A History of Israel: From the Rise of Zionism to Our Time* (New York: Knopf, 1970), pp. 309, 310 ("What will happen"). Donovan, *Conflict and Crisis*, p. 383 ("If the President"). Grose, *Israel in the Mind*, pp. 290–91, 292 ("I will cross that bridge"), 293 ("What do you mean"). "34 Jews are Slain in Hospital Convoy," *New York Times*, April 14, 1948. Larry Collins and Dominique Lapierre, *O Jerusalem* (New York: Simon & Schuster, 1972), p. 278 ("there were bodies"). The number of Arab victims of the Deir Yassin massacre remains a source of historical controversy. I have relied on Matthew Hogan, "The 1948 Massacre at Deir Yassin," in *Historian* 63, no. 2 (2001) .

27. Harmony and Hegemony

1. Brian Urquhart, *Ralph Bunche: An American Life* (New York: Norton, 1993), pp. 103, 122, 164. Charles P. Henry, *Ralph Bunche: Model Negro or American Other?* (New York: New York Univ., 1999), p. 145. Shabtai Rosenne, "Bunche at Rhodes: Diplomatic Negotiator," in Benjamin Rivlin, ed., *Ralph Bunche: The Man and His Times* (New York: Holmes & Meier, 1990), p. 178. Eytan Walter, *The First Ten Years: A Diplomatic History of Israel* (London: Weidenfeld & Nicolson, 1958), p. 31 ("Have a look").

2. Acheson, *Present at the Creation*, pp. 654–55. The CIA's support of the Free Officers is discussed in a number of sources. See, e.g., Miles Copeland, *The Game of Nations: The Amorality of Power Politics* (New York: Simon & Schuster, 1969), and Wilbur Crane Eveland, *Ropes of Sand: America's Failure in the Middle East* (New York: Norton, 1980). See also Anwar El Sadat, *Revolt on the Nile* (London: A. Windgate, 1957), pp. 117–18. Mohammad Naguib, *Egypt's Destiny: A Personal Statement* (London: Gollancz, 1955), p. 121. Sayed Ahmed, *Nasser and American Foreign Policy, 1952–1956* (London: LAAM, 1987), pp. 39–47. Holland, *America and Egypt*, p. 26 ("a Moslem Billy Graham").

3. Sources on Mossadegh and Operation Ajax abound. See, e.g., Rubin, *Paved with Good Intentions*, pp. 54–61, 62 ("Whether it is in Indo-China"), 63–90, and Mark Hamilton Lytle, *The Origins of the Iranian-American Alliance, 1941–1953*

(New York: Holmes & Meier, 1987), pp. 192–209. See also Stephen Kinzer, *All the Shah's Men: An American Coup and the Roots of Middle East Terror* (Hoboken, N.J.: John Wiley, 2003).

4. *FRUS*, 1955–57, vol. 18: NSC 5436/1 United States Policy on French North Africa, June 1, 1955, pp. 92–93 ("we cannot give"). Matthew Connelly, *A Diplomatic Revolution: Algeria's Fight for Independence and the Origins of the Post–Cold War Era* (New York: Oxford Univ. Press, 2002), pp. 45, 50 ("The French are operating"), 52–58, 123 ("having gone so far"), 153–54. Matthew F. Holland, *America and Egypt: From Roosevelt to Eisenhower* (Westport, Conn.: Praeger, 1996), p. 30. Frederick Quinn, *The French Overseas Empire* (New York: Praeger, 2000), p. 227 ("a vast conspiracy").

5. Dwight David Eisenhower Papers, White House Correspondence, box 3: Eisenhower to Dulles, June 16, 1953; Whitman File, International Series, box 15: Eisenhower to Churchill, April 7, 1953 ("From Foster's personal"). PRO, FO371/102732/14: Report of Lord Salisbury's Conversation with Mr. Dulles, July 11, 1953 ("The old colonial attitude"). Evelyn Shuckburgh, *Descent to Suez: Diaries, 1951–1956*, ed. John Charmley (New York: Norton 1986), p. 229. Hahn, *United States, Great Britain, and Egypt*, pp. 161–64.

6. I have written extensively on Alpha, Gamma, and the search for Arab-Israeli peace in the 1950s. See, e.g., *The Origins of the Second Arab-Israel War: Egypt, Israel, and the Great Powers* (London: Frank Cass, 1992); "Escalation to Suez: The Egypt-Israel Border War, 1949–56," *Journal of Contemporary History* 24, no. 3 (1989); "Secret Efforts to Achieve an Egypt-Israel Settlement prior to the Suez Campaign," *Middle Eastern Studies* 26, no. 3 (1990); "The Diplomatic Struggle for the Negev," *Studies in Zionism* 2, no. 1 (1989). On Omega, see *FRUS*, 1955–1957, vol. 15: Memorandum from the Secretary of State to the President, March 28, 1956, p. 410; Diary Entry by the President, March 28, 1956, p. 425. Salim Yaqub, *Containing Arab Nationalism: The Eisenhower Doctrine and the Middle East* (Chapel Hill: Univ. of North Carolina, 2004), pp. 42–45. On King Saud's visit to the United States, see Nathan J. Citino, *From Arab Nationalism to Opec: Eisenhower, King Sa'ūd, and the Making of U.S.-Saudi Relations* (Bloomington: Indiana Univ., 2002), pp. 122–23, 135, and Rachel Bronson, *Thicker Than Oil: America's Uneasy Partnership with Saudi Arabia* (Oxford: Oxford Univ., 2006), pp. 74–75.

7. PRO, CAB 128/30, July 27, 1956. USNA, 974.7301/7-2756: Paris to Department, July 27, 1956; 974.7301/6-158: Suez Canal Problem, 1954–58, June 1, 1958. Philip Ziegler, *Mountbatten* (London: Collins, 1985), pp. 537–38. Anthony Gorst and Scott W. Lucas, "Suez 1956: Strategy and the Diplomatic Process," *Journal of Strategic Studies* 23, no. 1 (1988): 399–400. Robert Rhodes James, *Anthony Eden* (London: Weidenfeld & Nicolson, 1986), p. 166 ("My object"). Bernard Ménager et al., eds., *Guy Mollet: Un camarade en république* (Lille: Presses Universitaires de Lille, 1987), p. 476 ("totally dependent").

8. DDE, Dulles Papers, Subject Series, Telephone Calls, box 5: Allen Dulles to Secretary Dulles, Oct. 30, 1956; Dulles to Eisenhower, Oct. 30, 1956; The Secretary

to Allen Dulles, Oct. 30, 1956. PRO, PREM 11/1105: Washington to Foreign Office Oct. 30, 1956. DDF, III, 1956, 93–95.

9. *British Broadcasting Company: Summary of World Broadcasts*, pt. 4, *The Arab World, Israel, Greece, Turkey, Persia*: Voice of the Arabs, Jan. 9, 1957; Voice of the Arabs, Jan. 18, 1957. Yaqub, *Containing Arab Nationalism*, pp. 71–90, 205–12, 221–23, 224, 225–36. Alan Dowty, *Middle East Crisis: U.S. Decision-Making in 1958, 1970 and 1973* (Berkeley: Univ. of California Press, 1984), pp. 27–35, 56, 80. See also Michael B. Oren, "Israel, the Great Powers, and the Middle East Crisis of 1958," *Studies in Zionism* 12, no. 2 (1992). For insights into the film *Ben-Hur*, I am indebted to one of my Harvard students, John Taylor Hebden.

10. Warren Bass, *Support Any Friend: Kennedy's Middle East and the Making of the U.S.-Israel Alliance* (Oxford: Oxford Univ. Press, 2003), pp. 4, 73, 79 ("immense satisfaction"), 100, 111, 128. Douglas Little, "The New Frontier on the Nile: JFK, Nasser, and Arab Nationalism," *Journal of American History* 75, no. 2 (1988): 500 ("somehow represented yesterday"), 502, 504, 510–13, 521–24. Robert Dallek, *An Unfinished Life: John F. Kennedy, 1917–1963* (Boston: Little, Brown, 2003), p. 222 ("The single most important"). Michael B. Oren, *Six Days of War: June 1967 and the Making of the Modern Middle East* (New York: Oxford Univ. Press, 2002), p. 14.

11. Bass, *Support Any Friend*, pp. 145–49, 158, 185–90. Avner Cohen, *Israel and the Bomb* (New York: Columbia Univ. Press, 1998), pp. 99–107, 108 ("A woman should not"), 155 ("seriously jeopardized"). Mordechai Gazit, *President Kennedy's Policy toward the Arab States and Israel: Analysis and Documents* (Tel Aviv: Tel Aviv Univ., 1983), pp. 18, 33, 42, 46–47. Spiegel, *Other Arab-Israeli Conflict*, pp. 110–12. Oren, *Six Days of War*, pp. 16–17. The transcript of the Kennedy–Ben-Gurion meeting at the Waldorf is available online at http://www .jewishvirtuallibrary.org/jsource/US-Israel/FRUS05_30_61.html.

12. William J. Burns, *Economic Aid and American Policy toward Egypt, 1955–1981* (Albany: State Univ. Press of New York, 1985), p. 159 ("go drink"). Richard B. Parker, *The Politics of Miscalculation in the Middle East* (Bloomington: Indiana Univ., 1993), p. 105. P. J. Vatikiotis, *Nasser and His Generation* (New York: St. Martin's, 1978), pp. 202–12. Mahmoud Riad, *The Struggle for Peace in the Middle East* (New York: Quartet Books, 1981), pp. 15–17.

13. Lyndon Baines Johnson Presidential Library, National Security file, Middle East, Israel boxes 140, 141: Conflicting U.S. Attitudes toward Military Aid to Israel, April 20, 1967; U.S.-Israel Relations, Nov. 3, 1967. USNA, Middle East Crisis files, 1967, Lot file 68D135, box 1: United States Statements on Israel: Johnson Statements, June 1, 1964. William B. Quandt, "The Conflict in American Foreign Policy," in Itamar Rabinovich and Haim Shaked, eds., *From June to October: The Middle East between 1967 and 1973* (New Brunswick: Transaction, 1978), pp. 5–6. I. L. Kenen, *Israel's Defense Line: Her Friends and Foes in Washington* (Buffalo: Prometheus, 1981), p. 173 ("You have lost"). Douglas Little, "The Making of a Special Relationship: The United States and Israel, 1957–68," *International Journal*

of Middle East Studies 25, no. 4 (Nov. 1993): 274–75. Michael Karpin, *The Bomb in the Basement: How Israel Went Nuclear and What That Means for the World* (New York: Simon & Schuster, 2006), p. 243 ("Take care of the Jews" and "If Israel is destroyed").

14. USNA, Middle East Crisis, Chronology June 4th–7th, box 15: Memorandum for the Middle East Task Force, May 29, 1967 ("Let us not forget"). LBJ, National Security File, History of the Middle East Conflict, box 17: Memorandum for the Record, The Arab-Israeli Crisis, May 27, 1967 ("If Israel fires first"); box 20: United States Policy and Diplomacy in the Middle East Crisis, May 15–June 10, 1967, pp. 56–59 ("Israel will not be alone" and "I failed"); History of the Middle East Conflict; box 19: Memorandum for the Record, Washington–Moscow "Hotline" Exchange, Oct. 22, 1968; Kosygin to Johnson, June 10, 1967 (10:00 a.m.); Johnson to Kosygin (10:58 a.m.); Movements of Sixth Fleet, June 10, 1967; The President in the Middle East Crisis, Dec. 19, 1968; Richard Helms Oral History; Llewellyn Thompson Oral History. Oren, *Six Days of War*, pp. 102–16, 164 ("Our goal"), 262–71.

15. Craig A. Daigle, "The Russians Are Going: Sadat, Nixon and the Soviet Presence in Egypt, 1970–1971," *Middle East Review of International Affairs* 8, no. 1 (March 2004): 3 ("The difference between"). William B. Quandt, *Peace Process: American Diplomacy and the Arab-Israeli Conflict since 1967*, 3d ed. (Washington, D.C.: Brookings Institution Press, 2005), pp. 67–68. Nadav Safran, *Israel: The Embattled Ally* (Cambridge: Belknap Press, 1978), p. 441. Thomas Wheelock, "Arms for Israel: The Limit of Leverage," *International Security* 3, no. 2 (1987): 124–26. *FRUS*, 1969–76, vol. E-5, Documents on Africa, 1969–72: Buchanan to the President, Feb. 18, 1970 ("Israel is the current"), on http://www.state.gov/r/pa/ho/frus/nixon/e5/54756.htm.

16. Quandt, *Peace Process*, pp. 77, 89–102. Daigle, "Russians Are Going," pp. 4 ("You would be mistaken"), 7 ("There is no reason"). Henry A. Kissinger, *Diplomacy* (New York: Simon & Schuster, 1994), pp. 738–39. Henry A. Kissinger, *White House Years* (Boston: Little, Brown, 1979), pp. 596, 603, 622–23, 626.

17. George Washington University, National Security Archive, "The October War and U.S. Policy," Document 63: Secretary's Staff Meeting, Oct. 23, 1973, p. 6 ("We could not make"), http://www.gwu.edu/~nsarchiv/NSAEBB/NSAEBB98/. Henry A. Kissinger, *Crisis: The Anatomy of Two Major Foreign Policy Crises* (New York: Simon & Schuster, 2003), pp. 43, 291, 317 ("It was a tremendous"), 340 ("We may have to take"). Alexander M. Haig Jr., with Charles McCarry, *Inner Circles: How America Changed the World: A Memoir* (New York: Warner, 1992), pp. 409, 411 ("Whatever it takes"), 412–17.

18. Anwar El Sadat, *In Search of Identity: An Autobiography* (New York: Harper & Row, 1977), pp. 292–95. Abba Eban, *Personal Witness: Israel through My Eyes* (New York: Putnam, 1992), pp. 570–72. Kenneth W. Stein, *Heroic Diplomacy: Sadat, Kissinger, Carter, Begin, and the Quest for Arab-Israeli Peace* (New York: Routledge, 1999), pp. 146–63, 175–79. George Washington University, National

Security Archive, "The October War and U.S. Policy," Document 63: Secretary's Staff Meeting, Oct. 23, 1973, p. 7 ("The Europeans behaved"), http://www.gwu.edu/~nsarchiv/NSAEBB/NSAEBB98/. Rashid Khalidi, *Resurrecting Empire: Western Footprints and America's Perilous Path in the Middle East* (Boston: Beacon, 2005), pp. 43 ("covert action"), 131.

19. Bill Adler, ed., *The Wit and Wisdom of Jimmy Carter* (Secaucus, N.J.: Citadel, 1977), pp. 68, 139 ("significant moral principle"). Jimmy Carter, *Living Faith* (New York: Three Rivers Press, 2001), pp. 22–24, 36 ("fellowship of faith"). Zbigniew Brzezinski, *Power and Principle: Memoirs of the National Security Adviser, 1977–1981* (New York: Farrar, Straus and Giroux, 1983), p. 27 ("After a couple of hours"). Douglas Brinkley, *The Unfinished Presidency: Jimmy Carter's Journey beyond the White House* (New York: Viking, 1998), p. 114. Seyom Brown, *The Faces of Power: Constancy and Change in United States Foreign Policy from Truman to Reagan* (New York: Columbia Univ., 1983), pp. 454–56. Jimmy Carter, *The Blood of Abraham: Insights into the Middle East*, new ed. (Fayetteville: Univ. of Arkansas Press, 1993), pp. 29, 193 ("The blood of Abraham").

20. Brown, *Faces of Power*, pp. 482–83, 489, 502. Quandt, *Peace Process*, pp. 188–90, 198–203. Brzezinski, *Power and Principle*, pp. 83, 87, 100, 105, 110–11, 117, 237–38, 242, 254–71, 284 ("You are probably"). Jimmy Carter, *Keeping Faith: Memoirs of a President* (New York: Bantam, 1982), pp. 279, 293, 296–97, 496 ("The Camp David Accords"). Saadia Touval, *The Peace Brokers: Mediators in the Arab-Israeli Conflict, 1948–1979* (Princeton: Princeton Univ. Press, 1982), pp. 291–314. Moshe Dayan, *Breakthrough: A Personal Account of the Egypt-Israel Peace Negotiations* (New York: Knopf, 1981), pp. 17, 89–99, 117, 126. On Carter's relationship with evangelical Christians, see Donald Wagner, "Evangelicals and Israel: Theological Roots of a Political Alliance," *Christian Century*, Nov. 4, 1998, p. 1024 ("The time has come").

21. The lyrics for "Midnight at the Oasis," written by David Nichtern, can be found at http://www.webfitz.com/lyrics/Lyrics/1974/131974.html. Said, *Orientalism*, pp. 27, 204, 59–60, 316, 319, 322. Edward W. Said, "Islam through Western Eyes," *Nation*, March 26, 1980. Meir Litvak and Joshua Teitelbaum, "Students, Teachers and Edward Said: Taking Stock of Orientalism," *Middle East Review of International Affairs* 10, no. 1 (March 2006): 3 ("to discover"). Bernard Lewis, *What Went Wrong: The Clash between Islam and Modernity in the Middle East* (New York: Perennial, 2003), pp. 151 ("Compared with its millennial"), 152–53. "Orientalism: An Exchange," *New York Review of Books*, Aug. 12, 1982, pp. 44 ("willful political assertions"), 46 ("beneath the umbrella"), 48 ("a genuine problem").

22. Mark Bowden, *Guests of the Ayatollah: The First Battle in America's War with Militant Islam* (New York: Atlantic Monthly, 2006), pp. 33, 38, 69 ("undermined the political"), 115 ("island of stability"), 125 ("The people of the United States"), 211, 218, 287, 313 ("Death to the Three"), 360, 479, 563, 564. Kenneth M. Pollack, *The Persian Puzzle: The Conflict between Iran and America* (New York: Random House, 2004), pp. 153–80. Brown, *Faces of Power*, pp. 515 ("Our rela-

tions with"), 524, 560 ("An attempt by"). Carter, *Keeping Faith*, pp. 458 ("It's almost impossible"), 466–67, 569.

28. The Thirty Years' War

1. Ronald Reagan, *Reagan, in His Own Hand*, ed. Kiron K. Skinner, Annelise Anderson, and Martin Anderson (New York: Simon & Schuster, 2001), p. 213. Ronald Reagan, *An American Life* (New York: Simon & Schuster, 1990), p. 518 ("He's not only a barbarian"). Alexander M. Haig Jr., *Caveat: Realism, Reagan, and Foreign Policy* (New York: Macmillan, 1984), pp. 182–84. "Israeli Jews Destroy Iraqi Atomic Reactor; Attack Condemned by U.S. and Arab Nations," *New York Times*, June 9, 1981, p. 1.

2. Reagan, *American Life*, pp. 442, 423 ("We're walking a tightrope"), 424 ("No matter how villainous"), 425–28, 430. Haig, *Caveat*, pp. 180–81, 186. Quandt, *Peace Process,* pp. 251, 252, 253–59. Spiegel, *Other Arab-Israeli Conflict*, pp. 416–26. Fred Lawson, "The Reagan Administration in the Middle East," *MERIP Reports*, no. 128 (Nov. 1984): 32. On the Arafat evacuation, see Barry Rubin and Judith Colp Rubin, *Yasir Arafat: A Political Biography* (Oxford: Oxford Univ., 2003), pp. 77, 86–89. On the role of the USS *New Jersey*, visit the battleship's website at http://www.battleshipnewjersey.org/history.html.

3. Reagan, *American Life*, pp. 496 ("Once again"), 497–507, 518 ("Any nation victimized"). Terry A. Anderson, *Den of Lions: Memoirs of Seven Years* (New York: Crown, 1993). Numerous websites document the terrorist attacks against the United States in the 1980s; see, e.g., "Target America," http://www.pbs.org/wgbh/pages/frontline/shows/target/etc/cron.html, and "Lebanon: The Hostage Crisis," http://www.country-data.com/cgi-bin/query/r-8105.html.

4. Lawrence E. Walsh, *Iran-Contra: The Final Report* (New York: Times Books, 1994), pp. 1–3, 10–24. Reagan, *American Life*, pp. 505–6 ("We wouldn't be shipping"), 516 ("I did not think"). Douglas A. Borer, "Inverse Engagement: Lessons from U.S.-Iraq Relations, 1982–1990," *Parameters* 33, no. 2 (2003): 52 ("No one had any doubts"), 53–56. Dana Priest, "Trip Followed Criticism of Chemical Arms' Use," *Washington Post*, Dec. 19, 2003, p. 42. Steve Coll, *Ghost Wars: The Secret History of the CIA, Afghanistan, and Bin Laden, from the Soviet Invasion to September 10, 2001* (New York: Penguin, 2005), p. 229 ("nation of beasts"). Numerous documents on American support for Saddam have been posted on the Web; see, e.g., "Saddam's Iron Grip: Intelligence Reports on Saddam Hussein's Reign," http://www.gwu.edu/~nsarchiv/NSAEBB/NSAEBB167/.

5. Kathleen Christison, "The Arab-Israeli Policy of George Shultz," *Journal of Palestine Studies* 18, no. 2 (1989): 29–47. Quandt, *Peace Process*, pp. 367–80. David Ignatius, "The Secret History of the U.S.-PLO Terror Talks," *Washington Post*, Dec. 4, 1988.

6. On Bush's comparisons of Saddam to Hitler and the protests they provoked from Jewish groups, see Allison Kaplan, "U.S Apologizes for Hitler Remark,"

Jerusalem Post, Nov. 7, 1991. Michael Kelly, *Martyrs' Day: Chronicle of a Small War* (New York: Vintage, 1993), pp. 120–21 ("I've been in the army"). H. Norman Schwarzkopf, with Peter Petre, *It Doesn't Take a Hero: The Autobiography* (New York: Bantam, 1992), p. 319 ("Saddam was what"). Colin Powell, with Joseph E. Persico, *My American Journey* (New York: Random House, 1995), pp. 461–71, 511–13. James Mann, *The Rise of the Vulcans: The History of Bush's War Cabinet* (New York: Penguin, 2004), pp. 185–91, 193 ("Our practical intention"). Coll, *Ghost Wars*, p. 229 ("It is not the world"). James A. Baker III and Thomas M. Defrank, *The Politics of Diplomacy: Revolution, War and Peace, 1989–1992* (New York: Putnam, 1995), pp. 262–63, 272–73, 277 ("What the President did"). "The Religion of George H. W. Bush," http://www.adherents.com/people/pb/George_HW_Bush.html ("Americans are the most religious"). Bush's "New World Order" speech is available online at "Bab—An Open Door to the Arab World," http://www.al-bab.com/arab/docs/pal/pa110.htm.

7. Dennis Ross, *The Missing Peace: The Inside Story of the Fight for Middle East Peace* (New York: Farrar, Straus and Giroux, 2004), pp. 68, 71–81. Baker and Defrank, *Politics of Diplomacy*, pp. 488 ("a rich tale"), 512 ("Like the walls"). David Horovitz, "Blunt Baker Urges Israel to Talk Peace," *Jerusalem Post*, June 14, 1990.

8. *Aladdin* lyrics, original and altered, appeared on http://www.angelfire.com/movies/disneybroadway/aladdin.html. Martin Kramer, *Ivory Towers on Sand: The Failure of Middle Eastern Studies in America* (Washington, D.C.: Washington Institute of Near East Policy, 2001), pp. 1, 5. Samuel P. Huntington, *The Clash of Civilizations and the Remarking of World Order* (New York: Simon & Schuster, 1996), pp. 217–18 ("The underlying problem").

9. Coll, *Ghost Wars*, pp. 249–56. "Text of Clinton Statement on Iraq, Feb. 17, 1998," http://www.cnn.com/ALLPOLITICS/1998/02/17/transcripts/clinton.iraq/ ("unholy axis"). Bill Clinton, *My Life: The Presidential Years* (Westminster, Md.: Knopf, 2005), p. 40 ("I was pleased"). Laurie Mylroie, "U.S. Policy toward Iraq," *Middle East Intelligence Bulletin* 3, no. 1 (Jan. 2001).

10. Clinton, *My Life: The Presidential Years*, pp. 78–79, 100–1 ("Now the horns"), 102–3, 104 ("Shalom, salaam, peace"), 244–45, 281 ("We had become friends"). Bill Clinton, *My Life: The Early Years* (Westminster, Md.: Knopf, 2005), p. 466 ("God will never"). David Horovitz, ed., *Yitzhak Rabin: Solider of Peace* (London: Peter Halban, 1996), pp. 115–22. Shimon Peres, *Battling for Peace: Memoirs*, ed. David Landau (London: Weidenfeld & Nicolson, 1995), pp. 335–37, 343–44. Dennis Ross, *Missing Peace*, pp. 101–21. Quandt, *Peace Process*, pp. 327–31. Connie Bruck, "The Wounds of Peace," *New Yorker*, Oct. 14, 1996.

11. Clinton, *My Life: The Presidential Years*, pp. 448–49 ("fanatics and killers"), 634–35 ("I am not a great man"), 642–46. Madeleine Albright, with Bill Woodward, *Madam Secretary* (New York: Miramax, 2003), pp. 289, 291, 294–95, 317, 490–91, 497. Douglas Waller, "A Frantic Hunt for Peace," http://www.cnn.com/ALLPOLITICS/time/2000/10/16/peace.html ("Close the gate!"). See also Robert

Malley and Hussein Agha, "Camp David: The Tragedy of Errors," *New York Review of Books*, Aug. 9, 2001. Coll, *Ghost Wars*, pp. 329, 376–77, 379, 380 ("Every Muslim"), 395–96, 405–15, 436 ("We are at war").

12. Richard Bernstein et al., *Out of the Blue: The Story of September 11, 2001, from Jihad to Ground Zero* (New York: Times Books, 2002), pp. 7, 25–26, 120–21, 131–39, 184 ("Please have fun"). CNN Breaking News, Sept. 11, 2001, Transcript # 091174CN, p. 4 ("these are Islamic terrorists").

13. Bob Woodward, *Plan of Attack* (New York: Simon & Schuster, 2004), pp. 26, 89, 112, 132, 154, 293, 317. Michael R. Gordon and Bernard E. Trainor, *Cobra II: The Inside Story of the Invasion and Occupation of Iraq* (New York: Pantheon, 2006), pp. 14–19, 36–40, 50–53, 93–94, 104, 108, 160–65. "Bush Delivers Graduation Speech at West Point," http://www.whitehouse.gov/news/releases/2002/06/20020601-3.html. Bush's statement on the Senate and House vote authorizing the war in Iraq can be found on the White House website, http://www.whitehouse.gov/news/releases/2002/10/20021016-11.html. Powell's Feb. 5 testimony to the Security Council appears on the U.S. State Department website, http://www.state.gov/secretary/former/powell/remarks/2003/17300.htm.

14. Gordon and Trainor, *Cobra II*, pp. 436–37. John Keegan, *Iraq War: The Military Offensive, from Victory in 21 Days to the Insurgent Aftermath* (Westminster, Md.: Knopf, 2005), pp. 204–10, 428, 448–50, 457–61, 475, 484–85, 493. L. Paul Bremer III, *My Year in Iraq: The Struggle to Build a Future of Hope* (New York: Simon & Schuster, 2006), pp. 14, 39–42, 57. "President Outlines Steps to Help Iraq Achieve Democracy and Freedom," http://www.whitehouse.gov/news/releases/2004/05/20040524-10.html. "Iraqi Smart Culture Card," http://cryptome.org/iraq-culture.htm. *A Short Guide to Iraq* (Washington, D.C.: War and Navy Departments, 1943), p. 5. Brian Turner, "What Every Soldier Should Know," *Here, Bullet* (Farmington, Me.: Alice James Books, 2005), reprinted with the permission of Alice James Books. Fouad Ajami, "Heart of Darkness," *Wall Street Journal*, Sept. 28, 2005. Francis Fukuyama, *America at the Crossroads: Democracy, Power, and the Neoconservative Legacy* (New Haven: Yale Univ. Press, 2006), p. 181 ("a self-fulfilling prophecy"). Christopher Hitchens, "The Perils of Withdrawal," *Slate*, Nov. 29, 2005. Thomas L. Friedman, "Budgets of Mass Destruction," *New York Times*, Feb. 1, 2004.

Bibliography

Archives and Libraries

Amin Rihani Papers, Library of Congress
Andrew Jackson Papers (microfilm) (Wilmington, Del.: Scholarly Resources, 1986)
Central Zionist Archives (CZA), Jerusalem
Cleveland Plain Dealer Archive
Cornelius Van H. Engert Papers, Georgetown Univ.
Cornell Univ. Library, Making of America Collection (MOA)
Franklin Delano Roosevelt Papers, Library of Congress
Harry S. Truman Presidential Museum and Library (online)
Henry Morgenthau Papers, Library of Congress
James M. Landis Papers, Library of Congress
Joel Barlow Papers, New York Public Library
John Fitzgerald Kennedy Presidential Library, Boston
John Jay Papers, Columbia Univ., New York
Karl S. Twitchell Papers, Princeton Univ.
Mariners' Museum Library, Washington, D.C.
New Hampshire Historical Society, Tuck Library
Oscar Straus Papers, Library of Congress
Papers of the American Board of Commissions for Foreign Missions (PABCFM), Bilkent Univ., Turkey
Public Record Office (PRO—British Foreign Office Documents), copies located at the Israel National Archives, Jerusalem
Thomas Jefferson Papers, American Memory Project, Library of Congress

Thomas Jefferson Papers, Princeton Univ.
United States National Archives (USNA)
William Blackstone Papers, Wheaton Univ.
William Eaton Papers (WEP), Huntington Library, San Marino, Calif.
William H. Seward Papers, Univ. of Rochester
William L. Westermann Paris Peace Conference Diaries, Columbia Univ.
William Tecumseh Sherman Papers, Notre Dame Univ.
William Yale Oral History, Columbia Univ.

Published Documents

The Adams-Jefferson Letters: The Complete Correspondence between Thomas Jefferson and Abigail and John Adams. Edited by Lester J. Cappon. Chapel Hill: Univ. of North Carolina Press, 1959.

Annals of the Congress of the United States: Third Congress. Washington, D.C.: Gales and Seaton, 1849.

Circular Letters of Congressmen to Their Constituents, 1789–1829. Edited by Noble Cunningham. Chapel Hill: Univ. of North Carolina Press, 1978.

The Conferences at Washington, 1941–1942, and Casablanca, 1943. Washington, D.C.: GPO, 1968.

The Debate on the Constitution. Edited by Bernard Bailyn. Washington, D.C.: Library of America, 1993.

Defending the West: The Truman-Churchill Correspondence, 1945–1960. Edited by G. W. Sand. Westport, Conn.: Praeger, 2004.

Diary and Autobiography of John Adams. Vol. 3, *Diary 1782–1804.* Cambridge: Harvard Univ. Press, Belknap Press, 1961.

The Documentary History of the Ratification of the Constitution. Edited by John Kaminksi and Gaspare Saladino. Madison: State Historical Society of Wisconsin, 2001.

Documents on British Foreign Policy, 1919–1939. Edited by Rohan Butler and J. P. T. Bury. London: Her Majesty's Stationery Office, 1963.

The Emerging Nation: A Documentary History of the Foreign Relations of the United States under the Articles of Confederation, 1780–1789. Edited by Mary Giunta. Washington, D.C.: National Historical Publications and Records Commission, 1996.

The Family Letters of Thomas Jefferson. Edited by Edwin Bettis and James Bear Jr. Columbia: Univ. of Missouri Press, 1966.

Foreign Relations of the United States (FRUS). Vols. from 1861 to 1948. Washington, D.C.: GPO.

The Intimate Papers of Colonel House. Edited by Charles Seymour. 4 vols. Boston: Houghton Mifflin, 1926–28.

Lafayette in the Age of the American Revolution. Edited by Stanley Idzerda and Robert Crout. Ithaca: Cornell Univ. Press, 1983.

Letters of Delegates to Congress, 1774–1789. Edited by Paul Smith. Washington, D.C.: Library of Congress, 1995.

The Letters of Louis D. Brandeis. Edited by Melvin I. Urofsky and David M. Levy. Albany: State Univ. of New York, 1973.

The Letters of Richard Henry Lee. Edited by James Ballagh. New York: Macmillan, 1914.

The Letters of Theodore Roosevelt. Edited by Elting Morison. Cambridge: Harvard Univ. Press, 1954.

The Life and Correspondence of Rufus King. Edited by Charles King. New York: Putnam, 1894.

Life and Letters of George Perkins Marsh. New York: Scribner, 1888.

Messages and Papers of the Presidents, 1789–1897. Edited by James D. Richardson. New York: Bureau of National Literature, 1917.

The Missionary Herald: Reports from Ottoman Syria, 1819–1870. Edited by Kamal Salibi and Yusuf Khoury. Amman: Royal Institute for Inter-faith Studies, 1995.

Naval Documents Related to the United States Wars with the Barbary Powers. 6 vols. Edited by Dudley Knox. Washington, D.C.: GPO, 1939–44.

New England Merchants in Africa: A History through Documents, 1802–1865. Edited by Norman Bennett and George Brooks. Boston: Boston Univ. Press, 1965.

Ninth Annual Report of the Smithsonian Institution. Washington, D.C.: Beverley Tucker, 1855.

Official Records of the Union and Confederate Navies in the War of the Rebellion. Washington, D.C.: GPO, 1894.

The Papers of Alexander Hamilton. Edited by Harold C. Syrett. 27 vols. New York: Columbia Univ. Press, 1961–87.

The Papers of Daniel Webster. Ser. 3, *Diplomatic Papers.* Vol. 1. Hanover: Univ. Press of New England, 1983.

The Papers of Dwight David Eisenhower. Edited by Alfred Chandler. Baltimore: Johns Hopkins Univ. Press, 1970.

The Papers of George Mason, 1725–1792. Edited by Robert Rutland. Chapel Hill: Univ. of North Carolina Press, 1970.

The Papers of George Washington. Edited by W. W. Abbit. Charlottesville: Univ. Press of Virginia, 1995.

The Papers of James Madison: Secretary of State Series 1801. Charlottesville: Univ. Press of Virginia, 1986.

The Papers of Jefferson Davis. Vol. 6, *1856–1860.* Edited by Lynda Crist and Mary Dix. Baton Rouge: Louisiana State Univ. Press, 1989.

The Papers of Josiah Bartlett. Edited by Frank Mevers. Hanover: Univ. Press of New England, 1979.

The Papers of Julia Dent Grant. Edited by John Simon. New York: Putnam, 1975.

The Papers of Woodrow Wilson. Edited by Arthur Link. 69 vols. Princeton: Princeton Univ. Press, 1966–94.

The Republic of Letters: The Correspondence between Thomas Jefferson and James Madison, 1776–1826. Edited by James Morton Smith. New York: Norton, 1995.

The Revolutionary War Diplomatic Correspondences of the United States. Edited by Francis Wharton. Washington, D.C.: GPO, 1889.

Selections from the Correspondence of Theodore Roosevelt and Henry Cabot Lodge, 1884–1918. New York: Scribner's, 1925.

Treaties and Other International Acts of the United States of America. Edited by Hunter Miller. Vol. 3. Washington, D.C.: GPO, 1933.

The White House Papers of Harry Hopkins. Edited by Robert Sherwood. London: Eyre and Spottiswoode, 1949.

The Writings of Albert Gallatin. Edited by Henry Adams. Vol. 1. New York: Antiquarian Press, 1960.

The Writings of Benjamin Franklin, 1789–1790. Edited by Albert Henry Smyth. New York: Macmillan, 1904. Reprint, New York: Haskell House, 1970.

The Writings of George Washington from the Original Manuscript Sources, 1745–1799. Edited by John C. Fitzpatrick. 39 vols. Washington, D.C.: GPO, 1931–44.

The Writings of Thomas Jefferson. Edited by Andrew A. Lipscomb. Washington, D.C.: Thomas Jefferson Memorial Association, 1905.

The Writings of Thomas Jefferson. Edited by Paul Ford. New York: Putnam, 1970.

Newspapers and Journals

Century Illustrated Monthly Magazine
Harper's New Monthly Magazine
Ladies' Magazine
Littell's Living Age
London Daily Mail
Los Angeles Times
New Englander and Yale Review
New York Daily Tribune
New York Times
Niles' Weekly Register
Princeton Review
Scribner's Monthly
Stars and Stripes (Cairo edition)
United States Democratic Review
Whig Review

Books

Aaronsohn, Alexander. *With the Turks in Palestine*. Boston: Houghton Mifflin, 1916.

Abraham, Sameer, ed. *Arabs in the New World: Studies in Arab-American Communities*. Detroit: Wayne State Univ., 1983.

Abu-Ghazaleh, Adnan. *American Missions in Syria: A Study of American Missionary Contributions to Arab Nationalism in 19th Century Syria*. Brattleboro, Vt.: Amana Books, 1990.

Acheson, Dean. *Present at the Creation: My Years in the State Department*. Toronto: George-McLeod, 1969.

Adler, Bill, ed. *The Wit and Wisdom of Jimmy Carter*. Secaucus, N.J.: Citadel, 1977.

Adler, Cyrus. *Jacob H. Schiff: His Life and Letters*. London: William Heinemann, 1929.

———. *Jews in the Diplomatic Correspondence of the United States*. Baltimore: Friedenwald, 1906.

Ahmad, Feroz. *The Making of Modern Turkey*. New York: Routledge, 1993.

Ahmed, Sayed. *Nasser and American Foreign Policy, 1752–1756*. London: LAAM, 1987.

Akçam, Taner. *A Shameful Act: The Armenian Genocide and the Question of Turkish Responsibility*. New York: Metropolitan Books, 2006.

Albright, Madeleine, with Bill Woodward. *Madam Secretary*. New York: Miramax, 2003.

Allen, Felicity. *Jefferson Davis: Unconquerable Heart*. Columbia: Univ. of Missouri Press, 1999.

Allen, Gardner W. *Our Navy and the Barbary Corsairs*. Boston: Houghton Mifflin, 1905.

Allibone, Samuel Austin. *A Critical Dictionary of English Literature, and British and American Authors*. Philadelphia: Lippincott, 1871.

Allison, Mary B. *Doctor Mary in Arabia: Memoirs*. Edited by Sandra Shaw. Austin: Univ. of Texas Press, 1994.

Allison, Robert J. *The Crescent Obscured: The United States and the Muslim World, 1776–1815*. New York: Oxford Univ. Press, 1995.

Amanat, Abbas, and Magnus T. Bernhardsson, eds. *The United States and the Middle East: Cultural Encounters*. New Haven: Yale Center for International and Area Studies, 2002.

Ambrosius, Lloyd E. *Woodrow Wilson and the American Diplomatic Tradition*. Cambridge: Cambridge Univ. Press, 1987.

The American Annual Register, 1827–1829. New York: Blunt, 1830.

American Geographical and Statistical Society. *Report and Memorial on Syrian Exploration*. New York: New York Univ., 1857.

The American in Algiers; or, The Patriot of Seventy-six in Captivity. New York: J. Buel, 1797.

Ammon, Harry. *James Monroe: The Quest for National Identity*. New York: McGraw-Hill, 1971.

Anderson, Irvine. *Aramco, the United States, and Saudi Arabia: A Study of the Dynamics of Foreign Oil Policy, 1933–1950*. Princeton: Princeton Univ. Press, 1981.

Anderson, R. C. *Naval Wars in the Levant, 1559–1853*. Princeton: Princeton Univ. Press, 1952.

Anderson, Terry A. *A Den of Lions: Memoirs of Seven Years*. New York: Crown, 1993.

Ani, Moukhtar. *Saudi Arabia: Its People, Its Society, Its Culture.* New Haven: HRAF Press, 1959.

Antonius, George. *The Arab Awakening.* London: Hamish Hamilton, 1938.

The Arabian Nights Entertainment: Consisting of One Thousand and One Stories, the First American Edition, Freely Transcribed from the Original Translation by Galland. Baltimore: H. & P. Rice and J. Rice, 1794.

Arberry, Arthur J. *The Koran Interpreted.* New York: Macmillan, 1955.

Ariel, Yaakov. *On Behalf of Israel: American Fundamentalist Attitudes toward Jews, Judaism, and Zionism, 1865–1945.* Brooklyn: Carlson, 1991.

Armerding, Paul L. *Doctors for the Kingdom: The Work of the American Mission Hospitals in the Kingdom of Saudi Arabia, 1913–1955.* Grand Rapids, Mich.: Eerdmans, 2003.

Armstrong, H. C. *Grey Steel: J. C. Smuts: A Study in Arrogance.* London: Arthur Barker, 1937.

Atkinson, Rick. *An Army at Dawn: The War in North Africa, 1942–1943.* New York: Henry Holt, 2002.

Auchincloss, Louis. *Woodrow Wilson.* New York: Penguin, 2000.

Augur, Helen. *Passage to Glory: John Ledyard's America.* Garden City, N.Y.: Doubleday, 1946.

Baepler, Paul, ed. *White Slaves, African Masters: An Anthology of American Barbary Captivity Narratives.* Chicago: Univ. of Chicago Press, 1999.

Baer, Gabriel, and Amnon Cohen, eds. *Egypt and Palestine: A Millennium of Association (868–1948).* New York: St. Martin's. 1984.

Bailey, Thomas A. *A Diplomatic History of the American People.* Englewood Cliffs, N.J.: Prentice-Hall, 1980.

———. *Woodrow Wilson and the Great Betrayal.* New York: Macmillan, 1947.

Baker, George E., ed. *The Life of William H. Seward, with Selections from His Works.* New York: J. S. Redfield, 1855.

Baker, James A., III, with Thomas M. DeFrank. *The Politics of Diplomacy: Revolution, War, and Peace, 1989–1992.* New York: Putnam, 1995.

Baker, John Martin. *A View of the Commerce of the Mediterranean.* Washington, D.C.: Davis and Force, 1819.

Baker, Ray Stannard. *Woodrow Wilson: Life and Letters, 1856–1890.* Garden City, N.Y.: Doubleday, 1927.

———. *Woodrow Wilson and World Settlement.* Garden City, N.Y.: Doubleday, Page, 1923.

Balakian, Peter. *The Burning Tigris: The Armenian Genocide and America's Response.* New York: HarperCollins, 2003.

Ballaster, Ros. *Fabulous Orients: Fictions of the East in England, 1662–1785.* Oxford: Oxford Univ. Press, 2005.

Bancroft, Frederic. *The Life of William H. Seward.* New York: Harper, 1899.

Baram, Phillip J. *The Department of State in the Middle East, 1919–1945.* Philadelphia: Univ. of Pennsylvania Press, 1978.

Barbour, Philip L. *The Three Worlds of Captain John Smith*. Boston: Houghton Mifflin, 1964.

Barclay, James Turner. *The City of the Great King; or, Jerusalem as It Was, as It Is, and as It Is to Be*. Philadelphia: James Challen, 1857.

Barnby, H. G. *The Prisoners of Algiers: An Account of the Forgotten American-Algerian War, 1785–1797*. New York: Oxford Univ. Press, 1966.

Barrell, George. *Letters from Asia: Written by a Gentleman of Boston, to His Friend in That Place*. New York: A. T. Goodrich, 1819.

Barrows, John D. *In the Land of Ararat*. New York: Revell, 1916.

Bartlett, Irving H. *Daniel Webster*. New York: Norton, 1978.

Bartlett, William H. *The Nile Boat; or, Glimpses of the Land of Egypt*. London: Arthur Hall, Virtue, 1850.

Barton, James. *Story of Near East Relief (1915–1930)*. New York: Macmillan, 1930.

———, ed. *"Turkish Atrocities": Statements of American Missionaries on the Destruction of Christian Communities in Ottoman Turkey, 1915–1917*. Ann Arbor: Gomidas Institute, 1998.

Bar-Zohar, Michael. *Ben-Gurion: A Biography*. Translated by Peretz Kidron. New York: Adama Books, 1977.

Bass, Warren. *Support Any Friend: Kennedy's Middle East and the Making of the U.S.-Israel Alliance*. Oxford: Oxford Univ. Press, 2003.

Beale, Howard K. *Theodore Roosevelt and the Rise of America to World Power*. Baltimore: Johns Hopkins Univ. Press, 1986.

Beaumont, Daniel. *Slave of Desire: Sex, Love, and Death in The 1,001 Nights*. Madison, N.J.: Fairleigh Dickinson Univ. Press, 2002.

Bellows, Henry W. *The Old World in Its New Face*. New York: Harper, 1869.

———. *Restatement of Christian Doctrines in 25 Sermons*. Boston: American Unitarian Association, 1869.

Belohlavek, John M. *Let the Eagle Soar!: The Foreign Policy of Andrew Jackson*. Lincoln: Univ. of Nebraska Press, 1985.

Bemis, Samuel Flagg. *John Quincy Adams and the Foundations of American Foreign Policy*. New York: Knopf, 1956.

Ben-Arieh, Yehoshua. *Painting the Holy Land in the 19th Century*. Jerusalem: Yad Izhak Ben-Zvi, 1997.

Benét, Stephen Vincent. *The Devil and Daniel Webster and Other Writings*. New York: Penguin, 2000.

Benson, Michael T. *Harry S. Truman and the Founding of Israel*. Westport, Conn.: Praeger, 1997.

Bernard, Stephane. *The Franco-Moroccan Conflict, 1943–1953*. New Haven: Yale Univ. Press, 1968.

Bernstein, Richard, et al. *Out of the Blue: The Story of September 11, 2001, from Jihad to Ground Zero*. New York: Times Books, 2002.

Beston, Henry. *The Book of Gallant Vagabonds*. New York: George H. Doran, 1925.

Bill, James. *The Eagle and the Lion: The Tragedy of American-Iranian Relations.* New Haven: Yale Univ. Press, 1988.

Bills, Scott L. *The Libyan Arena: The United States, Britain, and the Council of Foreign Ministers, 1945–1948.* Kent, Ohio: Kent State Univ. Press, 1995.

Bird, Isaac. *Bible Work in Bible Lands.* Philadelphia: Presbyterian Board of Publication, 1872.

Bishop, Jim. *FDR's Last Year.* New York: Morrow: 1974.

Black, Conrad. *Franklin Delano Roosevelt: Champion of Freedom.* London: Weidenfeld & Nicolson, 2003.

Blackstone, William E. *Jesus Is Coming.* Chicago: Revell, 1908.

Bliss, Daniel. *Letters from a New Campus: Written to His Wife Abby and Their Four Children during Their Visit to Amherst, Massachusetts, 1873–1874.* Beirut: American Univ. of Beirut, 1994.

———. *The Reminiscences of Daniel Bliss.* New York: Revell, 1920.

Bloom, Sol. *The Autobiography of Sol Bloom.* New York: Putnam, 1948.

Blyden, Edward Wilmot. *Christianity, Islam and the Negro Race.* Edinburgh: Edinburgh Univ. Press, 1967.

Bolotin, Norman, and Christine Laing. *The World's Columbian Exposition.* Urbana: Univ. of Illinois Press, 2002.

Bond, Alvan. *Memoir of the Rev. Pliny Fisk.* New York: Arno Press, 1977.

Bookin-Weiner, Jerome, and Mohamed El Mansour, eds. *The Atlantic Connection: 200 Years of Moroccan-American Relations.* Rabat: Edino Press, 1990.

Boorstin, Daniel. *The Americans: The National Experience.* New York: Random House, 1965.

Boot, Max. *The Savage Wars of Peace: Small Wars and the Rise of American Power.* New York: Basic Books, 2002.

Boudinot, Elias. *A Star in the West; or, A Humble Attempt to Discover the Long Lost Ten Tribes of Israel, Preparatory to Their Return to Their Beloved City, Jerusalem.* Trenton, N.J: Fenton, Hutchinson, and Dunham, 1816.

Bowden, Mark, *Guest of the Ayatollah: The First Battle in America's War with Militant Islam.* New York: Atlantic Monthly, 2006.

Bowen, Norman. *Lowell Thomas: The Stranger Everyone Knows.* Garden City, N.Y.: Doubleday, 1968.

Brackenridge, Hugh Henry, and Philip Freneau. *Father Bimbo's Pilgrimage to Mecca in Arabia, 1770.* Edited by Michael Davitt Bell. Princeton: Princeton Univ. Library, 1975.

Brandeis, Louis D. *The Jewish Problem: How to Solve It.* New York: Zionist Organization of America, 1919.

Brands, H. W. *Inside the Cold War: Loy Henderson and the Rise of the American Empire, 1918–1961.* New York: Oxford Univ. Press, 1991.

Brant, Irving. *James Madison.* Vol. 6. New York: Bobbs-Merrill, 1961.

Brecher, Frank W. *Reluctant Ally: United States Foreign Policy toward the Jews from Wilson to Roosevelt.* New York: Greenwood, 1991.

Brekus, Catherine A. *Strangers and Pilgrims: Female Preaching in America, 1740–1845.* Chapel Hill: Univ. of North Carolina Press, 1998.

Bremer, L. Paul, with Malcolm McConnell. *My Year in Iraq: The Struggle to Build a Future of Hope.* New York: Simon & Schuster, 2006.

Brewer, Josiah. *A Residence at Constantinople in the Year 1827, with Notes to the Present Time.* New Haven: Durrie and Peck, 1830.

Brinkley, Douglas. *The Unfinished Presidency: Jimmy Carter's Journey beyond the White House.* New York: Viking, 1998.

Brinton, Jasper Yeates. *The American Effort in Egypt: A Chapter in Diplomatic History in the Nineteenth Century.* Alexandria, Va.: Private printing, 1972.

Bronson, Rachel. *Thicker than Oil: America's Uneasy Partnership with Saudi Arabia.* Oxford: Oxford Univ. Press, 2006.

Brown, Anthony C. *Oil, God, and Gold: The Story of Aramco and the Saudi Kings.* Boston: Houghton Mifflin, 1999.

Brown, Cecil. *Suez to Singapore.* New York: Random House, 1942.

Brown, John. T., ed. *Churches of Christ.* Louisville: John P. Morton, 1904.

Brown, Michael. *The Israeli-American Connection: Its Roots in the Yishuv, 1914–1945.* Detroit: Wayne State Univ. Press, 1996.

Brown, Seyom. *The Faces of Power: Constancy and Change in United States Foreign Policy from Truman to Reagan.* New York: Columbia Univ. Press, 1983.

Browne, J. Ross. *Yusef, or, The Journey of the Frangi: A Crusade in the West.* New York: Harper, 1853.

Browne, Walter L. *The Political History of Lebanon, 1920–1950.* Vol. 2. Salisbury, N.C.: Documentary Publications, 1977.

Bruce, Michael. *The Nun of Lebanon.* London: Collins, 1951.

Bryson, Thomas A. *An American Consular Officer in the Middle East in the Jacksonian Era: A Biography of William Brown Hodgson, 1801–1871.* Atlanta: Resurgens Publications, 1979.

———. *American Diplomatic Relations with the Middle East, 1784–1975.* Metuchen, N.J.: Scarecrow Press, 1977.

———. *Seeds of the Mideast Crisis: The United States Diplomatic Role in the Middle East during World War II.* Jefferson, N.C.: McFarland, 1981.

———. *Tars, Turks, and Tankers: The Role of the United States Navy in the Middle East, 1800–1979.* London: Scarecrow, 1980.

———. *United States/Middle East Diplomatic Relations, 1784–1978: An Annotated Bibliography.* Metuchen, N.J.: Scarecrow, 1979.

Brzezinski, Zbigniew. *Power and Principle: Memoirs of the National Security Adviser, 1977–1981.* New York: Farrar, Straus and Giroux, 1983.

Buckingham, Clyde E. *Clara Barton: A Broad Humanity.* Alexandria, Va.: Mount Vernon Publishing, 1977.

Buhite, Russell. *Patrick J. Hurley and American Foreign Policy.* Ithaca: Cornell Univ. Press, 1973.

Burg, David. *Chicago's White City of 1893.* Lexington: Univ. Press of Kentucky, 1976.

Burnham, Daniel, ed. *Final Official Report of the Director of Works of the World's Columbian Exposition.* New York: Garland Publishing, 1989.

Burns, Edward McNall. *The American Idea of Mission: Concepts of National Purpose and Destiny.* New Brunswick: Rutgers Univ. Press, 1957.

Burns, James MacGregor. *Roosevelt: The Soldier of Freedom.* New York: Harcourt Brace Jovanovich, 1970.

Burns, James MacGregor, and Susan Dunn. *The Three Roosevelts: Patrician Leaders Who Transformed America.* New York: Grove Press, 2001.

Burns, William J. *Economic Aid and American Policy toward Egypt, 1955–1981.* Albany: State Univ. Press of New York, 1985.

Burton, David H. *Clara Barton: In the Service of Humanity.* Westport, Conn.: Greenwood, 1995.

———. *Theodore Roosevelt: Confident Imperialist.* Philadelphia: Univ. of Pennsylvania Press, 1968.

Bush, George. *The Life of Mohammed; Founder of the Religion of Islam, and of the Empire of the Saracens.* New York: Harper & Brothers, 1837.

———. *The Valley of Vision.* New York: Saxton and Miles, 1844.

Bush, George, and Brent Snowcroft. *A World Transformed.* New York: Knopf, 1998.

Calverley, Eleanor. *My Arabian Days and Nights.* New York: Crowell, 1958.

Caplan, Neil. *Futile Diplomacy.* Vol. 1. London: Frank Cass, 1983.

Carlton, Donna. *Looking for Little Egypt.* Bloomington, Ind.: IDD Books, 1994.

Carpenter, Teresa. *The Miss Stone Affair: America's First Modern Hostage Crisis.* New York: Simon & Schuster, 2003.

Carter, Jimmy. *The Blood of Abraham: Insights into the Middle East.* New ed. Fayetteville: Univ. of Arkansas Press, 1993.

———. *Keeping Faith: Memoirs of a President.* New York: Bantam, 1982.

———. *Living Faith.* New York: Three Rivers Press, 2001.

Casillas, Rex J. *Oil and Diplomacy: The Evolution of American Foreign Policy in Saudi Arabia, 1933–1945.* New York: Garland, 1987.

Cathcart, James Leander. *Tripoli.* LaPorte, Ind.: Herald Print, 1901.

Celleni, Joseph, ed. *Christian Protagonists for Jewish Restoration.* New York: Arno Press, 1977.

Chaillé-Long, Charles. *My Life in Four Continents.* Vol. 1. London: Hutchinson, 1912.

———. *The Three Prophets: Chinese Gordon, Mohammed-Ahmed (El Maahdi), Arabi Pasha.* New York: Appleton, 1884.

Charny, Israel, ed. *Encyclopedia of Genocide.* Santa Barbara: ABC-CLIO, 1999.

Chernow, Ron. *Alexander Hamilton.* New York: Penguin Press, 2004.

Cherry, Conrad, ed. *God's New Israel: Religious Interpretations of American Destiny.* Chapel Hill: Univ. of North Carolina Press, 1998.

Chidsey, Donald Barr. *The Wars in Barbary: Arab Piracy and the Birth of the United States Navy.* New York: Crown, 1971.

Chireau, Yvonne, and Nathaniel Deutsch. *Black Zion: African American Religious Encounters with Judaism*. New York: Oxford Univ. Press, 2000.

Christy, David. *King Cotton*. Cincinnati: Moore, Wilstach, Keys, 1855.

Citino, Nathan J. *From Arab Nationalism to OPEC: Eisenhower, King Sa'ūd, and the Making of U.S.-Saudi Relations*. Bloomington: Indiana Univ. Press, 2002.

Clark, Mark W. *Calculated Risk*. New York: Harper, 1950.

Cline, Myrtle. *American Attitude toward the Greek War of Independence, 1821–1828*. Atlanta: Higgins-McArthur, 1930.

Clinton, Bill. *My Life: The Early Years*. Westminster, Md.: Knopf, 2005.

———. *My Life: The Presidential Years*. Westminster, Md.: Knopf, 2005.

Clissold, Stephen. *The Barbary Slaves*. London: Paul Elek, 1977.

Cohen, Avner. *Israel and the Bomb*. New York: Columbia Univ. Press, 1998.

Cohen, Michael J. *Palestine and the Great Powers, 1945–1948*. Princeton: Princeton Univ. Press, 1982.

———, ed. *The Anglo-American Committee on Palestine, 1945–1946*. Vol. 35 of *The Rise of Israel: A Documentary Record from the Nineteenth Century to 1948*. Part 1. New York: Garland, 1987.

Cohen, Naomi Wiener. *A Dual Heritage: The Public Career of Oscar S. Straus*. Philadelphia: Jewish Publication Society of America, 1969.

———. *The Year after the Riots: American Responses to the Palestine Crisis of 1929–30*. Detroit: Wayne State Univ., 1988.

Cohen, Roger, and Claudio Gatti. *In the Eye of the Storm: The Life of General H. Norman Schwarzkopf*. New York: Farrar, Straus and Giroux, 1991.

Cole, Donald B. *The Presidency of Andrew Jackson*. Lawrence: Univ. Press of Kansas, 1993.

Coll, Steve. *Ghost Wars: The Secret History of the CIA, Afghanistan, and bin Laden, from the Soviet Invasion to September 10, 2001*. New York: Penguin, 2005.

Collins, Larry, and Dominique Lapierre. *O Jerusalem*. New York: Simon & Schuster, 1972.

Colton, Walter. *Visit to Constantinople and Athens*. New York: Leavitt, Lord, 1836.

Connelly, Matthew. *A Diplomatic Revolution: Algeria's Fight for Independence and the Origins of the Post–Cold War Era*. New York: Oxford Univ. Press, 2002.

Conrad, Lawrence I., ed. *The Formation and Perception of the Modern Arab World*. Princeton, N.J.: Darwin Press, 1990.

Cooley, James Ewing. *The American in Egypt, with Rambles through Arabia Petra and the Holy Land during the Years 1839–1840*. New York: Appleton, 1842.

Coon, Carleton. *A North Africa Story: The Anthropologist as OSS Agent*. Ipswich, Mass.: Gambit Press, 1980.

———, ed. *Daniel Bliss and the Founding of the American Univ. of Beirut*. Washington, D.C: Middle East Institute, 1989.

Cooper, John Milton. *The Warrior and the Priest: Woodrow Wilson and Theodore Roosevelt*. Cambridge: Harvard Univ. Press, 1983.

Copeland, Miles. *The Game of Nations: The Amorality of Power Politics*. London: Weidenfeld & Nicolson, 1969.

Cowdery, Jonathan. *American Captives in Tripoli*. Boston: Belcher & Armstrong, 1806.

Crabitès, Pierre. *Americans in the Egyptian Army*. London: Routledge, 1938.

Crafford, F. S. *Jan Smuts: A Biography*. Garden City, N.Y.: Doubleday, Doran, 1943.

Crawford, Kenneth G. *Report on North Africa*. New York: Farrar and Rinehart, 1943.

Cresson, Warder. *Jerusalem: The Center and Joy of the Universe*. Philadelphia: Self-published, 1844.

———. *The Key of David*. Philadelphia: Self-published, 1852.

———. *King Solomon's Two Women and the Living and Dead Child or Messiah*. Philadelphia: Self-published, 1852.

Cronon, David E., ed. *The Cabinet Diaries of Josephus Daniels, 1913–1921*. Lincoln: Univ. of Nebraska Press, 1963.

Curti, Merle. *American Philanthropy Abroad: A History*. New Brunswick: Rutgers Univ. Press, 1963.

Curtis, Jane, Will Curtis, and Frank Lieberman. *The World of George Perkins Marsh*. Woodstock: Countryman Press, 1982.

Dallek, Robert. *Franklin D. Roosevelt and American Foreign Policy, 1932–1945*. New York: Oxford Univ. Press, 1979.

———. *An Unfinished Life: John F. Kennedy, 1917–1963*. Boston: Little, Brown, 2003.

D'Alton, Martina. *The New York Obelisk*. New York: Metropolitan Museum of Art, 1993.

Davis, John. *The Landscape of Belief: Encountering the Holy Land in Nineteenth-Century American Art and Culture*. Princeton: Princeton Univ. Press, 1996.

Davis, Leslie A. *The Slaughterhouse Province: An American Diplomat's Report on the Armenian Genocide, 1915–1917*. New Rochelle, N.Y.: Aristide D. Caratzas, 1989.

Davis, Moshe, ed. *With Eyes toward Zion*. Vol. 2, *Themes and Sources in the Archives of the United States, Great Britain, Turkey and Israel*. New York: Praeger, 1986. Vol. 3 (with Yehoshua Ben-Arieh), *Western Societies and the Holy Land* (1991). Vol. 4, *America and the Holy Land* (1995). Vol. 5 (with Yehoshua Ben-Arieh), *Jerusalem in the Mind of the Western World, 1800–1948* (1997).

Davis, Robert. *Christian Slaves, Muslim Masters*. New York: Palgrave Macmillan, 2003.

Dawisha, Adeed. *Arab Nationalism in the Twentieth Century: From Triumph to Despair*. Princeton: Princeton Univ. Press, 2003.

Dawn, Ernest C. *From Ottomanism to Arabism: Essays on the Origins of Arab Nationalism*. Urbana: Univ. of Illinois Press, 1973.

Dawson, Nelson, ed. *Brandeis and America*. Lexington: Univ. Press of Kentucky, 1989.

Dayan, Moshe, *Breakthrough: A Personal Account of the Egypt-Israel Peace Negotiations.* New York: Knopf, 1981.

Dearborn, Henry A. S. *The Life of William Bainbridge, Esq., of the United States Navy.* Princeton: Princeton Univ. Press, 1931.

Dearden, Seton. *A Nest of Corsairs.* London: Butler and Tanner, 1976.

DeConde, Alexander. *A History of American Foreign Policy.* New York: Scribner, 1971.

De Kay, James Tertius. *A Rage for Glory: The Life of Commodore Stephen Decatur.* New York: Free Press, 2004.

De Leon, Edwin. *Thirty Years of My Life on Three Continents.* London: Ward and Downey, 1890.

DeNovo, John A. *American Interests and Policies in the Middle East, 1900–1939.* Minneapolis: Univ. of Minnesota Press, 1963.

D'Este, Carlo. *Eisenhower: A Soldier's Life.* New York: Henry Holt, 2002.

Diebels, Mary Chrysostom. *Peter Markoe (1752–1792): A Philadelphia Writer.* Washington, D.C.: Catholic Univ. of America Press, 1944.

Dillman, Richard, ed. *The Major Essays of Henry David Thoreau.* Albany: Whitston, 2001.

Dobkin, Marjorie Housepian. *Smyrna 1922: The Destruction of a City.* Kent, Ohio: Kent State Univ. Press, 1988.

Dobson, John M. *America's Ascent: United States Becomes a Great Power, 1880–1914.* DeKalb: Northern Illinois Univ. Press, 1978.

Dockrill, Michael, ed. *The Paris Peace Conference, 1919: Peace without Victory.* New York: Palgrave, 2001.

Dodwell, Henry H. *The Founder of Modern Egypt: A Study of Muhammad 'Ali.* Cambridge: Cambridge Univ. Press, 1931. Reprint, New York: AMS Press, 1977.

Dolmetsch, Carl. *"Our Famous Guest"—Mark Twain in Vienna.* Athens: Univ. of Georgia Press, 1992.

Donovan, Robert J. *Conflict and Crisis: The Presidency of Harry S. Truman, 1945–1948.* New York: Norton, 1977.

Dorr, David F. *A Colored Man round the World by a Quadroon.* Printed for the author, 1858.

Douglass, Frederick. *Autobiographies.* New York: Library of America, 1994.

Doumato, Eleanor A. *Getting God's Ear: Women, Islam, and Healing in Saudi Arabia and the Gulf.* New York: Columbia Univ. Press, 2000.

Dowty, Alan. *Middle East Crisis: U.S. Decision-making in 1958, 1970 and 1973.* Berkeley: Univ. of California Press, 1984.

Duncan, Dayton, and Geoffrey C. Ward. *Mark Twain: An Illustrated Biography.* New York: Knopf, 2001.

Dupuy, E. *Américains et Barbaresques.* Paris: R. Roger et F. Chernoviz, 1910.

Dye, William. *Moslem Egypt and Christian Abyssinia.* New York: Negro Universities Press, 1969.

Dyer, Brainerd. *The Public Career of William M. Evarts.* Berkeley: Univ. of California Press, 1933.

Eaton, William. *Interesting Detail of the Operations of the American Fleet in the Mediterranean, Communicated in a Letter from W.E. Esq. to His Friend in the County of Hampshire.* Springfield, Mass.: Bliss & Brewer, 1804.

Eban, Abba. *Personal Witness: Israel through My Eyes.* New York: Putnam, 1992.

Eddy, William A. *F.D.R. Meets Ibn Saud.* New York: American Friends of the Middle East, 1954.

Einstein, Lewis. *Inside Constantinople.* London: John Murray, 1917.

Elliot, Charles. *Remarkable Characters and Places in the Holy Land.* Hartford: J. B. Burr, 1867.

Ellis, Joseph J. *American Sphinx. The Character of Thomas Jefferson.* New York: Vintage, 1998.

———. *Founding Brothers: The Revolutionary Generation.* New York: Vintage, 2002.

Ellison, James. *The American Captive; or, The Siege of Tripoli: A Drama in Five Acts.* Boston: Joshua Belcher, 1812.

Elon, Amos. *Herzl.* New York: Holt, Rinehart and Winston, 1975.

Elsbree, Oliver Wendell. *The Rise of the Missionary Spirit in America, 1790–1815.* Williamsport, Pa.: Williamsport Printing and Binding Co., 1928.

Elton, Godfrey. *Gordon of Khartoum.* New York: Knopf, 1955.

Emerson, Everett. *Puritanism in America, 1620–1750.* Boston: Twayne, 1977.

English, George Bethune. *The Grounds of Christianity Examined by Comparing the New Testament with the Old.* Boston: A.M., 1813.

———. *A Narrative of the Expedition to Dongola and Sennaar under the Command of His Excellence Ismael Pasha Undertaken by Order of His Highness Mehemmed Ali Pasha, Viceroy of Egypt.* Boston: Wells and Lilly, 1823.

Esthus, Raymond A. *Theodore Roosevelt and the International Rivalries.* Claremont: Regina Books, 1970.

Evans, Laurence. *United States Policy and the Partition of Turkey, 1914–1924.* Baltimore: Johns Hopkins Press, 1965.

Eveland, Wilbur Crane. *Ropes of Sand: America's Failure in the Middle East.* New York: Norton, 1980.

Eytan, Walter. *The First Ten Years: A Diplomatic History of Israel.* London: Weidenfeld & Nicolson, 1958.

Eytinge, Rose. *The Memoirs of Rose Eytinge.* New York: Frederick A. Stoker, 1905.

Fairbank, John, ed. *The Missionary Enterprise in China and America.* Cambridge: Harvard Univ. Press, 1974.

Farman, Elbert. *Along the Nile with General Grant.* New York: Grafton Press, 1904.

———. *Egypt and Its Betrayal.* New York: Grafton Press, 1908.

Faulk, Odie B. *The U.S. Camel Corps.* New York: Oxford Univ. Press, 1976.

Fawcett, Louise L. *Iran and the Cold War: The Azerbaijan Crisis of 1946*. Cambridge: Cambridge Univ. Press, 1992.

Fein, Isaac M. *The Making of an American Jewish Community: The History of Baltimore Jewry from 1773 to 1920*. Philadelphia: Jewish Publication Society, 1971.

Feingold, Henry L. *The Politics of Rescue: The Roosevelt Administration and the Holocaust, 1938–1945*. New Brunswick: Rutgers Univ. Press, 1970.

———. *Zion in America: The Jewish Experience from Colonial Times to the Present*. New York: Twayne, 1974.

Feinstein, Martin. *American Zionism, 1884–1904*. New York: Herzl Press, 1965.

Fellman, Michael. *Citizen Sherman: A Life of William Tecumseh Sherman*. New York: Random House, 1995.

Felton, Harold W. *Uriah Phillips Levy*. New York: Dodd, Mead, 1978.

Fick, Nathaniel. *One Bullet Away: The Making of a Marine Officer*. Boston: Houghton Mifflin, 2005.

Field, Henry M. *From Egypt to Japan*. 19th ed. New York: Scribner, 1905.

Field, James A., Jr. *America and the Mediterranean World, 1776–1882*. Princeton: Princeton Univ. Press, 1969.

Finkelstein, Dorothee Metiltsky. *Melville's Orienda*. New Haven: Yale Univ. Press, 1961.

Finley, John H. *A Pilgrim in Palestine*. New York: Scribner, 1919.

Finnie, David H. *Pioneers East: The Early American Experience in the Middle East*. Cambridge: Harvard Univ. Press, 1967.

Fisher, Sir Godfrey. *Barbary Legend: War, Trade and Policy in North Africa, 1415–1830*. Oxford: Oxford Univ. Press, 1957.

Fitzpatrick, Donovan, and Saul Saphire. *Navy Maverick: Uriah Phillips Levy*. Garden City, N.Y.: Doubleday, 1963.

Forrestal, James. *The Forrestal Diaries*. New York: Viking, 1951.

Foss, John. *A Journal of the Captivity and Sufferings of John Foss*. Newburyport, Mass.: Angier March, 1798.

Fowler, William M. *Jack Tars and Commodores: The American Navy, 1783–1815*. Boston: Houghton Mifflin, 1984.

Frankel, Jonathan. *The Damascus Affair: "Ritual Murder," Politics, and the Jews in 1840*. Cambridge: Cambridge Univ. Press, 1997.

Frankfurter, Felix. *Felix Frankfurter Reminisces: Recorded in Talks with Harlan B. Phillips*. New York: Reynal, 1960.

Freely, John. *A History of Robert College*. Istanbul: Y.K.Y., 2000.

Freeman, John. *Herman Melville*. New York: Macmillan, 1926.

Friedman, Isaiah. *The Question of Palestine: British-Jewish-Arab Relations, 1914–1918*. New Brunswick: Transaction, 1992.

Fromkin, David. *A Peace to End All Peace: The Fall of the Ottoman Empire and the Creation of the Modern Middle East*. New York: Avon, 1989.

Fukuyama, Francis. *America at the Crossraods: Democracy, Power, and the Neoconservative Legacy*. New Haven: Yale Univ. Pres, 2006.

Gaddis, John Lewis. *The Cold War: A New History*. New York: Penguin, 2005.

———. *Surprise, Security, and the American Experience*. Cambridge: Harvard Univ. Press, 2004.

———. *The United States and the Origins of the Cold War*. New York: Columbia Univ. Press, 1992.

Gal, Allon. *David Ben-Gurion and the American Alignment for the Jewish State*. Bloomington: Indiana Univ. Press, 1991.

Gale, Robert L. *A Herman Melville Encyclopedia*. Westport, Conn.: Greenwood, 1995.

Ganin, Zvi. *Truman, American Jewry, and Israel, 1945–1948*. New York: Holmes & Meier, 1979.

Gazit, Mordechai. *President Kennedy's Policy toward the Arab States and Israel: Analysis and Documents*. Tel Aviv: Tel Aviv Univ., 1983.

Gelfand, Lawrence E. *The Inquiry: American Preparations for Peace, 1917–1919*. New Haven: Yale Univ. Press, 1963.

Gendzier, Irene L. *Notes from the Minefield: United States Intervention in Lebanon and the Middle East, 1945–1958*. Boulder: Westview Press, 1999.

Gibbons, Helen Davenport. *The Red Rugs of Tarsus: A Woman's Record of the Armenian Massacre of 1909*. New York: Century, 1917.

Gibbons, Herbert A. *The Blackest Page of Modern History*. New York: Putnam, 1916.

Gibran, Gibran Khalil. *The Prophet*. New York: Knopf, 1952.

Gidney, James B. *A Mandate for Armenia*. Kent, Ohio: Kent State Univ. Press, 1967.

Gilbert, Martin. *Israel: A History*. London: Black Swan, 1998.

Gilner, Elias. *War and Hope: A History of the Jewish Legion*. New York: Herzl Press, 1969.

Godfried, Nathan. *Bridging the Gap between Rich and Poor: American Economic Development Policy toward the Arab East, 1942–1949*. New York: Greenwood, 1987.

Goetzmann, William. *New Lands, New Men*. New York: Viking, 1986.

———. *When the Eagle Screamed: America and the Second Great Age of Discovery*. Norman: Univ. of Oklahoma Press, 2000.

Goldberg, Isaac. *Major Noah: American-Jewish Frontier*. Philadelphia: Jewish Publication Society of America, 1936.

Goldman, Shalom. *God's Sacred Tongue: Hebrew and the American Imagination*. Chapel Hill: Univ. of North Carolina Press, 2004.

———, ed. *Hebrew and the Bible in America: The First Two Centuries*. Hanover: Brandeis Univ. Press and Dartmouth College, 1993.

Goodell, William. *Forty Years in the Turkish Empire*. New York: Robert Carter, 1883.

Goodwin, Charles. A. *Narrative of Joshua Gee of Boston, Mass., While He Was Captive in Algeria of the Barbary Pirates, 1680–1687*. Hartford: Wadsworth Atheneum, 1943.

Gordon, Leland James. *American Relations with Turkey, 1830–1930: An Economic Interpretation.* Philadelphia: Univ. of Pennsylvania Press, 1932.

Gordon, Michael R., and Bernard E. Trainor. *Cobra II: The Inside Story of the Invasion and Occupation of Iraq.* New York: Pantheon, 2006.

Goren, Arthur, ed. *Dissenter in Zion: From the Writings of Judah L. Magnes.* Cambridge: Harvard Univ. Press, 1982.

Gowing, Lawrence. *Paintings of the Louvre.* London: Stewart, Tabori, & Chang, 1987.

Grabill, Joseph L. *Protestant Diplomacy and the Near East: Missionary Influence on American Policy, 1810–1927.* Minneapolis: Univ. of Minnesota Press, 1969.

Grant, Ulysses S. *Personal Memoirs of U.S. Grant.* New York: C. L. Webster, 1885.

Grayson, Benson Lee. *Saudi-American Relations.* Washington, D.C.: Univ. Press of America, 1982.

Greene, Frederick Davis. *Armenian Massacres, or, The Sword of Mohammed.* Philadelphia: National Publishers Co., 1896.

Greenville, John A. S., and George B. Young. *Politics, Strategy, and American Diplomacy: Studies in Foreign Policy, 1873–1917.* New Haven: Yale Univ. Press, 1966.

Grenville, Vernon. *Yankee Doodle-Doo: A Collection of Songs of the Early American Stage.* New York: Payson & Clarke, 1927.

Grose, Peter. *Israel in the Mind of America.* New York: Knopf, 1983.

Grosrichard, Alain. *The Sultan's Court: European Fantasies of the East.* Translated by Liz Heron. London: Verso, 1998.

Guelzo, Allen C. *Abraham Lincoln: Redeemer President.* Grand Rapids, Mich.: Eerdmans, 1999.

Gurock, Jeffrey S., ed. *American Jewish History: The Colonial and Early National Periods, 1654–1840.* New York: Routledge, 1998.

Guthrie, Grace D. *Legacy to Lebanon.* Richmond, Va.: Self-published, 1984.

Habachi, Labib. *The Obelisks of Egypt.* Cairo: American Univ. in Cairo Press, 1984.

Haddawy, Husain, trans. *The Arabian Nights.* New York: Norton, 1990.

Hagan, Kenneth J. *This People's Navy: The Making of American Sea Power.* New York: Free Press, 1991.

Hahn, Peter L. *Caught in the Middle East: U.S. Policy toward the Arab-Israeli Conflict, 1945–1961.* Chapel Hill: Univ. of North Carolina Press, 2004.

———. *The United States, Great Britain, and Egypt, 1945–1956: Strategy and Diplomacy in the Early Cold War.* Chapel Hill: Univ. of North Carolina Press, 1991.

Haig, Alexander M., Jr. *Caveat: Realism, Reagan, and Foreign Policy.* New York: Macmillan, 1984.

Haig, Alexander M., Jr., with Charles McCarry. *Inner Circles: How America Changed the World: A Memoir.* New York: Warner, 1992.

Haight, Sarah Rogers. *Letters from the Old World by a Lady of New York.* New York: Harper, 1840.

Hall, Luella J. *The United States and Morocco, 1776–1956.* Metuchen, N.J.: Scarecrow Press, 1971.

Halperin, Samuel. *The Political World of American Zionism*. Detroit: Wayne State Univ. Press, 1961.

Halpern, Ben. *A Clash of Heroes: Brandeis, Weizmann, and American Zionism*. New York: Oxford Univ. Press, 1987.

Halpern, Ben, and Jehuda Reinharz. *Zionism and the Creation of a New Society*. New York: Oxford Univ. Press, 1998.

Hamby, Alonzo L. *Man of the People: A Life of Harry S. Truman*. New York: Oxford Univ. Press, 1995.

Hamilton, Alexander, John Jay, and James Madison. *The Federalist Papers*. Cutchogue, N.Y.: Buccaneer Books, 1992.

Hamlin, Cyrus. *Among the Turks*. New York: Robert Carter, 1878.

———. *My Life and Times*. Boston: Pilgrim Press, 1893.

Handy, Robert T. *The Holy Land in American Protestant Life, 1800–1948*. New York: Arno Press, 1981.

Hanson, Joseph. *The Musselmen Humbled; or, A Heroic Poem in Celebration of the Bravery Displayed by the American Tars, in the Contest with Tripoli*. New York: Southwick and Hardcastle, 1806.

Harbord, James G. *Conditions in the Near East: American Military Mission to Armenia*. Washington, D.C.: GPO, 1920.

Hargreaves, Mary W. M. *The Presidency of John Quincy Adams*. Lawrence: Univ. Press of Kansas, 1985.

Harris, David. *Britain and the Bulgarian Horrors of 1876*. Chicago: Univ. of Chicago Press, 1939.

Harris, Thomas. *The Life and Services of Commodore William Bainbridge, United States Navy*. Philadelphia: Carey Lea and Blanchard, 1837.

Harrison, Paul W. *Doctor in Arabia*. London: Robert Hale, 1943.

Harrison, Thomas Skelton. *The Homely Diary of a Diplomat in the East, 1897–1899*. Boston: Houghton Mifflin, 1917.

Hart, Parker T. *Saudi Arabia and the United States: Birth of a Security Partnership*. Bloomington: Indiana Univ. Press, 1998.

Hart, Robert A. *The Great White Fleet*. Boston: Little, Brown, 1965.

Hattis, Susan L. *The Bi-national Idea in Palestine during Mandatory Times*. Haifa: Shikmona, 1970.

Hawes, Louisa. *Memoir of Mrs. M. E. Van Lemep, by Her Mother*. Hartford: Belknap and Hamersley, 1849.

Heckscher, August. *Woodrow Wilson*. New York: Scribner, 1991.

Hedges, William H. *The Old and New World Romanticism of Washington Irving*. New York: Greenwood, 1986.

Hellman, George S. *Washington Irving, Esquire: Ambassador at Large from the New World to the Old*. New York: Knopf, 1925.

Helmreich, Paul C. *From Paris to Sèvres: The Partition of the Ottoman Empire at the Peace Conference of 1919–1920*. Columbus: Ohio State Univ. Press, 1974.

Henry, Charles P. *Ralph Bunche: Model Negro or American Other?* New York: New York Univ. Press, 1999.

Hertzberg, Arthur, ed. *The Zionist Idea: A Historical Analysis and Reader*. New York: Atheneum, 1972.

Hesseltine, William B., and Hazel Wolf. *The Blue and the Gray on the Nile*. Chicago: Univ. of Chicago Press, 1961.

Hietala, Thomas. *Manifest Design: Anxious Aggrandizement in Late Jacksonian America*. Ithaca: Cornell Univ. Press, 1985.

Hillman, William, and Harry Truman. *Mr. President: The First Publication from the Personal Diaries, Private Letters, Papers, and Revealing Interviews of Harry S. Truman, Thirty-second President of the United States of America*. New York: Farrar, Straus and Young, 1952.

Hirsch, H. N. *The Enigma of Felix Frankfurter*. New York: Basic Books, 1981.

Hirshson, Stanley. *The White Tecumseh: A Biography of General William T. Sherman*. New York: John Wiley, 1997.

Hitti, Philip. *Lebanon in History from the Earliest Times to the Present*. London: Macmillan, 1962.

Hobsbawm, E. J. *The Age of Empire, 1875–1914*. New York: Pantheon, 1987.

Hodson, Joel. *Lawrence of Arabia and American Culture*. Westport, Conn.: Greenwood, 1995.

Holden, Edith. *Blyden of Liberia*. New York: Vantage Press, 1966.

Holland, Matthew F. *America and Egypt: From Roosevelt to Eisenhower*. Westport, Conn.: Praeger, 1996.

Holmes, Oliver Wendell. *Ralph Waldo Emerson*. Boston: Houghton Mifflin, 1885.

Holmes, Reed M. *The Forerunners*. Independence, Mo.: Herald, 1981.

Hoover, Herbert. *The Memoirs of Herbert Hoover*. New York: Macmillan, 1957.

Hopwood, Derek. *The Russian Presence in Syria and Palestine, 1843–1914: Church and Politics in the Near East*. Oxford: Clarendon Press, 1969.

Horovitz, David, ed. *Yitzhak Rabin: Soldier of Peace*. London: Peter Halban, 1996.

Horton, George. *The Blight of Asia: An Account of the Systematic Extermination of Christian Populations by Mohammedans. . . .* 1926. Reprint, Indianapolis: Bobbs-Merrill, 1953.

Hourani, Albert. *Arabic Thought in the Liberal Age, 1798–1939*. Cambridge: Cambridge Univ. Press, 1962.

House, Edward, ed. *What Really Happened at Paris*. New York: Scribner, 1921.

Howard, Harry N. *The King-Crane Commission: An American Inquiry in the Middle East*. Beirut: Khayats, 1963.

Howe, George F. *Northwest Africa: Seizing the Initiative in the West*. Washington, D.C.: Center of Military History, 1991.

Howe, Samuel G. *An Historical Sketch of the Greek Revolution*. New York: n.p., 1828.

Hull, Cordell. *The Memoirs of Cordell Hull*. 2 vols. New York: Macmillan, 1948.

Huntington. Samuel P. *The Clash of Civilizations and the Remaking the World Order*. New York: Simon & Schuster, 1996.

Hurewitz, J. C., ed. *The Middle East and North Africa in World Politics: A Documentary Record*. Vol. 1, *European Expansion, 1535–1914*. 2d ed. New Haven: Yale Univ. Press, 1975.

———. *The Struggle for Palestine*. New York: Greenwood, 1968.

Iriye, Akira. *From Nationalism to Internationalism: U.S. Foreign Policy to 1914*. London: Routledge and Kegan Paul, 1977.

Irving, Washington. *Alhambra*. Boston: Ginn, 1902.

———. *The Conquest of Granada*. New York: Putnam, 1850.

———. *Mahomet and His Successors*. Chicago: Belford, Clarke, 1973.

Irving, Washington, William Irving, and James Paulding. *Salmagundi*. Chicago: Belford, Clarke, 1807.

Irwin, Ray. *The Diplomatic Relations of the United States with the Barbary Powers, 1776–1816*. New York: Russell & Russell, 1970.

Irwin, Robert. *For Lust of Knowing: The Orientalists and their Enemies*. London: Penguin, 2007.

Isaacson, Walter, and Evan Thomas. *The Wise Men: Six Friends and the World They Made*. New York: Touchstone, 1986.

Israel, John, and Henry Lundt. *Journal of a Cruize in the U.S. Ship* Delaware *74 in the Mediterranean in the Years 1833 & 34*. 1835. Reprint, New York: Arno Press, 1977.

James, Lawrence. *The Golden Warrior*. New York: Paragon, 1993.

James, Robert Rhodes. *Anthony Eden*. London: Weidenfeld & Nicolson, 1986.

Jampoler, Andrew C. A. *Sailors in the Holy Land: The 1848 American Expedition to the Dead Sea and the Search for Sodom and Gomorrah*. Annapolis: Naval Institute Press, 2005.

Jefferson, Thomas. *Autobiography*. New York: Capricorn, 1959.

Jessup, Henry Harris. *Fifty-three Years in Syria*. Vol. 2. New York: Revell, 1910.

———. *The Setting of the Crescent and the Rising of the Cross: or, Kamil Abdul Messiah, a Syrian Convert from Islam to Christianity*. Philadelphia: Westminster Press, 1898.

Johannsen, Robert W., et al. *Manifest Destiny and Empire: American Antebellum Expansionism*. Edited by Sam Haynes and Christopher Morris. Arlington: Univ. of Texas Press, 1997.

Johnson, Sarah Barclay. *Hadji in Syria*. New York: Arno Press, 1977.

Jones, George, A. M. *Excursions to Cairo, Jerusalem, Damascus, and Balbec from the United States Ship* Delaware, *during Her Recent Cruise: With an Attempt to Discriminate between Truth and Error in Regard to the Sacred Places of the Holy City*. New York: Van Nostrand and Dwight, 1836.

Jones, Kenneth V., ed. *Adams, John Quincy, 1767–1848: Chronology, Documents, Bibliographical Aids*. New York: Oceana Publications, 1970.

Joyce, Miriam. *Kuwait, 1945–1956: An Anglo-American Perspective*. London: Frank Cass, 1998.

Kaplan, Justin. *Mr. Clemens and Mr. Twain*. New York: Simon & Schuster, 1966.

Kaplan, Robert D. *The Arabists: The Romance of an American Elite.* New York: Free Press, 1993.

Karabell, Zachary. *Parting the Desert: The Creation of the Suez Canal.* New York: Knopf, 2003.

Kark, Ruth. *American Consuls in the Holy Land, 1832–1914.* Jerusalem: Magnes Press, Hebrew Univ., 1994.

Karpin, Michael. *The Bomb in the Basement: How Israel Went Nuclear and What That Means for the World.* New York: Simon & Schuster, 2006.

Kaufman, Menahem. *The Magnes-Philby Negotiations, 1929: The Historical Record.* Jerusalem: Magnes Press, 1998.

Kaufman, Menahem, and Mira Levine, eds. *Guide to America–Holy Land Studies, 1620–1948.* Vol. 4, *Resource Material in British, Israeli and Turkish Repositories.* New York: Praeger, 1984.

Keegan, John. *Iraq War: The Military Offensive, from Victory in 21 Days to the Insurgent Aftermath.* Westminster, Md.: Knopf, 2005.

Kelly, Michael. *Martyrs' Day: Chronicle of a Small War.* New York: Vintage, 1993.

Kenen, I. L. *Israel's Defense Line: Her Friends and Foes in Washington.* Buffalo: Prometheus, 1981.

Kennedy, Charles Stuart. *The American Consul: A History of the United States Consular Service, 1776–1914.* New York: Greenwood, 1990.

Keyal, Philip, and Joseph Keyal. *The Syrian-Lebanese in America.* Boston: Twayne, 1975.

Khalaf, Samir. *Persistence and Change in 19th Century Lebanon.* Beirut: American Univ. of Beirut, 1979.

Khalidi, Rashid, ed. *The Origins of Arab Nationalism.* New York: Columbia Univ. Press, 1991.

———. *Western Footprints and America's Perilous Path in the Middle East.* Boston: Beacon Press, 2005.

Kheirallah, George. *Arabia Reborn.* Albuquerque: Univ. of New Mexico Press, 1952.

Kinross, Lord. *The Ottoman Centuries: The Rise and Fall of the Turkish Empire.* New York: Morrow Quill, 1977.

Kinzer, Stephen. *All the Shah's Men: An American Coup and the Roots of Middle East Terror.* Hoboken, N.J.: Wiley, 2003.

Kirakossian, Arman, ed. *The Armenian Massacres, 1894–1896: U.S. Media Testimony.* Detroit: Wayne State Univ. Press, 2004.

Kirk, George. *The Middle East in the War.* Survey of International Affairs, 1939–1946, Royal Institute of International Affairs. London: Oxford Univ. Press, 1952.

Kirkland, Elizabeth Cabot. *Letters.* Cambridge: Massachusetts Historical Society, 1905.

Kirshner, Ralph. *The Class of 1861: Custer, Ames, and Their Classmates after West Point.* Carbondale: Southern Illinois Univ. Press, 1999.

Kissinger, Henry A. *Crisis: The Anatomy of Two Major Foreign Policy Crises*. New York: Simon & Schuster, 2003.

———. *Diplomacy*. New York: Simon & Schuster, 1994.

———. *White House Years*. Boston: Little, Brown, 1979.

Kitzen, Michael L. S. *Tripoli and the United States at War: A History of America's Relations with the Barbary States, 1785–1805*. Jefferson, N.C.: McFarland, 1962.

Kloian, Richard. *The Armenian Genocide: News Accounts from the American Press*. Berkeley: Anto Press, 1985.

Kloman, Erasmus. *Assignment Algiers: With the OSS in the Mediterranean Theater*. Annapolis: Naval Institute Press, 2005.

Knightley, Phillip, and Colin Simpson. *The Secret Lives of Lawrence of Arabia*. London: Thomas Nelson, 1969.

Knock, Thomas J. *To End All Wars: Woodrow Wilson and the Quest for a New World Order*. Princeton: Princeton Univ. Press, 1992.

Korn, Bertram. *American Jewry and the Civil War*. New York: Jewish Publication Society of America, 1951.

Kramer, Martin. *Ivory Towers on Sand: The Failure of Middle Eastern Studies in America*. Washington, D.C.: Washington Institute of Near East Policy, 2001.

Krieger, Barbara. *Divine Expectations: An American Woman in 19th Century Palestine*. Athens: Ohio Univ. Press, 1999.

Krout, Marty H., ed. *Lew Wallace, An Autobiography*. New York: Harper, 1906.

Kruger, James R. *Turning On Water with a Shovel: The Career of Elwood Mead*. Albuquerque: Univ. of New Mexico Press, 1992.

Kuklick, Bruce. *Puritans in Babylon: The Ancient Near East and American Intellectual Life, 1880–1930*. Princeton: Princeton Univ. Press, 1996.

Kuniholm, Bruce R. *The Origins of the Cold War in the Near East: Great Power Conflict and Diplomacy in Iran, Turkey, and Greece*. Princeton: Princeton Univ. Press, 1980.

Kurzer, Dan. *Ben-Gurion: Prophet of Fire*. New York: Simon & Schuster, 1983.

Kurzman, Dan. *Genesis 1948: The First Arab-Israeli War*. New York: Da Capo Press, 1970.

Lacroix-Riz, Annie. *Les Protectorats d'Afrique du Nord entre la France et Washington: Du débarquement à l'indépendance, Maroc et Tunisie, 1942–1956*. Paris: L'Harmattan, 1988.

LaFeber, Walter. *The Cambridge History of American Foreign Relations*. Vol. 2, *The American Search for Opportunity, 1865–1913*. Cambridge: Cambridge Univ. Press, 1993.

———. *The New Empire: An Interpretation of American Expansion, 1860–1898*. Ithaca: Cornell Univ. Press, 1998.

Lane, Edward, and Edward Stanely Poole, eds. *The Thousand and One Nights: Commonly Called, in England, the Arabian Nights' Entertainments*. London: Bell Press, 1883.

Langer, William L., and S. Everett Gleason. *The Undeclared War, 1940–1941*. Gloucester: P. Smith, 1968.

Lansing, Robert. *The Big Four and Others of the Peace Conference*. Boston: Houghton Mifflin, 1921.

Laqueur, Walter. *A History of Zionism*. New York: Simon & Schuster, 1989.

Larsen, Peter. *Theodore Roosevelt and the Moroccan Crisis, 1904–1906*. Princeton: Princeton Univ. Press, 1984.

Larson, Deborah Welch. *Origins of Containment: A Psychological Explanation*. Princeton: Princeton Univ. Press, 1985.

Larson, Erik. *The Devil in the White City: Murder, Magic, and Madness at the Fair That Changed America*. New York: Vintage, 2003.

Lash, Joseph P. *From the Diaries of Felix Frankfurter*. New York: Norton, 1975.

Latourette, Kenneth. *Missions and the American Mind*. Indianapolis: National Foundation Press, 1949.

Laurie, Thomas. *The Ely Volume; or, The Contributions of Our Foreign Missions to Science and Human Well-Being*. Boston: American Board of Commissioners for Foreign Missions, 1881.

Lavsky, Hagit. *Before Catastrophe: The Distinctive Path of German Zionism*. Detroit: Wayne State Univ. Press, 1996.

Lawlor, Laurie. *Magnificent Voyage: An American Adventurer on Captain James Cook's Final Expedition*. New York: Holiday House, 2002.

Ledyard, John. *A Journal of Captain Cook's Last Voyage to the Pacific Ocean*. Hartford: Nathaniel Patten, 1783.

Leeson, Marc. *Saving Monticello: The Levy Family's Epic Quest to Rescue the House That Jefferson Built*. New York: Free Press, 2001.

Leff, Laurel. *Buried by the Times: The Holocaust and America's Most Important Newspaper*. New York: Cambridge Univ. Press, 2005.

Leiner, Frederick C. *The End of Barbary Terror: American's 1815 War against the Pirates of North Africa*. Oxford: Oxford Univ. Press, 2006.

Lenczowksi, George. *The Middle East in World Affairs*. Ithaca: Cornell Univ. Press, 1980.

Leo, Africanus. *The History and Description of Africa, and of All the Notable Things Therein Contained*. London: Hakluyt Society, 1896.

Lesch, David. *Syria and the United States: Eisenhower's Cold War in the Middle East*. Boulder: Westview Press, 1992.

———, ed. *The Middle East and the United States*. Boulder: Westview Press, 1999.

Lewis, Bernard. *The Arabs in History*. London: Hutchinson's Univ. Library, 1950.

———. *The Crisis of Islam: Holy War and Unholy Terror*. New York: Modern Library, 2003.

———. *The Emergence of Modern Turkey*. London: Oxford Univ. Press, 1968.

———. *What Went Wrong: The Clash between Islam and Modernity in the Middle East*. New York: Perennial, 2003.

Liebling, A. J. *The Road Back to Paris*. Garden City, N.Y.: Doubleday, Doran, 1944.

Life of Mohammad. Bombay: American Mission Press, 1851.

Lindsay, Rao H. *Nineteenth-Century American Schools in the Levant: A Study of Purposes*. Ann Arbor: Univ. of Michigan School of Education, 1965.

Link, Arthur S. *Wilson: The Struggle for Neutrality*. Princeton: Princeton Univ. Press, 1960.

Lippman, Thomas W. *Inside the Mirage: America's Fragile Partnership with Saudi Arabia*. Boulder: Westview Press, 2004.

Little, Douglas. *American Orientalism: The United States and the Middle East since 1945*. Chapel Hill: Univ. of North Carolina Press, 2002.

Lodge, Henry Cabot. *The Senate and the League of Nations*. New York: Scribner, 1925.

Lohbeck, Don. *Patrick J. Hurley*. Chicago: H. Regnery, 1956.

Long, David. *Nothing Too Daring: A Biography of Commodore David Porter, 1780–1843*. Annapolis: U.S. Naval Institute, 1970.

———. *The United States and Saudi Arabia*. Boulder: Westview Press, 1985.

Longrigg, Stephen Hemsley. *Oil in the Middle East: Its Discovery and Development*. London: Oxford Univ. Press, 1954.

Loring, William. *A Confederate Soldier in Egypt*. New York: Dodd, Mead, 1884.

Lothrop, Thornton Kirkland. *William Henry Seward*. Boston: Houghton Mifflin, 1896.

Louis, William R. *The British Empire in the Middle East, 1945–1951*. New York: Oxford Univ. Press, 1984.

———. *Imperialism at Bay, 1941–1945: The United States and the Decolonization of the British Empire*. Oxford: Clarendon Press, 1977.

Love, Donald M. *Henry Churchill King of Oberlin*. New Haven: Yale Univ. Press, 1956.

Lowdermilk, Walter C. *Conquest of the Land through Seven Thousand Years*. 1948. Reprint, Washington, D.C.: U.S. Department of Agriculture, Soil Conservation Service, 1953.

———. *Palestine: Land of Promise*. New York: Harper, 1944.

Lowenthal, David. *George Perkins Marsh: Versatile Vermonter*. New York: Columbia Univ. Press, 1958.

Lowenthal, Marvin. *Henrietta Szold, Life and Letters*. New York: Viking, 1942.

Lynch, William F. *Commerce and the Holy Land (A Lecture)*. Philadelphia: King and Baird, 1860.

———. *Narrative of the United States' Expedition to the River Jordan and the Dead Sea*. Philadelphia: Blanchard and Lea, 1853.

———. *Naval Life, Observations on Shore and Afloat the Midshipman*. New York: Scribner, 1851.

Lytle, Mark Hamilton. *The Origins of the Iranian-American Alliance, 1941–1953*. New York: Holmes & Meier, 1987.

Macintyre, Ben. *The Man Who Would Be King: The First American in Afghanistan*. New York: Farrar, Straus and Giroux, 2004.

Mack, John E. *A Prince of Our Disorder: The Life of T. E. Lawrence.* Oxford: Oxford Univ. Press, 1990.

MacMillan, Margaret. *Paris 1919: Six Months That Changed the World.* New York: Random House, 2002.

Madison, James. *Notes of Debates in the Federal Convention of 1787.* Athens: Ohio Univ. Press, 1966.

Mahan, Alfred Thayer. *The Problem of Asia.* Boston: Little, Brown, 1900.

———. *Retrospect and Prospect.* Boston: Little, Brown, and Company, 1902.

Malachy, Yona. *American Fundamentalism and Israel: The Relation of Fundamentalist Churches to Zionism and the State of Israel.* Jerusalem: Graph Press, 1978.

Malloy, William M. *Treaties, Conventions, International Acts, Protocols and Agreements between the United States of American and Other Powers, 1779–1909.* Washington, D.C.: GPO, 1910.

Malone, Dumas. *Jefferson the President: First Term, 1801–1805.* Boston: Little, Brown, 1970.

Mandel, Neville. *The Arabs and Zionism before World War I.* Berkeley: Univ. of California Press, 1976.

Mann, James. *The Rise of the Vulcans: The History of Bush's War Cabinet.* New York: Penguin, 2004.

Mantel, S. G. *Explorer with a Dream, John Ledyard.* New York: Julian Messner, 1969.

Manuel, Frank E. *The Realities of American-Palestine Relations.* 1949. Reprint, Westport, Conn.: Greenwood, 1975.

Markoe, Peter. *The Algerine Spy in Pennsylvania; or, Letters Written by a Native of Algiers on the Affairs of the United States in America, from the Close of the Year 1783 to the Meeting of the Convention.* Philadelphia: Prichard and Hall, 1787.

Marks, Frederick W., III. *Velvet on Iron: The Diplomacy of Theodore Roosevelt.* Lincoln: Univ. of Nebraska Press, 1979.

———. *Wind over Sand: The Diplomacy of Franklin Roosevelt.* Athens: Univ. of Georgia Press, 1988.

Marlowe, John. *Spoiling the Egyptians.* New York: St. Martin's, 1975.

Marrs, K. Ray. *I Was There When the World Stood Still.* Bloomington: 1st Books, 2003.

Marsot, Afaf Lutfi al-Sayyid. *Egypt in the Reign of Muhammad Ali.* Cambridge: Cambridge Univ. Press, 1984.

Martin, Maria. *History of the Captivity and Sufferings of Maria Martin.* Philadelphia: Jacob Meyer, 1811.

Martin, Marty E. *Pilgrims in Their Own Land: 500 Years of Religion in America.* Boston: Little, Brown, 1984.

Martin, Ralph G. *Golda: Golda Meir, the Romantic Years.* New York: Scribner, 1988.

Mason, Alfred DeWitt, and Frederick J. Barny. *History of the Arabian Mission.* New York: Board of Foreign Missions Reformed Church in America, 1926.

Mattar, Philip. *The Mufti of Jerusalem: Al-Hajj Amin al-Husayni and the Palestinian National Movement*. New York: Columbia Univ. Press, 1988.

Matthews, Franklin. *Back to Hampton Roads*. New York: B. W. Huebsch, 1909.

May, Ernest. *Imperial Democracy: The Emergence of America as a Great Power*. Chicago: Imprint Publications, 1961.

McCarthy, Justin. *Death and Exile: The Ethnic Cleansing of Ottoman Muslims, 1821–1922*. Princeton, N.J.: Darwin Press, 1995.

McCloy, Drew R. *The Last of the Fathers: James Madison and the Republican Legacy*. Cambridge: Cambridge Univeristy Press, 1989.

McCullough, David. *John Adams*. New York: Simon & Schuster, 2001.

———. *Truman*. New York: Simon & Schuster, 1992.

McDaniel, Robert A. *The Shuster Mission and the Persian Constitutional Revolution*. Minneapolis: Bibliotheca Islamica,1974.

McDougall, Walter A. *Promised Land, Crusader State: The American Encounter with the World since 1776*. New York: Mariner Books, 1997.

McFeely, William. *Grant: A Biography*. New York: Norton, 1981.

McGilvary, Margaret. *The Dawn of a New Era in Syria*. New York: Revell, 1920.

Mckee, Christopher. *Edward Preble: A Naval Biography, 1761–1807*. Annapolis: Naval Institute Press, 1972.

Meacham, Jon. *American Gospel: God, the Founding Fathers, and the Making of a Nation*. New York: Random House, 2006.

Mead, Walter Russell. *Special Providence: American Foreign Policy and How It Changed the World*. New York: Routledge, 2002.

Medoff, Rafael. *Baksheesh Diplomacy: Secret Negotiations between American Jewish Leaders and Arab Officials on the Eve of World War II*. Lanham, Md.: Lexington Books, 2001.

———. *Zionism and the Arabs: An American Jewish Dilemma, 1898–1948*. Westport, Conn.: Praeger, 1997.

Meir, Golda. *My Life*. New York: Putnam, 1975.

Melman, Yossi, and Dan Raviv. *Friends in Deed: Inside the U.S.-Israel Alliance*. New York: Hyperion, 1994.

Melton, Jeffrey Alan. *Mark Twain, Travel Books, and Tourism: The Tide of a Great Popular Movement*. Tuscaloosa: Univ. of Alabama Press, 2002.

Melville, Herman. *Clarel: A Poem and Pilgrimage to the Holy Land*. Chicago: Northwestern Univ. Press, 1991.

———. *Journals*. Edited by Howard C. Horsford and Lynn Horth. Chicago: Northwestern Univ. Press, 1989.

———. *Moby Dick*. New York: Hendrick's House, 1952.

———. *Redburn*. New York: Literary Classics of the United States Inc., 1983.

———. *White-Jacket; or, The World in a Man-of-War*. Oxford: Oxford Univ. Press, 1990.

Ménager, Bernard, et al., eds. *Guy Mollet: Un camarade en république*. Lille: Presses Universitaires de Lille, 1987.

Merk, Frederick. *Manifest Destiny and Mission in American History.* New York: Knopf, 1963.

Merkley, Paul Charles. *The Politics of Christian Zionism, 1891–1948.* London: Frank Cass, 1998.

Merriam, Eve. *The Voice of Liberty: The Story of Emma Lazarus.* New York: Farrar, Straus and Cudahy, 1959.

Meryon, Charles Lewis, and Hester Lucy Stanhope. *The Travels of Lady Hester Stanhope.* London: H. Colburn, 1846.

Meyer, Isadore, ed. *Early Zionism in America.* Philadelphia: American Jewish Historical Society, 1958.

Miller, Aaron. *Search for Security: Saudi Arabian Oil and American Foreign Policy, 1939–1949.* Chapel Hill: Univ. of North Carolina Press, 1980.

Miller, Ellen Clare. *Eastern Sketches.* New York: Arno Press, 1977.

Miller, H., ed. *Treaties and Other International Acts of the United States of America* Washington, D.C.: GPO, 1933.

Miller, Merle. *Plain Speaking: An Oral Biography of Harry S. Truman.* New York: Putnam, 1974.

Miller, Nathan. *Theodore Roosevelt: A Life.* New York: Morrow Quill, 1992.

Miller, Roman J. *Around the World with the Battleships.* Chicago: A. C. McClurg, 1909.

Millspaugh, Arthur C. *Americans in Persia.* Washington, D.C.: Brookings Institution, 1946.

Minor, Clorinda. *Meshullam!; or, Tidings from Jerusalem: From the Journal of a Believer Recently Returned from the Holy Land.* Philadelphia: Self-published, 1851.

Mitchell, Timothy. *Colonising Egypt.* Berkeley: Univ. of California Press, 1988.

Monaghan, Jay. *Diplomat in Carpet Slippers: Abraham Lincoln Deals with Foreign Affairs.* Indianapolis: Bobbs-Merrill, 1945.

Monroe, Elizabeth. *Britain's Moment in the Middle East, 1914–1956.* Baltimore: Johns Hopkins Univ. Press, 1963.

Montague, Edward P. *Narrative of the Late Expedition to the Dead Sea.* Philadelphia: Carey and Hart, 1849.

Morgan, James Morris. *Recollections of a Rebel Reefer.* Boston: Houghton Mifflin, 1917.

Morgenthau, Henry. *All in a Life-Time.* Garden City, N.Y.: Doubleday, Page, 1922.

———. *Ambassador Morgenthau's Story.* Garden City, N.Y.: Doubleday, 1918.

———. *The Murder of a Nation.* New York: Armenian General Benevolent Union of America, 1974.

Morgenthau, Henry, III. *Mostly Morgenthau: A Family History.* New York: Ticknor & Fields, 1991.

Morley, Bertha B. *Marsovan 1915: The Diaries of Bertha B. Morley.* Ann Arbor: Gomidas Institute, 2000.

Morris, Edmund. *The Rise of Theodore Roosevelt.* New York: Modern Library, 2001.

————. *Theodore Rex*. New York: HarperCollins, 2003.

Morris, Edward Joy. *Notes of a Tour through Turkey, Greece, Egypt, Arabia Petrea, to the Holy Land*. Philadelphia: Carey and Hart, 1842.

Morse, Arthur D. *While Six Million Died*. London: Martin Secker and Warburg, 1968.

Mott, Thomas Bentley. *Twenty Years as Military Attaché*. 1937. Reprint, New York: Arno Press, 1979.

Mott, Valentine. *Travels in Europe and the East*. New York: Harper and Brothers, 1842.

Motter, T. H. Vail. *The Persian Corridor and Aid to Russia*. Washington, D.C.: Office of the Chief of Military History, 1952.

Muccigrosso, Robert. *Celebrating the New World: Chicago's Columbian Exposition of 1893*. Chicago: Ivan R. Dee, 1993.

Munford, Kenneth. *John Ledyard: An American Marco Polo*. Portland: Binfords and Mort, 1939.

Munro, John M. *A Mutual Concern: The Story of the American University of Beirut*. Delmar, N.Y.: Caravan Books, 1977.

Murphy, Robert. *Diplomat among Warriors*. Garden City, N.Y.: Doubleday, 1964.

Muslih, Muhammad Y. *The Origins of Palestinian Nationalism*. New York: Columbia Univ. Press, 1988.

Naff, Alixa. *The Arab Americans*. Philadelphia: Chelsea House, 1999.

Naguib, Mohammad. *Egypt's Destiny: A Personal Statement*. London: Gollancz, 1955.

Neider, Charles, ed. *The Complete Essays of Mark Twain*. Garden City, N.Y.: Doubleday, 1963.

Newcomb, Harvey. *Cyclopedia of Missions*. New York: Scribner, 1854.

Nicholson, Thomas. *An Affecting Narrative of the Captivity and Suffering of Thomas Nicholson Who Has Been Six Years a Prisoner among the Algerines*. Boston: N. Coverly, 1818.

Noah, Mordecai Manuel. *Correspondence and Documents Relative to the Attempt to Negotiate for the Release of the American Captives at Algiers, including Remarks on Our Relations with that Regency*. Washington, D.C.: n.p., 1816.

Nolte, Richard H., ed. *The Modern Middle East*. New York: Atherton Press, 1963.

North, Michael. *Reading 1922: A Return to the Scene of the Modern*. New York: Oxford Univ. Press, 1999.

Notter, Harley. *The Origins of the Foreign Policy of Woodrow Wilson*. Baltimore: Johns Hopkins Univ. Press, 1937.

Noveck, Simon, ed. *Great Jewish Personalities in Modern Times*. Washington, D.C.: B'nai B'rith Department of Adult Jewish Education, 1960.

Obenzinger, Hilton. *American Palestine: Melville, Twain, and the Holy Land Mania*. Princeton: Princeton Univ. Press, 1999.

Offner, Arnold. *Another Such Victory: President Truman and the Cold War, 1945–1953*. Palo Alto: Stanford Univ. Press, 2002.

Oldroyd, Osborn. *The Assassination of Abraham Lincoln.* Union, N.J.: Lawbook Exchange, 2001.

Olin, Stephen. *Travels in Egypt, Arabia Petra and the Holy Land.* New York: Harper, 1844.

Oren, Michael B. *The Origins of the Second Arab-Israel War: Egypt, Israel, and the Great Powers, 1952–56.* London: Frank Cass, 1992.

———. *Six Days of War: June 1967 and the Making of the Modern Middle East.* New York: Oxford Univ. Press, 2002.

Orfalea, Gregory, ed. *Grape Leaves: A Century of Arab American Poetry.* Salt Lake City: Univ. of Utah Press, 1988.

Osborn, Henry S. *Palestine, Past and Present.* Philadelphia: James Challen and Son, 1859.

Owen, E. R. J. *Cotton and the Egyptian Economy: 1820–1914.* London: Oxford Univ. Press, 1969.

Packer, George. *The Assassin's Gate: America in Iraq.* New York: Farrar, Straus and Giroux, 2005.

Paine, Albert Bigelow. *Mark Twain: A Biography: The Personal and Literary Life of Samuel Langhorne Clemens.* New York: Harper, 1912.

Palmer, Frederick. *Bliss, Peacemaker.* New York: Dodd, Mead, 1934.

Palmer, Michael A. *Guardians of the Gulf: A History of America's Expanding Role in the Persian Gulf, 1833–1992.* New York: Free Press, 1992.

Paludan, Phillip Shaw. *The Presidency of Abraham Lincoln.* Lawrence: Univ. Press of Kansas, 1994.

Panitz, Esther L. *Simon Wolf: Private Conscience and Public Image.* Rutherford: Fairleigh Dickinson Univ. Press, 1987.

Parker, Richard B. *The Politics of Miscalculation in the Middle East.* Bloomington: Indiana Univ. Press, 1993.

Parrish, Michael E. *Felix Frankfurter and His Times: The Reform Years.* New York: Free Press, 1982.

Parker, Richard B. *Uncle Sam in Barbary: A Diplomatic History.* Gainesville: Univ. Press of Florida, 2004.

Parsons, Levi. *The Dereliction and Restoration of the Jews: A Sermon, Preached in Park-Street Church Boston, Sabbath, Oct. 31, 1819, Just before the Departure of the Palestine Mission.* Boston: Samuel T. Armstrong, 1819.

———. *The Memoir of Rev. Levi Parsons.* Compiled by Daniel Oliver Morton. New York: Arno Press, 1977.

Patai, Raphael, ed. *Herzl Year Book 7.* New York: Herzl Press, 1971.

Patton, George S. *War as I Knew It.* Boston: Houghton Mifflin, 1995.

Paullin, Charles Oscar. *Diplomatic Negotiations of American Naval Officers, 1778–1883.* Baltimore: Johns Hopkins Univ. Press, 1912.

Pears, Sir Edwin. *Forty Years in Constantinople, 1873–1915.* New York: Appleton, 1916.

Pellew, George. *American Statesmen: John Jay.* Cambridge, Mass: Riverside Press, 1890.

Peltier, Jean G. *World War II Diary of Jean Gordon Peltier.* Groveland: Perfect Art, 2000.

Pendar, Kenneth. *Adventures in Diplomacy: The Emergence of General de Gaulle in North Africa.* London: Cassell, 1966.

Penrose, Stephen. *That They May Have Life: The Story of the American University of Beirut, 1866–1941.* Princeton: Princeton Univ. Press, 1941.

Peres, Shimon. *Battling for Peace: Memoirs.* Edited by David Landau. London: Weidenfeld & Nicolson, 1995.

Perkins, Bradford. *The Cambridge History of American Foreign Relations.* Vol. 1, *The Creation of a Republican Empire, 1776–1865.* Cambridge: Cambridge Univ. Press, 1993.

Perret, Geoffrey. *Ulysses S. Grant.* New York: Random House, 1997.

Peterson, Merrill D. *"Starving Armenians": America and the Armenian Genocide, 1915–1930 and After.* Charlottesville: Univ. of Virginia Press, 2004.

Philby, H. St. John. *Arabian Oil Ventures.* Washington, D.C.: Middle East Institute, 1964.

———. *Saudi Arabia.* London: Ernest Benn, 1955.

Philipson, David. *My Life as an American Jew.* Cincinnati: John G. Kidd, 1941.

Phillips, Clifton Jackson. *Protestant America and the Pagan World: The First Half Century of the American Board of Commissioners for Foreign Missions, 1810–1860.* Cambridge: Harvard Univ. Press, 1969.

Pletcher, David M. *The Awkward Years: American Foreign Relations under Garfield and Arthur.* Columbia: Univ. of Missouri Press, 1962.

A Pocket Guide to North Africa. Washington, D.C.: War and Navy Department, 1942.

Poe, Edgar Allan. *The Works of the Late Edgar Allan Poe.* Vol. 4. New York: Arthur Gordon Pym, 1856.

Pollack, Kenneth M. *The Persian Puzzle: The Conflict between Iran and America.* New York: Random House, 2004.

Porch, Douglas. *The Path to Victory: The Mediterranean Theater in World War II.* New York: Farrar, Straus and Giroux, 2004.

Powell, Colin L., with Joseph E. Persico. *My American Journey.* New York: Random House, 1995.

Power, Samantha. *A Problem from Hell: America and the Age of Genocide.* New York: Basic Books, 2002.

Price, Willadene. *Bartholdi and the Statue of Liberty.* Chicago: Rand McNally, 1959.

Prideaux, Humphrey. *The True Nature of Imposture Fully Displayed in the Life of Mahomet.* Fairhaven, Vt.: James Lyon, 1798.

Prime, William C. *Tent Life in the Holy Land.* New York: Harper, 1857.

Pulson, W. D. *The Life and Work of Captain Alfred Thayer Mahan.* New Haven: Yale Univ. Press, 1939.

Pyle, Ernie. *Here Is Your War.* New York: Henry Holt, 1943.

Quandt, William B. *Peace Process: American Diplomacy and the Arab-Israeli Conflict since 1967.* 3d ed. Washington, D.C.: Brookings Institution Press, 2005.

Quinn, Frederick. *The French Overseas Empire.* New York: Praeger, 2000.

Raab, James. *W. W. Loring.* Manhattan, Kan.: Sunflower Univ. Press, 1997.

Rabinowitz, Ezekiel. *Justice Louis D. Brandeis: The Zionist Chapter of His Life.* New York: Philosophical Library, 1968.

Raider, Mark A. *The Emergence of American Zionism.* New York: New York Univ. Press, 1998.

Rame, David. *Road to Tunis.* New York: Macmillan, 1944.

Randall, Willard Sterne. *Alexander Hamilton: A Life.* New York: Perennial, 2003.

Range, Willard. *Franklin D. Roosevelt's World Order.* Athens: Univ. of Georgia Press, 1959.

Rapoport, Louis. *Shake Heaven and Earth: Peter Bergson and the Struggle to Rescue the Jews of Europe.* Jerusalem: Gefen, 1999.

Ratzabi, Shalom. *Between Zionism and Judaism: The Radical Circle in Brith Shalom, 1925–1933.* Leiden: Brill, 2002.

Reagan, Ronald. *An American Life.* New York: Simon & Schuster, 1990.

———. *Reagan, in His Own Hand.* Edited by Kiron K. Skinner, Annelise Anderson, and Martin Anderson. New York: Free Press, 2001.

Reckner, James A. *Teddy Roosevelt's Great White Fleet.* Annapolis: Naval Institute Press, 1988.

Reinharz, Jehuda. *Chaim Weizman: The Making of a Statesman.* New York: Oxford Univ. Press, 1993.

Reinharz, Shulamit, and Mark A. Raider, eds. *American Jewish Women and the Zionist Enterprise.* Waltham, Mass.: Brandeis Univ. Press, 2004.

Remini, Robert V. *Andrew Jackson and the Course of American Freedom, 1822–1832.* Vol. 2. New York: Harper & Row, 1981.

Riad, Mahmoud. *The Struggle for Peace in the Middle East.* New York: Quartet Books, 1981.

Richter, Julius. *History of Protestant Missions in the Near East.* 1910. Reprint, New York: AMS Press, 1970.

Riggs, Henry H. *Days of Tragedy in Armenia.* Ann Arbor: Gomidas Institute, 1917.

Rihani, Ameen. *The Fate of Palestine.* Beirut: Rihan House, 1967.

———. *The Path of Vision.* Beirut: Rihani House, 1970.

Riley, James. *Sufferings in Africa: Captain Riley's Narrative.* New York: Potter, 1965.

Riley, Henry A. *The Restoration at the Second Coming of Christ: A Summary of Millenarian Doctrines.* Philadelphia: Lippincott, 1868.

Rippy, J. Fred. *Joel R. Poinsett: Versatile American.* Durham: Duke Univ. Press, 1935.

Ritchie, Donald A. *James M. Landis: Dean of the Regulators*. Cambridge: Harvard Univ. Press, 1980.

Rizk, Salom. *Syrian Yankee*. Garden City. N.Y.: Doubleday, Doran, 1943.

Robbins, Thomas. *Diaries, 1796–1854*. Boston: Thomas Todd, 1886.

Roberts, Edmund. *Embassy to the Eastern Courts of Cochin-China, Siam, and Muscat, in the U.S. Sloop-of-War* Peacock, *during the Years 1832–3–4*. New York: Harper, 1837.

Robinson, Edward. *Biblical Researches in Palestine, Mount Sinai and Arabia Petraea: A Journal of Travels in the Year 1838 by E. Robinson and E. Smith, Undertaken in Reference to Biblical Geography*. 3 vols. Boston: Crocker & Brewster, 1841.

———. *Later Biblical Researches in Palestine and Adjacent Regions: A Journal of Travels in the Year 1852*. London: John Murray, 1856.

Robotti, Frances Diane, and James Vescovi. *The USS* Essex *and the Birth of the American Navy*. Holbrook, Mass.: Adams Media Corp., 1999.

Roosevelt, Elliott. *As He Saw It*. New York: Duell, Sloan and Pierce, 1946.

Roosevelt, Theodore. *An Autobiography*. New York: Da Capo Press, 1985.

———. *Theodore Roosevelt's Diaries of Boyhood and Youth*. New York: Scribner, 1928.

Ross, Dennis. *The Missing Peace: The Inside Story of the Fight for Middle East Peace*. New York: Farrar, Straus and Giroux, 2004.

Roth, Philip. *The Plot Against America*. Boston and New York: Houghton Mifflin, 2004.

Rowson, Susanna. *Slaves in Algiers; or, The Struggle for Freedom*. Philadelphia: Wrigley and Berriman, 1794.

Rubin, Barry. *Paved with Good Intentions: The American Experience and Iran*. New York: Viking, 1981.

———. *The Great Powers in the Middle East, 1941–1947*. London: Cass, 1980.

Rubin, Barry, and Judith Colp Rubin. *Yasir Arafat: A Political Biography*. Oxford: Oxford Univ. Press, 2003.

Rubinger, Naphtali J. *Abraham Lincoln and the Jews*. New York: Jonathan David, 1962.

Rusk, John. *The Authentic Life of T. DeWitt Talmage*. New York: L. G. Stahl, 1902.

Rutland, Robert A. *The Presidency of James Madison*. Lawrence: Univ. Press of Kansas, 1990.

Sachar, Howard M. *The Emergence of the Middle East, 1914–1924*. New York: Knopf, 1969.

———. *A History of Israel: From the Rise of Zionism to Our Time*. New York: Knopf, 1970.

Sadat, Anwar el-. *In Search of Identity: An Autobiography*. New York: Harper & Row, 1977.

———. *Revolt on the Nile*. Translated by Thomas Graham. London: A. Wingate, 1957.

Safran, Nadav. *Israel: The Embattled Ally*. Cambridge: Belknap Press, 1978.

Said, Edward. *Orientalism*. New York: Vintage, 1979.

Saikal, Amin. *The Rise and Fall of the Shah*. Princeton: Princeton Univ. Press, 1980.

Sampson, Anthony. *The Seven Sisters: The Great Oil Companies and the World They Shaped*. New York: Bantam, 1991.

Sandys, George. *Description of the Ottoman Empire*. Amsterdam: Theatrum Orbis Terrarum, 1973.

Sarna, Jonathan D. *Jacksonian Jew: The Two Worlds of Mordecai Noah*. New York: Holmes & Meier, 1981.

Savary, Claude Etienne. *Letters on Egypt, Containing a Parallel between the Manners of Its Ancient and Modern Inhabitants*. London: G. G. J. and J. Robinson, 1787.

Schachner, Nathan. *Thomas Jefferson: A Biography*. New York: Thomas Yoseloff, 1951.

Schaff, Philip. *Through Bible Lands: Notes of Travel in Egypt, the Desert, and Palestine*. New York: American Tract Society, 1878.

Scherer, George H. *Mediterranean Missions, 1808–1870*. Beirut: Bible Lands Union for Christian Education, n.d.

Schlesinger, Arthur M., Jr. *The Age of Jackson*. Boston: Little, Brown, 1950.

Scholes, Walter, and Marie Scholes. *The Foreign Policies of the Taft Administration*. Columbia: Univ. of Missouri Press, 1970.

Schroeder, Seaton. *Fifty Years of Naval Service*. New York: Appleton, 1922.

Schueller, Malini Johar. *U.S. Orientalisms*. Ann Arbor: Univ. of Michigan Press, 1998.

———, ed. *David F. Dorr: A Colored Man round the World*. Ann Arbor: Univ. of Michigan Press, 1999.

Schuldiner, Michael, and Daniel J. Kleinfeld. *The Selected Writings of Mordecai Noah*. London: Greenwood, 1999.

Schwarzkopf, H. Norman, with Peter Petre. *It Doesn't Take a Hero: The Autobiography*. New York: Bantam, 1992.

Seeger, Robert. *And Tyler Too: A Biography of John and Julia Gardiner Tyler*. New York: McGraw-Hill, 1963.

Seward, Olive Risley. *Around the World Stories*. Boston: D. Lothrop, 1889.

———, ed. *William H. Seward's Travels around the World*. New York: Appleton, 1873.

Shaban, Fuad. *Islam and Arabs in Early American Thought: Roots of Orientalism in America*. Durham, N.C.: Acorn Press, 1991.

Shaler, William. *Sketches of Algiers*. Boston: Cummings, Hillard, 1826.

Sharafuddin, Mohammed. *Islam and Romantic Orientalism: Literary Encounters with the Orient*. London: I. B. Tauris, 1994.

Sharif, Regina S. *Non-Jewish Zionism: Its Roots in Western History*. London: Zed Press, 1983.

Shaw, George Bernard. *The Complete Plays of Bernard Shaw*. London: Constable Press, 1931.

Shaw, Stanford. *History of the Ottoman Empire and Modern Turkey*. Vol. 1, *Empire of the Gazis: The Rise and Decline of the Ottoman Empire, 1280–1808*. Cambridge: Cambridge Univ. Press, 1976.

Sheehan, Michael K. *Iran: The Impact of United States Interests and Policies, 1941–1943*. Brooklyn: Theo Gaus' Sons, 1968.

Shepherd, Naomi. *The Zealous Intruders: The Western Rediscovery of Palestine*. London: Collins, 1987.

Shimoni, Gideon. *The Zionist Ideology*. Hanover: Univ. Press of New England, Brandeis Univ. Press, 1995.

Shire, Michael. *The Jewish Prophet: Visionary Words from Moses to Heschel*. London: Frances Lincoln, 2002.

Schoenbaum, David. *The United States and the State of Israel*. New York: Oxford Univ. Press, 1993.

Shotwell, James. *At the Paris Peace Conference*. New York: Macmillan, 1937.

Shpiro, David. *From Philanthropy to Activism: The Political Transformation of American Zionism in the Holocaust Years, 1933–1945*. Oxford: Pergamon Press, 1994.

Shuckburgh, Evelyn. *Descent to Suez: Diaries, 1951–1956*. Edited by John Charmley. New York: Norton, 1986.

Shwadran, Benjamin. *The Middle East, Oil, and the Great Powers*. Jerusalem: Israel Univ. Press, 1973.

Silberman, Neal Asher. *Digging for God and Country: Archeology and the Secret Struggle for the Holy Land, 1799–1917*. New York: Knopf, 1982.

Silverberg, Robert. *If I Forget Thee, O Jerusalem: American Jews and the State of Israel*. New York: Morrow, 1970.

Silverstein, Gordon. *Imbalance of Powers: Constitutional Interpretation and the Making of American Foreign Policy*. Oxford: Oxford Univ. Press, 1997.

Simmes, Raphael. *Memoirs of a Service Afloat*. Baltimore: Baltimore Publishing Co., 1887.

Simons, Geoff. *Libya and the West: From Independence to Lockerbie*. Oxford: Centre for Libyan Studies, 2003.

Smelser, Marshall. *The Democratic Republic*. New York: Harper & Row, 1968.

Smith, Gaddis. *American Diplomacy during the Second World War, 1941–1945*. New York: Knopf, 1985.

Sobel, Samuel. *Intrepid Soldier*. Philadelphia: Cresset, 1980.

Southgate, Horatio. *Narrative of a Tour through Armenia, Kurdistan, Persia, and Mesopotamia*. London: Appleton, 1840.

Sparks, Jared. *The Life of John Ledyard, the American Traveller*. Cambridge: Hillard and Brown, 1828.

Spiegel, Steven L. *The Other Arab-Israeli Conflict: Making America's Middle East Policy, from Truman to Reagan*. Chicago: Univ. of Chicago Press, 1985.

Stagg, J. C. A. *Mr. Madison's War: Politics, Diplomacy, and Warfare in the Early American Republic, 1783–1830*. Princeton: Princeton Univ. Press, 1983.

Steers, Edward. *Blood on the Moon: The Assassination of Abraham Lincoln*. Lexington: Univ. Press of Kentucky, 2001.

Stegner, Wallace. *Discovery: The Search for Arabian Oil*. Beirut: Export Press, 1971.

Stein, Kenneth W. *Heroic Diplomacy: Sadat, Kissinger, Carter, Begin, and the Quest for Arab-Israeli Peace*. New York: Routledge, 1999.

Stein, Leonard. *The Balfour Declaration*. London: Vallentine, Mitchell, 1961.

Steiner, Franklin. *The Religious Beliefs of Our Presidents: From Washington to F.D.R.* New York: Prometheus, 1995.

Stephens, John Lloyd. *Incidents of Travel in Egypt, Arabia Petraea, and the Holy Land*. New York: Harper, 1855.

Sternlicht, Sanford V. *Uriah Phillips Levy: The Blue Star Commodore*. Norfolk, Va.: Norfolk Jewish Community Council, 1961.

Stevens, James. *An Historical and Geographical Account of Algiers*. Philadelphia: Hogan and McElroy, 1797.

Stevens, Marcia, and Malcolm Stevens. *Against the Devil's Current: The Life and Times of Cyrus Hamlin*. Lanham, Md.: Univ. Press of America, 1988.

Stevens, Mark. *Six Months at the World's Fair*. Detroit: Detroit Free Press, 1895.

Stevens, Mrs. Mark. *A Lecture on What You Missed in Not Visiting the World's Fair*. Flint: n.p., 1895.

Still, William N. *American Sea Power in the Old World: The United States Navy in European and Near Eastern Waters, 1865–1917*. Westport, Conn.: Greenwood, 1980.

St. John, Ronald Bruce. *Libya and the United States: Two Centuries of Strife*. Philadelphia: Univ. of Pennsylvania Press, 2002.

Strong, Douglas H. *Dreamers and Defenders: American Conservationists*. Lincoln: Univ. of Nebraska Press, 1988.

Strong, Josiah. *Our Country: Its Possible Future and Its Present Crisis*. New York: American Home Mission Society, 1885.

Strout, Cushing. *The American Image of the Old World*. New York: Harper & Row, 1963.

Studies in the National Military Victories of Egypt [Arabic]. Cairo: Ministry of Information, 1984.

Sumner, Charles. *White Slavery in the Barbary States*. Boston: J. P. Jewett, 1853.

Swift, John. *Going to Jericho*. New York: A. Roman, 1868.

Sykes, Christopher. *Crossroads to Israel, 1917–1948*. Bloomington: Indiana Univ. Press, 1973.

Symonds, Craig L. *Navalist and Antinavalists: The Naval Policy Debate in the United States, 1785–1827*. Newark: Univ. of Delaware Press, 1980.

Talmage, T. DeWitt. *New Tabernacle Sermons*. New York: George Munro, 1886.

———. *Talmage on Palestine: A Series of Sermons*. New York: W. D. Rowland, 1890.

Tauber, Eliezer. *The Emergence of the Arab Movements*. London: Frank Cass, 1993.

Taylor, Baynard. *The Lands of the Saracen; or, Pictures of Palestine, Asia Minor, Sicily, and Spain.* New York: Putnam, 1855.

Teveth, Shabtai. *Ben Gurion: The Burning Ground, 1886–1948.* Boston: Houghton Mifflin, 1987.

Thackery, William Makepeace. *From Cornhill to Grand Cairo.* London: George Routledge, 1888.

Thomas, Benjamin P. *Abraham Lincoln: A Biography.* New York: Random House, 1968.

Thomas, Evan. *John Paul Jones: Sailor, Hero, Father of the American Navy.* New York: Simon & Schuster, 2003.

Thomas, Lowell. *Good Evening Everybody.* New York: Morrow, 1976.

———. *With Lawrence in Arabia.* London: Hutchinson, n.d.

Thomas, Nancy, ed. *The American Discovery of Ancient Egypt.* New York: Abrams, 1995.

Thomson, William. *The Land and the Book; or, Biblical Illustrations Drawn from the Manners and Customs,the Scenes and Scenery, of the Holy Land.* Vol. 1. New York: Harper, 1886.

Tibawi, A. L. *American Interests in Syria, 1800–1901.* Oxford: Clarendon Press, 1966.

Tibi, Bassam. *Arab Nationalism: Between Islam and the Nation-State.* New York: St. Martin's, 1997.

Tocqueville, Alexis de. *Democracy in America.* New York: Appleton, 1901.

Touval, Saadia. *The Peace Brokers: Mediators in the Arab-Israeli Conflict, 1948–1979.* Princeton: Princeton Univ. Press, 1982.

Trachtenberg, Marvin. *The Statue of Liberty.* New York: Penguin, 1986.

Trask, Robert. *The United States Response to Turkish Nationalism and Reform, 1914–1939.* Minneapolis: Univ. of Minnesota, 1971.

Truman, Harry S. *Memoirs.* Vol. 2, *Years of Trial and Hope.* Garden City, N.Y.: Doubleday, 1956.

Tuchman, Barbara W. *Bible and Sword: England and Palestine from the Bronze Age to Balfour.* New York: Ballantine, 1956.

Tucker, Glenn. *Dawn like Thunder: The Barbary Wars and the Birth of the U.S. Navy.* New York: Bobbs-Merrill, 1963.

Turnbull, Archibald Douglas. *Commodore David Porter, 1780–1843.* New York: Century, 1929.

Turner, Brian. *Here, Bullet.* Farmington, Me.: Alice James Books, 2005.

Turner, Frederick Jackson. *The Frontier in American History.* 1920. Reprint, New York: Henry Holt, 1947.

Twain, Mark. *The Innocents Abroad; or, The New Pilgrims' Progress Being Some Account of the Steamwhip Quaker City's Pleasure Excursion to Europe and the Holy Land.* Pleasantville, N.Y.: Reader's Digest, 1990.

Tyler, Royall. *The Algerine Captive; or, The Life and Adventures of Doctor Updike Underhill, Six Years a Prisoner among the Algerines.* Hartford: Peter B. Gleason, 1816.

Urofsky, Melvin I. *American Zionism from Herzl to the Holocaust*. Garden City, N.Y.: Anchor, 1975.

———. *The Levy Family and Monticello*. Monticello: Thomas Jefferson Foundation, 2001.

———. *A Voice That Spoke for Justice: The Life and Times of Stephen S. Wise*. Albany: State Univ. of New York Press, 1982.

Urquhart, Brian. *Ralph Bunche: An American Life*. New York: Norton, 1993.

U.S. Department of the Army, the United States Army in World War II: The Middle East Theater. Washington, D.C.: GPO, 1953.

Ussher, Clarence, and Grace Knapp. *An American Physician in Turkey*. Boston: Houghton Mifflin, 1917.

Van der Meulen, D. *The Wells of Ibn Saud*. New York: Praeger, 1957.

Van Deusen, Glyndon. *William Henry Seward*. New York: Oxford Univ. Press, 1967.

Vandewalle, Dirk. *A History of Modern Libya*. Cambridge: Cambridge Univ. Press, 2006.

Van Dyke, Henry. *Out-of-Doors in the Holy Land: Impressions of Travel in Body and Spirit*. New York: Scribner, 1908.

Vatikiotis, P. J. *The History of Egypt: From Muhammad Ali to Sadat*. Baltimore: Johns Hopkins Univ. Press, 1980.

———. *Nasser and His Generation*. New York: St. Martin's, 1978.

Vester, Bertha Spafford. *Our Jerusalem: an American Family in the Holy City, 1881–1949*. 1950. Reprint, New York: Arno Press, 1977.

Vogel, Dan. *Mark Twain's Jews*. Jersey City, N.J.: KTAV Publishing House, 2006.

Vogel, Lester I. *To See a Promised Land: Americans and the Holy Land in the Nineteenth Century*. University Park: Pennsylvania State Univ. Press, 1993.

Volney, Constantin-François. *Voyage en Syrie et en Egypte, pendant les années 1783, 1784, et 1785*. Paris: Desenne et Volland, 1787.

Wagenknecht, Edward. *Daughters of the Covenant: Portraits of Six Jewish Women*. Amherst: Univ. of Massachusetts Press, 1983.

Walker, Charles T. *A Colored Man around the World: What He Saw and Heard in the Holy Land and Europe*. Augusta, Ga.: John M. Weigle, 1892.

Wallace, Edwin S. *Jerusalem the Holy: A Brief History of Ancient Jerusalem, with an Account of the Modern City and Its Conditions, Political, Religious and Social*. New York: Revell, 1898.

Walsh, Lawrence E. *Iran Contra: The Final Report*. New York: Times Books, 1994.

Walworth, Arthur. *Woodrow Wilson*. New York: Norton, 1978.

Warner, Charles Dudley. *Mummies and Moslems*. Toronto: Belford Brothers, 1876.

———. *My Winter on the Nile*. Hartford: American Publishing Co., 1876.

Warren, Henry White. *Sights and Insights; or, Knowledge by Travel*. New York: Nelson and Phillips, 1874.

Washburn, George. *Fifty Years in Constantinople*. Boston: Houghton Mifflin, 1909.

Washington, Joseph, ed. *Jews in Black Perspective*. Rutherford: Fairleigh Dickinson Univ. Press, 1984.

Watrous, Stephen D., ed. *John Ledyard's Journey through Russia and Siberia 1787–1788: The Journal and Selected Letters*. Madison: Univ. of Wisconsin Press, 1966.

Watts, Martin. *The Jewish Legion and the First World War*. London: Palgrave Macmillan, 2004,

Weinberg, Albert K. *Manifest Destiny: A Study of Nationalist Expansionism in American History*. 1935. Reprint, Chicago: Quadrangle, 1963.

Weisberger, Bernard A. *Statue of Liberty: The First Hundred Years*. Boston: Houghton Mifflin, 1985.

Weizmann, Chaim. *Trial and Error: The Autobiography of Chaim Weizmann*. Philadelphia: Jewish Publication Society of America, 1949.

Wert, Jeffrey D. *General James Longstreet*. New York: Simon and Schuster, 1993.

Wessels, William. *Born to Be a Soldier: The Military Career of William Wing Loring*. Fort Worth: Texas Christian Univ. Press, 1971.

Wharton, Edith. *In Morocco*. New York: Scribner, 1920.

Wheelan, Joseph. *Jefferson's War: America's First War on Terror, 1801–1805*. New York: Carroll & Graf, 2003.

Whipple, A. B. C. *To the Shores of Tripoli: The Birth of the U.S. Navy and Marines*. New York: Morrow, 1991.

Whitehead, Ernest D. *World War II: An Ex-Sergeant Remembers*. Kearney, N.J.: Morris Publishing, 1996.

Williams, Stanley T., ed. *Journal of Washington Irving, 1828 and Miscellaneous Notes on Moorish Legend and History*. New York: American Book Co., 1937.

Williams, William Appleman. *The Shaping of American Diplomacy: Readings and Documents in American Foreign Policy, 1750–1955*. Chicago: Rand McNally, 1956.

Willis, Nathaniel Parker. *Summer Cruise in the Mediterranean on an American Frigate*. New York: Scribner, 1853.

Wilmington, Martin W. *The Middle East Supply Centre*. Albany: State Univ. of New York Press, 1971.

Wilson, J. Christy. *Apostle to Islam: A Biography of Samuel M. Zwemer*. Grand Rapids, Mich.: Baker Book House, 1952.

Winter, Jay, ed. *America and the Armenian Genocide of 1915*. Cambridge: Cambridge Univ. Press, 2003.

Wissa, Hanna F. *Assiout: The Saga of an Egyptian Family*. Sussex: Book Guild, 1994.

Wolf, Simon. *The Presidents I Have Known from 1860–1918*. Washington, D.C.: Byron S. Adams, 1918.

———. *Selected Addresses and Papers of Simon Wolf*. New York: Bloch, 1926.

Woodruff, Samuel. *Journal of a Tour to Malta, Greece, Asia Minor, Carthage, Algiers, Port Mahon, and Spain*. Hartford: Cooke, 1831.

Woodward, Bob. *Plan of Attack*. New York: Simon & Schuster, 2004.

Wortham, H. E. *Chinese Gordon*. Boston: Little, Brown, 1933.

Wriggins, Howard. *Picking Up the Pieces from Portugal to Palestine: Quaker Refugee Relief in World War II*. Lanham, Md.: Univ. Press of America, 2004.

Wright, L. C. *United States Policy toward Egypt, 1830–1914*. New York: Exposition Press, 1969.

Wright, Louis B., and Julia H. Macleod. *The First Americans in North Africa: William Eaton's Struggle for a Vigorous Policy against the Barbary Pirates, 1799–1805*. New York: Greenwood, 1945.

Wyman, David S., and Rafael Medoff. *A Race against Death: Peter Bergson, America, and the Holocaust*. New York: New Press, 2004.

Wynn, Humphrey. *Desert Eagles*. Osceola, Wis.: Motorbooks International, 1993.

Yale, William. *The Near East: A Modern History*. Ann Arbor: Univ. of Michigan Press, 1958.

Yaqub, Salim. *Containing Arab Nationalism: The Eisenhower Doctrine and the Middle East*. Chapel Hill: Univ. of North Carolina Press, 2004.

Yeselson, Abraham. *United States–Persia Diplomatic Relations, 1883–1921*. New Brunswick: Rutgers Univ. Press, 1956.

Young, John Russell. *Around the World with General Grant: A Narrative of the Visit of General U.S. Grant, Ex-President of the United States, to Various Countries in Europe, Asia and Africa, in 1877, 1878, 1879*. New York: American News Co., 1879.

Zacks, Richard. *The Pirate Coast: Thomas Jefferson, the First Marines, and the Secret Mission of 1805*. New York: Hyperion, 2005.

Zakaria, Fareed. *From Wealth to Power: The Unusual Origins of America's World Role*. Princeton: Princeton Univ. Press, 1996.

Zeine, Zeine N. *The Emergence of Arab Nationalism*. 3d ed. Delmar, N.Y.: Caravan Books, 1973.

Ziegler, Philip. *Mountbatten*. London: Collins, 1985.

Ziff, Larzer. *Return Passages: Great American Travel Writing, 1780–1910*. New Haven: Yale Univ. Press, 2000.

Zilversmit, Arthur. *The First Emancipation: The Abolition of Slavery in the North*. Chicago: Univ. of Chicago Press, 1967.

Zimmerman, Walter. *First Great Triumph: How Five Americans Made Their Country a World Power*. New York: Farrar, Straus and Giroux, 2002.

Zug, James. *American Traveler*. New York: Basic Books, 2005.

Zwemer, A. E., and S. M. Zwemer. *Zigzag Journeys in the Camel Country: Arabia in Picture and Story*. New York: Revell, 1911.

Zwemer, Samuel, and James Cantine. *The Golden Milestone: Reminiscences of Pioneer Days Fifty Years Ago in Arabia*. New York: Revell, 1938.

Articles

Adler, Selig. "The Palestine Question in the Wilson Era." *Jewish Social Studies* 10, no. 4 (Oct. 1948).

Allen, John. "Inventing the Middle East." *On Wisconsin* (Winter 2004).

Almond, Philip. "Western Images of Islam, 1700–1900." *Australian Journal of Politics and History* 49, no. 3 (2003).

Amann, Peter. "Prophet in Zion: The Saga of George J. Adams." *New England Quarterly* 37 (Dec. 1964).

An American. "An Audience with Sultan Abdul Mejud." *Knickerbocker* 19 (June 1842).

Audenreid, J. C. "General Sherman in Europe and the East." *Harper's New Monthly Magazine* 47, no. 280 (Sept. 1873).

Baram, Phillip. "Undermining the British: Department of State Policies in Egypt and the Suez Canal before and during World War II." *Historian* 40, no. 4 (Aug. 1978).

Ben Rejeb, Lotfi. "America's Captive Freemen in North Africa: The Comparative Method in Abolitionist Persuasion." *Slavery and Abolition* 9 (1988).

Berge, William H. "Voices for Imperialism: Josiah Strong and the Protestant Clergy." *Border States*, no. 1 (1973).

Biger, Gideon. "The American View of the Tel Hai Affair." *Journal of Israeli History* 19, no. 1 (1998).

Blumberg, Arnold. "William Seward and Egyptian Intervention in Mexico." *Smithsonian Journal of History* 1 (Winter 1966–67).

Borer, Douglas A. "Inverse Engagement: Lessons from U.S.-Iraq Relations, 1982–1990." *Parameters* 33, no. 2 (2003).

Bornstein, George. "A Forgotten Alliance: Africans, Americans, Zionists and Irish." *Times Literary Supplement*, March 4, 2005.

Breitman, Richard. "The Allied War Effort and the Jews, 1942–1943," *Journal of Contemporary History* 20, no. 1 (Jan. 1985).

Brekus, Catherine A. "Harriet Livermore, the Pilgrim Stranger: Female Preaching and Biblical Feminism in Early Nineteenth-Century America." *Journal of the Early Republic* 65 (Sept. 1996).

Brier, Bob. "Saga of Cleopatra's Needles," *Archaeology* 55, no.6 (Nov.–Dec. 2002).

Bruck, Connie. "The Wounds of Peace." *New Yorker*, Oct. 14, 1996.

Buel, Clarence Clough. "Preliminary Glimpses of the Fair." *Century* 45, no. 4 (Feb. 1893).

"Bush on Ezekiel's Vision." *Princeton Review* 16, no. 3 (1844).

Cantor, Milton. "Joel Barlow's Mission to Algiers." *Historian* 25 (1963).

Caplan, Dennis. "John Adams, Thomas Jefferson, and the Barbary Pirates: An Illustration of Relevant Costs for Decision Making." *Issues in Accounting Education* 18, no. 3 (2003).

Christison, Kathleen. "The Arab-Israeli Policy of George Schultz." *Journal of Palestine Studies* 18, no. 2 (1989).

Cohen, Michael J. "American Influence on British Policy in the Middle East during World War Two: First Attempts at Coordinating Allied Policy on Palestine." *American Jewish Historical Quarterly* 67, no. 1 (Sept. 1977).

———. "Secret Diplomacy and Rebellion in Palestine, 1936–1939." *International Journal of Middle East Studies* 8, no. 3 (July 1977).

Cox, Frederick J. "Arabi and Stone: Egypt's Military Rebellion, 1882." *Cahiers d'Histoire Egyptienne* 8 (April 1956).

———. "The American Naval Mission in Egypt." *Journal of Modern History* 26, no. 2 (June 1954).

Daigle, Craig A. "The Russians Are Going: Sadat, Nixon and the Soviet Presence in Egypt, 1970–1971." *Middle East Review of International Affairs* 8, no. 1 (March 2004).

Daniel, Robert L. "The Armenian Question and American-Turkish Relations, 1914–1927." *Mississippi Valley Historical Review* 46 (Sept. 1959).

DeMott, Robert. "Steinbeck's Other Family: New Light on East of Eden?" *Steinbeck Newsletter* 7, no. 1 (Winter 1994).

Dunn, John, "Egypt's Nineteenth-Century Armaments Industry." *Journal of Military History* 61 (April 1997).

Earle, Edward M. "American Interest in the Greek Cause, 1821–1827," *American Historical Review* 33, no. 1 (Oct. 1927).

———. "Early American Policy concerning Ottoman Minorities." *Political Science Quarterly* 42, no. 3 (Sept. 1927).

———. "Egyptian Cotton and the American Civil War." *Political Science Quarterly* 41, no. 4 (Dec. 1926).

Efimenco, Marbury N. "American Impact upon Middle East Leadership." *Political Science Quarterly* 69, no. 2 (June 1954).

Eidelberg, Shlomo. "The Adams Colony in Jaffa (1866–1868)." *Midstream* 3 (Autumn 1957).

Eiselein, Gregory. "Emotion and the Jewish Historical Poems of Emma Lazarus." *Mosaic* 37 (2004).

Farman, Elbert Eli. "Negotiating for the Obelisk." *Century Illustrated Monthly Magazine* 24 (Oct. 1882).

Ford, Alexander Fume. "Our American Colony at Jerusalem." *Appleton's Magazine* 8 (1906).

Fox, Frank. "Quaker, Shaker, Rabbi: Warder Cresson: The Story of a Philadelphia Mystic." *Pennsylvania Magazine of History and Biography* 95 (1971).

Frazier, Robert. "Acheson and Formulation of the Truman Doctrine." *Journal of Modern Greek Studies* 17, no. 2 (1999).

Fromkin, David. "The Importance of T. E. Lawrence." *New Criterion* 10, no. 1 (Sept. 1995).

Funk, Arthur L. "Negotiating the 'Deal with Darlan.'" *Journal of Contemporary History* 8, no. 2 (April 1973).

Gelvin, James L. "Zionism and the Representation of Jewish Palestine at the New York World's Fair, 1939–40." *International History Review* 22, no. 1 (2000).

Gillespie, Joanna. "Mary Briscoe Baldwin (1811–1877), Single Woman Missionary and 'Very Much My Own Mistress.'" *Anglican and Episcopal History* 57 (March 1988).

Goldman, Shalom. "Professor George Bush: American Hebraist and Proto-Zionist." *American Jewish Archives* 43, no.1 (1991).

Gorst, Anthony, and Scott W. Lucas. "Suez 1956: Strategy and the Diplomatic Process." *Journal of Strategic Studies* 23, no. 1 (1988).

Grabill, Joseph. "Cleveland H. Dodge, Woodrow Wilson, and the Near East." *Journal of Presbyterian History* 48 (Winter 1970).

Grant, Jonathan. "The Sword of the Sultan: Ottoman Arms Imports, 1854–1914." *Journal of Military History* 66 (Jan. 2002).

Hale, William Harlan. "'General' Eaton and His Improbable Legion." *American Heritage* 11, no. 2 (Feb. 1960).

Halpern, Ben. "The Americanization of Zionism." *American Jewish History* 69, no. 1 (1979).

Hamdani, Abbas. "Columbus and the Recovery of Jerusalem." *Journal of the American Oriental Society* 99, no. 1 (1979).

Hamlin, Cyrus. "American Educatin in the Ottoman Empire." *Arena* 22, no. 1 (Dec. 1899).

Herbert, T. Walter. "The Force of Prejudice: Melville's Attack on Missions in Typee." *Border States*, no. 1 (1973).

Herzl, Theodore. "Mark Twain and the British Ladies: A Feuilleton." *Commentary* 28, no. 3 (Sept. 1959).

Hogan, Matthew. "The 1948 Massacre at Deir Yassin Revisited." *Historian* 63, no. 2 (Winter 2001).

"The Holy Land Appropriated: The Careers of Selah Merrill, Nineteenth Century Christian Hebraist, Palestine Explorer, and U.S. Consul in Jerusalem." *American Jewish History* 85, no. 2 (June 1997).

Howard, Harry N. "President Lincoln's Minister Resident to the Sublime Porte." *Balkan Studies* 5 (1964).

Hoxie, Elizabeth F. "Harriet Livermore: Vixen and Devotee." *New England Quarterly* 18 (March 1945).

Isaacs, Abram S. "Will the Jews Return to Palestine." *Century Illustrated Monthly Magazine* 26, no. 1 (May 1883).

J.L.C. "Trade to the Black Sea." *National Register* 5, no. 12 (May 23, 1818).

Kaplan, Lawrence S. "The Monroe Doctrine and the Truman Doctrine: The Case of Greece." *Journal of the Early Republic* 13, no. 1 (Spring 1993).

Keating, John S. "Cruise of the USS *Flying Carpet.*" *True* 33, no. 199 (Dec. 1953).

Kedourie, Elie. "The American University of Beirut." *Middle Eastern Studies* 3 (1966).

Kennedy, David M. "What 'W' Owes to 'WW.'" *Atlantic Monthly*, March 2005.

Kirkland, John Thornton. "Letter on the Holy Land." *Christian Examiner and General Review* 23, no. 2 (1842).

Klingelhofer, Herbert E. "Abolish the Navy!" *Manuscripts* 33, no. 4 (Fall 1981).

Knee, Stuart. "Anglo-American Relations in Palestine, 1919–1925: An Experiment in Realpolitik." *Journal of American Studies of Turkey* 5 (1997).

Kobbe, Gustav. "Sights at the Fair." *Century Illustrated Monthly Magazine* 46, no. 6 (Sept. 1893).

Kotzin, Daniel P. "An Attempt to Americanize the Yishuv: Judah L. Magnes in Mandatory Palestine." *Israel Studies* 5, no. 1 (2000).

Langley, Lester D. "Jacksonian America and the Ottoman Empire." *Muslim World* (Duncan Black Macdonald Center, Hartford Seminary Foundation), 1978.

Lawson, Fred. "The Reagan Administration in the Middle East." *MERIP Reports*, no. 128 (Nov. 1984).

Lazarus, Emma. "Epistle to the Hebrews." *American Hebrew* 13 (Feb. 2, 1883).

———. "The Jewish Problem." *Century Illustrated Monthly Magazine* 36, no. 6 (Feb. 1883).

Lebow, Richard. "The Morgenthau Peace Mission of 1917." *Jewish Social Studies* 32, no. 4 (Oct. 1970).

———. "Woodrow Wilson and the Balfour Declaration." *Journal of Modern History* 40, no. 4 (Dec. 1968).

Lewis, James R. "Savages of the Seas: Barbary Captivity Tales and Images of Muslims in the Early Republic." *Journal of American Culture* 13, no. 2 (Summer 1990).

Little, Douglas. "The Making of a Special Relationship: The United States and Israel, 1957–68." *International Journal of Middle East Studies* 25, no. 4 (Nov. 1993).

———. "The New Frontier on the Nile: JFK, Nasser, and Arab Natinalism." *Journal of American History* 75, no. 2 (Sept. 1988).

Litvak, Meir, and Joshua Teitelbaum. "Students, Teachers and Edward Said: Taking Stock of Orientalism." *Middle East Review of International Affairs* 10, no. 1 (March 2006).

Louis, William Roger. "American Anti-colonialism and the Dissolution of the British Empire." *International Affairs* 61, no. 3 (Summer 1985).

Macleod, Julia H. "Jefferson and the Navy: A Defense." *Huntington Library Quarterly* 8 (Feb. 1945).

Malley, Robert, and Hussein Agha. "Camp David: The Tragedy of Errors." *New York Review of Books*, Aug. 9, 2001.

Malone, Joseph J. "America and the Arabian Peninsula: The First Two Hundred Years." *Middle East Journal* 30, no. 3 (Summer 1976).

Manela, Erez. "Friction from the Sidelines: Diplomacy, Religion and Culture in American-Egyptian Relations, 1919–1939." *The United States and the Middle East: Diplomatic and Economic Relations in Historical Perspective*. New Haven: Yale Center for International and Area Studies (2000).

Marom, Daniel. "Who Is the 'Mother of Exiles'?: Jewish Aspects of Emma Lazarus's *The New Colossus.*" *Prooftexts* 20, no. 3 (2000).

Mayer, David N. "By the Chains of the Constitution: Separation of Powers Theory and Jefferson's Conception of the Presidency." *Perspectives on Political Science* 26 (1997).

McCarthy, W. Barry. "Ibn Saud's Voyage." *Life*, March 19, 1945.

McClellan, George B. "The Bombardment of Alexandria." *North American Review* 142, no. 355 (June 1886).

———. "The War in Egypt." *Century Illustrated Monthly Magazine* 24, no. 5 (Sept. 1882).

———. "A Winter on the Nile." *Scribner's Monthly* 13, nos. 3–4 (Jan.–March 1877).

McMurty, Gerald. "Influences of Riley's *Narrative* upon Abraham Lincoln." *Indiana Magazine of History* 30, no. 2 (June 1934).

Mead, Elwood. "The New Palestine." *American Review of Reviews* 70, no. 6 (Dec. 1924).

Milani, Abbas. "Hurley's Dream." *Hoover Digest*, no. 3 (2003).

Miller, Rory. "Bible and Soil: Walter Clay Lowdermilk, the Jordan Valley Project and the Palestine Debate." *Middle Eastern Studies* 39, no. 2 (April 2003).

Mylroie, Laurie. "U.S. Policy toward Iraq." *Middle East Intelligence Bulletin* 3, no. 1 (Jan. 2001).

Novelists Magazine. Vol. 18 (Containing The Arabian Nights Entertainment). London: Harrison, 1785.

Omer-Sherman, Ranen. "Emma Lazarus, Jewish American Poetics, and the Challenge of Modernity." *Journal of American Women Writers* 19 (2003).

Oren, Michael B. "The Diplomatic Struggle for the Negev." *Studies in Zionism* 2, no. 1 (1989).

———. "Escalation to Suez: The Egypt-Israel Border War, 1949–56." *Journal of Contemporary History* 24, no. 3 (July 1989).

———. "Israel, the Great Powers, and the Middle East Crisis of 1958." *Studies in Zionism* 12, no. 2 (1992).

———. "Secret Efforts to Achieve an Egypt-Israel Settlement prior to the Suez Campaign." *Middle Eastern Studies* 26, no. 3 (1990).

Ozick, Cynthia. "Mark Twain and the Jews." *Commentary* 99, no. 5 (May 1995).

Quandt, William B. "The Conflict in American Foreign Policy." In *From June to October: The Middle East between 1967 and 1973*, edited by Itamar Rabinovich and Haim Shaked. New Brunswick: Transaction, 1978.

Perry, Yaron. "John Steinbeck's Roots in Nineteenth-Century Palestine," *Steinbeck Studies* 15, no. 1 (Spring 2002).

Peskin, Lawrence A. "The Lessons of Independence: How the Algerian Crisis Shaped Early American Identity." *Diplomatic History* 28, no. 3 (June 2004).

Pollack, Josh. "Saudi Arabia and the United States, 1931–2002." *Middle East Review of International Affairs* 6, no. 3 (Sept. 2002).

Priest, Dana. "Trip Followed Criticism of Chemical Arms' Use." *Washington Post*, Dec. 19, 2003.

Prince, Elaine B. "The Patrilineal Descent of Vice-President Bush." *NEXUS: The Bimonthly Newsletter of the New England Genealogical Society* 3 (1986).

Rihani, Ameen. "Palestine and the Proposed Arab Federation." *Annals of the American Academy of Political and Social Science* 164 (Nov. 1932).

Rivlin, Benjamin. "The United States and Moroccan International Status, 1943–1956: A Contributory Factor in Morocco's Reassertion of Independence from France." *International Journal of African Historical Studies* 15, no. 1 (1982).

Rook, Robert E. "An American in Palestine: Elwood Mead and Zionist Water Resource Planning, 1923–1936." *Arab Studies Quarterly* 22, no. 1 (Winter 2000).

Rosenne, Shabtai. "Bunche at Rhodes: Diplomatic Negotiator." In *Ralph Bunche: The Man and His Times*, edited by Benjamin Rivlin. New York: Holmes & Meier, 1990.

Said, Edward. "Islam through Western Eyes." *Nation*, March 26, 1980.

———. "Orientalism: An Exchange." *New York Review of Books*, Aug. 12, 1982.

———. "Taking Stock of Orientalism." *Middle East Review of International Affairs* 10, no. 1 (March 2006).

Sangmuah, Egya N. "Sultan Mohammed ben Youssef's American Strategy and the Diplomacy of North African Liberation, 1943–61." *Journal of Contemporary History* 27, no. 1 (Jan. 1992).

Satloff, Robert. "In Search of 'Righteous Arabs.'" *Commentary* 118, no. 1 (July 2004).

Satterthwaite, Joseph C. "The Truman Doctrine: Turkey." *Annals of the American Academy of Political and Social and Science* 401 (May 1972).

Schueller, Malini Johar. "Performing Whiteness, Performing Blackness: Dorr's Cultural Capital and the Critique of Slavery." *Criticism* 41, no. 2 (1999).

Shargel, Baila Round. "American Jewish Women in Palestine: Bessie Gotsfeld, Henrietta Szold, and the Zionist Enterprise." *American Jewish History* 90, no. 2 (June 2002).

Smith, Simon. "Piracy in Early British America." *History Today* 46 (May 1996).

Stone, Charles P. "Stone Pacha and the Secret Dispatch." *Journal of the Military Service Institution of the United States* 8, no. 29 (March 1887).

Stone, Fanny. "The Diary of an American Girl in Cairo during the War of 1882." *Century Illustrated Monthly Magazine* 28, no. 2 (June 1883).

Tichi, Cecelia. "The Puritan Historians and Their New Jerusalem." *Early American Literature* 6 (1971).

Tuchman, Barbara. "The Assimilationist Dilemma: Ambassador Morgenthau's Story." *Commentary* 63, no. 5 (May 1977).

Turgay, A. Uner. "Ottoman-American Trade during the Nineteenth Century." *Journal of Ottoman Studies* 3, no. 1 (1982).

Turner, Robert F. "The War on Terrorism and the Modern Relevance of the Congressional Power to 'Declare War.'" *Harvard Journal of Law & Public Policy* 25 (2002).

Vitalis, Robert. "The New Deal in Egypt: The Rise of Anglo-American Commercial Competition in World War II and the Fall of Neocolonialism." *Diplomatic History* 20, no. 2 (Spring 1996).

Wagner, Donald. "Evangelicals and Israel: Theological Roots of a Political Alliance." *Christian Century*, Nov. 4, 1998.

Weiner, Jerome B. "Foundations of U.S. Relations with Morocco and the Barbary States." *Hespris-Tamuda* [Morocco] 20–21 (1982–83).

Wheelock, Thomas. "Arms for Israel: The Limit of Leverage." *International Security* 3, no. 2 (1987).

Yale, William. "Ambassador Henry Morgenthau's Special Mission of 1917." *World Politics* 1, no. 3 (April 1949).

Young, Bette Roth. "Emma Lazarus and Her Jewish Problem." *American Jewish History* 84 (Dec. 1996).

Younis, Adele L. "The Arabs Who Followed Columbus." *Arab World* 12, no. 3 (March 1966).

Yousuff, Sheikh Ali. "Egypt's Reply to Colonel Roosevelt." *North American Review* 191 (June 1910).

Zirinsky, Michael. "American Presbyterian Missionaries at Urmia during the Great War." *Journal of Assyrian Academic Studies* 12, no. 1 (April 1998).

Unpublished Dissertations

Antakly, George. "American Protestant Educational Missions: Their Influence on Syria and Arab Nationalism, 1820–1923." American Univ., 1976.

Bartur, Ron. "American Consular Assistance to the Jewish Community of the Land of Israel at the End of the Ottoman Period to the Outbreak of World War I, 1856–1914." [Hebrew]. Hebrew Univ., 1984.

Conn, Cary Corwin. "John Porter Brown, Father of Turkish-American Relations: An Ohioan at the Sublime Porte, 1832–1872." Ohio State Univ., 1973.

Cook, Ralph Elliot. "The United States and the Armenian Question, 1894–1924." Tufts Univ., 1957.

Hourihan, William James. "Roosevelt and the Sultans: The United States Navy in the Mediterranean, 1904." Univ. of Massachusetts, 1975.

Kerner, Howard. "Turko-American Diplomatic Relations, 1860–1880." Georgetown Univ., 1948.

Laffey, Robert. "United States Policy toward and Relations with Syria, 1941–1947." Univ. of Notre Dame, 1981.

Larsen, Peter. "Theodore Roosevelt and the Moroccan Crisis, 1904–1906." Princeton Univ., 1984.

Marr, Timothy Worthington. "Imagining Ishmael: Studies of Islamic Orientalism from the Puritans to Melville." Yale Univ., 1997.

Metwalli, Ahmed Mohamed. "The Lure of the Levant: The American Literary Experience in Egypt and the Holy Land, 1800–1865." State Univ. of New York at Albany, 1971.

Najjar, Nada. "The Space In-between: The Ambivalence of Early Arab-American Writers." Univ. of Toledo, 1999.

Nance, Susan. "Crossing Over: A Cultural History of American Engagement with the Muslim World, 1830–1940." Univ. of California, Berkeley, 2003.

Oder, Irwin. "The United States and the Palestine Mandate, 1920–1948: A Study of the Impact of Interest Groups on Foreign Policy." Columbia Univ., 1956.

Rook, Robert Edward. "Blueprints and Prophets: Americans and Water Resource Planning for the Jordan River Valley, 1860–1970." Kansas State Univ., 1996.

Walt, Joseph W. "Saudi Arabia and the Americans: 1928–1951." Northwestern Univ., 1960.

Wright, Walter Livingston. "American Relations with Turkey to 1831." Princeton Univ., 1928.

Websites

Adams, Roger C. "Meet Lew Wallace: American Minister to Turkey, 1881–1885." http://www.ben-hur.com/meet_ambassador.html (accessed Sept. 8, 2005).

Anderson, Amy. "Thy Kingdom Come: Jonathan Edwards and the Millennium." Department of Philosophy and Religion Pages. Aug. 26, 2003. Hillsdale College. http://www.hillsdale.edu/oldacademics/phil&rel/JE/Papers/98/AndersonA.html (accessed July 8, 2004).

Autry, Jaxon B. "Lynch's Holy Expedition to the Dead Sea and the Surrounding Area." Biography of William Francis Lynch. Dec. 2001. Colorado State Univ., Pueblo. http://chass.colostate-pueblo.edu/history/seminar/lynch/autry.htm (accessed July 8, 2004).

"Beth Aram—The Aramean homepage in Germany." http://www.beth-aram.de/dokumente3.html.

Blyden, Eluemuno-Chukuemeka. "Edward Wilmot Blyden and Africanism in America." Edward Wilmot Blyden Virtual Museum. 1992. Columbia Univ. http://www.columbia.edu/~hcb8/EWB_Museum/EWB1.html (accessed July 11, 2004).

Bushrui, Suheil B. "The Thoughts and Works of Ameen Rihani." http://www.alhewar.com/Bushrui_Rihani.html (accessed March 25, 2005).

Chryssis, George C. "American Philhellenes and the War for Independence." AHEPA Family Websites. March 20, 2002. Order of AHEPA. http://www.ahepafamily.org/d5/Grk%20Inde-mar02.htm (accessed July 11, 2004).

Crocker, John. "The Book of the Thousand and One Nights." Arabian Nights Resource Center. n.d. Arabian Nights Entertainments. http://www.crock11.freeserve.co.uk/arabian.htm (accessed July 8, 2004).

"Declaration of War against Germany, 1917." http://www.classbrain.com/artteenst/publish/article_86.shtml (accessed May 18, 2004).

"Defining the Common Good: Oman as a Model for Global Citizenship." History of Oman. 2001. Maryland Center for the Study of History. http://www.geocities .com/CollegePark/Union/8191/mcsh/Omanncss.html (accessed July 11, 2004).

"Documenting the American South." http://docsouth.unc.edu/nc/helper/helper.html.

Egyptian State Information Service. "Orabi Pasha." Aug. 2004. http://216.239.41 .104/search?q=cache:O8sDNNWobzsJ:www.sis.gov.eg/calendar/html/c1310397 .htm+orabi&hl=en&start=2.

The First Farmers of Oregon. http://www.gesswhoto.com/centennial-farmers.html.

Friedman, S. Morgan. "The Inflation Calculator." Dec. 11, 2000. Morgan S. Fried-man. http://www.westegg.com/inflation/infl.cgi (accessed July 11, 2004).

Gawalt, Gerard W. "America and the Barbary Pirates: An International Battle Against an Unconventional Foe." Thomas Jefferson Papers. Oct. 29, 2001. Library of Congress. http://memory.loc.gov/ammem/mtjhtml/mtjprece.html (accessed July 8, 2004).

Gibran Khalil Gibran Homepage. http://leb.net/gibran (accessed March 24, 2005).

"Henry Eckford." Virtual American Biographies. 2000. Virtualogy. http://www .famousamericans.net/henryeckford/ (accessed July 11, 2004).

Howell, Karen E. Smith. "Down East Tales IX." A Maine Family's History. June 6, 2004. Calais Alumni. http://www.calaisalumni.org/Maine/tales9.htm (accessed July 12, 2004).

Icenogle, David. "Americans in the Egyptian Army." http://www.home.earthlink .net/~atomic_rom/officers.htm.

———. "The Expeditions of Chaille-Long." http://www.saudiaramcoworld.com/ issue/197806/the.expeditions.of.chaille-long.htm.

"John Ledyard." Meeting of Frontiers: Mutual Perceptions- Travel Accounts- John Ledyard. n.d. Meeting of Frontiers. Library of Congress. http://memory.loc.gov/ intldl/mtfhtml/mfpercep/perceptledyard.html (accessed July 8, 2004).

"Judah Magnes." http://www.wzo.org.il/en/resources/view.asp?id=1349&subject=70.

"JWA-Henrietta Szold—Building the Yishuv." Jewish Women's Archive, http://www .jwa.org/exhibits/wov/szold/yishuv.html.

Karp, Abraham J. "Judaic Treasures of the Library of Congress: Mordecai Manuel Noah." 1991. Jewish Virtual Library. American-Israeli Cooperative Enterprise. http://www.us-israel.org/jsource/loc/noah.html (accessed July 8, 2004).

Kidwai, A. R. "Translating the Untranslatable: A Survey of English Translations of the Quran." July 12, 2003. Quranic Studies. http://www.quranicstudies.com/ article32.html (accessed July 11, 2004).

"Mark Twain and His Times." http://etext.lib.virginia.edu/railton/about/srchmtf .html.

Papazian, Dennis R. "Misplaced Credulity: Contemporary Turkish Attempts to Refute the Armenian Genocide." http://www.umd.umich.edu/dept/armenian/ papazian/misplace.html.

"Profiles in Caring: Clara Barton." http://www.nahc.org/NAHC/Val/Columns/ SC10-1.html (accessed Nov. 30, 2004).

Railton, Stephen. "Search MT's Works." Mark Twain in His Times and in His Texts. 2004. Univ. of Virginia Library. http://etext.lib.virginia.edu/railton/about/srchmtf.html (accessed July 12, 2004).

Robert College. "The History of Robert College." n.d. http://www.robcol.k12.tr/admin/headmaster/history.htm (accessed July 12, 2004).

Said, Edward. "Thoughts about America." *Counterpunch*, March 5, 2002. http://www.counterpunch.org/saidamerica.html.

"Senate Salaries since 1789." http://www.senate.gov/artandhistory/history/common/briefing/senate_salaries.htm.

Shrine of North America. "A Short History of the Shrine." http://www.shrinershq.org/shrine/shorthistory.html (accessed Sept. 8, 2005).

"Sir Joseph Banks Biography, Bt, KCB, FRS." Australian National Botanic Gardens. n.d. Australian Government Department of the Environment and Heritage. http://www.anbg.gov.au/biography/banks.biography.html (accessed July 8, 2004).

Strong, Josiah. "Anglo-Saxon Predominance (1891)." http://xroads.virginia.edu/~DRBR/strong.html (accessed Jan. 15, 2005).

"Warder Cresson (1798–1860)." Jewish Virtual Library. 2004. American-Israeli Cooperative Enterprise. http://www.us-israel.org/jsource/biography/Cresson.html (accessed July 11, 2004).

Wood, Dr. Clanance Ashton. "John Ledyard the Traveler." Long Island Genealogy. Dec. 6, 2003. Long Island Historical and Genealogical Research Resource. http://longislandgenealogy.com/Ledyard/two.htm (accessed July 8, 2004).

———. "Southhold's John Ledyard." Long Island Genealogy. Dec. 6, 2003. Long Island Historical and Genealogical Research Resource. http://longislandgenealogy.com/Ledyard/one.htm (accessed July 8, 2004).

Woodbury, Chuck. "U.S. Camel Corps Remembered in Quartzite Arizona." The Army's Bold Experiment with the U.S. Camel Corps. 2003. Out West Newspaper. http://www.outwestnewspaper.com/camels.htm (accessed July 12, 2004).

"The World's Columbian Exposition: Idea, Experience, Aftermath." Aug. 1, 1996. http://xroads.virginia.edu/~MA96/WCE/title.html.

Acknowledgments

THE LIST OF ACKNOWLEDGMENTS, LIKE THE JORDAN RIVER of the American imagination, is long and wide. It begins with Princeton Professor L. Carl Brown, who, during a course on modern Middle Eastern history twenty years ago, mentioned that Civil War veterans had helped modernize Egypt's army and set up literacy schools. The lecture introduced me to the fascinating but scantily researched subject of America in the Middle East. Shortly after 9/11, when my close friend and editor Robert Weil asked me what was the one book on the Middle East that had yet to be written but that must be, I had no difficulty in responding.

Since then, my journey through the history of America in the Middle East has been assisted by a great number of friends, colleagues, and students. My first thanks are to the Shalem Center in Jerusalem, to its president, Dan Polisar, and its founder, Yoram Hazony, and to the Shalem board, headed by Roger Hertog, whom I regard as a mentor. Gratitude is due to David Hazony, the sage editor of Shalem's journal, *Azure*, and to Shalem's incomparable spokeswoman, Stefanie Pearson. I can scarcely express my appreciation—and affection—for my personal staff at Shalem, for Meira Zoloff, Leora Peters, Noa Harnik, and my longtime assistant, Noa Bismuth.

Among the exceptional people at Shalem who contributed their time and talents to this book were Yishai Haetzni, Rachel Cavits, Marina Pilipodi, Galina Tocker, Anat Altman, Karen Brunwasser, and Aharon Horwitz. In addition, I would like to acknowledge the generous research grant from Michael Moskowitz, a good friend of Shalem, which was made in the memory of his father, Zeide Yoel Moskowitz.

Through Shalem's college internship program, I was honored to work with a number of young and devoted researchers who assisted me in locating book sources and culling relevant passages and quotations. My ardent thanks go to Sarah Ronis, Rachel Isaacs, Frederick Meiton, Ben Green, Bari Weiss, Ariel Beery, Jonah Fruchter, Allison Gordon, Jennifer Feinberg, Cecile Zweibach, Sol Adelsky, Jason Silberman, Rafi Feingold, Shaun Hoffman, Rebecca Bornstein, Joe Grant, Michele Margolis, Avigail Sugarman, Jeffrey Yoskowitz, Rebecca Harris, Jacob Victor, Aaron Rothstein, Mordechai Levy-Eichel, Ayalon Eliach, Noam Kutler, David Feith, Matthew Louchheim, Batya Nadler, Paul Kandel, Rebecca Rohr, and Zvika Krieger. I am especially grateful to the young people who applied their remarkable editing skills to the manuscript, to William Feldman, Jeremy Ershow, Andrew Steinberg, Gabe Scheinmann, Adelia Malmuth, Ariana Kroshinsky, and Alieza Salzberg.

I want to thank Yael Hartman, Evelyn Emers, Eleanor Burgess, Ali Yaycioglu, and Seth Robinson, who at various times served as my research assistants in the United States. Singular thanks go to Eitan Goldstein, my indefatigable, resourceful, and brilliant chief assistant, who is destined to become one of the great scholars of American diplomacy.

I have been blessed with numerous friends who have backed me throughout this project and offered greatly valued comments on the text. Thanks go to Matthew Miller, Marty Peretz, Ruth Yudekovitz, Anne Louise Antonoff, Rose Schwartz, Stuart Hershkowitz, Sharon Friedman, Naomi and Jonathan Price, Tova Hartman, Marshall Huebner, Helen Katz, John Krivine, Mark Gerson, Dan Klionsky, Jerome and Ellen Stern, Michael and Susan Ashner, and to my father-in-law, Burt Edelstein.

A special note of thanks is reserved for Professor John Gaddis,

Robert A. Lovett Professor of Diplomatic History at Yale, for his help in probing the Middle East policies of John Quincy Adams, and Walter Russell Mead, the Henry A. Kissinger Senior Fellow in U.S. Foreign Policy at the Council of Foreign Relations, for his insights on the impact of the Middle East on the making of the U.S. Constitution and on American missionary movements. I am grateful to the Yale and Harvard students who offered fresh feedback on the lectures and readings of the course derived from this study.

My sincerest thanks go to Jeannie Luciano, the publishing director of W. W. Norton, and to her dedicated team, including Tom Mayer, Louise Brockett, Rachel Salzman, Nancy Palmquist, Julia Druskin, Otto Sonntag, Bill Rusin, and Eleen Cheung. Above all, I am indebted to Bob Weil, whose wisdom and insights permeate this book.

No mere acknowledgment could suffice to express my gratitude for the love and constant encouragement I received throughout this project from my parents and from my wife and our children, Yoav, Noam, and Lia. To you, especially, thank you.

Illustration Credits

Frontispiece: From the Collection of William Stewart. Part III opener: "Zouave Regiment Marching Up Pennsylvania Ave., Washington, D.C., in 1861," Courtesy of West Point Museum Art Collection, United States Military Academy, West Point, New York. As most part opening images are repeated in the inserts, the credits for the other part openers are listed below.

Insert One: John Ledyard, Courtesy of Ledyard Bank, New Hampshire; George Bush, Courtesy of the Library of Congress; Joel Barlow, Courtesy of the British Library; George Sandys, Courtesy of Myles Sandys; Joel Roberts Poinsett, The Granger Collection, New York; William Bainbridge, Courtesy of the Mariners' Museum, Newport News, Virginia; Commodore Edward Preble, Courtesy of the Massachusetts Historical Society; Stephen Decatur, Courtesy of the Mariners' Museum, Newport News, Virginia; Mordechai Manuel Noah, Courtesy of the American Jewish Archives; Harriet Livermore, Courtesy of the Whittier Home, Amesbury, Massachusetts, photograph by Tom Hardiman; Cyrus Hamlin, Cyrus Hamlin Collection, George J. Mitchell Dept. of Special Collections & Archives, Bowdoin College Library, Brunswick, Maine; Eli Smith, Courtesy of *Reminiscences of Bureau*

County, Part Two by N. Matson, published by Republican Book and Job Office. Princeton, Illinois, 1872; Warder Cresson, Courtesy of the American Jewish Historical Society, Newton Center, Massachusetts, and New York; James Turner Barclay, Courtesy of the Scottsville Museum; George Perkins Marsh, Courtesy of the Hood Museum of Art; Haji Ali, Courtesy of Cate Mueller / Mueller Media; William Francis Lynch, Courtesy of the Naval Historical Center; Ismail Pasha, Thaddeus Mott, William Wing Loring, Charles Pomeroy Stone, James Morris Morgan, Charles Chaillé-Long, and Erastus Sparrow Purdy, Courtesy of William B. Hesseltine and Hazel C. Wolf, *The Blue and the Gray on the Nile*, The University of Chicago Press, 1961; Rolla Floyd, Courtesy of Ariel Publishing House and the American Colony Photograph Archive; "American Tourists," reprinted from the July 26, 1890, edition of *Graphic Magazine*, Courtesy of the New York Public Library; Ulysses and Julia Grant, Image provided by the President and Fellows of Harvard College: from HOLLIS #002333836; Edward Wilmot Blyden and Lew Wallace, Courtesy of Corbis / Visual Photos Israel; "Innocents Abroad," Courtesy of the Mark Twain Project, Bancroft Library, University of California, Berkeley; Elbert Eli Farman, Courtesy of the Warsaw Historical Society, Warsaw, New York.

Insert Two: "Egypt Bringing Light to Asia," Courtesy of Musée Bartholdi–Colmar, reproduction Chr. Kempf; Emma Lazarus, The Granger Collection, New York; Samuel Marinus Zwemer, Courtesy of the Western Theological Seminary Collection at the Joint Archives of Holland; Clara Barton, Alfred Thayer Mahan, Theodore Roosevelt, Henry Morgenthau, Louis Dembitz Brandeis, and Gibran Khalil Gibran, Courtesy of Corbis / Visual Photos Israel; Ameen Rihani, Courtesy of the Ameen Rihani Organization; Charles Crane, Courtesy of the Oberlin College Archives, Oberlin, Ohio; Wilson and Balfour, from *Panorama de la Guerre* volume 7–La Victoire, page 298, published by 'Librairie Illustrée Jules Tallandrier, Paris, 1919; T. E. Lawrence and Lowell Thomas, Courtesy of Corbis / Visual Photos Israel; Golda Meir, University of Wisconsin–Milwaukee, Archives Department; Henrietta Szold, Courtesy of Hadassah, The Women's Zionist Organization of America, Inc; Judah Leib

Index

Society for the Suppression of Vice, 303
SOCONY, 410
Somalia, 573
 Chaillé-Long's expedition to, 203–4
Somers, Richard, 61
Son of Ali Baba, The (film), 507
Son of the Sheikh (film), 403
Sons of Liberty, 82
Sous, Reis Muhammad, 56
South Yemen, 529
Soviet Union, xxii, 382, 394, 410, 425,
 449, 460, 498, 507, 509, 510, 516,
 524, 529, 531, 537, 548, 550–51,
 552, 554, 561, 568, 585, 600
 Afghanistan invaded by, 547,
 560–61, 601
 German invasion of, 443, 448
 Hurley's Iran mission and, 455–56
 Iran and, 477, 479–81, 600
 Palestine partition debate and,
 491–92
 Six-Day War and, 525–26
 U.S.-Libya clash and, 478–79
 Yom Kippur War and, 533–34
Spafford, Anna, xix, 227, 280, 282,
 400
Spafford, Horatio, xix, 227, 280–81,
 282, 400
Spain, 24, 293, 310, 316, 556, 557
Spanish Inquisition, 337
Spark, USS, 107
Spence, Robert T., 61
Sperry, Charles, 291
Sphinx, 236–37
Spiegel, Steven L., 11
Spring of the Judge (Ein HaShofet),
 365–66
Stacey, May, 170–71
Stalin, Joseph, 456, 467, 479, 480,
 492
Standard Oil Company of California
 (SOCOL), 413, 415
Standard Oil Company of New Jersey,
 326, 364, 394
Stanhope, Hester, 144, 157–58

Star of America (*Kawbab Amerika*),
 370
Stark, USS, 560
Star Spangled Banner, 10
Stars and Stripes, 465–66
State Department, U.S, 11, 105, 119,
 143, 144, 166, 184, 190, 214, 248,
 259, 279, 282, 289, 290, 321, 349,
 373, 377, 417, 419, 443, 445, 452,
 455, 456, 461, 468, 473, 478, 479,
 511, 513, 523, 562
 Adams colony and, 225–26
 Arabists of, 423–26, 428, 489
 Armenian massacre and, 331–332,
 338
 Cleopatra's Needle and, 250–53
 division of Near Eastern Affairs
 (NEA) of, xx, 320, 364, 407–8,
 477, 481, 483
 French invasion of Mexico and, 187
 Jewish State opposed by, 494–95,
 497–98
 Palestine partition opposed by,
 493–95, 497–98
 Truman and deceptive document of,
 494–95
 U.S.-Saudi relations and, 408, 416,
 418
Statue of Liberty, 10, 269–70, 272, 597
 Lazarus verse inscribed on, 273
steam technology, 152
Stegner, Wallace, 417
Steinbeck, John, 166
Stephens, John Lloyd, xviii, 152–54,
 156–60, 161, 182, 464
Stethem, Robert Dean, 556
Stettinius, Edward, 468
Stevens, James, 180
Stevens, Mrs. Mark, 301–4
Stiles, Ezra, 85, 89
Stimson, Henry L., 425
stock market crash of 1929, 426
Stone, Charles Pomeroy, 194–97, 198,
 208, 234, 269, 603
 Urabi revolt and, 265–67, 268

The Contemporary
Middle East

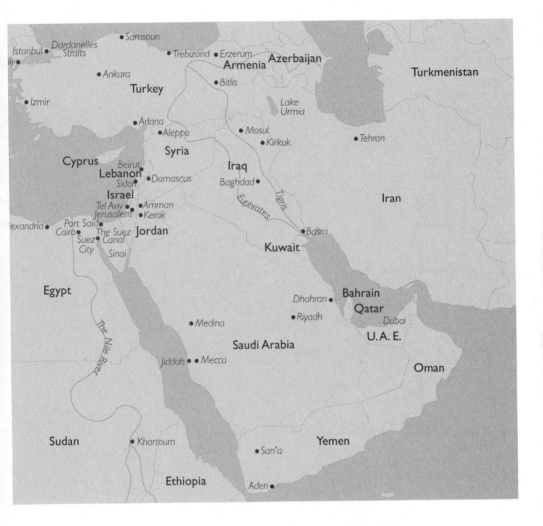